Principles and Practice of

PSYCHOPHARMACOTHERAPY

Principles and Practice of
PSYCHOPHARMACOTHERAPY

PHILIP G. JANICAK, MD

Chief, Research Unit
Illinois State Psychiatric Institute
Professor, Department of Psychiatry
College of Medicine
University of Illinois at Chicago
Chicago, Illinois

JOHN M. DAVIS, MD

Director of Research
Illinois State Psychiatric Institute
Gilman Professor, Department of Psychiatry
College of Medicine
University of Illinois at Chicago
Chicago, Illinois

SHELDON H. PRESKORN, MD

Director, Psychiatric Research Institute
Professor and Vice Chairman, Department of Psychiatry
University of Kansas School of Medicine—Wichita
Wichita, Kansas

FRANK J. AYD, Jr., MD

Editor, International Drug Therapy Newsletter
Emeritus Director, Professional Education and Research
Taylor Manor Hospital
Ellicott City, Maryland

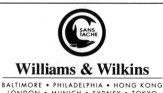

Williams & Wilkins

BALTIMORE • PHILADELPHIA • HONG KONG
LONDON • MUNICH • SYDNEY • TOKYO

A WAVERLY COMPANY

Editor: David C. Retford
Managing Editor: Molly L. Mullen
Copy Editor: S. Gillian Casey
Designer: Norman W. Och
Illustration Planner: Wayne Hubbel
Production Coordinator: Barbara J. Felton
Manuscript Editor/Indexer: Nijole Beleska Grazulis, M.S.

Library of Congress Cataloging-in-Publication Data
Principles and practice of psychopharmacotherapy / Philip G. Janicak . . . [et al.]. —
1st ed.
     p.   cm.
    Includes index.
    ISBN 0-683-04373-0
    1. Mental illness—Chemotherapy.   2. Psychopharmacology.
  I. Janicak, Philip G.
    [DNLM: 1. Psychotropic Drugs—metabolism.   2. Psychotropic Drugs—
therapeutic use.   3. Mental Disorders—drug therapy.   Wm 402 P957 1993]
RC483.P74   1993
616.8′918—dc20
DNLM/DLC
for Library of Congress   93-21771
                                              CIP
                                              Rev.

94   95   96   97
2   3   4   5   6   7   8   9   10

Josephine, Edward, Mary, and Matthew,
For the gift of a life filled with love.

Our patients and their families.
If this endeavor alleviates your suffering in any way,
our efforts will have been rewarded a thousand-fold.

Philip G. Janicak

To my family with love and thanks:
Deborah, Richard, Kathy, Markey, Jody, and Rob.

To the international community of Physicians and Scientists
dedicated to developing better ways of treating mental illness.

John M. Davis

Belinda and Ericka,
For your love, understanding, and patience.

Marie and Sister Sylvia,
For your support and encouragement.

Sheldon H. Preskorn

My wife and my family,
For their love, support, and understanding.

My patients, who have taught me so much.
My colleagues, who have shared their knowledge with me.

Frank J. Ayd, Jr.

It is indeed fitting that *Principles and Practice of Psychopharmacotherapy* should be published in the year in which health care reform has assumed priority on the United States domestic policy agenda, with mental health care a central component of reform proposals.

For more than three decades now, research on mental disorders has owed much of its energy and focus to the scientific and clinical use of psychoactive medications. Arguably, the "psychopharmacology revolution" has been the principal driving force behind the explosion of information about brain and behavior, and refinements in our capacity to treat mental disorders. Beginning in the early 1960s, specific and often dramatic responses of major mental disorders to medications afforded evidence of a biological component to these conditions. This evidence triggered a gradual ideologic shift in the perceptions of mental disorders held by professionals and, eventually, the public. Researchers working with major mental illnesses were invigorated, and those who had dismissed major mental disorders as reflecting characterological flaws or environmental causes, exclusively, were forced to reconsider.

The psychopharmacology revolution—and, specifically, clinical psychopharmacologic research—launched a derivative revolution in clinical methodologies. Put simply, this demanding field required reliable diagnoses and behavioral rating instruments, and thus the research diagnostic criteria were developed, leading eventually to the American Psychiatric Association's Diagnostic and Statistical Manual of Mental Disorders, third edition (DSM-III) and, soon, DSM-IV. This system, based on observable symptoms and behaviors, yields diagnoses for the major mental disorders that today are as reliable as any in medicine. This tool enabled, in turn, a new era of epidemiologic research, exemplified in the National Institute of Mental Health (NIMH) Epidemiologic Catchment Area (ECA) study. Documentation provided by the ECA and related research of the high community prevalence of mental disorders has been an influential factor in the decision to include mental illness in the nation's health care reform efforts.

Another critically important outcome of the psychopharmacology revolution was the rapid expansion of neuroscience. While mental health scientists continue to make very substantial contributions to molecular neuroscience, their special contribution has been a commitment to integrating behavioral science and neuroscience— that is, to understand how the brain functions as an integrated whole, with respect to specific behaviors and in response to the impact of environmental factors. At another level, the tools and questions inspired by psychopharmacologic research have fostered a growing integration of basic and clinical neuroscience, seen, for example, in neuroimaging.

In spite of economic pressures to the contrary (i.e., medication is cheaper to administer than are psychosocial therapies), medications should never be perceived as a singular solution to the age-old enigma of mental illnesses that touch upon every facet of human existence. Indeed, research inspired by the psychopharmacology revolution has enriched our awareness of the awesome complexity of human behavior and, specifically, of the intricate interactions of biology and environment, broadly defined, as they impact on the pathogenesis and treatment of mental disorders. In reinforcing our appreciation of the centrality and impact of psychological and social factors on the biology of the mental state, our achievements in psychopharmacology have redirected attention to fundamental requisites of mental health treatment and all other medical practice: a comprehensive clinical assessment; a focus on the longitudinal course of illness; and, most critically, a willingness to devote *time*, not just procedural interventions, to patients.

Indeed, given the yet-emanating ripples of the psychopharmacology revolution on work to elucidate the ubiquity and connectedness of neurochemical systems—work that today is rewriting principles of clinical care throughout medicine—psychopharmacology clearly has been a leader in highlighting the limitations, no less than the benefits, of all high-technology medicine.

It is reassuring to see that these and other hard-won lessons of 30 years of psychopharmacologic research and clinical practice serve as the keystone of this impressive volume. The authors state seven unambiguous *principles* at the outset, and

never let the reader forget that improved patient care is the ultimate objective of the formidable scientific and regulatory enterprise described herein.

Adherence to the human element of psychopharmacotherapy is only enhanced by the fact that *Principles and Practice of Psychopharmacotherapy* is an authored rather than edited text. In the age of Medline, science bulletins via facsimile machine, and the tsunami of specialty journals and symposia proceedings that threatens to engulf us all, the wholeness of a text written jointly by a small team of authors is as welcome as it is needed. Drs. Janicak, Davis, Preskorn, and Ayd remind us that, collectively, they bring 100 years of experience to their *interpretive* explication of the principles and practice of psychopharmacotherapy. Knowing the authors as I do, I am certain that they have thought, discussed, and, no doubt, vigorously challenged and debated among themselves the interpretations and clinical recommendations presented here. "Technology transfer" gains a soul. It is readily apparent that we are not being offered a bound computer printout, but an engaging and important contribution to the literature on the art, no less than the science, of medicine.

While the breadth of the work defies summarization, I will comment on a few points in *Principles and Practice of Psychopharmacotherapy* that were particularly interesting, or gratifying, from my own perspective as a clinician-investigator and science administrator.

Foremost is the emphasis given to thorough clinical assessment. As a physician and, especially, as a consulting psychopharmacologist, I am continually impressed by how easily a failure to assess every aspect of a patient's medical, family, and behavioral history can lead to failures of treatment. The most important time investment the physician can make to an episode of care, whether a one-time visit or the first of many as physician and patient work together to manage a chronic or recurrent illness, is the pretreatment evaluation. The information is needed "up front," as this phrase refers both to time and candor. Tough and often difficult questions must be addressed: the pattern and duration of symptoms, the patient's exposure to possibly stressful life events, suicidal potential, substance use, and any painful aspects of personal and family history.

As the authors make clear, the quality of the assessment sets the tone for and exerts a profound, lasting impact on the quality of the therapeutic alliance that must ensue. Psychopharmacotherapy, so easily—and often—denigrated as the epitome of "mindless" mental health practice is, in fact, laden with psychological demands and opportunities. Too few of our critical observers appreciate the extent to which the psychopharmacology revolution mobilized a renaissance in psychotherapy. This is certainly true of my own specialty area of manic-depressive illness; substantially freed of the disruptions of mania and the profound withdrawal of depression, patient and therapist can sustain their focus on the many psychological issues related to the illness and also confront basic developmental tasks. With the introduction and refinement of novel new compounds that at last promise to lift the biochemical barriers that inhibit and prohibit expressiveness and connectedness in severe disorders such as schizophrenia, it is abundantly clear that opportunities for time-intensive therapeutic alliances will only increase in the future.

Still, exquisite balance must be maintained between empathy on the one hand and efficiency and efficacy, on the other. Thus, I particularly appreciate the meta-analyses undertaken in a variety of areas by the authors. While our science advances by thesis and diathesis, clinical success requires some level of synthesis. Informed meta-analyses constitute a bridge from the research literature to a type of practical guidance that permits and promotes coherent clinical judgments. Among the priorities of the ongoing NIMH Treatment Research Initiative are studies examining the long-term treatment of chronic and recurrent disorders. Integration of biological, psychosocial, and rehabilitative therapies, particularly for mental disorders with a long-term course, will include research on combined treatments and also will examine the benefits of potential medication "cocktails," a topic discussed by the authors.

One can only be pleased by the attention given to the special issues presented by childhood disorders. Young people under the age of 20 years are in the peak age range for development of depression, manic-depressive illness, phobias, and substance abuse. As indicated in the *National Plan for Research on Child and Adolescent Mental Disorders*, childhood and adolescent disorders cost America $1.5 billion in treatment expenses each year, even though less than one-fifth of afflicted children receive the treatment they desperately need. The NIMH is committed to advancing the research base as broadly and as flexibly as each new piece of information about the onset and treatment of these disorders dictates. Basic research, as well as growing emphasis on the development of effective, science-based preventive strategies, will serve to accelerate the need for treatment research—psychopharmacologic and psychosocial—alone and in combination. This book shows appropriate sensitivity to both the nuance and the imperative of psychopharmacotherapy in childhood disorders.

Principles and Practice of Psychophar-macotherapy is in step, too, with the promising, needed level of attention that recently has been directed to women's health concerns. The NIMH is looking intensively at ways in which the field can take advantage of recent Food and Drug Administration policies that have begun to remove some of the barriers to the conduct of clinical trials involving women. This is an issue of special concern to readers given the gender distribution seen in many mental disorders.

As a final note, I commend the authors not only for the attention devoted to "special patient populations," but also for their efforts to make this text accessible to a diverse array of health care providers and related professionals. Mental illness is increasingly understood not to exist on a separate plane, as it were, but to occur in—and often as a part of—general medical illness. Major depression is among the most common clinical problems that primary care physicians are called upon to diagnose and treat in adult patients. Yet while a majority of all patients with depression—74%—are seen in the general medical sector during the course of an episode of illness, the depression is recognized and treated effectively in only one in

four individuals! Inadequate treatment of mental disorders, moreover, is not limited to the general medical practice sector. The NIMH Collaborative Program on the Psychobiology of Depression, a large, multi-site study, has provided evidence that, despite availability of effective psychopharmacologic treatments, these may not be applied appropriately, even in the hands of psychiatrists and other mental health specialists. In this study involving patients with severe, protracted depression, nearly one in three of those admitted as inpatients to university medical centers received either *no* somatic antidepressant therapy or clearly inadequate doses.

In this Decade of the Brain, *Principles and Practice of Psychopharmacotherapy* lucidly and comprehensively makes available to a diverse readership one of the most powerful and promising knowledge bases in 20th century medicine. One can be confident that this volume will do much to ensure that the power and the promise will be available to our patients well into the 21st century.

Frederick K. Goodwin, M.D.
Director
National Institute of Mental Health

Over the last three decades there has been an explosion of information about drug therapies for the management of mental disorders. This phenomenon closely parallels the expansion of ever more sophisticated technologies that subserve the field of neuroscience. As a result, pathophysiology has become an increasingly more appropriate foundation upon which to diagnose these disorders as well as to develop more effective biological remedies. A further development has been the growing number of well-conceived and carefully executed clinical drug trials, making assimilation of this expansive literature a daunting task.

The goal of *Principles and Practice of Psychopharmacotherapy* is to provide a clinical logic that incorporates contemporary knowledge about drug therapies into the overall management of the mentally ill. The intended audience includes: residents in psychiatry and family practice, as well as the general practitioners of these medical specialties; psychiatric nurses, psychologists, and social workers; and other mental health professionals who are involved with patients taking psychotropic medications.

We would like to highlight what we believe to be the unique strengths of this work. **First, this book has been conceived and written by four authors only.** Each is a professor of psychiatry, and in combination we bring to this effort *over 100 years of research and clinical experience*. This work has truly been a team effort, with multiple and extensive meetings and phone discussions, as well as careful reviews and critiques of original and subsequent drafts by each author over the last two years. Further, expert opinion has also been sought and graciously given in the form of detailed critiques by such recognized leaders as Max Fink, M.D., Ghanshyam Pandey, Ph.D., and Donald Klein, M.D.

The results are:

- A work characterized by a comprehensive *summarization of the literature* (e.g., about 2000 references, most since 1985)
- A uniformity and succinctness of style and organization throughout the text
- The development of *treatment strategies* based on the best scientific data available and tempered by our combined clinical experience.

In Chapter 1 we **formulate seven guiding principles** that clearly demarcate the role of drug therapy within the context of a comprehensive, often lifelong, treatment approach. Next, to help guide therapeutic choices, **we provide statistical summarizations, by means of meta-analyses,** of the extensive, ever more methodologically rigorous, literature comparing various drug and somatic therapies to placebo or each other.

To set the stage for such an exercise, we discuss in Chapter 2 the **qualities that characterize a well-designed study** and the issues critical to appreciating the strengths and the weaknesses of combining the outcomes of multiple trials to derive a "bottom-line" conclusion on relative efficacy.

In Chapter 2 we also explore **the role of drug therapy from the patient-consumer's perspective.** Thus, such issues as informed consent, the cost of treatment, and labelled versus nonlabelled uses for FDA-approved medications are carefully considered.

In Chapter 3 we discuss **the relevant pharmacokinetic principles,** particularly as they apply to the treatment recommendations rendered throughout the text.

In Chapters 4 through 12 **we deal with the major classes of psychotropics** as well as the pertinent diagnostic issues related to various drug therapies. This constitutes the core of our work, and includes the:

- Antipsychotics
- Antidepressants
- Somatic therapies
- Mood stabilizers
- Anxiolytics/sedative-hypnotics.

Our approach to each of these drug groups and related somatic therapies begins with a consideration of the possible mechanisms of action, followed by a comprehensive literature review on efficacy and adverse effects. These discussions then serve as the basis for the development of a **clinical therapeutic strategy.** Knowing that many patients fail standard treatment recommendations, either because of insufficient efficacy or intolerance to adverse effects, led us to emphasize the latter's importance.

The book concludes with two chapters (Chapters 13 and 14) on **disorders that require separate consideration.** The first group includes *Panic, Obsessive-Compulsive, Post-Traumatic Stress, Somatoform, and Dissociative disorders.* Although traditionally these are classified as anxiety disorders, their symptoms and varied treatment responsivity require a separate series of discussions. Finally, certain groups of patients are considered in light of their specialized needs when contemplating psychotropic drug therapy. They include the *pregnant patient, children and adolescents, the elderly, the personality disordered, as well as patients whose conditions are complicated by medical problems* (e.g., the alcoholic patient; the HIV-infected patient).

Throughout the book an attempt is made to create a "reader-friendly" compendium. Thus, for any given topic one can quickly peruse the *introductory* and *conclusionary* statements; the *critical points* in the text as indicated by italics, bulleting of information, and/or bolding; the *tabular data* (e.g., statistical summaries of the comparative efficacy of a new agent versus placebo and/or a standard drug therapy); and the *treatment strategy diagrams,* all of which succinctly outline our suggested approach to a given disorder. This allows the reader to quickly assimilate the most important information, while also providing a more in-depth discussion to be reviewed as time permits. Illustrative *case examples* are also provided to underscore a particular clinical issue.

As "no man is an island," no author (or group of authors) could presume to take sole credit for such an endeavor as we now put forth. Therefore, it is with gratitude that we wish to acknowledge the editorial assistance of Nijole Beleska Grazulis,

M.S., who also indexed this work. We thank Dave Retford, Barbara Felton, Molly Mullen, Jonathan Pine, Gillian Casey, and Wayne Hubbel of Williams & Wilkins for their guidance and expertise. Further, Drs. Janicak and Davis wish to sincerely thank Rajiv P. Sharma, M.D., Javaid I. Javaid, Ph.D., Subash Pandey, Ph.D., Mark Watanabe, Ph.D., Pharm D., Sheila Dowd, Alan Newman, and Jane Retallack for their efforts on behalf of this enterprise. Dr. Preskorn would like to thank Sharon Hickok for her assistance in making this textbook a reality, and his mentors, colleagues, residents, medical students, and patients, who have provided insights and intellectual stimulation throughout the years. Dr. Ayd would like to thank Mary Ann Ayd and Ann Lovelace.

Finally, good night, Michael Fisher, wherever you are.

Philip G. Janicak, M.D.
John M. Davis, M.D.
Sheldon Preskorn, M.D.
Frank Ayd, Jr, M.D.

CONTENTS

14. Assessment and Treatment of Special Populations 481

CHAPTER 1
General Principles

The art and the science of psychopharmacotherapy have expanded rapidly in the past decade, creating both an opportunity and a challenge. As a result, while improved therapies to ease a patient's suffering are inevitable, this requires the practitioner to continually assimilate new information about recent advances, including: *novel agents* targeted to impact specific components of various neurotransmitter systems; *combination strategies; alternative uses* of existing agents; and the *specialized requirements* of a growing number of identified diagnostic subtypes. Throughout this book, we will provide a **decision-making method** that incorporates this growing data base for the optimal utilization of drug therapies in clinical practice.

Our model is grounded on a scholarly review and summation of the critical, supporting research. Beginning with a discussion of the major principles underlying our approach, we follow with chapters on specific psychiatric disorders and their related therapies. **The goal is to provide a logical treatment strategy that can be readily applied and easily adapted to an ever-increasing body of relevant, scientific data.**

This approach is based on several underlying assumptions:

- The *medical model* serves as the foundation for the treatment of psychiatric disorders.
- A *nontheoretical approach* is advocated in considering etiology/pathogenesis
- An *empirically based foundation*, derived from scientific investigation, is used to guide treatment decisions.

All modalities, from electroconvulsive therapy (ECT) to psychotherapy, can be incorporated into our approach when empirical data supports their utility. When sufficient data are lacking, we will offer suggestions based on the cumulative clinical and research experience of the authors.

Principles of Psychopharmacotherapy

PRINCIPLE ONE

The diagnostic assessment, subject to revisions, is fundamental to our model (Table 1.1).

Patients present with symptoms. The clinician's goal is to formulate these problems within the context of the highest level of diagnostic sophistication (Table 1.2) based upon the subjective and objective

Table 1.1.
Principles of Psychopharmacotherapy

Principle One	The diagnostic assessment, subject to revisions, is fundamental to our model.
Principle Two	Pharmacotherapy alone is generally insufficient for complete recovery.
Principle Three	The phase of an illness (e.g., acute, maintenance, prophylaxis) is of critical importance in terms of the initial intervention and the duration of treatment.
Principle Four	The risk to benefit ratio must always be considered when developing a treatment strategy.
Principle Five	Prior personal (and possibly family) history of a good or a bad response to a specific agent usually dictates the first line choice for a subsequent episode.
Principle Six	It is important to target specific symptoms that serve as markers for the underlying psychopathology and monitor their presence or absence over an entire course of treatment.
Principle Seven	It is necessary to observe for the development of adverse effects throughout the entire course of treatment. Such monitoring often involves the use of the laboratory to insure safety as well as optimal efficacy.

Table 1.2.
Levels of Diagnostic Sophistication

Diagnostic Level	Description	Example	Diagnostic Impression
Symptomatic	Isolated symptom(s)	Auditory hallucinations	Psychosis, NOS[a]
Syndromic	Constellation of signs and symptoms Inclusion/exclusion criteria	Irritability Pressured, irrelevant speech Insomnia Poor judgment	Bipolar disorder, manic phase, with mood incongruent psychotic features
Pathophysiologic	Demonstrable structural or biochemical changes	Elevated TFTs[a] Lowered TSH[a]	Hyperthyroidism
Etiologic	Known causative factor(s)	Positive for thyroid antibodies Diffuse toxic goiter on ultrasonogram	Thyrotoxicosis secondary to Graves' hyperthyroidism

[a]NOS, not otherwise specified; TFTs, thyroid function tests; TSH, thyroid-stimulating hormone.

components of the evaluation (1, 2). To accomplish this task, the clinician must realize that behavioral symptoms in psychiatry are analogous to localizing signs to the neurologist. Such symptoms as depressed mood or auditory hallucinations are mediated through the function or dysfunction of specific brain regions. Different etiologically determined disorders can cause dysfunction in the same brain region, leading to similar phenomenological presentations. For example, a brain tumor, a stroke, or demyelinating plaque can all affect the frontal lobe, culminating in similar behavioral symptoms.

The increased specificity of a syndromic, as compared to a symptomatic, diagnosis comes from the utilization of both inclusion criteria (i.e., a constellation of symptoms and signs present for a set interval of time) and exclusion criteria (i.e., conditions that may mimic the syndrome under consideration but have a known, alternate pathophysiologic or etiologic basis) (3). Currently, most psychiatric diagnoses are at the syndromic level, with similar presentations often representing substantially different underlying mechanisms. Therefore, it is not surprising that considerable variability is found in the treatment outcome of patients diagnosed with the same syndrome. Further, patients with the same pathophysiology may be erroneously separated into different categories because of differences in their syndromic presentation. A classic example is multiple sclerosis (MS), which typically presents with signs and symptoms separated in time and space. Another example is tertiary syphilis, known as the great mimic, due to its myriad clinical presentations. For this reason, clinicians must be ready to alter their diagnosis, as well as treatment plans, if dictated by changes in the course of illness.

Although such criteria-based syndromes have certain limitations, we would emphasize that they have been a useful first step in developing an empirical approach to psychopharmacologic and somatic therapies. Systematic studies of the effects of psychotropics on such syndromes permit investigators to:

- Conduct *sequential investigations* in different groups of patients with the same signs and symptoms with reasonable confidence that they are treating patients with similar disorders
- Perform *replication studies*, as well as *multisite clinical trials*
- Be more *confident in the results* from such studies, since they employ the same criteria
- *Clarify the effectiveness* of a specific treatment
- Compare the *relative effectiveness* of one treatment to another when assessing the outcome in patients with similar syndromic diagnoses
- Clarify which particular symptoms may be *critical variables in predicting a drug versus placebo difference* (e.g., neurovegetative symptoms of depression)
- Clarify *atypical or specific types of presentations that may not benefit from standard treatments* (e.g., atypical or psychotic depressive disorders).

Finally, diagnoses based on etiology or pathophysiology are superior to symptomatic or syndromic diagnoses in terms of their specificity and usefulness (4). As in other areas of medicine, the likelihood of a successful outcome increases based on the level of diagnostic specificity, since treatment can then be targeted to the underlying factor(s).

PRINCIPLE TWO

Pharmacotherapy alone is generally insufficient for complete recovery.

While drug therapy may be the cornerstone of recovery, there is almost always a need for some type of educational and psychosocial intervention, as well as psychotherapy when indicated. Examples include the use of anxiolytic agents in combination with behavior modification for phobic disorders or the use of interpersonal psychotherapy plus antidepressants for depressive disorders. Further, since there is often a delayed onset of action with many of the psychotropics, early counseling may avoid premature discontinuation by a patient, as well as provide hope and reassurance during this lag phase. In addition to communicating in an understandable fashion the nature of the symptoms and disorder, and incorporating the patient and the family as active participants in the treatment plan, the clinician must generally be prepared to respond to the following questions:

- What do I have?
- Will I get better?
- What will it take?
- What are the limitations?
- What will it cost?

Simple, straightforward explanations of a patient's condition and the rationale for a specific course of action are generally well received. For those unable to benefit because of cognitive disruption, reassurance and expressions of empathy and concern are often therapeutic. A thorough, brief review of what is known about the cause of the patient's disorder should be communicated, while dispelling common myths about their condition (e.g., the problem is related to a lack of discipline or traumatic life experiences). A patient's prognosis should be realistically, and to the extent possible, optimistically explained. Various options should also be discussed, as noted in the section on informed consent (see Informed Consent in Chapter 2).

While the clinician should always take the role of counselor and advisor, the ultimate course of action should be left to the patient, except in those few instances when the patient cannot make a rational, prudent, and informed decision on his/her own behalf. Bringing the patient into the process as an active, informed participant is beneficial to self-esteem and improves compliance. There are, however, two instances when the clinician should not defer to the patient's wishes: if the illness significantly affects the ability to make an informed decision; or when a treatment is requested (e.g., a drug of abuse) that cannot be provided in good faith.

The educational process should continue throughout the entire treatment relationship and often involves clarifying issues as they arise. When a patient does not respond to the first line of treatment, the process should address the possible reasons this has occurred, as well as the rationale for attempting second and subsequent treatment strategies. Finally, since many psychiatric disorders are recurrent, educating the patient and the family as to the early warning symptoms of a relapse may allow for earlier intervention and perhaps even prevention. In this way, a patient may suffer less sequelae, often avoiding unnecessary hospitalizations and prolonged recovery phases from subsequent, repeated exacerbations.

Other, more specific forms of therapy may also be indicated. These may include cognitive or interpersonal psychotherapy, or specific forms of behavior desensitization and biofeedback. Some patients may benefit from insight-oriented psychotherapy and/or group, family, or marital counseling. Finally, in more chronic disorders, patients often benefit from vocational rehabilitation in addition to adequate pharmacotherapy. A knowledgeable clinician realizes that these disorders do not occur in a vacuum, and regardless of diagnosis, each patient requires an individualized treatment plan to optimize outcome.

PRINCIPLE THREE

The phase of an illness (e.g., acute, relapse, recurrence) is of critical importance in terms of the initial intervention and the duration of treatment.

Ideally, after an acute episode, some patients should receive indefinite prophylaxis on the assumption that recurrence is inevitable. But, since it is difficult to accurately predict which patients will have subsequent episodes, there is a reluctance to expose those who will not relapse to the adverse effects of long-term therapy.

The course of an illness also dictates the need for and duration of maintenance and prophylactic therapy. In particular, prophylaxis may not be indicated for an uncomplicated first episode depending on the specific disorder and the patient's response to standard interventions. Conversely, patients with histories of multiple relapses, positive family histories, prolonged durations of or particularly severe acute episodes, and delayed rate of response to treatment intervention are candidates for ongoing prophylaxis.

Some medications are clearly indicated during an acute phase of treatment but not for maintenance or prophylactic purposes. Conversely, certain drugs may not be very useful for acute management, but are exceptionally beneficial for maintenance or prophylaxis. For example, in an acute manic episode, adjunctive benzodiazepines may rapidly sedate patients; however, they are infrequently used as maintenance strategies once the acute symptoms are under control. With early signs of breakthrough and possible relapse, however, they may again play a role in preventing a recrudescence of the full manic phase. Another example is lithium, which is relatively ineffective with more severe, manic exacerbations, such as stage 2 or stage 3 mania. But once the acute symptoms have been controlled with other drug or somatic interventions, lithium is effective for maintenance and prophylaxis.

PRINCIPLE FOUR

The risk to benefit ratio must always be considered when developing a treatment strategy.

Specific factors to consider are both psychiatric and physical contraindications. For example, bupropion might be contraindicated in a psychotically depressed patient because of its structural similarity to diethylpropion, an agent known to induce psychotic symptoms in certain patients. Conversely, it may be the drug of choice for a bipolar disorder with intermittent depressive episodes that is otherwise under good control with standard mood stabilizers. This is based on the assumption that bupropion is less likely to induce manic swings in comparison to standard heterocyclic antidepressants. Another example would be the avoidance of benzodiazepines for the treatment of panic disorder in a patient with a history of alcohol or sedative-hypnotic abuse, due to the increased risk of misuse or dependency.

Physical as well as psychiatric status is also critically important. The presence of intercurrent medical disorders increases the likelihood of an adverse outcome in an otherwise appropriate medication. With a recent history of myocardial infarction, certain tricyclic antidepressants or low potency antipsychotics might be contraindicated due to potential adverse effects on cardiac function. Another example would be the avoidance of carbamazepine in a bipolar patient with a persistently low white blood cell count. Finally, β-blockers are typically contraindicated in a patient with asthma.

A related issue is the patient's ability to adequately metabolize and eliminate drugs. For example, lithium is excreted entirely by the kidneys, and if a patient suffers from significantly impaired renal function, high and potentially toxic levels could develop on standard doses. While the dose could be adjusted to compensate for the decrease in drug clearance, it might be more appropriate to choose another mood stabilizer, such as valproic acid or carbamazepine, since they are primarily metabolized through the liver.

A final consideration is the cost of treatment, which not only includes financial issues but also the inconvenience and potential for adverse effects (see Cost of Treatment in Chapter 2).

PRINCIPLE FIVE

Prior personal (and possibly family) history of a good or a bad response to a specific agent usually dictates the first line choice for a subsequent episode.

Given the development of new drugs with more refined mechanisms of action, patients' responses to therapeutic interventions become increasingly critical sources of data. With poor or inadequate response to a previous trial of a given medication, the choice of drug can be made more difficult. Whether desirable or undesirable, however, response provides insights into the underlying pathophysiology. Therefore, the careful monitoring of outcome can provide information for modifying previously suboptimal therapies. If initial or prior response is inadequate, common issues to consider include:

- Appropriate *diagnosis*
- Adequacy of *treatment* (e.g., sufficient dose, blood concentration, or duration)
- *Noncompliance*
- Intercurrent *substance or alcohol abuse; medical problems;* the concomitant use of *prescription or over-the-counter medications*
- Lack of adequate or appropriate *social support*

- The presence of a diagnosis is on *Axis II* (see Appendix).

PRINCIPLE SIX

It is important to target specific symptoms that serve as markers for the underlying psychopathology and monitor their presence or absence over an entire course of treatment.

For example, in a bipolar patient, reduction of the amplitude of mood swings may be the focus of acute therapy. During the maintenance phase, however, the most sensitive predictor of an impending relapse might be excessive jocularity, decreased need for sleep, or rapidity of speech. Careful attention to the onset of such symptoms might permit early treatment, preventing a full-blown recurrence.

It is also important to recognize that certain symptoms may respond before others. In a depressive episode, vegetative symptoms such as sleep and appetite disturbances will often respond early in the course of treatment, whereas mood may take several weeks to improve. Cognizant of these different temporal patterns of response, the clinician may be encouraged to continue with a certain approach. Also, educating the patient regarding the differential time course to response for various symptoms may facilitate compliance. Subsequently, during the maintenance/prophylactic phase, the clinician should monitor how effectively a treatment prevents the re-emergence of the acute symptoms.

PRINCIPLE SEVEN

It is necessary to observe for the development of adverse effects throughout the entire course of treatment. Such monitoring often involves the use of the labora-

tory to insure safety as well as optimal efficacy.

First, it is important to confirm that the adverse effects are actually due to a specific treatment. Since patients in clinical studies often experience a wide range of adverse effects while on placebo, one should not prematurely conclude that such events are due to medication.

With the development of new, more specific agents, it is increasingly crucial to note and report undesirable behavioral effects as well as physical reactions. For example, if a patient becomes excessively passive, there is a chance that the behavior will be missed or attributed to the underlying psychiatric condition. In fact it might be a previously unrecognized effect of a new medication. The identification of previously unknown adverse effects (while undesirable in themselves) can be the basis for the next round of serendipitous discoveries about the underlying pathophysiology of a given disorder.

The first role of the laboratory is to detect specific adverse effects to target organs (see Role of the Laboratory later in this chapter). Monitoring will generally be tailored to the specific therapy because of its known potential for causing certain problems. Examples include periodic *blood counts with carbamazepine or clozapine,* and *thyroid and renal function studies with long-term maintenance or prophylactic lithium.*

Another use of the laboratory is for therapeutic drug monitoring (TDM) of psychotropics with defined optimal ranges and/or narrow therapeutic indices. While TDM is not needed for many psychotropics, it is important to insure safety and efficacy in others, including lithium; several tricyclic antidepressants; carbamazepine; valproic acid; and certain antipsychotics.

Since many of these drugs have wide interindividual concentration ranges on the same dose, various factors must be considered. Elimination rates can vary to a clinically significant degree among different patients on the same dose, such that some will develop subtherapeutic concentrations, others concentrations in the therapeutic range, and still others toxic concentrations. In this instance, TDM provides the necessary information on how rapidly a patient eliminates the drug so the dose can be adjusted to maximize safety and efficacy.

REFERENCES

1. Kendell RE. The role of diagnosis in psychiatry. Oxford: Blackwell Scientific, 1975.
2. Lee S, Chow CC, Wang YK et al. Mania secondary to thyrotoxicosis. Br J Psychiatry 1991;159:712–713.
3. Goodwin WG, Preskorn SH. DSM-III and pharmacotherapy. In: Turner SM, Hersen M, eds. Adult psychopathology and diagnosis. New York: John Wiley, 1984:453–464.
4. Preskorn S. The future of psychopharmacology: potentials and needs. Psychiatr Ann 1990;20:625–633.

Role of Neuroscience

Psychopharmacotherapy is still an empirically based approach. Advances in the neurosciences, however, are occurring at an increasingly rapid pace and will ultimately provide a much more complete understanding of cerebral structure and function, as well as guide clinical drug therapies in the future.

One important example is the use of *brain imaging,* such as positron emission tomography (PET), single photon emission computerized tomography (SPECT), and magnetic resonance imaging (MRI). These techniques are allowing us to localize brain regions underlying many behavioral symptoms (e.g., anxiety, vigilance, sadness), while at the same time enabling us to attain greater levels of diagnostic sophistication.

Perhaps most critical to a discussion on psychotropics is the explosion of knowledge about the fundamental biochemical processes subserving psychiatric disorders. At the ultrastructural level we can isolate and study biologically important substances (e.g., neurotransmitters; receptor subtypes; various components of the post ligand-receptor interface, including second messenger systems). Once characterized, they can become the target for specific drug development. Concurrently, observing how new drugs interact with these cellular components, enhances our knowledge of their functional role in mediating specific behavioral symptoms. Newer agents can then serve as probes to test whether these components are relevant to a given psychiatric disorder.

MECHANISM OF ACTION

Psychotropic drugs affect specific biochemical processes, most often enzymes, their receptors, or ion channels. When a given drug's action on such a process produces a physiological response (whether intended or otherwise), that is termed the "mechanism of action." **It is axiomatic that central effects mediate the clinical actions of psychotropic medications. But, for any given drug, the effects on known processes may not be the mechanism mediating response. Instead, the clinical outcome may be the result of some as yet unrecognized central action.** This is due in part to the limited understanding of the pathophysiology underlying specific psychiatric disorders. When the fundamental biology underlying a disorder is unknown, it is impossible to state how a drug is correcting a given syndrome. Typically, proposed "mechanisms of action" for behavioral effects are simply the actions of the drug in question on known central biochemical processes. Whether these actions are truly the mechanisms underlying the behavioral effect (e.g., amelioration of depression), must be viewed with healthy skepticism.

With the rapid developments in neuroscience, we are likely to see further reliance on drug probes to test the functional integrity of neurotransmitter systems in specific disorders. An ever-increasing number of biochemical processes are being unraveled that may mediate specific psychotropics' effects. Such processes include:

- *Enzymes* responsible for the synthesis and degradation of an expanding list that includes neurotransmitters, neuropeptides, neurohormones, etc.
- The process involved in the *delivery of neurotransmitters into vesicles* within the cytoplasm
- *Release mechanisms*
- *Reuptake pumps*
- Subtypes of pre- and postsynaptic *receptors*
- *Receptor subcomponents*
- *Second messenger* systems.

As these various processes are better characterized, they will increasingly become the targets for future drug development.

DRUG DEVELOPMENT AND ITS IMPLICATIONS

The first psychotropics of the modern era (e.g., lithium, neuroleptics, tricyclics, monoamine oxidase inhibitors) were primarily discovered by serendipity. Therefore, these agents were not engineered to have selective actions, but instead have a wide range of central biochemical effects, as well as affecting more than one neurotransmitter system simultaneously.

This situation has multiple repercussions:

- *Such drugs can be helpful in more than one condition* since they act by more than one mechanism.
- *Any one of these drugs' actions could be responsible for the clinical effect;* therefore, such drugs provide limited insight into the pathophysiology of a given condition.
- Generally, due to their multiplicity of effects, *these "broad spectrum" medications are more poorly tolerated* than agents with fewer biochemical interactions.

Attempts to customize agents can greatly reduce the "signal to noise ratio" and enhance the development of more specific treatments.

While there are many problems with the first generation of modern psychotropics, they have been extremely effective, while providing insights into the underlying pathophysiology. Studying the effects of these agents on specific biochemical functions has had great heuristic value, leading to the generation of numerous hypotheses that have guided subsequent drug development. One set of hypotheses deals with the possible mechanisms underlying the clinical efficacy of these agents, and includes:

- The *dopamine theory,* based on the actions of neuroleptics
- The *catecholamine and indoleamine theories,* based on the actions of various antidepressants

- The *permissive, adrenergic-cholinergic balance, and bidimensional hypotheses,* based not only on the effects of antidepressants but also on the modulating interactions among various neurotransmitter systems.

Concurrently, hypotheses were also developed regarding the undesirable or toxic effects associated with the various biochemical actions of these agents. Examples include:

- *Orthostatic hypotension* secondary to α_1-adrenergic receptor blockade
- *Cardiotoxicity* secondary to membrane stabilization
- *Central anticholinergic syndrome* due to the potent anticholinergic effects of many psychotropics.

Chemists can now better define the structure/activity relationship of these early psychotropics to guide the development of newer drugs. Such relationships are refined by in vitro testing to determine whether newly synthesized compounds have the desired biochemical effect on specific targets, such as enzyme inhibition or receptor blockade. Simultaneously, these agents are tested for any undesirable effects. Where such effects exist, modifications can be made to the chemical structure to eliminate or reduce such unwanted qualities. When a new psychotropic drug meets the desired inclusion and exclusion criteria, it is then tested in the clinic to determine whether it possesses the desired therapeutic effect. Results from these clinical studies provide critical feedback regarding the mechanism(s) of action, which will guide the development of future generations of agents.

Selective serotonin reuptake inhibitors (e.g., fluoxetine, sertraline, paroxetine) and bupropion represent the first examples marketed in the United States of

agents engineered to eliminate many of the earlier side effects. First introduced in the late 1980s, they had important research and clinical implications. From the research standpoint, they advanced our understanding of the pathophysiology of various disorders, while providing a way to test for the existence of putative biochemically distinct subtypes. Such attempts were unsuccessful with earlier generation psychotropics, in part due to their lack of specific action. For example, the tricyclic antidepressants are effective in depressive disorders, enuresis, and panic attacks, but different mechanisms are believed to be responsible for these varied efficacies. In a similar way, all tricyclics have effects on both the norepinephrine and serotonin reuptake systems within the clinically relevant concentration range. Attempts in the past to distinguish between "serotonergic" versus "adrenergic" depressive disorders with such agents were unsuccessful, due to the nonspecific nature of these drugs' effects, even if two such forms of depressive disorders exist. Newer agents, however, are orders of magnitude different in their affinity for one system versus another and can be used as probes to expand our understanding of the relevant neurobiology.

Clinically these agents also have several advantages since they:

- Are generally *safer and better tolerated*
- Have *more specific pharmacological actions*
- *Can test the functional integrity* of a given neurotransmitter system.

Thus, the first era of modern psychopharmacotherapy (i.e., serendipitous discovery) is giving way to the second era, which is the refinement of drugs based upon known biochemical effects. This will eventually lead to the next era, which will be the synthesis of compounds with specific interactions at newly discovered subcomponents of the neuron. The existence of such agents will also permit the development of an empirically based hierarchical treatment plan that will define the agent of first choice and then which agent(s) is most likely to help when the first choice is unsuccessful or poorly tolerated. Our approach will allow the reader to both anticipate such developments and incorporate them as they occur.

Diagnostic Assessment

Diagnosis is critical to understanding a patient's presenting complaints, as well as serving as the basis for developing treatment strategies. For this reason, each treatment section is preceded by introductory discussions of the major psychiatric diagnostic categories (see Appendix A). We further refine this organization by incorporating factors that often affect presentation and response to treatment. Such variables include:

- *Phase of the illness* being treated (e.g., acute, prevention of relapse, prevention of recurrence)
- *Confounding issues* such as other psychiatric or medical conditions
- *Psychosocial stressors*, to the extent that they impact on symptom presentation and effectiveness of treatment.

Our model recognizes that the current understanding of pathophysiology and etiology is at a rudimentary stage. **Therefore, diagnostic assessment of any patient is an ongoing process that must be continuously updated throughout treatment.** Such revisions are based upon information acquired from the patient during followup, including response, partial response, or lack of response to specific interventions, as well as the emergence of new knowledge from subsequent scientific investigations.

The diagnostic assessment consists of several stages, including:

- A *subjective account* of the pertinent information, including personal and family history
- *Objective parameters*, including the mental status exam
- The *initial impression*, culminating in a preliminary diagnosis
- *Treatment planning*, including further diagnostic workup, first line treatment strategies, and education of the patient and the family.

SUBJECTIVE COMPONENT

This aspect of a psychiatric evaluation incorporates several sources of information, including the individual's own account, family and friends' reports, the referral source(s), and any earlier data base, such as the chart from a previous hospitalization. Basic identifying information such as age, sex, race, marital status, present family situation, living circumstances, work skills, present work situation, and sources of income is essential. The individual's communication of the basic problem(s), or the "chief complaint," will set the stage for an elucidation of the chronology of precipitating events that culminated in seeking help. Next is an exploration of any prior psychiatric history and/or treatment, either personally or in other family members; serious past or ongoing medical problems, either personally or in family members; and the use or abuse of medications, illicit drugs, or alcohol.

OBJECTIVE COMPONENT

Objective data include a thorough physical-neurological evaluation, supplemented by laboratory data, such as routine blood work, urinalysis, chest x-ray, electrocardiogram (ECG), and drug screen (see Role of the Laboratory later in this chapter). All this information is routinely collected when a person first enters the hospital, but on an outpatient basis, the clinician may select only those tests deemed appropriate at the time.

The mental status examination is the most important aspect of this phase and scrutinizes how an individual is feeling, acting, and thinking at the time of the interview (i.e., a cross-sectional versus longitudinal evaluation). The clinician begins with a basic observation of *overt appearance* and *motoric behavior,* including *affect* (i.e., overt emotional reactions, in terms of intensity, quality, appropriateness, and continuity), and *mood* (i.e., underlying feeling tone). It is important to note that affect and mood may not always be synonymous, and this discrepancy can complicate the diagnostic assessment.

Thought processes, including memory and orientation, reflect one's ability or inability to collect and communicate ideas in a logical and coherent fashion. *Thought content* explores the substance of one's ideation, and typical aberrations such as obsessions, phobias, illusions, delusions, or hallucinations may be elicited. Evaluation of *memory and orientation* is critical to the differentiation of a psychiatric versus nonpsychiatric medical disorder. Memory for immediate, recent, and remote events can be readily tested, as well as orientation to time, place, person, space, and situation. Assuming the level of anxiety is not sufficient to impair responses to questions in these areas, deficits usually imply some impairment of brain functioning, which may or may not be reversible.

Intellectual capacity is considered in the context of an individual's social, cultural, and educational opportunities. The presentation of problem-solving situations congruent with one's life circumstances is an excellent way to determine intellect and capacity to make sound *judgments*. *Insight* has many levels of meaning. It may simply refer to a basic appreciation of how and why an individual finds himself in his present situation, or it can refer to a person's appreciation of a more complex set of causal relationships that have culminated in the present problem. One's *abstractive ability* is the capacity to perceive a conceptual commonality in otherwise distinct or separate entities. This ability can be tested by similarities, proverbs, and appreciation of humor.

To summarize, the mental status exam highlights several aspects of cognitive functioning. Each succeeding component requires that earlier aspects be intact for adequate reality testing, as well as the optimal expression of one's personality, as subjectively perceived and objectively observed, in terms of emotions, thoughts, and behavior.

INITIAL IMPRESSION

Having obtained the necessary information from subjective and objective sources, the next step is the development of a preliminary diagnostic assessment, including commentary when possible on the five major axes (Diagnostic and Statistical Manual of Mental Disorders, 3rd ed, revised (DSM-III-R)), as well as other differential diagnostic considerations (see Appendix). The diagnostic assessment serves many purposes:

- It is *a shorthand way of labelling and referring* to patients' complaints.
- It *provides a way of conceptualizing complaints* within the framework of our current knowledge, so that appropriate treatment can be instituted.
- It *facilitates research* by allowing data to be systematically collected from different patients with the same condition.
- It is important for *billing*.

The most basic assessment is a *description of the phenomena* (e.g., anxiety, etiology undetermined). An assessment also takes the additional form of an *"initial impression"* (e.g., phobic disorder) *and a differential diagnosis* of other possible categories that need further exploration (e.g., rule out hyperthyroidism, rule out an agitated depression). As such, diagnosis serves an analogous function in medicine as does hypothesis formulation in science. The value of a given diagnosis (or hypothesis) is determined by the degree to which it explains the facts of the case (i.e., the presentation, the course, and response to treatment). If the diagnosis does not lead to an acceptable treatment outcome based on these criteria, it must be revised, just as a hypothesis is revised in science.

TREATMENT PLANNING

The last step (and obvious culmination) of the diagnostic assessment is formulation of the initial treatment plan, including the potential role of pharmacotherapy. The first consideration is to decide what other diagnostic workup is necessary. Typical procedures include the obtaining of corroborative history from spouse and family; psychological testing; and other physical and neurological evaluation as dictated by the initial findings. These steps should further refine the working diagnostic impression. Often there is also the need to consider and treat more than one problem. The course of treatment in a hospitalization may simply consist of separating the individual from recent environmental stresses and allowing his/her own restorative resources to stabilize in the protective and supportive milieu of an inpatient setting. Other treatments are often necessary, however, and may include:

- *Psychotherapy* (e.g., individual, family)
- *Sociotherapy* (e.g., recreational, occupational, and activities therapy)
- *Pharmacotherapy* (e.g., anxiolytics, antidepressants, antipsychotics)
- *Somatic therapy* (e.g., electroconvulsive treatment).

While the focus of this work is pharmacotherapy, incorporating these other modalities is often critical to a successful outcome and is also discussed.

Diagnostic Approaches

While the ideal course would be to consider the symptoms as the behavioral manifestation(s) of an underlying cerebral pathology and formulate subsequent treatment plans on this assumption, for now, most treatments are dictated by a specific diagnosis.

This text will attempt to develop a hierarchical framework for considering first-line treatment choices and subsequent options, if initial interventions fail. We begin with treatment recommendations from the standpoint of our current diagnostic nosology. We will also present cases of pa-

tients who do not easily fit into a single major diagnostic category, or in whom treatment based upon syndromic constellations proves unsuccessful. When possible we will then suggest a strategy based on data about the underlying pathophysiology. These working strategies will be drawn from the presenting behavioral symptoms and quality of response to earlier therapeutic trials.

A hypothetical vignette may serve to illustrate such a paradigm shift from a syndromic to a pathophysiologic approach in patients who do not respond adequately to standard therapeutic trials.

> *Case Example.* The patient's presenting problems are anger and impulse control, symptoms that may not fit well into an Axis I or II diagnostic category. The clinician may conceptualize these symptoms as cyclothymia and begin treatment with a mood stabilizer such as lithium. If unsuccessful, a reasonable second approach might be a trial with divalproex sodium or carbamazepine. If symptoms persist one might consider dysthymia because of the presence of persistent dysphoric symptoms, and initiate treatment with a serotonergic reuptake inhibitor. However, in this scenario, the patient not only remains symptomatic but also evidences some worsening of impulsivity and anger.

At this point, having exhausted therapeutic approaches based on empirical data, it may be useful to shift paradigms. Whereas previously trial and error may have been the only recourse, we are now approaching the point when a pathophysiologic paradigm may help guide the selection of subsequent drug therapies. There is considerable evidence that impulsivity in various mammalian species is mediated in part through serotonin mechanisms. More specifically, serotonin may influence the function of the amygdaloid and septal-hippocampal formations, perhaps through 5-HT_{1A} receptors located in these regions.

There is also evidence of low cerebrospinal fluid (CSF) 5-hydroxyindoleacetic acid (5-HIAA) in impulsive individuals. In a non-responsive impulsive patient we might hypothesize that diminished serotonin plays a role in the pathophysiology. This hypothesis could now be tested and simultaneously serve as the foundation for a pathophysiologically based treatment by choosing therapies specific for various components of this system. Use of a 5-HT$_{1A}$ agonist (e.g., buspirone) might be the next step, since there is limited evidence from open trials that it has antiaggressive properties.

Education

Educating a patient as well as the family is of the utmost importance for any treatment plan to succeed. Good clinicians, like good teachers:

- *Communicate* at a level appropriate to the individual's ability to comprehend.
- Convey their suggestions in the context of a working *theoretical framework* (be it right or wrong!).
- Encourage the patient to become an *active participant* in treatment.

Role of the Laboratory

Interest in the neurobiologic substrates of psychiatric disorders parallels the increase in effective somatic therapies, which in turn have extended the laboratory's role in evaluating patients. Though the laboratory can never replace clinical acumen (whether in psychiatry or any other medical specialty), it can play a significant role in:

- Elucidating and quantifying *biological factors* associated with various psychiatric disorders
- Determining the *choice of treatment*
- Monitoring *clinical response*.

This chapter reviews the standard medical assessment for the psychiatric patient; summarizes specific tests frequently employed in the clinical and research setting; and discusses the laboratory's role in treatment evaluation (e.g., therapeutic drug monitoring) (1–3).

MEDICAL ASSESSMENT

General principles for assessment include:

- A *detailed physical examination*, which may reveal medical problems previously missed; new, unrelated medical problems; incorrect diagnoses; or complications associated with various psychiatric treatments
- The *avoidance of wasteful screening batteries with limited clinical utility.* Instead, specific lab tests based on a careful assessment and integration of the history and physical examination are the ideal
- Recognition of *presenting signs and/or symptoms that dictate the need for further medical evaluation* (e.g., a known history of recurring or chronic medical illness; prominent physical symptoms; evidence of an organic mental disorder

on the Mini-Mental State Examination; substance abuse disorder, etc.)

- In specific cases, the utilization of *treatment options that require lab testing* (e.g., lithium, ECT, etc.).

ADMISSION ASSESSMENT FOR INPATIENTS

A screening battery to evaluate the general physical condition of the patient is outlined in Table 1.3. Supplementary lab and diagnostic tests may be required when specific clues from the history, physical examination, or initial lab screen suggest a physical disturbance (Table 1.4). Finally, Table 1.5 lists tests often utilized for very specific clinical circumstances.

Table 1.3.
Inpatient Screening Battery

Complete blood count (CBC)
Blood chemistries (SMAC)
Thyroid function tests
B12, folate levels
Screening tests for syphilis
Urinalysis
Electrocardiogram (ECG)
Chest x-ray

Table 1.4.
Supplementary Tests

Skull films, CT scan, MRI
EEG, evoked potentials
Drug screen, heavy metal screen, blood levels of medications, blood/breath alcohol levels
Erythrocyte sedimentation rate
Lumbar puncture with CSF studies
Serum ceruloplasmin
HIV testing
Anti-nuclear antibodies
Monospot test
Blood culture
Pregnancy tests
Skin tests for tuberculosis/brucellosis
Urine: porphyrins, osmolality
Stool: occult blood
Arterial blood gases
Polysomnography, nocturnal penile tumescence

LABORATORY TESTS

Demonstrable lab abnormalities in psychiatric disorders are not sufficiently specific or sensitive to identify with certainty the correct diagnosis or appropriate treatment. They can, however, indicate an association between a given disorder and a

Table 1.5.
Batteries for Specific Clinical Circumstances[a]

ELDERLY PSYCHIATRIC PATIENTS
  Complete blood count (including serum hemoglobin; erythrocyte sedimentation rate determination; total and differential white blood cell count)
  Serum B12 and folate level determinations
  Complete biochemical profile (including serum electrolytes—sodium, potassium, bicarbonate; blood urea nitrogen, serum creatinine; serum calcium and phosphorus; blood glucose)
  Liver function tests
  Thyroid function tests
  Serological test for syphilis
  Urinalysis
  Lumbar puncture
  Chest x-ray
  ECG
  Skull x-ray; EEG, if necessary
  CT scan, if indicated
SUSPECTED SUBSTANCE ABUSE
  Breath alcohol tests
  Blood alcohol levels
  Urine drug screens
  Gas chromatography-mass spectroscopy (GC-MS)
PRE-LITHIUM WORK UP
  Complete blood count
  Serum electrolytes
  Blood urea nitrogen; serum creatinine
  Thyroid function tests
  Urinalysis
  ECG
  Pregnancy test
PRE-ECT WORK UP
  Complete blood count (including hemoglobin)
  Blood chemistries (e.g., SMA-20)
  Chest x-ray; spinal x-rays (if indicated)
  Urinalysis
  ECG

[a]Tables 1.3, 1.4, and 1.5 are adapted from reference 1.

specific measure which may or may not be relevant to its pathogenesis or etiology. Biological markers may be *"state-dependent,"* serving as aids in the diagnosis of a specific psychiatric illness with which they are associated, as well as useful for following treatment response. On the other hand, *"trait"* markers may help in identifying vulnerable individuals.

Neuroendocrine Tests

Given that the seat of hormonal modulation is in the limbic-hypothalamic-pituitary-axis, endocrine changes serve as important correlates to major psychiatric disorders. This includes basal hormone concentrations, as well as responses to pharmacological challenges. It is equally important to note that endocrine disorders may present with psychiatric symptoms (e.g., manic symptoms in hyperthyroidism, severe depression in hypercortisolism, psychotic symptoms associated with Cushing's syndrome). Several commonly employed neuroendocrine tests include the following.

The Dexamethasone Suppression Test

The dexamethasone suppression test (DST) procedure typically involves an oral dose of 1.0 mg of dexamethasone, taken at 11:00 PM. For inpatients, blood samples are typically drawn the next day at 8:00 AM, 4:00 PM, and 11:00 PM, while for outpatients, a single 4:00 PM sample is usually collected. These are then analyzed for plasma cortisol concentrations. *Normally, the single 1.0 mg dose of dexamethasone at 11:00 PM will suppress plasma cortisol secretion, resulting in concentrations below 5 g/dl for the next 24 hours. Levels higher than this indicate non-suppression, or a positive test result.* Due to variation in assay methods, however, any concentration in

the 4–7 g/dl range must be interpreted with caution. An abnormal DST (non-suppression) increases the probability of a major depressive episode or at least an affective component to the illness. It cannot, however, be used as a diagnostic test because of its low specificity (i.e., identifies only about 45–50% of patients with major depression); nor can it serve as an adequate screening device since almost 7% of normal controls and approximately 19% of acute schizophrenic patients may be non-suppressors (4, 5). Some studies have indicated that failure of the DST to normalize after somatic treatment for depression might indicate a higher likelihood of relapse (6). If confirmed, this may have greater application in clinical psychiatry. Table 1.6 lists causes of false positive and false negative results on the DST.

Thyrotropin-Releasing Hormone Stimulation Test. After an overnight fast, an intravenous line is started around 8:30 AM. At 8:59 AM, blood samples are collected for baseline thyroid indices, including thyroid-stimulating hormone (TSH). At 9:00 AM, synthetic TRH is administered i.v. (usually a dose of 500 µg given over 30 seconds). Transient side effects include:

- Gastrointestinal or genitourinary symptoms
- A sensation of warmth
- Dryness of mouth or metallic taste
- Tightness in the chest.

Plasma samples for TSH concentrations are then collected 15, 30, 60, and 90 minutes after the TRH infusion.

A normal response is an increase in plasma TSH of 5–15 micro-units/ml above baseline. A response of less than 5 micro-units/ml above baseline is generally considered to be blunted (some labs consider a response below 7 micro-units/ml to be blunted) and may be consistent with a

Table 1.6.
Causes of False Positives or Negatives on DST

False Positives	False Negatives
Pregnancy	Addison's disease
Obesity	Hypopituitarism
Weight loss or malnutrition	Slow metabolism of dexamethasone
Alcohol abuse/withdrawal	Drugs
Infection	Exogenous corticosteroids
Trauma	Indomethacin
Diabetes mellitus	High doses of benzodiazepines
Carcinoma	High doses of cyproheptadine
Cushing's syndrome	
Anorexia nervosa	
Renal/cardiac disease	
Cerebrovascular disease	
Antipsychotic withdrawal	
Temporal lobe epilepsy	
Drugs	
Estrogens	
Narcotics	
Sedative-hypnotics	
Anticonvulsants	

Adapted from Kirch DG. Medical assessment and lab testing in psychiatry. In: Kaplan HI, Sadock BJ, eds. Comprehensive textbook of psychiatry, 5th ed. Baltimore: Williams & Wilkins, 1989:525–533.

major depression. An abnormal test is found in approximately 25% of patients with depression. A blunted TSH response (especially in conjunction with an abnormal DST) may help in confirming the differential diagnosis of a major depressive episode and support continued antidepressant treatment. An increased baseline TSH or an "augmented" TSH response (higher than 30 micro-units/ml), in conjunction with other thyroid indices, might identify patients with hypothyroidism, mimicking a depressive disorder. These patients may benefit from thyroid replacement therapy.

Other Neuroendocrine Tests

These include:

- *Blunted growth hormone response* to various stimuli, such as insulin-induced hypoglycemia, L-dopa, 5-hydroxytryptamine, apomorphine, d-amphetamine, clonidine, growth hormone releasing hormone (GHRH), and TRH. The growth hormone response to clonidine is one challenge test that has been consistently reported to be positive by several different research groups. This test measures the responsiveness of postsynaptic α_2-adrenergic receptors and may be a "trait" marker for depression
- *Blunted prolactin response* to such agents as fenfluramine, methadone, and L-tryptophan is based on a possible serotonin deficiency in depression
- Plasma *melatonin levels* and urinary levels of its primary metabolite, *6-hydroxy melatonin* are used in research as indices of noradrenergic functioning before and after treatment with antidepressants.

Biochemical Markers

Although research on neurotransmitters and/or their metabolites has found numerous abnormalities, no routine lab test has been developed to reliably enhance diagnosis or treatment (see Mechanism of Action in Chapter 7). Some consistent findings include:

- An association between suicidal behavior and impulsive aggression with decreased levels of the serotonin metabolite *5-HIAA in CSF*
- Low 24-hr *urinary 3-methoxy-4-hydroxyphenylglycol (MHPG)* (metabolite of norepinephrine (NE)), primarily in bipolar disorders (i.e., depressed phase).

Peripheral tissue markers include high-molecular weight complex biomolecules (receptors), and enzyme systems that can be obtained from outside the central nervous system (CNS) (e.g., in platelets, lymphocytes, skin fibroblasts, and erythrocytes) and are thought to reflect or parallel central neuronal activity. Some noteworthy findings are:

- *Increased platelet α_2-adrenergic receptors* in depression
- *Decreased* β-adrenergic receptor binding sites on lymphocytes in affective disorders
- Significantly *decreased ^{3}H-imipramine binding sites in platelets* from depressed and obsessive-compulsive disorder (OCD) patients.

Genetic Markers

Gross *chromosomal abnormalities* can be used to identify various types of mental retardation, as in the case of Down's Syndrome (i.e., Trisomy 21) or the Fragile X Syndrome. Molecular genetics examines specific deoxyribonucleic acid (DNA) sequences or restriction fragment length polymorphisms (RFLPs) in the genes of patients with psychiatric disorders and normal controls, as well as specific *human lymphocyte antibody (HLA) subtypes*. Genetic *linkage studies* attempt to establish the chromosomal locus of certain disorders

(e.g., chromosome 4 in Huntington's Disease, chromosomes 14, 19, and 21 in Alzheimer's Disease). Further, there have been conflicting results from studies of the X-chromosome or chromosome 11 in bipolar disorder. High lithium erythrocyte/plasma ratios and high muscarinic acetylcholine receptor density, which have been reported in mood disorders, may be potential markers for candidate genes, particularly when the gene's locus on its chromosome is known.

Brain Imaging Techniques

In clinical psychiatry, brain imaging offers a modest amount of information, chiefly useful in differential diagnosis (7). In research, however, it has proved invaluable in clarifying the relationship between neuroanatomic loci and pathophysiology.

Computerized Tomography

Computerized tomography (CT) is used in the clinical setting primarily to rule out organic lesions that might underlie and/or contribute to a psychiatric disorder. Specific indications may include:

- *First episode after age 40* of a psychotic, mood, or personality disorder
- *Abnormal motoric movements*
- *Delirium or dementia* of unknown etiology
- Persistent *catatonia*
- *Anorexia* nervosa.

Indications, for contrast, include the presence of focal signs and symptoms, and/or any lesion noted on a non-contrast scan. Findings include:

- *Reversed cerebral asymmetry* in schizophrenics
- *Cerebellar atrophy*, third *ventricle en-*

largement, and *high ventricle-to-brain ratios* in chronic schizophrenic patients
- A negative correlation between *ventricular enlargement and antipsychotic treatment-response* in chronic schizophrenics
- *Cortical atrophy,* as evidenced by sulcal widening, in chronic schizophrenia.

In addition, abnormalities have been reported in depression, alcoholism, Alzheimer's disease, and multi-infarct dementia. It is important to note that these are statistical findings in the psychiatric research setting, however, and CT is not sufficiently sensitive or specific to be used as a routine diagnostic test.

Magnetic Resonance Imaging

MRI uses a magnetic field to detect the frequencies at which substructures of chemical elements in body tissue resonate. The characteristic frequencies of various brain tissues are recorded to create an exquisitely detailed picture of brain structures. The established clinical utility of MRI is in the diagnosis of primary degenerative dementias (e.g., Alzheimer's and Pick's diseases). In addition, recent studies of schizophrenia have demonstrated smaller frontal lobe size, ventricular enlargement (especially in the frontal horns), and temporolimbic abnormalities, including complete or partial agenesis of the corpus callosum.

Possible advantages of MRI over CT include:

- *Imaging in all planes,* including sagittal and coronal, in addition to transverse
- *Higher resolution* of tissue structures
- *Better differentiation* of gray matter from white matter
- *Better definition of lesions* in demyelinating disorders (e.g., multiple sclerosis) and therefore, early identification

- Excellent *visualization of the posterior fossa and pituitary* regions
- Potential for measuring *physiological variables.*

In clinical practice, however, the CT scan is generally preferred, as it is convenient, safe, relatively comfortable, less expensive, and especially helpful as a diagnostic tool in patients with a history of cerebral concussion or subarachnoid hemorrhage.

Other Imaging Techniques

These are primarily research tools and lack general applicability in routine psychiatric diagnosis or treatment, and include the following.

Positron Emission Tomography. PET provides functional images of the brain and is particularly promising in the study of neurotransmitter systems. A positron-emitting element (e.g., fluorine-18, carbon-14, carbon-ll) is incorporated into a biologically significant compound (e.g., D-glucose), which is then administered intravenously. The distribution of the compound in different regions of the brain when the patient is at rest or engaged in a specific task is then mapped. This technique can also be used to measure receptor density in a given location.

Important PET scan findings include:

- Reduced prefrontal metabolism
- High metabolic rates in the orbital frontal cortex and basal ganglia of OCD patients.
- Neuroleptic blockade of D_2 receptors in schizophrenia

Single Photon Emission Computed Tomography. SPECT is a method that allows the measurement of cerebral blood flow when certain designated brain areas are activated by having the subjects perform specific experimental tasks (e.g., cognitive challenge tests like Wisconsin Card-Sorting). As in PET, SPECT, too, can visualize both cortical as well as subcortical structures. Though the pictures are not as clear as those produced by PET scan, SPECT offers a less expensive alternative to study brain activity.

Both SPECT and PET studies have revealed a characteristic pattern of hypoperfusion in posterior temporoparietal regions in Alzheimer's Disease.

Regional Cerebral Blood Flow Mapping Techniques. Such mapping techniques use radioactive probes (e.g., Xenon-13) to delineate perfusion of cortical structures. They have generally confirmed prefrontal cortex dysfunction in schizophrenia.

Neurophysiological Testing

Electroencephalogram

The electroencephalogram (EEG) procedure is useful in differentiating some organic mental disorders from idiopathic psychiatric syndromes as well as to help identify focal structural lesions in the cortex (8, 9). In some patients with episodic, paroxysmal behavioral disturbances and a presumptive diagnosis of schizophrenia, a sleep-deprived EEG with nasopharyngeal leads may help rule out an epileptiform disorder contributing to or underlying psychotic behavior. In general, an EEG is indicated in patients who are younger (especially under 25) and presenting with their first psychotic episode, or in patients with a history of possible cerebral injury or neurological disturbance (e.g., accidents, unconsciousness, infections, perinatal complications, seizures). It has the advantages of safety, being a relatively inexpensive procedure, and relative freedom from discomfort to the patient.

Limitations of the EEG are numerous, however, and include:

- An apparently *normal EEG does not exclude organic disease* or epilepsy.
- *ECT and psychotropics* affect the EEG, making interpretation difficult at times.
- *Sampling error* is possible because the paroxysmal electrical activity may not have occurred during the time of recording. In such cases, a sleep-deprived EEG or a 24-hr ambulatory recording might be helpful.

Sometimes, a video camera is also used to help define the seizure type (e.g., epileptic or psychogenic) and quantify the abnormal behavior that accompanies the aberrant electrical activity.

In the search for specific neurophysiological markers of idiopathic psychiatric syndromes (e.g., schizophrenia, major mood disorders), studies have reported various nonspecific EEG abnormalities. In addition, psychiatric patients appear more sensitive to activation procedures like:

- Sleep-deprivation
- Provocative stimuli (e.g., photic stimulation with flashing strobe light)
- Hyperventilation.

Thus far, however, no specific EEG patterns have been identified that can accurately aid in the diagnosis of a particular psychiatric condition.

Computed Topographic Mapping of the Electroencephalogram

CT mapping of the EEG (CTM/EEG), also referred to as brain electrical activity mapping (BEAM), involves the recording of cortical electrical activity in certain specified frequencies, which a computer then graphically visualizes in two-dimensional, color-coded maps. This procedure is chiefly used in psychopharmaco-logic and neuropsychological research.

Polysomnography

Polysomnography (PSG) refers to sleep recordings that simultaneously monitor various physiological parameters (usually nighttime). The tests that may be carried out include EEG, electromyogram (EMG), electro-oculogram (EOG), ECG, rapid eye movement (REM), nocturnal penile tumescence (NPT), respiratory air flow, and vital signs. In a typical sleep laboratory, a 12- to 16-channel polygraph recording is made. Uses include:

- Investigation and diagnosis of *sleep dis-orders,* especially, sleep apnea and nar-colepsy
- Research in *depression* (REM density and latency; total sleep time)
- *Drug/alcohol* withdrawal studies
- Nocturnal penile tumescence in the dif-ferentiation of functional from organic causes of *impotence.*

Evoked Potentials

These are electrophysiological record-ings (on the order of milliseconds, as op-posed to minutes in other brain-imaging techniques like PET) evoked from specific cortical areas (e.g., visual, auditory, soma-tosensory) using discrete types of sensory stimulation (e.g., flashes of light). They can differentiate between certain organic and functional disorders (e.g., visual evoked potentials (VEP), in suspected hys-terical blindness), as well as evaluate de-myelinating disorders, such as multiple sclerosis. At this time, however, evoked potentials are mainly employed in the study of biological markers. For example, several studies have found low-amplitude, late (greater than 250 milliseconds) brain-

stem auditory evoked potentials (BSAEPs) in schizophrenic patients, suggesting at-tentional impairment.

Other Techniques

Electroretinogram (ERG) reflects cen-tral dopaminergic function. Abnormalities in *smooth pursuit eye tracking movements (SPEM)* may represent vulnerability mark-ers for psychosis in general. *EMG* and *nerve conduction studies* may help in cases where myopathies or peripheral neuropa-thies are suspected. *Magnetoencepha-lography (MEG)* is a noninvasive tech-nique that measures the weak magnetic fields generated by the electrical activity of the brain (including the deeper subcor-tical areas) and converts them back into electric signals, which are then recorded. It holds great promise for neuroscience research.

Therapeutic Drug Monitoring

The ideal drug treatment strategy achieves maximum therapeutic response with a minimum of side effects. In many branches of medicine, monitoring plasma levels, rather than dose of a drug, is often the optimal way to reach this goal (10). While not a routine procedure in psychia-try, this approach is used for lithium, car-bamazepine, and valproic acid, as well as for some antidepressants; however, for most psychoactive drugs this approach re-mains experimental. The best use of this technique remains for those circumstances when response is not adequate or unex-pected adverse events occur. In this chap-ter we will review the clinical utilization of therapeutic drug monitoring as follows:

- State the **theoretical basis** of the blood level-clinical response relationship.
- Note the **methodological issues** that

complicate the interpretation of results from plasma level-clinical response studies.

- Integrate results from existing valid studies to emphasize the **clinical applicability** of therapeutic drug monitoring.

Theoretical Basis

If a drug produced immediate pharmacologic effects, then the monitoring of plasma levels would be unnecessary. For example, one can directly observe the clinical stages of anesthesia and adjust the anesthetic dosage by simply monitoring its effects. On the other hand, if there is a long interval between clinical response and drug administration, weeks may be required to achieve the desired effect. In such situations, if the plasma concentrations required for clinical response are known, doses can be adjusted more rapidly to achieve the proper levels. Such monitoring is also useful when there are large interindividual differences in response to the same dose for the same diagnosis. Given that there are also large interindividual variations in plasma levels with the same dose of a psychotropic, knowledge of the potential therapeutic range for a given agent could provide more precise guidelines for individualized dose adjustment.

For example, the half-time to response with antipsychotics is about 2 weeks, so increasing the dose every few days can overrun this lag period, often leading to doses much higher than required. While dose is usually adjusted based on clinical response, knowing the minimally effective level may avoid greater than necessary drug exposure. The primary data in determining the minimally effective dose come from dose-response trials. Plasma level studies can also supplement these data since there is a positive correlation be-

tween levels achieved and the dose required. Thus, one can estimate the average dose needed to produce a certain concentration. In another sense, plasma levels can be thought of as a fine tuning of the dose.

The basic assumptions that underlie the relationship between plasma levels and clinical response are:

- An *optimum concentration* exists at which maximum pharmacologic response will occur.
- A relationship exists between the drug *concentration in plasma and the site of action.*
- *Pharmacogenetic and environmental factors* vary the quantity of antipsychotic that reaches the receptor site in different individuals.

At low concentrations there will be no response, followed by an increased response as levels rise. After the maximum pharmacologic response is achieved, further increases in concentration will not enhance response. Thus, a plasma level-response relationship may show the typical sigmoidal shape. Further, at higher concentrations, various side effects of a drug may be more prominent, defining the relationship between its plasma level and these side effects. Thus, a composite plot of the clinical benefit versus drug plasma level will result in an inverted U-shaped relationship that defines the range (or "therapeutic window") to achieve optimum benefit. For most drugs, the upper end of the therapeutic window represents toxicity. Hypothetically, some drugs could actually lose their clinical effectiveness as a result of their action on different receptors at higher concentrations. The only agent for which there is evidence to support this contention, however, is the antidepressant nortriptyline. Even here, the data are limited. For a drug that does not have serious toxic effects at higher concentrations, the blood level-clinical benefit relationship will eventually plateau.

Methodological Issues

A number of methodological issues have confounded the interpretation of results, thus minimizing the clinical utility of the plasma level-therapeutic response relationship (11). These issues can be grouped as follows:

- *Dose* strategy
- *Assay* method
- Patient *population*
- Study *design*.

Dose Strategy. The most insidious methodological error in plasma level/clinical response studies is the systematic confound of raising the dose when a patient fails to respond. This frequently misses the lower end of the therapeutic window because patients are not kept at the lower dose for a sufficient time to document ineffectiveness. Additionally, because patients respond at a slower rate than the rate of dose increases, some considered responders at a higher dose may have actually improved at a lower dose, had it been maintained for a longer period of time.

To illustrate, consider two examples of patients with inadequate clinical response. In the first, poor response is due to a low plasma level. When the clinician increases the dose, the plasma level also rises, and although there may be a response at the higher plasma level, frequent repeated dose increases can obscure the low end of a possible therapeutic window or the threshold level for response. In the second example there is an adequate plasma level but in a refractory patient. When the dose is increased, the plasma level rises; however, the patient will remain nonresponsive at any concentration.

In research trials, one experimental design to solve this confound is to nonrandomly assign a fixed dose based on the patient's clinical condition at admission and then hold it constant throughout the rest of the study. The investigator may initially preassign patients to high, medium, or low doses based on his/her clinical judgment; but this is done before treatment starts and is usually based on the severity of the symptoms present. In the absence of a large number of well-designed studies, this method is less rigorous but usable in the interpretation of dose/response studies.

A more effective trial design to define the plasma level-clinical response relationship is to use a constant (or fixed) dose design, regardless of clinical status. It can be a single fixed dose or random assignment to several different fixed doses (perhaps low, medium, and high) to investigate the low and the high end of a potential therapeutic window. When data from several fixed-dose studies indicate a possible therapeutic range for a specific drug, prospectively targeting patients to various plasma levels can then be a useful method. In this design patients are maintained in a predetermined fixed plasma level range during the trial period.

Assay Methods. Analytical techniques can broadly be divided into *chemical* or *biological* assays. Chemical methods primarily utilize physicochemical characteristics of a drug, in conjunction with some instrumentation, and are generally individualized for each compound or a group of similar compounds. Biological methods, on the other hand, are based upon some biological activity of the drug. In general, they do not quantitate the specific drug concentration, but rather the activity of the drug is transformed into a concentration equivalent. As a result, these methods cannot distinguish between compounds that have similar biological activities. This problem is highlighted by studies involving antipsychotics, since many laboratories have utilized radioreceptor assay (RRA) for drug measurements. Javaid et al. (1980) have shown that in the same plasma sample, chemical assay and RRA resulted in substantially different levels for various antipsychotics (12) (Table 1.7). Since RRA also measures pharmacologically active metabolites, this outcome was not surprising. A brief description of the principles of these methods along with their utility is given in Table 1.8. **Currently, gas liquid chromatographic (GLC or GC) and high pressure liquid chromatographic (HPLC) methods are the most commonly used for such analyses.**

In earlier studies the method of blood collection and sample handling prior to analysis could also have resulted in variable plasma level measurements. For example, it has been reported that during blood collection of tricyclic antidepressants and phenothiazines contact with rubber stoppers for extended periods of time could result in spuriously low plasma levels (12, 13).

Patient Population. *Patient population* issues include:

- The presence of *refractory* patients
- *Nonhomogeneous* patient samples

- Patient *noncompliance*, particularly in outpatient studies
- Small patient *sample sizes*.

Study Design. Important issues relating to study design are the following:

- Inadequate evaluation of clinical response
- Concurrent, *multiple drug treatments*
- Too-brief an *observation period*
- Variable time of *blood sampling*.

As noted earlier, the interpretation of plasma level versus clinical response data even in well-designed studies is further complicated by the presence of multiple **active metabolites** formed by biotransformation, the major route of elimination for most psychotropics.

Clinical Applicability

Substantial data indicating large differences in plasma levels among patients treated with the same dose of a psychotropic provide one rationale for adjusting the dose based on blood levels to achieve the optimal clinical effect. However, the putative therapeutic range must be established for each individual drug. It is also necessary for valid studies to define clinically meaningful limits. Thus, a large body of information is required before even an approximation of the therapeutic range can be determined.

Table 1.7.
Antipsychotic Levels by Gas-Liquid Chromatography and Radioreceptor Assay[a]

Drug	Number of Subjects	Gas-Liquid Chromatography (ng/ml)	Radioreceptor Assay (ng/ml)
Haloperidol	20	7.2	10.1
Butaperazine	10	152.0	201.0
Fluphenazine	20	0.97	7.1
Trifluoperazine	35	0.7	5.7

[a]Same plasma sample was analyzed by the two methods.
From reference 11.

Table 1.8.
Various Techniques Used for Therapeutic Drug Monitoring[a]

Method	Principle	Comments
CHEMICAL ASSAYS		
Spectrometric	Drug is extracted into organic solvent and subsequently measured by colorimetric reaction or fluorescence.	At therapeutic concentrations, sensitivity fair to poor for potent antipsychotics; specificity—poor to fair; rarely used at present.
GLC	Compounds are separated between moving gas phase and stationary liquid phase and detected by different detectors; the method is individualized for each compound or a group of similar compounds after extraction.	The use of specific detectors, such as electron capture (ECD) and nitrogen/phosphorus (NPD), gives good-to-excellent sensitivity and specificity; commonly used in many labs for routine measurements.
HPLC	Compounds are separated between moving liquid phase and a stationary phase and detected by different detectors; the method is individualized for each compound or a group of similar compounds after extraction.	The use of special detectors, such as fluorescence or electrochemical detectors, results in good-to-excellent sensitivity and specificity; commonly used in many labs for routine measurements.
GC-MS	After extraction, the compounds are separated by GC and fragmented by MS; each compound gives specific mass fragments.	Very specific, with good-to-excellent sensitivity; not economical for routine analysis; generally used to establish specificities for other techniques.
BIOLOGICAL ASSAYS		
RRA	Radiolabelled drug bound to receptors can be displaced by unlabelled compounds with similar binding characteristics; the plasma can be used without extraction.	This method measures the inhibitory activity of the sample; although simple, with fair sensitivity, the method has poor specificity; some labs use in clinical studies.
RIA	Antibodies are prepared against the drug linked to a protein; the displacement by the sample of radiolabelled drug from antibody-antigen complex is determined; the sample can be used without extraction.	The method is sensitive and simple; however, the specificity is poor to fair and depends on the cross reactivity of structurally related compounds; generally restricted to the labs that have specific antibodies because currently they are not commercially available.

[a]From reference 11.

Plasma levels of various psychotropics differ widely among individuals due to differences in their rates of metabolism. Therefore, the clinician must adjust each patient's dosage to achieve maximum benefit with minimal side effects. We believe the best way to understand plasma levels is not through arbitrarily selected numbers defining the upper or lower limits of the therapeutic window, but by assessing the utility of a given plasma level in the clinical context of a specific patient, including:

• To determine *compliance*
• To establish *adequacy* of the pharmacotherapy in nonresponders
• To *maximize the clinical response* where the drug plasma level-response relationship is elucidated

- To help define the *dose-response relationship*
- To clarify when potential *drug interactions* may alter steady-state concentration levels
- To avoid *toxicity* due to unnecessarily high plasma levels
- To be used as a safeguard for the clinician in potential *medical-legal* situations.

Lithium.   For most psychiatrists, this is the area of lab testing with which they are most familiar. Lithium has a well-defined, narrow serum concentration range (14). For acute mania, therapeutic lithium levels fall between a range of 0.5 mEq/liter on the low end and an upper range around 1.5 mEq/liter. There may be individual patients with idiosyncratic responses outside this range or who exhibit adverse effects or toxicity at lower levels. It is recommended that blood levels be drawn about 4–5 half-lives (i.e., 4–6 days) after an adjustment in dose, or more frequently if unexpected reactions occur. Blood should be collected 10–12 hours after the last dose.

After resolution of the acute phase, maintenance levels of at least 0.8 mEq/liter are necessary for adequate coverage, and should be obtained once every 3–4 months, or more often if clinically indicated. Other follow-up tests include periodic thyroid function tests, blood urea nitrogen (BUN), serum creatinine, serum calcium (since lithium may cause hypoparathyroidism), and an ECG. Thyroid function tests (TFTs) and renal function should be monitored approximately every 6–12 months (see Maintainance/Prophylactic Treatment in Chapter 10).

Anticonvulsants.   The plasma levels of anticonvulsants used to treat psychiatric disorders have not been established. Because there are data on their usefulness to treat seizure disorders, monitoring of blood levels has increased the safety of anticonvulsants (and indirectly their efficacy), while also verifying compliance and determining the cause of toxicity when more than one medication is concurrently administered (see Alternate Treatment Strategies in Chapter 10).

The anticonvulsant therapeutic range for plasma concentrations of *carbamazepine* is 4–12 g/ml. Strict guidelines for hematological investigations in patients on carbamazepine therapy need to be followed since aplastic anemia and agranulocytosis have been reported in association with its use.

A good correlation has not yet been established between daily dose, serum level, and therapeutic effect of *divalproex sodium;* however, therapeutic serum levels for most patients will range from 50 to 120 g/ml. Patients should be monitored closely for nonspecific symptoms like malaise, weakness, lethargy, facial edema, anorexia, and vomiting—indicative of hepatotoxicity. Liver function tests (LFTs) should be performed prior to therapy and at frequent intervals thereafter, especially during the first 6 months.

Antidepressants.   Indications for ordering antidepressant (AD) blood levels include:

- Questionable patient compliance
- Poor response to an "adequate" dose, raising doubts about unusual pharmacokinetics, such as excessively slow or fast metabolism, leading to unusually low or high blood levels
- Side effects at a low dose
- Medically ill; children and adolescents; elderly patients
- Patients for whom treatment is urgent and it is imperative to achieve therapeutic levels as soon as possible. Thus, a

test dose may identify a fast metabolizer, who may require a higher dose; however, there is no evidence that this approach could accelerate response, an issue that needs to be tested in controlled trials. Further, there is no evidence that high doses will shorten the lag period for any psychotropic agent.

These issues are discussed in greater detail in Chapter 7, Pharmacokinetics.

Antipsychotics. Clear guidelines for measuring therapeutic serum concentrations of antipsychotics have not yet been established. There may, however, be specific situations in which they may be of some value (e.g., monitoring of haloperidol levels might be useful in patients on concurrent carbamazepine therapy, since carbamazepine is known to reduce serum concentrations of haloperidol). These issues are discussed in greater detail in Chapter 5, Pharmacokinetics/Plasma Levels.

Antianxiety/Sedative-Hypnotics. Because of their large therapeutic index, measurement of anxiolytic or sedative-hypnotic serum concentrations is not usually necessary in clinical practice, unless abuse, overdose, or inadvertent toxicity are suspected (see Adverse Effects of Anxiolytics/Sedative-Hypnotics in Chapter 12).

Summary

Historically, many of the pioneers in psychiatry attempted to correlate "mental" symptoms with identifiable brain pathology. This tradition continues by using "state-of-the-art" techniques to search for biological correlates of psychopathology. This, in turn, may lead to a better understanding of pathogenesis and causation, culminating in more specific treatment strategies.

The laboratory plays as important a role in clinical psychiatry as it does in other medical specialties. Use of the lab is most helpful in:

- Identifying medical disorders that present with cognitive, affective, and behavioral changes, or when psychiatric disorders mimic medical/neurological syndromes
- Medical workup prior to specialized treatment options
- The selective use of drug concentrations to enhance efficacy and minimize toxicity.

It is important that clinicians appreciate the need for the judicious choice of lab tests for a particular individual, while being sensitive to economic realities, degree of discomfort, and risk of adverse effects. They must also be cognizant of the nuances in interpreting lab data (i.e., their specificity, sensitivity, and predictive value). Finally, they need to integrate lab data with the history, interview, and physical examination to formulate the most accurate diagnosis and appropriate treatment plan.

CONCLUSION

In summary, clinicians should be prepared to take advantage of an ever-increasing number of newer, more specific agents. They can accomplish this by:

- Adopting a *medical model* when evaluating the patient's complaints
- Taking a *stepwise, empirically based approach to treatment* selection
- Adopting the stance of a *behavior psychopharmacologist* when evaluating a patient's response, recognizing that any reaction to medication (intended or otherwise) could provide useful information

• *Keeping current with recent, relevant developments* in the neurosciences.

The application of our principles should help clinicians to incorporate new developments in psychopharmacology into their practice. The end result will be improved patient care and further insights into pathophysiology, which can serve as the basis for our next generation of therapies.

REFERENCES

1. Israni TH, Janicak PG. Laboratory assessment in psychiatry. In: Flaherty J, Davis JM, Janicak PG, eds. Psychiatry: Diagnosis and therapy. Norwalk, Connecticut: Appleton and Lange, 1993:30–39.
2. Rose RB, Morihisa JM. Lab and other diagnostic tests in psychiatry. In: Talbott JA, Hales RE, Yudofsky SC, eds. The American Psychiatric Press textbook of psychiatry. Washington, D.C.: American Psychiatric, 1988.
3. Kirch DG. Medical assessment and lab testing in psychiatry. In: Kaplan HI, Sadock BJ, eds. Comprehensive textbook of psychiatry. 5th ed. Baltimore: Williams & Wilkins, 1989:525.
4. The APA Task Force on lab tests in psychiatry. The DST: an overview of its current status in psychiatry. Am J Psychiatry 1987;144(10):1253–1262.
5. Sharma RP, Pandey GN, Janicak PG, Peterson J, Comaty JE, Davis JM. The effect of diagnosis and age on the DST: a meta-analytic approach. Biol Psychiatry 1988;24:555–568.
6. Arana GW, Baldessarini RJ, Ornstein M. The DST for diagnosis and prognosis in psychiatry. Arch Gen Psychiatry 1985; 42:1193–1204.
7. Andreasan NL. Brain imaging: applications in psychiatry. Science 1988;239:1381–1388.
8. Lishman WA. Organic psychiatry. The psychological consequences of cerebral disorder. 2nd ed. London: Blackwell Scientific, 1987.
9. Cummings JL. Clinical neuropsychiatry. Orlando: Grune & Stratton, 1985.
10. Preskorn SH, Fast GA. Therapeutic drug monitoring for antidepressants: efficacy, safety, and cost effectiveness. J Clin Psychiatry 1991;52(6):23–33.
11. Javaid JI, Janicak, PG, Holland, D. Blood level monitoring of antipsychotics and antidepressants. Psychiatr Med 1991;9(1):163–187.
12. Javaid JI, Pandey GN, Duslak B, et al. Measurement of neuroleptic concentrations by GLC and radioreceptor assay. Commun Psychopharmacol 1980;4:467–475.
13. Cochran E, Carl J, Hanin I, et al. Effect of vacutainer stoppers on plasma tricyclic levels: a reevaluation. Commun Psychopharmacol 1978;2:495–503.
14. Janicak PG, Davis JM. Clinical usage of lithium in mania. In: Burrows GD, Norman, Davies, eds. Antimanics, anticonvulsants and other drugs in psychiatry. New York: Elsevier Science, 1987:21–34.

CHAPTER 2

Assessment of Drug Efficacy and Relevant Clinical Issues

A series of related issues is pertinent to the decision-making process a clinician employs in the application of drug therapy. The first section of this chapter considers the quality of the research data on drug efficacy by classifying studies based on predetermined criteria for methodological rigor. The companion section on meta-analysis reviews the rationale and potential complications inherent in statistically summarizing the data across several studies that assess drug efficacy. While mindful of the inherent shortcomings in this statistical approach, we believe such summarizations provide the clinician with a meaningful quantitative statement about a specific drug's clinical value.

The next section addresses issues relevant to the clinician-patient relationship during the assessment, initial treatment, and maintenance/prophylactic phases of psychopharmacotherapy.

The final two discussions explore various aspects related to the Food and Drug Administration (FDA) regulatory process and the cost of treatment. The latter issue not only includes the expenses associated with the assessment and treatment components, but more importantly, the total impact of a mental disorder on patients, their families, and society.

Evaluation of Drug Study Designs

To give the reader an accurate understanding of the literature on psychotropic drug efficacy, we have provided two perspectives. The first statistically summarizes the existing drug outcome studies, producing a "bottom-line" quantitative assessment of the difference between an experimental drug and placebo or other standard agent (see Drug Management later in this chapter). Secondly, we have classified studies (i.e., Class I, II, III) based on their methodological rigor so the reader can judge the quality of the data used to arrive at our statistical summaries (Table 2.1). These two perspectives are provided so practitioners can make the best informed decision about specific drug choices for their patients. The classification of studies is the topic of this section.

The most crucial issue in evaluating a drug study is the extent to which the design allows the investigator to adequately test the hypothesis in question. In addition to a proper blind, there are sev-

Table 2.1.
Classification of Study Designs

Classification	Criteria
Class I: At least the first nine criteria	Random assignment (prospective)
	No concomitant active medication
	Parallel (or appropriate crossover) design
	Double-blind, placebo control
Class II: Six of the ten criteria	Adequate sample
	Appropriate population
	Standardized assessments
	Either clear presentation of data or appropriate statistics
Class III: Five of the ten criteria	Adequate dose of medication
	Active controls[a]

[a]Desirable in all classes.

eral other important elements in a well-controlled study, including:

- *Random assignment* in a parallel or crossover design
- No "active" concomitant *medications*
- An adequate *sample*
- The use of *objective measures*
- Proper presentation of the *data*.

Without adequate controls and appropriate methodology, the ability to generalize is compromised, bringing into question a study's validity and/or the interpretation of its results.

RANDOM ASSIGNMENT

Random assignment under double-blind conditions is the most important element of a controlled trial. Without it, patients most likely to respond could be preferentially assigned to one treatment arm, and any difference in efficacy would be secondary to this bias. Further, the degree of improvement in the control group provides the measure by which the experimental group's outcome is compared.

Crossover and ABA (placebo-drug-placebo) designs should not be confused. In crossover studies, patients are randomly assigned to one of the two arms, so that generally a placebo is given first, then

the active drug, or vice versa. The usual design is a placebo lead-in period, then active drug A or B, succeeded by a placebo period again, and then the "crossover" from A to B or B to A. There should be a washout period, during which placebo is administered between the first and the second active drug phases, unless B is a placebo. Such designs often have an adequate sample size, objective evaluation, random assignment, and quantitative statistical analysis, with individual patients serving as their own controls.

If patients are maintained on placebo and the crossover to active treatment is not randomized (or in some other way controlled), they may be switched concurrent with a spontaneous change in clinical state. Any coincidental improvement or deterioration might then be due to the cyclic nature of the disorder and not the drug's effect. Other nonpharmacological interventions may also be introduced at this juncture. For example, if staff become concerned about a patient, they may intervene with more intensive milieu, family, or individual therapy.

CONCOMITANT MEDICATIONS

Avoidance of active concomitant medication is the next most important requirement. Such medication constitutes a major artifact because it can markedly weaken the drug/placebo difference. Thus, comparison treatments may be equally efficacious due to the concomitant medication and not any inherent efficacy of the experimental agent. Some studies have used multiple agents, in different doses, with some known to be specifically effective for the disorder under investigation. For example, in some studies comparing carbamazepine or divalproex sodium to placebo or lithium, patients also received adjunctive antipsychotics, making firm conclusions difficult (see Alternate Treatment Strategies in Chapter 10).

Concomitant medication should not be confused with rescue medications. The latter are nonspecific agents (or potentially effective drugs used in subtherapeutic doses) employed so that patients can remain in the study for an adequate time, thus allowing for a valid comparison between the experimental agent and placebo (or standard drug).

SAMPLE ADEQUACY

Equally critical to a properly designed study is sample adequacy (i.e., size and appropriateness). It is hard to make definitive conclusions with very small sample sizes, (e.g., five per group), since variation is too great. The minimum sample size needed to make inferences also depends on how large the experimental drug/placebo effect size is (i.e., the larger the effect size, the smaller the sample needed).

The population should also be appropriate to the disorder, so that patients included have the typical manifestations of the condition under investigation. Thus, if one were studying an antibiotic for the treatment of pneumococcal pneumonia, the selected patients should have this dis-

ease and not a viral pneumonitis. The same applies for an antipsychotic as regards chronic, treatment-resistant, or agitated, developmentally disabled patients. Conversely, if studying an agent thought to benefit treatment resistance, one might deliberately select a patient population that satisfied such criteria.

A related issue is complicated *entrance criteria* that may be counterproductive, in that many patients who have a classic presentation and would be excellent for study are excluded because they fail to meet one or more minor criteria. This results in too small a sample size and can lead to the inclusion of patients who technically fit the criteria but are not the most appropriate. This is particularly true with an uncommon disorder and/or with patients who are difficult to enroll in clinical trials (e.g., acutely manic).

Another issue is patients who volunteer for an advertised study. Undoubtedly some will have the true disorder, but others, although responding to an advertisement, may only minimally meet symptom criteria and may not have spontaneously sought help otherwise.

Some symptomatic volunteers may include newly recognized classic cases; patients referred to a tertiary referral center may be an atypical, treatment-resistant population, however.

RATING SCALES

Another important element is the use of reliable and valid rating instruments. To establish whether a drug is more effective than placebo, a global assessment of clinical improvement is often adequate; however, a valid rating scale(s) can also establish the qualitative nature of a response. *What is important is that symptom degree and change are quantified.* In an open study, patients are often evaluated by the investigator's global impression, an approach obviously subject to bias. The use of adequately normed and standardized quantitative scales to assess patients at baseline and during treatment provides an element of objectivity. A reliably trained rater using valid instruments anchored by clear operational definitions makes it much harder for bias to enter, even if the study is not double-blind.

DATA ANALYSIS

The presentation of data and the statistical analysis are two critical factors. The inclusion of baseline and final ratings on each patient from a standardized (or even a simple global, semiquantitative) scale, allows for useful comparisons between those on active treatment or placebo. Even if formal analyses are not done, findings from such studies are often impressive, and skeptical readers can always perform their own statistics.

Raw numbers depicting those who respond to an active drug or placebo provide the clinician with a "feel" for what actually happened, whereas the mean change scores on some abstract scale may have little meaning to the clinician. It is best to have the data speak directly to the reader in an uncomplicated fashion, and such presentations should always be included.

Equally important is the use of suitable quantitative statistical analyses, including more complicated models, since they can hold certain variables constant, control for artifacts, and provide supplementary information. Whatever statistics are used, they should be explicitly described in sufficient detail so the reader knows exactly what was done and can make a judgment about their appropriateness. For example, there are many different types of analyses of variance (ANOVA), and some may not be appropriate to the task at hand. ANOVAs, or multivariate analyses of variance (MANOVAs), or analyses of covariance (ANCOVAs) are familiar statistics, but are often imprecisely described. If only the results of an ANOVA with a $p < 0.001$ are provided, the reader may be justifiably dubious, since this model may not be the most proper (p is an estimate of the probability that the results occurred by chance). Consequently, sufficient details are required to clarify which model was used.

DOUBLE-BLIND TECHNIQUES

In a double-blind study, neither the patient nor the evaluator knows who is receiving active experimental medication or placebo. If enough patients are available for three or more groups, an active control medication group can also be used.

A standard active drug control serves two important purposes. First, it validates the experiment by demonstrating that the standard drug is clearly superior to placebo in this population. Second, it serves as a benchmark, since it has a known efficacy. Hence, an effective new drug could be equal to or better than a standard drug, and both should be better than placebo. Alternatively, the new drug could be less effective than the standard drug but more efficacious than placebo. Defining a dose-response relationship can help identify the optimal dose, which in turn can then be used to validate the experiment.

STUDY DESIGNS

Optimal

Studies differ in their quality. The authors feel that several features should be considered when classifying study designs. Though our classification is arbitrary, it is intended as a device to focus on all important criteria, not just one (e.g., "blinding").

A *Class I* controlled study satisfies at least the first nine of the following criteria:

1. *Random* assignment
2. No *concomitant active medications*
3. *Parallel* (or appropriate crossover) design
4. Double *blind,* placebo control
5. *Sample size* adequacy
6. Appropriate *population*
7. Standardized treatment *assessments*
8. Clear, descriptive *presentation of data* or use of suitable, quantitative *statistical analyses*
9. Adequate *dose* of medication
10. *Active controls* (e.g., active standard drug).

The last criterion is a plus factor that enhances the value of any given study.

Class II studies are those that satisfy at least six of the 10 criteria. For example, a *single-blind study* allows for some bias, but if the other criteria (e.g., random assignment, parallel groups, etc.) are met, then the data may still be valid. An AB design with no randomization or statistical analyses may still have many excellent features. A mirror-image design, such as Baastrup and Schou's study of lithium's prophylactic effects would be a good example (1) (see Maintenance/Prophylaxis with Mood Stabilizers in Chapter 10). Such studies may have many elements of a better controlled design, including:

• Patients have a *classic presentation.*
• *Objective, quantifiable, and meaningful measures* are used to evaluate important clinical factors.
• A *large sample* is used.
• There is a *longer period of observation.*

A *Class III* study is one that meets at least five of the 10 criteria. While these studies have some important elements of a controlled trial, many aspects are uncon-trolled. Because a bias can exist, however, does not mean it does. Since every question cannot be answered by a Class I design for reasons of practicality or cost, Class II and Class III studies are often used to at least partially resolve questions that would not otherwise be addressed.

An example of a Class III study is the ABA design. A variable-length placebo lead-in period, drug period, and post-drug placebo period are suspect, however, since many nonrandom variables can influence their length. The choice of when to start active drug may correspond to a worsening of the patient's condition, while the choice to stop treatment may foreshadow discharge, with its own stresses. Such nonrandom events constitute a major artifact. With such a design, the staff can guess early and late in the hospitalization that patients are on placebo, and are on active treatment in the middle of the study, making the blind more illusionary than real.

While there are many confounds with such a design, it does provide important information about whether a patient relapses when switched to placebo after an active drug. It is often not possible to do a meaningful statistical analysis on an ABA design, since there is no control group for comparison. The fact that some patients improve more on a drug in period B than in the placebo period A, may be a factor of time and rater bias. Since there is no control group, one cannot say that this improvement is better than what would have occurred in the natural course of the illness. Relapse in the second placebo period, however, can provide valuable information, since some patients improve with placebo, but this improvement fluctuates over time.

ABA designs may also answer another scientific question (i.e., once the disease process is "turned off," will patients relapse when placebo is substituted?). For most psychotropics, we do not know whether relapse will occur immediately after a drug is stopped within a few days of achieving remission. The active disease may only have been suppressed, with relapse likely after discontinuation. Since there is limited information on the distinction between maintenance and prophylaxis for most drugs, this type of data makes a valuable contribution.

A mirror-image study (i.e., a design in which the time period on a new treatment is compared retrospectively to a similar time period without the new therapy) is often more like the "real world" of clinical practice, and hence, its results may be easier to generalize.

There is bias in mirror-image studies, however, given the absence of a blind and nonrandom assignment. Since the control group represents the prospective phase, other variables could have changed in the interim. Without blinding, there is no way to avoid an evaluator's enthusiasm for a given treatment. Careful assessment by objective measurements can minimize the bias, but not all such studies include this.

Less Definitive Designs

Uncontrolled studies are the most biased, with concomitant medication the source of greatest error. For example, a patient started on drug A who fails to immediately respond is then given drug B, but drug A could have a delayed effect on the patient, which is falsely attributed to drug B. Some case reports may attribute coincidental events to a specific drug. Thus, the critical reader should always clarify the role of concomitant medication as an artifact. Sometimes clinical myths can develop from several case reports on the efficacy of a specific drug when all patients were also on concomitant medication! Rare side effects can be defined by

case reports, but the writer should always warn of coincidence, thus providing an honesty of purpose to the report.

Open designs can differ dramatically in their quality. Some report on a variety of patients given different concomitant medications, diagnosed without the use of inclusion or exclusion criteria, and have outcome determined by the clinical investigator's opinion, based only on memory. By contrast, others include specified diagnostic criteria, with patients who are excellent examples of the disorder under study; use only one treatment; and are evaluated quantitatively and concurrently. Often the most important ingredient in an open study is the investigator's clinical judgment, which is, in fact, the measuring instrument. While a more clinically experienced investigator may remain unbiased, those with less experience may unknowingly err in this regard. Designs that incorporate quantitative evaluation of the medical record are superior to those that rely on clinician recall.

Finally, early in a drug's career it is important to distinguish which conditions are benefitted and which are not. The spectrum of disorders for which a drug is beneficial is important information, particularly in developing new indications for existing agents, such as imipramine for panic attack or clomipramine for obsessive-compulsive disorder (OCD). Since we cannot do Class I, II, or III studies addressing all possible variables, good open studies are valuable.

Systematic case-controlled studies (e.g., a non-randomized control group) can also provide useful information, but unfortunately they are rarely employed in psychopharmacology research. Some conditions are rare or pose an imminent danger to the patient (e.g., neuroleptic malignant syndrome (NMS)), making it impossible to conduct prospective, controlled trials. In these situations, case-controlled methodology can provide some degree of rigor. Since these studies are not random-assignment, however, the outcome can be substantially biased.

CONCLUSION

We will apply our classification of study designs throughout the text to help the clinician interpret the quality of results from clinical trials. Further, we hope to give the critical reader a perspective on the depth and validity of the available data. Most studies in our analyses of drug efficacy will be Class I or II; and if not, we will discuss accordingly.

REFERENCES

1. Baastrup P, Schou M. Lithium as a prophylactic agent. Arch Gen Psychiatry 1967;16: 162–172.

Statistical Summarization of Drug Studies

Meta-analysis is a statistical method that combines data from individual drug studies to obtain a quantitative summary of their results. This statistical model includes:

- The *overall effect* (i.e., how effective is a drug)
- The probability that this overall effect is *statistically significant*
- The *statistical confidence limits* on the overall effect
- The extent of *variability among all studies*, as well as the degree to which it is accounted for by discrepant results from a small fraction of the total number of studies
- The possible effect(s) of methodological or substantive *variables that could alter the outcome.*

When possible, meta-analyses were computed to summarize the overall effects from controlled clinical trials of commonly used psychotropics. This summarized data is used to compute an effect size and to calculate the probability that a given drug is different from placebo and/or equivalent to or more effective than standard drug treatments. The goal is to estimate the extent of clinical improvement with a specific treatment as an aid to therapeutic decision-making.

Unfortunately, efficacy is often assumed on the basis of clinical lore or by uncritically accepting the results of a given study. An article may review several highly publicized references to support a certain position, but the careful reader may find that many of the studies quoted are poorly controlled or report duplicate data. A good example is the literature on clonazepam as a treatment for acute mania. Many review articles quote numerous references to support its efficacy. But a careful scrutiny of the literature reveals only one small, controlled study, whose interpretation is limited by the use of active concomitant medication (see Lithium plus Benzodiazepines in Chapter 10). Ideally, to make an informed judgment about a new drug, one should critically consider each individual study before drawing any conclusions. While the numbers of uncontrolled trials vastly exceed those of their better-designed counterparts, a surprisingly large number of controlled reports are published (i.e., approximately 8,000 in over 25,000 general medical or subspecialty journals each year). *Meta-analysis can provide a systematic estimate of this data.*

OMNIBUS METHODS VERSUS META-ANALYSIS

Meta-analysis is not simply counting the number of studies that find a significant difference or taking an average of their mean improvement. Hedges and Olkin refer to such statistical models as omnibus or "vote counting methods," noting that they have a number of methodological problems (1). For example, they do not weight studies according to a standard criteria, such as the number of subjects in a report. Furthermore, such methods only calculate one statistical parameter indicating the probability that the studies considered together show a statistically significant difference.

An important difference between this method and meta-analysis is the ability to clarify whether all studies included show a consistent effect size (i.e., estimate homogeneity). For example, if a few studies find a large difference and the majority none, an omnibus method might still produce a statistically significant difference. The appropriate conclusion, however, is that the results across studies are highly inconsistent. Thus, with omnibus methods, errors in a few small studies can disproportionately contribute to the final results, a phenomenon Gibbons, Janicak, and Davis (1987) have illustrated with simulations (2). The meta-analytic methods in this text will always compare experimental with control groups and do not employ omnibus methods.

With meta-analysis the statistical significance of the combined results can be overwhelming when all the differences are in the same direction. For example, when the authors performed a meta-analysis on the probability that maintenance antipsychotics produced a lower relapse rate in schizophrenics than placebo (53% relapsed on placebo and 20% on maintenance antipsychotics), the difference was significant to 10^{-100}! Typically, when multiple studies have the same outcome, the results of a meta-analysis will be markedly statistically significant. By contrast, p values of 0.05 or 0.01 are very difficult to interpret, since an artifact from a single study could produce such "nonsignificant" significant levels.

One of the major purposes of meta-analysis is to demonstrate that findings are consistently and overwhelmingly statistically significant when studies are combined. When there is a consistent finding, with some studies clearly significant and others having strong trends, a box score method may misleadingly show some positive and some negative outcomes. Frequently, large studies are positive, but some of the smaller, ostensibly negative studies, show a strong trend that does not reach statistical significance due to their limited sample size.

META-ANALYTIC STATISTICAL METHOD

Throughout this book, the authors have employed a computer-assisted literature search for all studies on a given psychotropic; reviewed the bibliography of each report to identify other pertinent articles; and also obtained translations of the relevant non-English language articles, whenever possible. All double-blind, random-assignment studies in the world literature that tested a given drug against placebo or other standard agent(s) were systematically identified. Next, the standard techniques recommended by Hedges and Olkin (1985) for continuous data or the Mantel-Haenszel model for discontinous data were employed (1). Since continuous are more statistically powerful than discrete data, they were preferentially used, when available, to derive the effect size. The sample size (N), mean ($\bar{x}$), and standard deviations (SDs), were extracted, as well as how many patients had a good or poor response by deriving a cut-off point to separate responders from nonresponders. When a semiquantitative scale was provided, patients with moderate improvement or more were classified as "responders" and those with minimal improvement, no change, or worse as "nonresponders." For most medication studies, the majority of patients on placebo were usually rated only minimally improved, making this particular choice for a cut-off point the optimal way to distinguish drug versus placebo differences. We note here the importance of having an a priori working definition of response threshold, since choosing the best cut-off point in each individual study would bias the outcome (2).

Graphic Inspection of Results

The essence of meta-analysis is inspection of the data. Thus, this approach produces a visual representation of each study in the context of all the others. A review of the actual rating scale scores gives the critical reader a feel for the data, as well as an index of suspicion if there is undue variability. This is far more important than any statistical parameter.

Studies in the literature often present a wide variety of data obtained with different rating scales, measuring instruments, and statistical techniques. This makes it difficult to compare and contrast these studies holding constant results expressed in a wide variety of units. In statistics, actual scores are often converted to standardized scores by subtracting a given

value for each subject from the mean and dividing the result by the standard deviation. This creates a new value in **Z** *score units*, with a mean of zero and a standard deviation of 1 (i.e., standard scores). In meta-analysis the mean of the control group is subtracted from the mean of the experimental group and divided by the pooled group standard deviation. This is similar to the concept of percentages. Thus, data is expressed in uniform units rather than in actual means and standard deviations, which often vary substantially between studies. With meta-analysis, if a given study is discrepant (e.g., has a high placebo response rate or an unusually high drug efficacy rate), it will stand out; and this can be expressed graphically, using Z units derived from effect sizes; or percent response versus percent nonresponse; or the odds ratio (a statistical term used as an alternate to chi square). One can look down the list and observe the drug-placebo difference, as well as the variability between studies (e.g., see Table 7.16). The reader can then note if the finding is similar in all studies, or conversely, whether there is a big effect in some but not others.

Therefore, meta-analysis abstracts results from each study and expresses them in a common unit, so one can easily compare and contrast. This allows us to focus on the hypothesis under examination rather than be distracted by the myriad differences among studies.

When the results from several studies are converted into similar units, a simple inspection of a graph or table readily reveals which studies have different outcomes from the majority. Such discrepancies can also be examined by a variety of statistical indices. For example, one can calculate a statistical index of homogeneity, remove the most discrepant study, and recalculate, revealing that all but one study is homogenous. If two studies are discrepant, one could remove both and again reexamine the indices of homogeneity, and so on. For an example, the authors summarize the relative efficacy of unilateral nondominant versus bilateral electrode placement for the administration of electroconvulsive therapy (ECT). Here, 10 studies had one result, and two others a different outcome (see Tables 8.10 and 8.11).

Effect Size

Effect size defines the magnitude of the difference between the experimental and the control groups. This is quite different from the statistical significance, which is the probability that such a finding may occur by chance, leading to rejection of the null hypothesis. Statistical significance is primarily determined by the sample size, so studies with a large number of subjects may find a highly significant result. By contrast, effect size is independent of sample size. Thus, in a 6-person study, if 2 out of 3 patients are benefitted by an antipsychotic and 1 out of 3 improve on placebo, this result would not be statistically significant. But, if 200 out of 300 patients benefit from an antipsychotic while only 100 out of 300 benefit from placebo, this would be highly statistically significant. While the effect size, (i.e., 67% on drug and 33% on placebo improving) is the same in both studies, only the results of the second study are clearly statistically significant because of its larger sample size.

The effect size of a *continuous variable* is frequently expressed as the difference between the mean of the experimental minus the mean of the control group divided by the pooled standard deviation. For example, in Chapter 5, data from the National Institute of Mental Health (NIMH) collaborative study demonstrated that antipsychotic-treated patients averaged a 4.2-point increase on a 6-point improvement scale, whereas the placebo patients averaged only a 2.2-point increase (i.e., an average difference of 2 points). The standard deviation of this data was approximately 1.7, so in effect size units, the improvement was approximately 1.2 (i.e., 2.0/1.7) standard deviation units. For *discontinuous data,* the effect size for a drug-placebo comparison is usually expressed as the difference between the percent improvement with the experimental drug and the percent improvement with placebo.

Examples of meta-analyses in this text that determined the effect size of various psychotropics include (see Tables in Chapters 5 and 7):

- Maintenance antipsychotics versus placebo
- Depot versus oral maintenance antipsychotics
- Maintenance antipsychotics with or without psychosocial therapy
- Several individual antidepressants versus placebo for acute treatment
- Combined cyclic and combined monoamine oxidase inhibitor (MAOI) antidepressants versus placebo for acute treatment
- Maintenance antidepressants versus placebo

Interpretation of Effect Size

When there are a number of double-blind studies, the question of efficacy is usually readily determined. If the probability of a drug's superiority over placebo is significant (e.g., 10^{100} to 10^{20}), and the effect size is consistent, the possibility of a false positive outcome is nil. The only possible exception is a major qualitative defect in the methodology.

Effect Size of Medical Drug Therapies

To provide a more general context in which to evaluate the effect sizes for various psychotropics, it is helpful to consider the data on the efficacy of various medical treatments, such as penicillin and streptomycin for pneumococcal pneumonia. At the time penicillin was discovered, double-blind methodology was not frequently used, and the standard therapy was sulfa drugs. In open studies penicillin reduced the death rate from pneumonia by about 50%. When streptomycin was introduced, double-blind, random-assignment designs were being utilized, and the British conducted a multi-sanatorium study. They established an effect size for streptomycin, which can be expressed as a continuous variable (i.e., 0.8 effect size units) or as a discontinuous variable (i.e., 69% of patients improved with streptomycin versus 36% with placebo). We have tabulated all drug therapies used as adjuncts to surgery to determine relative efficacies (Table 2.2). Since the results ranged from completely ineffective to substantially beneficial, this represents an unbiased sample of effect sizes.

These examples quantitate the beneficial effects of an unbiased selection of standard antibiotics used as adjunctive treatments. The purpose is to give the clinician an appreciation for the magnitude of improvement, while also allowing us to place recent psychotropics in the context of other drugs' efficacy for general medical and surgical disorders. In general, psychotropics met or exceeded the effect of these medical drug treatments.

Confidence Interval

An important question in meta-analysis is the consistency of the results (i.e., its confidence interval). Thus, we not only want to know how much more effective a drug is, but do all the clinical trials agree on the size of the therapeutic effect.

Table 2.2.
Effectiveness of New Drug *Adjunctive Therapies* after Surgery in Comparison to Standard Non drug Treatments (1964–1972)

Treatment	Patients Who Developed a Complication or Died (%)		Decrease in Morbidity or Mortality (%)
	Standard Treatment	Standard plus Adjunct	
Ampicillin for colon surgery	41	3	38
Neomycin-erythromycin for colon surgery	30	0	30
Antibiotics before heart surgery	33	26	7
Antibiotics after heart surgery	30	15	15
Heparin to prevent venous thrombosis	22	4	18
Chlorhexidine in contaminated wounds	13	13	0
Antibiotics after appendectomy	50	43	7
Vinblastine for cancer of lung	94	92	2
HATG with kidney transplant	34	31	3
Prednisone for cirrhosis	42	41	1
TSPA for cancer of colon	48	55	−7
Chemotherapy for cancer of breast	38	32	6
Average	40%	30%	10%

CRITICAL ISSUES IN META-ANALYSIS

There are several issues that must be considered when interpreting the results of a meta-analysis, including:

- Choice of studies
- Selection of patients who enter clinical trials
- The "file drawer" problem
- Pattern of results
- Continuous versus dichotomous data
- Reporting of standard deviations
- Crossover designs
- Redundant data.

Choice of Studies: the Need for a Control Group

A critical methodological issue for a proper meta-analysis is the choice of studies. It is important that all studies meet reasonable criteria; otherwise, there is a potential bias introduced. The authors chose only those studies that had an appropriate control group which provided a standard by which a drug's effects could be measured. By contrast, there have been meta-analyses of multiple studies on psychotherapy, all done without comparison groups, or with invalid comparison groups. Combining the effect size of these studies only reflects the enthusiasm of the investigator rather than any true effect, since there is no valid comparison.

Patients Who Enter Clinical Trials

Most clinical trials study newly admitted, "voluntary" patients who enter a research setting and are kept drug-free for 1 or more weeks. More severely disturbed patients, however, are usually not candidates for research. Also, since symptomatic volunteers are often used in outpatient studies, it may be more difficult to confirm the presence of a given disorder, especially given the frequent lack of valid and reliable diagnostic tests. Thus, this brings into question the generalizability of the studies' results.

File Drawer Problem

One of the most important pitfalls in meta-analysis was labelled the "file drawer" problem by Easterbrook et al., 1991 (3). In a recent survey they indicated that studies with positive outcomes were twice as likely to be published (and usually in more prestigious and therefore higher profile journals). Thus, there is a systematic tendency for positive results to be reported and negative results to be "filed away" and go unreported.

Given the tendency not to publish negative data, we have attempted to include double-blind, random-assignment trials from meeting presentations; reports of symposia; exhibits; or available unpublished data from the individual author(s), pharmaceutical industry, or government.

This problem goes beyond unpublished papers, with some investigators performing multiple statistical analyses and emphasizing the most favorable outcome. Indeed, we have found single reports of detailed statistical discussions for a positive aspect of a study, with only passing reference to a negative aspect that was not statistically significant. An example of this is a report on the benefit of lithium in treating alcohol dependence (4). Here, the negative result in nonaffectively disordered alcoholics is not adequately presented for comparison with their mood disordered counterparts (see The Alcoholic Patient in Chapter 14).

Reviewing the actual numbers of patients allows one to eliminate duplicate publications of the same data, since positive results are much more likely to be published more than once. The methodological rigor of a good meta-analysis guards against biases, fortuitous results, and most important, being overly influenced by a few positive reports.

The file drawer problem also has implications for interpretation in meta-analysis. Certain techniques, particularly the vote counting or omnibus methods, carry forward any positive result to the final summary statistics. Also, with a vote counting (or omnibus) method, one often tabulates the vote according to the most positive rating outcome, usually emphasized by the study's author.

Another safeguard is to calculate the number of patients whose negative results (hypothetically hidden in the file drawer) would result in converting a positive to a negative meta-analysis.

We believe the file drawer issue is less of a problem in meta-analysis than in the narrative review, which often lists only those publications that support a particular conclusion. When the "original" documents are read, however, they often prove to be reviews of other references! Thus, the reference list gives a false impression of more studies than were actually done. Other problems include:

- Studies listed as *"controlled"* do not include random-assignment or a valid control group.
- Studies are *misquoted*.
- A conclusion or abstract is quoted but this is *not consistent* with the data in the article.
- The same data appears in *multiple publications*.

Interpretation of the Pattern of Results

The pattern and consistency of results across all studies are very important. For example, if there are a few small-sample-size positive studies and many large-sample negative studies, it is likely that the smaller studies were aberrations. If the results between individual studies are highly discordant, it is a mistake to conclude that the overall effect is significant. Rather, the conclusion is that some studies show a drug effect and others do not, requiring one to explain the discrepancy. It is preferable to evaluate studies by some a priori criteria for methodological rigor and then examine whether there is an equal effect size in the more versus less rigorous studies.

Continuous versus Categorical Data

For the most part, the meta-analyses used in this text are based on fourfold contingency tables, which include the number of responders or nonresponders to a given treatment. An advantage of dichotomous data is that information from individual subjects can be abstracted (i.e., the results come from actual patients). In one sense this is not strictly a meta-analysis, since calculations are not done on summary parameters but on observations of individual subjects. Such an approach has the advantage of directness, however, since the percent of patients who respond or do not respond to a new treatment, standard treatment, or placebo is intuitively meaningful to clinicians; whereas, a change of 0.8 standard deviation units may not be.

Reporting of Standard Deviations

A meta-analysis cannot be calculated unless the pertinent standard deviations are known. Unfortunately, clinical reports often give the sample size and mean ratings for the various groups, but do not report the standard deviations (or standard error of the mean (SEM)), which are necessary for effect size calculations. Thus, investigators should always report the indices of variability (e.g., confidence intervals, standard deviations) for the critical variables related to their primary hypothesis.

Crossover Designs

Crossover trials play an important role in psychopharmacological research. Since there was no method for doing a meta-analysis with such designs, the authors have developed a method (a variation on Hedges' method for uncrossed designs), with suitable modification for paired data (5).

Redundant Data

It is inappropriate to statistically evaluate a patient studied with two different measures as if that patient were two different subjects (i.e., each patient can only be counted once). For example, investigators may initially report on the first 20 subjects, and in a second paper, report on a total of 60, including the original 20 subjects. The same patient counted twice (or more), will magnify any finding. Additionally, it introduces a bias by giving undue weight to the findings of groups who report their data in multiple publications, as opposed to those reporting their findings only once.

CONCLUSION

The information presented in this chapter provides the background for later sections, which will quantitatively summarize the controlled literature for the various classes of psychotropics. In all cases, the data were obtained from controlled, clinical trials comparing a new (or experimental) treatment to placebo or a standard agent. The goal of these summations is to give a reader the critical "bottom line," devoid of our subjective bias, as well as the bias from isolated publications inconsistent with the trend seen when the controlled data is combined.

REFERENCES

1. Hedges LV, Olkin I. Statistical methods for meta-analysis. Orlando, Florida: Academic Press, 1985.
2. Gibbons RD, Janicak PG, Davis JM. A response to Overall and Rhoades regarding their comment on the efficacy of unilateral vs. bilateral ECT [Letter to the Editor]. Convulsive Ther 1987;3(3):228–237.
3. Easterbrook P, Berlin JA, Gopalan R, Matthews DR. Publication bias in clinical research. Lancet 1991;337:867–872.
4. Reynolds RN, Mercy J, Coppen A. Prophylactic treatment of alcoholism by lithium carbonate: an initial report. Alcohol Clin Exp Res 1977;1(2):109–111.
5. Gibbons R, Hedeker DR, Davis JM. Estimation of effect size from a series of experiments involving paired comparisons. J Educ Stat (in press).

Patient Issues

INFORMED CONSENT

Assessment of Capacity to Consent

Treatment always implies a contract between the patient (consumer) and clinician (provider). Any contract assumes a patient has both the capacity to give consent, as well as the willingness to do so. Clinicians who treat patients decide a question of capacity (either explicitly or implicitly) each time they hospitalize, perform surgery, or treat with drugs (1). There is an imperative embodied in the law which states that, with only certain exceptions, a valid consent is a necessary prerequisite in any clinical decision to provide treatment. There is an analogy to be drawn between capacity and mental illness. Clinicians often do not agree on the definition of a mental disorder, but it is a concept that is of constant practical significance. Persons are committed as a result of a mental disorder that significantly impairs their judgment, or are released if found not to have one. When insanity is an issue, persons will or will not be held responsible for their actions because of a mental disorder. With great difficulty and appreciable limitations, psychiatrists have developed standards for recognizing and categorizing these disorders. Though acceptance of the standards is not unanimous, they are at least consensual.

With psychiatric outpatients who are legally competent, issues of consent are not usually problematic. These patients can simply refuse their medication and/or seek help from another therapist, and there is little doubt that they are acting competently and voluntarily. By contrast, in the hospital setting (especially the public sector) there are a number of involuntary patients for whom legal issues are very relevant. Thus, the involuntarily committed patients often do not have the same options as their outpatient counterparts, and issues regarding their legal rights become a critical factor in treatment planning.

We advocate a consumer-oriented approach to the clinician-patient relationship. Thus, a therapist should be an educator and advisor, rather than dictate treatment. Since patients must live with their disease, as well as tolerate the prescribed treatments, they should play an active part in related decisions. Ideally, different options are examined for their relative merits, and then the clinician recommends a treatment plan. In the typical outpatient practice, the two parties agree with the assessment and the treatment plan, with the patient always having the final say. If there is disagreement, a compromise can often be reached that is satisfactory to both. A third scenario occurs when a compromise cannot be reached. In most instances, the patient seeks care elsewhere, since clinicians, in good conscience, cannot comply with a treatment plan inconsistent with their professional judgment and/or solely dictated by the patient. Examples include the paranoid individual who declines medication based on delusional ideation, but is not committable; and the drug-seeking patient who demands medication that the physician cannot ethically prescribe.

The one exception to this approach involves the patients who are unable to make an informed decision on their own behalf and/or pose an immediate danger by virtue of their mental disorder. In this instance, the patient is protected by both the legal and medical systems. The laws of most states allow commitment when patients are an imminent danger to self and/or others due to their mental disorder. When there was no active treatment, confinement was the only option available. Now, with the availability of very effective drug therapies, hospitalization lasts typically no more than a few weeks. Thus, treatment should be the focus of the medical-legal dialogue, and confinement only a vehicle to insure its adequacy.

The authors will suggest specific procedures for the clinical assessment of capacity to consent, as well as permissible courses of action that logically follow such assessments (2) (see Figure 2.1).

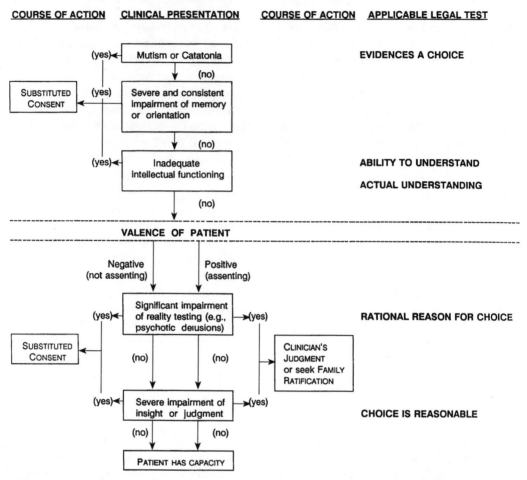

Figure 2.1. Assessment of capacity to consent. Adapted from Janicak PG, Bonavich, PR. The borderland of autonomy: medical-legal criteria for capacity to consent. J Psychiatry & Law 1980;8:379.

Mental Status Exam

Ability to Communicate. The mental status exam is critical to the determination of a patient's capacity to consent, and the ability to communicate is an absolute prerequisite (see Diagnostic Assessment in Chapter 1). Psychomotor impairments such as *mutism* or *catatonia* (withdrawn type) would severely affect an individual's fundamental ability to communicate any appreciation of the issues involved and their ramifications. Although an individual may actually be well oriented, intellectually appreciate, and even later remember, events that occurred and the issues involved, that individual is not capable of consenting if unable to demonstrate these faculties.

Memory. If able to communicate, the next factor to consider is *memory*. Most commonly recent recall is impaired, but in an acute situation (e.g., drug-induced delirium), immediate memory may also be disrupted. Frequently, immediate and recent memory impairment are superimposed on a more chronic organic state (e.g., degenerative dementia), with additional problems in remote memory. The more memory components involved, and the greater the severity of impairment in any one, the less able an individual will be to adequately register, retain, and recall information necessary to give consent. The most critical memory components involve the immediate-recent spectrum of functioning. Gross dysfunction of these memory processes can usually be tested in the standard mental status examination. **Intact immediate-recent memory components are also a prerequisite to giving informed consent.**

Orientation. In acute biological derangements, such as phencyclidine (PCP) intoxication or an electrolyte imbalance, *disorientation* can occur to all spheres (e.g., person, place, time, situation), including spatial relationships. A person severely disoriented to a situation clearly lacks capacity, being unable to appreciate the nature of the interaction. One may be disoriented to other spheres, however, and still be capable of consenting. The clinician should ascertain which spheres are affected, as well as the severity of dysfunction in each. If there is a significant impairment of both memory and orientation, capacity should be regarded as at least diminished, if not entirely lacking. Since these problems may have a fluctuating course, intermittently improving and deteriorating, repeated assessment over time is necessary to reach a valid conclusion. **In summary, both memory and orientation must be substantially intact to**

support a conclusion that the patient can give consent.

Intellectual Functioning. The quality of a patient's *intellectual functioning* in the context of that person's educational, social, and cultural experiences must also be considered. Minimally, a patient should demonstrate the ability to express an understanding of issues on a level comparable to the majority of those with average intelligence. This cognitive process can be tested by asking the patient to summarize or to reformulate and express a concept, question, or situation posed by the examiner. This exercise obviously calls for clinical judgment in choosing the items to which the patient responds, as well as in evaluating the intellectual level shown by the responses. The likelihood of clinical bias is generally greater, the "higher" the cognitive process under examination. In a sense, the clinician may be able to do no better than conscientiously apply the clinician's own "reasonable man" standard. **The threshold for adequate intellectual function is a response which provides evidence that abstract and logical processing are intact.**

Reality Testing. Next to be evaluated are *perception of reality* and the quality of *thought content*. An example would be a severely depressed patient who expresses feelings of guilt and worthlessness, at times to the extent of misperceiving the explanation of a treatment that is prescribed. From the clinician's point of view, the presented recommendation is a means of alleviating the vegetative signs of depression; however, from the distorted viewpoint of a severely depressed patient, this may be interpreted as a justifiable punishment. A careful explanation of the mode and purpose of a proposed treatment should be followed by attempts to elicit feedback from patients that will reveal the extent of their reality testing.

Insight and Judgment. Issues of *insight* and *judgment* are particularly difficult to assess, since a clinician's view is biased by that person's own value system. Furthermore, these processes are much more complicated aspects of cognitive functioning, and in fact, can be conceptualized as the culmination of the previously discussed factors.

At the very least, patients should manifest a basic awareness of the relationship between specific events in their life and the condition for which treatment is proposed. This would define the minimum insight necessary to give consent.

Although generally assessed together, intact insight does not imply sound judgment, which also involves an awareness of the current condition (i.e., a comprehension of both the problem and the process by which its alleviation may be accomplished). Since the assessment of judgment is complicated by the inevitable involvement of the clinician's value system, this assessment should be made in light of the patient's own expressed values—setting aside any conflicts between the value system of the patient and that of the examiner. This process is best accomplished by eliciting the premises that underlie the patient's decision(s). These premises may or may not have the quality of "reasonableness," but if they are regarded as such by the clinician (though perhaps, in the clinician's opinion, erroneous), it should be concluded that the patient has capacity. If they are not "reasonable," the inquiry should continue, with one possibility being that the premises are the product of the patient's illness. This conclusion would mitigate against a finding of capacity, though it should not be conclusive. It is only when the basis for a decision is clearly the result of

the illness that the unreasonableness of the decision may indicate a lack of capacity. Thus, if the decision is unreasonable, but is not the product of the illness, there should be a finding of capacity.

Age Factor. A final question is the issue of *age,* which may also play a significant role. In addressing this factor, Stanley et al. (1984) compared elderly (mean age = 69.2 ± 5.3) to younger medical patients (mean age = 33.7 ± 6.6) for capacity to consent (3). While both groups tended to make reasonable decisions, the elderly patients demonstrated poorer comprehension for various elements of the informed consent process.

Tests of Capacity

To develop more precise operational guidelines, the authors have related the major components of a psychiatric evaluation (especially those deemed most important in the assessment of capacity) to various tests formulated by the courts.

In a review of the literature, Roth et al. (1977) concluded that there are five categories for tests of competency (i.e., capacity) (4):

- *"Evidencing a choice,"* which verifies the presence or absence of a decision by a patient for or against treatment
- The *"reasonable outcome of choice" test,* which evaluates the patient's ability to reach the "reasonable," the "right," or the "responsible" decision
- The *"choice based on rational reasons" test,* which attempts to ascertain the quality of a patient's thinking and whether it is a product of mental illness
- The *"ability of the patient to understand"* the risks, benefits, and alternatives to treatment (including no treatment)

- The *"actual understanding,"* which defines competence based on the accuracy of the patient's perceptions.

Roth and colleagues assert that in practice, competency is usually determined by the interplay of one or more of these tests and two other variables: *the risk/benefit ratio of treatment* and *the valence of the patient's decision* (i.e., consent to or refusal of treatment) (4). We include valence as a factor in our guidelines, since agreement or lack of agreement between the patient and the clinician may dictate different courses of action, given the overriding preference to be in accord with the expressed wishes of the patient. We exclude the risk-benefit ratio as a factor, however, since ideally this consideration should occur before or after an assessment of capacity, but not as part of the actual determination.

Algorithm for Assessing the Capacity to Consent

This schema assumes an adult patient, not under legal guardianship, who presents with a non-emergent disorder. First, components of the psychiatric evaluation are listed in the order they should be considered. Second, we indicate the various courses of action the clinician may take in response to specific situations (e.g., seek court determination of capacity to consent). Finally, the various tests of capacity are related to those clinical factors most pertinent to each test (Fig. 2.1).

Informed Consent

Once capacity has been assured, a patient's decision to accept or refuse treatment must be ascertained as being informed and freely given. The information conveyed in a one-to-one, personal inter- action with the patient should have the following characteristics:

- *Accurate*
- *Adequate* (complete in necessary detail, such as name, nature and purpose of treatment)
- *Comprehensible* to the patient, and include the opportunity for the patient to ask questions
- *Appropriate*
  - Describe potential *benefit(s)*, including the likelihood of success
  - Indicate potential *risks* (e.g., side effects and complications)
- Present *alternatives*, if reasonable ones exist
- Explain *anticipated results without treatment*.

The use of booklets, video cassettes, or audio tapes should never take the place of a personal encounter with the patient. A dated and signed progress note, including the above details is usually considered sufficient documentation.

The Right to Treatment

One of the more controversial, if not paradoxical, developments in mental health law has been the establishment of a patient's right to treatment, followed by its legal counterpoint—the right to refuse treatment (5). While some contend there is no conflict between these two rights, the reality is that they are often at odds. The problem is most obvious with involuntarily committed patients, where the right to refuse treatment contradicts the reason for their hospitalization.

While the principle of personal inviolability requires us to respect a patient's decisions about treatment in all ordinary situations, exceptions are necessary in extraordinary circumstances. The possibility of serious harm is the determining factor here, precluding an absolute right to make one's own health choices.

We would propose that all mentally ill persons, whether adjudicated or presumed incompetent, retain the right to articulate their objection to or refusal of treatment and that any such concerns must be heard. The critical factor regarding treatment refusals by the mentally ill is whether, when, how, and by whom such a refusal can be overridden. In the authors' opinion, the decision to override a treatment refusal is best made by medical personnel rather than the legal system; the override decision can be made in all circumstances, not just emergencies; and it can and should be made expeditiously (6).

Consequences of Refusal of Treatment. The translation of the abstract right-to-refuse issue into real-world outcomes reveals serious consequences that are more complicated than may be assumed. For example, there is reliable research showing that psychotherapy without medication is not effective in treating such severe disorders as schizophrenia (7, 8). Therefore, there is often no effective alternate, less-restrictive treatment, and the only real option is no treatment.

Judicial override has proven to be very harmful to the patients, often taking many months (4 on the average). During this medication-free period, serious harm may befall a patient, other patients, and their care givers; as well as markedly lengthening the hospitalization. When the law requires that a patient's refusal can be overridden only by judicial process, critical treatment time is lost, and it is important to consider whether this delay has any effect on recovery.

While most controlled trials lasted only weeks, the longitudinal study of the effect of psychotherapy versus drugs by the previously noted work of May and his cowork-

ers is particularly germane (7, 8). Schizophrenic patients were randomly assigned to either antipsychotics or no medication. After 6 months or more, the initial nonmedication group was then given active drug. Those patients who did not receive medication for the first 6 months did substantially worse during the following 3 to 5 years, spending twice as much time in the hospital as the initially medicated group. **Thus, this study documents the potential harmful consequences that may occur when patients do not receive early effective treatment.**

The Need for Periodic Review. Protected both as to the need for and the right to treatment, how can a patient be safeguarded subsequently? First, the course of treatment should be periodically reviewed, as already mandated by law or administrative regulation in the majority of states and their institutions. Second, a patient-initiated review mechanism should be formalized in the hospital setting, so that questions and concerns about the course of treatment can be voiced. Finally, on an informal basis, patients are always free to object, discuss, or openly voice complaints about treatment.

Conclusion

The initial step in obtaining informed consent requires a careful assessment of the capacity to give such consent. The authors provide guidelines for appropriate action when such competence cannot be verified (see Figure 2.1). Once the examiner has initially confirmed capacity, the necessary information must be conveyed in a personal interaction and repeated at appropriate intervals throughout the entire treatment relationship. Finally, the clinician must carefully consider the delicate balance concerning a patient's right to treatment, right to refuse treatment, and the clinically relevant risk/benefit ramifications inherent in the ultimate course of action.

COMPLIANCE

Once capacity has been assured and informed consent given to a treatment plan, compliance becomes the next crucial issue.

Compliance is defined as adherence to the recommended treatment plan of a health care professional. Typically, it is partial at best, in that medications prescribed are taken less often than recommended, irregularly, and at times excessively. There are various reasons for noncompliance, which can be categorized as follows:

* Rational
* Capricious
* Absolute refusal
* Confusion
* Iatrogenic.

Thus, no matter how astute a diagnostician or how brilliant the treatment recommendations, frequently these efforts are merely academic exercises and never actualized due to noncompliance.

Factors Decreasing Compliance

A greater appreciation and recognition of the issues that enter into decreased compliance may minimize its impact. The stigma of a mental disorder; the frequent denial of illness; and the disruption in cognitive processes that is often a part of the illness all play a significant role. Side effects of medications, often not recognized as such by patients or inadequately inquired about by the clinician, also complicate adherence to therapy. The delay or time lag in the onset of action of many

psychotropics, as well as a delayed time course for a recurrence after stopping medication, also contribute. In this regard, the concept of prevention and prophylaxis must be carefully reviewed with the patient. Finally, the impact of treatment "cost" on compliance needs to be explored and the means to circumvent such impediments sought (see Cost of Treatment later in this chapter).

Strategies to Increase Compliance

Since noncompliance occurs frequently, it is important to recognize this reality; inquire directly about the issue; and sometimes indirectly evaluate it by using medication diaries, counting medications, and/or therapeutic drug monitoring (TDM).

Most important is an understanding and promotion of those factors which can increase compliance. The most critical factor in enhancing compliance is to encourage *active patient participation*, to the extent possible, in treatment planning and implementation. This includes *adequate communication* so that there is a working understanding of the rationale for a given treatment. Interactions around treatment recommendations should always be done in the context of an *empathic approach* and *trusting* relationship. *Family and community involvement and support* is often a critical determining factor. Finally, *emphasis on the positive effects of medication* for a patient's quality of life should be emphasized, and when at all possible, the most *simplified drug regimen* utilized.

TREATMENT TERMINATION

Termination of treatment may be initiated by the patient, the clinician, or by mutual agreement. At this juncture, the potential for recurrence should be clearly discussed in the context of the risk to benefit ratio (e.g., diminished side effects or toxicity from drug discontinuation versus a recurrence of the disorder). Part of this process should be the identification of possible prodromal symptoms, which should alert the patient to return for a reevaluation of status and the possible resumption of medication to preclude a full episode (e.g., decreased sleep as a prodrome to a manic phase). Prediction of an impending episode, however, may not be a useful strategy in all disorders (see discussion on intermittent antipsychotic maintenance strategy in Chapter 5).

CONCLUSION

Adequate compliance with treatment is a major issue impacting on the potential for a successful outcome. As noted in this section, several factors may contribute to a patient's willingness to persist with treatment as prescribed. Perhaps foremost is the clinicians' ability to communicate their approach in an empathetic and understandable manner.

REFERENCES

1. Appelbaum PS, Grisso T. Assessing patients' capacities to consent to treatment. N Engl J Med 1988;319:1635–1638.
2. Janicak PG, Bonavich, PR. The borderland of autonomy: medical-legal criteria for capacity to consent. J Psychiatry & Law 1980: 8;361–387.
3. Stanley B, Guido J, Stanley M, Shortell D. The elderly patient and informed consent: empirical findings. JAMA 1984;252:1302–1306.
4. Roth LH, Meisel A, Lidz CW. Tests of competency to consent to treatment. Am J Psychiatry 1977;134:279–284.
5. Appelbaum PS. The right to refuse treatment with antipsychotic medications: retrospect and prospect. Am J Psychiatry 1988; 145:413–419.
6. Brakel J, Davis JM. Taking harms seriously: involuntary mental patients and the right to refuse treatment. Indiana Law Review 1991; 25(2):429–473.
7. May PRA. Treatment of schizophrenia: a comparative study of five treatment methods. New York: Science House, 1968.
8. May PRA. Rational treatment for an irrational disorder: what does the schizophrenic patient need? Am J Psychiatry 1976;133: 1008–1012.

Drug Management

ACUTE, MAINTENANCE, AND PROPHYLACTIC THERAPY

Since most psychiatric disorders are recurrent and chronic in nature, appropriate management always requires the consideration of three phases of treatment:

- *Acute,* or the control of a current episode
- *Maintenance,* or the prevention of relapse once an acute episode has been alleviated and it is assumed that the disease process has been suppressed
- *Prophylactic,* or the prevention of future episodic exacerbations.

Acute intervention(s) may produce a full response, partial response, or no response. The last outcome is usually due to problems such as:

- Intolerance due to side effects
- Refractoriness
- Discontinuation (i.e., cessation of treatment for any reason other than intolerance or refractoriness).

As emphasized earlier, adequacy and appropriateness of drug therapy should always be reviewed in the event of unsatisfactory results. If a patient has been properly diagnosed but only responds partially to an adequate drug trial, a more difficult clinical decision-making process then ensues. The two major options are to switch to a different subgroup of drug (e.g., from a phenothiazine to a butyrophenone neuroleptic); or alternatively, to augment the initial medication (e.g., adding lithium to an antipsychotic regimen). In patients who are not helped by one drug treatment, switching to a different class within the same family is usually the approach that is most successful (e.g., from a heterocyclic antidepressant (HCA) to a serotonin reuptake inhibitor (SRI) or MAOI). Regardless of the outcome with subsequent drug treatment trials, the same sequential logic can be applied.

The patient who manifests full remission should be continued on adequate *maintenance therapy* for periods of at least 4 to 12 months, with the exact duration determined by the particular disorder, as well as the prior history of severity and frequency of relapses.

Prophylactic therapy beyond the first 4–12 months should be dictated by several factors:

- *Chronicity* of illness
- Frequency and severity of *relapses*
- Associated *"comorbidity"*, such as other medical conditions, concurrent substance or alcohol abuse, or other psychiatric disorders (e.g., dysthymia with major depressive disorder).

In general, the more of these factors that are present, the more likely that an indefinite maintenance/prophylactic medication regimen will be required.

During all phases of treatment, education, supportive therapy, and at times, more specific types of psychotherapy are essential for a satisfactory outcome. Thus, sociotherapies can enhance the beneficial effects of antipsychotics in schizophrenia,

reducing rehospitalizations (see Role of Psychosocial Therapies in Chapter 5); interpersonal therapy (IPT) can complement adequate maintenance antidepressant treatment, possibly diminishing the frequency of episodes (see Psychosocial Therapies in Chapter 7); and cognitive-behavioral techniques in combination with anti-obsessive agents (e.g., clomipramine) can improve the quality of life for OCD patients, minimizing time spent on disabling rituals (see Obsessive-Compulsive Disorder in Chapter 13).

MONOTHERAPY, COPHARMACY, AND POLYPHARMACY

As emphasized in Chapter 1, a major principle of drug therapy is the value of *monotherapy* (i.e., using only one medication). The rationale includes:

- Ease of administration
- Enhanced compliance
- Minimization of side effects
- Avoidance of drug-drug interactions
- Easier assessment of the benefit or lack of benefit with a particular drug.

Copharmacy is the concurrent use of two agents to improve results. At times it is necessary (e.g., an antiparkinsonian agent plus an antipsychotic to control extrapyramidal side effects (EPS)) or desirable (e.g., an antipsychotic plus an antidepressant to alleviate a psychotic depressive episode). The rational combination of medications is widely used in medicine if there is a sound pharmacological principle; empirical data to support a greater efficacy; reduced side effects; or enhanced safety. Examples include lithium potentiation of antidepressants; and oral antipsychotics to supplement depot intramuscular preparations while establishing a new steady state plasma level or managing a sudden relapse.

If this strategy is required, the authors would discourage the use of fixed-ratio combinations (e.g., amitriptyline plus perphenazine) and instead recommend the use of these or other similar agents independently. The primary reason is to afford more flexibility in the choice of specific agents and relative dosing of each drug.

When using more than one agent, it is important to make adjustments with a single agent at any given time. If more than one drug is increased, reduced, or switched concurrently, it will be difficult to identify which alteration was responsible for any significant change in status (whether good or bad).

A second area of concern, when using two or more agents concurrently, is the potential for clinically relevant and possibly deleterious *drug-drug interactions*. Thus, as noted in subsequent chapters, the addition or elimination of an agent may significantly alter the activity of the concurrent drug treatment (e.g., carbamazepine lowering haloperidol plasma levels; see Anticonvulsants in Chapter 10).

Polypharmacy is the simultaneous use of more than one agent from the same class or more than two drugs from different classes, and is rarely warranted. While there are some exceptions (e.g., low doses of trazodone given at bedtime for its sedative hypnotic effects during the early phases of treatment with fluoxetine; or the concurrent use of an SRI and 5-HT$_{1a}$ agonist), this practice is more likely to increase the risk of toxicity (via additive or synergistic effects); and/or adverse drug-drug interactions, while adding little to enhance clinical efficacy.

Role of the Food and Drug Administration

The Food and Drug Administration (FDA) was established in the 1930s by federal law to ensure the relative safety of food, cosmetics, and medicinals, as well as to regulate the marketing of such products, due to ongoing abuses in promotional claims. Since then, its scope of responsibilities has been revised often in response to specific incidents, such as the tragedy of thalidomide in the 1960s. In terms of medicinals, the FDA oversees drug development, including the extensive clinical trials that must be conducted to establish efficacy and safety for a defined indication. The focus of its activity is to ensure that:

• A medication is not marketed in which the *risk outweighs the benefit* likely to be derived.

• The *promotion of the medication* does not encourage uses for which the manufacturer has not received approval.

Confusion can arise when a medication is generally deemed useful by the medical profession in a condition for which its use has not been approved; thus, no one has the right to promote such use. This scenario is common, since marketed drugs are frequently found helpful for disorders beyond the formal labelled indications. Part of the reason for this situation is the long and expensive process needed to produce sufficient data to obtain FDA labelling approval, which in the early 1990s is estimated to cost as much as $200,000,000. Frequently, there is not sufficient monetary incentive to warrant such expenditure, yet a compound is often found to be effective by researchers and clinicians in a given medical discipline.

The FDA has taken a position that the individual physician is in the best position to determine whether a medication may be helpful for a specific patient based upon that physician's reading of the literature, as well as clinical experience. Otherwise, many patients would be denied effective treatment because of insufficient commercial incentive to carry out the costly process needed to receive marketing approval. A case in point is lithium, which languished in the United States for years, despite extensive use in the rest of the world for bipolar disorder. The reasons were two-fold: (*a*) there had been several deaths earlier when lithium was used as a salt substitute in individuals on a fluid-restricted diet; and (*b*) since lithium is a naturally occurring substance, no company could receive a patent for exclusive marketing rights. As a result, there was no way to recoup a sponsor's expenditure to receive marketing approval. Thus, for almost 2 decades, bipolar patients in the United States were denied the single most effective form of treatment. This situation could not be allowed to continue, given the personal, family, and societal cost of untreated bipolar disorder, and ultimately the federal government itself sponsored the research needed to achieve the appropriate labelling of lithium.

APPROVED VERSUS LABELLED

The words "approved" and "labelled" have different definitions and implications, and the failure to recognize this distinction can lead to erroneous descriptions about a medication and its use. A medication is "approved" for marketing if its database supports its benefit for a recognized condition and its risks are suffi-

ciently offset by its efficacy for a particular indication. The term "labelling" refers to the indications for which a medication can be promoted by the company marketing the compound. When a physician uses a drug for indications beyond the package insert, then an "approved" drug is being prescribed for an "unlabelled" indication. The physician must critically and carefully weigh the evidence supporting the drug's efficacy and balance the potential benefit against the potential risks for the indication in question. As with any treatment, the patient needs to be informed about these variables in a balanced manner so as to give an informed decision about accepting or rejecting a treatment.

To have a "labelled" indication, the marketing company has to make a formal submission to the FDA, documenting a compound's usefulness (and safety) for a specific condition. The submission is referred to as a new drug application (NDA). To support labelling as an antidepressant for example, a company must submit at least two unequivocal studies demonstrating the superiority of their drug over placebo (or appropriate control condition). Typically, an NDA is considerably more extensive than just two pivotal studies. The extent of the application also depends on whether the drug is new to the market or whether the company is seeking an additional indication for which it can promote the sale of an existing approved drug.

Even a modest NDA will require a substantial investment in money and time. The financial expenditure includes the outlay for clinical trials to collect the data and to assemble the application. Time is also a crucial variable, since the only way to justify the expenditure is through sales of the product, making the remaining patent life an important variable in such a decision. If it is short, then the patent may expire before the NDA can be assembled, submitted, and reviewed to receive "labelling" for that indication.

There are many worthwhile uses for medications that have not received formal "labelling" due to an economic decision. The data supporting such uses typically comes from clinical experience in individual patients, then a series of case reports, and finally, controlled studies. The latter are typically funded by government grants to university-based researchers who have no commercial interest in the medication. Results from such studies are published in medical journals but are generally not assembled into a formal NDA to the FDA. Therefore, such an indication cannot be promoted by the marketing company, although physicians are free to prescribe the drug if they are convinced that the medical literature and their clinical experience support such a use.

Research Studies versus Clinical Application

To put this matter in perspective, the use of most FDA-approved drugs in clinical practice usually goes beyond the clinical database, even when the drug is being prescribed for the "labelled" indication. A major reason is the difference between patients who enter clinical trials and those whom most clinicians treat. To enter a clinical trial, a patient must meet rigorous inclusion and exclusion criteria, leading to a narrow subgroup who will actually receive the drug once marketed. Some of the most important differences include:

- The absence of patients on *concomitant psychotropics*
- The absence of patients with *serious medical conditions*
- The absence of patients with concomitant *substance abuse*
- The absence of patients with *central*

nervous system disease or trauma (e.g., previous history of seizures, closed head trauma, or dementia)
- The limited, if any, experience with *hospitalized patients*
- The *underrepresentation of patients younger than 18* and *older than 65.*

In reality, patients whose conditions are complicated by these issues are the most frequent recipients of medications, yet they are usually excluded from the clinical trials used for the approval process.

Furthermore, most psychiatric disorders are chronic, although some may go through intervals of apparent quiescence (e.g., major depressive disorder), while others are persistent but relatively asymptomatic (e.g., schizophrenia) with effective treatment. Hence, treatment with psychotropics is best considered in terms of months or years of continuous or intermittent therapy, rather than a few days or weeks. By contrast, the vast majority of the clinical trials involve short-term use. Thus, a typical database for the approval of a new antidepressant is usually based on the experience with 2000–8000 patients (carefully selected as described above), with the majority exposed to the medication for less than 2 months. Often less than 25% will have received medication for more than 4 months, and less than 10% for more than 6 months. When a drug is marketed, most patients will be exposed to it for a minimum of 4–6 months. Yet, when treatment goes beyond 2 months, the database on the safety and continued efficacy of a medication is modest at best. Thus, while clinicians commonly use psychotropics for both maintenance and prophylactic purposes, an approved drug only has to be shown effective in the acute phase.

Only after a drug has been on the market for several years has sufficient experience been achieved so that many of these issues can be addressed with confidence. Even then most of that experience is nonsystematic. Problems may be detected in several ways:

- Clinicians are encouraged to send to the *FDA adverse experience reporting forms* when a patient develops a problem during treatment.
- The FDA may mandate specific *post-marketing surveillance programs* when a concern about the safety or efficacy of a new medication is suggested by either the preclinical or clinical database used for marketing approval.
- *A researcher may detect a problem* when studying patients treated with a medication, whether or not the primary focus is safety or efficacy.

Conclusion

This discussion is not intended to be critical of the approval process nor of the way physicians use medications. Rather it is meant to put the matter of using "approved" medications for "unlabelled" indications in perspective. While some have criticized such uses, the reality is that the application of many medications in clinical practice goes beyond the package insert. Further, to produce the data needed to address these clinical uses would add an enormous burden on the system in terms of costs and time. Even with such revisions, new drug development would become an even more risky enterprise, so that research and development would be curtailed, especially innovative efforts critical to advances in patient care. The expense of new medications would rise even higher, adding further to the percentage of the gross national product covering health care expenses. The end result would likely be the even slower development of inno-

vative treatments, with new products becoming cost prohibitive to many patients, especially those who are dependent upon the government and health maintenance organizations. Even now patients under such plans are often excluded from receiving the latest developments, unless empirical trials with older treatments have failed. Thus, these patients may be treated with agents that are less effective and more toxic than their successors. From this perspective, the current system seems to be a reasonable compromise, ensuring that new agents are safe and effective for a specific condition and then dependent on clinicians to carefully monitor outcome. From such clinical experience, the safe and effective use of "approved" medications can then be extended to a broader population for uses beyond those "labelled" in the package insert.

INVESTIGATIONAL DRUGS

An investigational drug is typically one that has not been approved for marketing by the FDA for human use (1). This designation may also refer to agents approved by the FDA for a specific indication, but employed otherwise (i.e., a nonlabelled use). Examples of the latter may include:

- A different *preparation or formulation*
- A higher than approved *dosage*
- A different *patient* population.

The Belmont Report (1979), in considering differences between the research and the clinical setting, noted that departure from commonly accepted drug practice for individual patients should not be considered research (2). Innovative strategies, however, should be developed in research protocols as quickly as possible to assure safety and efficacy of such a practice.

A general rule is that if there is any element of research involved (e.g., large number of subjects; systematic data collection; intent to publish), the entire proposal should be submitted in writing and reviewed by the local institutional review board (IRB). These entities are committees formally designated by a research institution to review, approve, and monitor research on human subjects (3).

Investigational drugs may also be used on an emergency (i.e., life-threatening) basis, but should be reported to an IRB within 5 working days. Subsequent use in other patients should have the institution's IRB approval.

Compassionate use provisions have allowed the limited employment of investigational drugs in the past (e.g., treatment INDs). More recently, the controversy surrounding acquired immunodeficiency syndrome (AIDS) and other life-threatening diseases has increased the pressure on the FDA to expand this program. Clozapine was also initially administered under such a program. Patients under the care of a responsible physician may now bring unapproved drugs into the United States or have them sent under specified conditions.

As required when using a marketed drug for FDA-labelled or nonlabelled indications, an important responsibility in the use of an investigational drug is the reporting of adverse effects to the FDA.

CONCLUSION

In this book, we will critically review both the formal FDA "labelled" indications, as well as those indications accepted by experts in the field of psychopharmacotherapy. In terms of the latter, meta-analysis will be used when possible to formally assess the size and quality of the database which supports the usefulness of a drug for a clinically accepted, but not formally "labelled," indication. These analyses can then aid the clinician in the decision to use a given drug for an "unlabelled" indication in a specific patient.

REFERENCES

1. Teuting P. Investigational drugs and research. Janicak PG, Davis JM, guest eds. Psychiatr Med. 1991;9(2):333–347.
2. The Belmont Report: ethical principles and guidelines for the protection of human subjects of research. [Report of the National Commission for the Protection of Human Subjects of Biomedical and Behavioral Research]. OPRR Reports. April 18, 1979.
3. Kessler DA. The regulation of investigational drugs. N Engl J Med 1989;320:281–288.

Cost of Treatment

Cost, in this context, implies more than just the price of the medication and the services of the treating clinician. Since most psychiatric disorders are chronic conditions, the cost of treatment must take into consideration the acute, maintenance, and prophylactic phases.

When calculating the total cost incurred by initiating therapy, one should consider:

- The *medication itself*
- *Ancillary procedures* to start and monitor therapy (e.g., preliminary and follow-up laboratory tests)
- Managing *adverse outcomes* (e.g., drug-drug interactions that may require medical attention)
- Cost of *outpatient versus inpatient* treatment

- The comparative cost of *alternate therapies* (e.g., ECT versus medication for psychotic depression).

If such costs are prohibitive, it may be appropriate to select an alternate option, so that compliance and overall outcome can be better assured.

Fortunately, for most psychotropics side effects are minimal, usually involving nuisance complaints. With some agents, such as clozapine, however, the potential for more serious adverse effects does exist and must be carefully explained to the patient and family. As importantly, one should always factor in the cost of not providing adequate treatment, including:

- The mortality risk
- The morbidity risk and related costs such as:
  - Adverse sequelae
  - Lost productivity
  - Disruption in socioeconomic relationships.

PRICE OF PSYCHOTROPICS

In general, the price on a per-milligram basis decreases as the dosage of the capsule or tablet increases, or as the lot size increases (e.g., 1000 versus 100). The cost of generic substitutes is usually considerably less than that for the trade name psychotropic; but issues of bioequivalence must also be factored in (see The Four Primary Pharmacokinetic Phases in Chapter 3). Using the fewest tablets to achieve a targeted dose level is always less expensive

(e.g., a 5-mg tablet of Navane is about 50 cents, versus 85 cents for 5 1-mg tablets). Unit dose systems, sustained release preparations, and concentrate forms all increase the cost (1).

The cost of medication ranges from a few cents to several dollars a day. The cost of providing outpatient treatment can amout to several hundred dollars a week, depending on the frequency of visits and therapist charges. The cost of hospitalization can be as high as $700 or $800 a day. The cost to the patient in terms of the social consequences can be incalculable. The use of a slightly more effective medication that prevents even one hospitalization could pay for several years of drug treatment. One side effect avoided, particularly if it results in hospitalization, will quickly pay for any increased difference in medication expense. Thus, the cost to society for not providing the best medication can be quite substantial. More expensive but safer medications are preferable because of the high cost of treating adverse effects. A drug that causes fewer side effects also translates into better compliance. Most importantly, when one provides optimal total care (i.e., inpatient, outpatient, drug management), this also improves the patient's quality of life.

REFERENCES

1. Jurman RJ, Davis JM. Comparison of the cost of psychotropic medications: an update. Janicak PG, Davis JM, guest eds. Psychiatr Med 1991;9(2):349–359.

CHAPTER 3

Pharmacokinetics

General Principles

Pharmacokinetics describes what the body does to a drug. It is characterized by four primary phases:

- Absorption
- Distribution
- Metabolism
- Elimination.

One of the first steps in the development of a new drug is determining its pharmacokinetics so that a dose most appropriate for clinical trials can be selected (1, 2). Initially, pharmacokinetic parameters are frequently established by the use of radioisotope-tagged drugs. In such studies, the tagged compound is administered and blood, urine, and stool samples are collected to measure the radioactivity, rather than using a chemical technique to identify a specific structure. Total radioactivity in blood, urine, and feces permits an initial determination of how an agent is excreted. Most psychotropics are primarily excreted in the urine, with a smaller percentage in the bowel.

Pharmacodynamics describes what a drug does to the body (i.e., both desirable and undesirable effects). It depends on critical drug concentrations at sites of action such as:

- Enzymes
- Receptors
- Second messengers.

The steps involved in reaching that critical concentration are in the realm of pharmacokinetics. Once present in adequate concentrations, drugs recognize and bind to a site of action, thereby activating or inactivating it. These interactions produce a cascade of events involving changes in subcellular components of a target neuron or group of neurons, ultimately culminating in clinically relevant, behavioral effects (3–7). The most important pharmacokinetic factors are described in Table 3.1.

HALF-LIFE

Half-life is the time needed to clear 50% of a drug from the plasma. It also determines the length of time necessary to reach steady state. The general rule is that the time to reach steady state concentration or virtual clearance of a drug is five times the half-life (not five times the dos-

Table 3.1.
Pharmacokinetic Factors

Absorption	Process by which a drug proceeds from the site of administration to the site of measurement (generally plasma or whole blood)
First-pass effect	Hepatic extraction of orally administered drugs prior to reaching the systemic circulation
Volume of distribution (V_D)	How much drug is distributed throughout the body
Steady state concentration (C_{SS})	The drug concentration achieved when the amount administered per unit time equals the amount eliminated per unit time
Biological half-life ($t_{1/2}$)	Time required for the drug concentration in plasma (or blood) to fall by one-half
Elimination rate constant (K_e)	Percent of drug in the body eliminated per unit time
Clearance (Cl)	A measure of a drug's elimination from the body (i.e., the amount of drug in the body times the elimination rate constant)
First order kinetics	The amount of drug eliminated per unit time is directly proportional to its plasma concentration
Zero order kinetics	Only a fixed amount of drug is eliminated per unit time regardless of plasma concentration

ing interval). The reason is that during every half-life period, a patient either clears or accumulates 50% of the eventual concentration produced by that dosing rate. Therefore, in one half-life a patient will have reached 50% of the concentration that will eventually be achieved. In two half-lives, a patient achieves the initial 50% plus half of the remaining 50%, for a total of 75%. With three half-lives, a patient achieves the initial 50% and the next 25% plus half of the remaining 25%, for a total of 87.5%. At 97% (i.e., 5 half-lives), the patient is essentially at steady state, which is the rationale behind the general rule.

Steady State

Steady state concentration (C_{SS}) means that the total concentration of a drug in plasma will not change as long as the dosing rate (i.e., dose and dose schedule) remains unchanged or other factors do not alter the rate of metabolism or elimination. Once plasma steady state is reached, the drug concentration in various body compartments (e.g., adipose tissue, the brain) is at equilibrium. In this instance the amount excreted every 24 hours will equal the amount taken every 24 hours, as long as disease, personal habits, the physician, or the patient do not alter the regimen.

Another general rule is that the longer the half-life, the longer the interval between starting the drug and seeing its full effects, whether beneficial or adverse. Figure 3.1 demonstrates two different curves of drugs with half-lives of 72 and 6 hours, respectively. Assuming a once-a-day dosing schedule, such as with a sedative-hypnotic at bedtime, drugs with these respective half-lives will accumulate in various tissues at two different rates and to different extents. In the case of the drug with a 72-hour half-life, the trough concentration before the next dose will be substantial relative to the peak concentration produced by the next dose. In the case of the drug with a 6-hour half-life, it will be

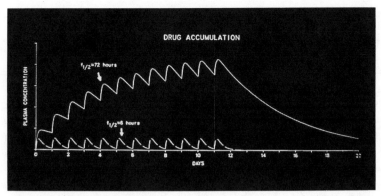

Figure 3.1.   Plasma drug concentration versus time curve for two model drugs: one with a half-life of 6 hours and one with a half-life of 72 hours.

trivial relative to the peak concentration produced by the next dose.

The length of the half-life determines the time needed to assess response as well as to clear a drug. For example, fluraze-pam, a benzodiazepine (BZD) sedative-hypnotic, may not achieve C_{SS} for several weeks after it is started (8–10). Therefore, if 2 weeks earlier a prn sedative was ordered and a patient has been taking it daily since then, declining cognitive function may actually be the result of a drug initially prescribed 2–3 weeks previously! Conversely, if a patient at steady state becomes pregnant, it will take an equal length of time to clear a potentially terato-genic drug after its cessation.

ZERO AND FIRST ORDER KINETICS

Zero order kinetics occurs when only a fixed amount of drug is eliminated for a given interval of time, since enzymes for biotransformation and elimination are saturated (5, 6). Alcohol is the classic example, where blood levels rise exponentially with increased amounts, because elimination mechanisms are saturated and only a certain fraction of the total dose can be eliminated.

First order kinetics means that the amount eliminated per unit of time is directly proportional to the amount ingested, so there is a linear relationship between dose change and plasma level change (i.e., 1:1). In contrast, with zero order kinetics, there is a proportionally larger increase in the plasma concentration for each dose increment because the elimination mechanism is saturated. As an example, one-third of patients on tricyclic antidepressants (TCAs) demonstrate zero order kinetics when concentrations exceed about 200 ng/ml (11, 12). Thus, they experience proportionally greater increases in drug plasma levels at the high end of the curve because of enzyme saturation.

Most psychotropics exhibit first order kinetics over the clinically relevant dose range, but some, such as alcohol, fluoxetine, and paroxetine, do not (13–15). **The reason for concern is the less-predictable relationship between dose changes and plasma drug level changes.** When prescribing drugs with zero order kinetics, the clinician knows that levels will be higher with each dose escalation, but does not know how much higher.

Role of Pharmacokinetics

Pharmacokinetics determines the minimum requirement for a drug's onset or offset of action. A drug cannot have an onset prior to reaching a critical concentration at the effector site (that is, the minimum requirement). Nonetheless, reaching that critical concentration may not temporally coincide with the clinical onset of action. For many psychotropic medications, the drug initiates a cascade of events that requires further time before the desired clinical effect is observed (e.g., antidepressant or antipsychotic effect.)

Knowing the differential pharmacokinetics for a class of drugs allows the clinician to choose specific members to hasten or delay onset or offset of action (8, 10, 16, 17). For example, lorazepam is rapidly absorbed from the gastrointestinal (GI) tract into the systemic circulation and from there distributed into the brain by all routes of administration (i.e., oral, intramuscular, or intravenous). In contrast, oxazepam, the most polar BZD, is slowly absorbed from the GI tract. Even after oxazepam is in the systemic circulation, it slowly enters tissue compartments, including the brain, during the distribution phase. Unlike lorazepam, oxazepam is not available in either the intramuscular or intravenous formulations. Thus, lorazepam would be preferable to achieve acute control of alcohol withdrawal (e.g., delirium tremens), while oxazepam would better stabilize a dependency-prone patient on sedative-hypnotics, since it does not cause the euphoria seen with rapid absorption. Such euphoria can also be seen with diazepam, not due to its rapid absorption, but rather to its rapid distribution into fat tissue. Oxazepam's short half-life is a dis-

advantage when used for this purpose, however. While most of our data came from studies with the BZDs (rather than the antidepressants or antipsychotics) even here the issues are more complex than simple pharmacokinetic explanations.

Pharmacokinetics determines how long a drug's action will persist. For drugs that induce *tolerance,* knowledge of their elimination half-life may predict the timing of a withdrawal syndrome after discontinuation. Again, a good example is the benzodiazepines, since the principal difference among them is pharmacokinetic rather than pharmacodynamic (8, 9). Thus, all these agents produce sedative-hypnotic tolerance that may cause a minor (e.g., sleeplessness, increased anxiety) or a major (e.g., withdrawal delirium) abstinence syndrome when discontinued. When given in bioequivalent doses (i.e., adjusting the dose to compensate for differences in potency), the major determinant of an abstinence syndrome is their half-life. Longer acting BZDs (e.g., clonazepam) have their own *built-in taper* due to slow clearance, allowing time for readjustment of compensatory changes in the brain that eliminate or blunt withdrawal symptoms. By contrast, short-lived BZDs (e.g., alprazolam) are more likely to produce withdrawal syndromes (10, 18–21). This pharmacokinetic fact is the rationale for switching dependent patients to an equipotent dose of a long-lived BZD, which can then be tapered more safely.

Differences in the biological half-life ($t_{1/2}$) determine how frequently drugs must be taken to maintain the desired effect. The knowledgeable practitioner will choose an agent from a class of similar compounds based in part on how well its pharmacokinetics meet the need(s) for which it is prescribed. When a clinician wants an immediate, but short-lived effect, the ideal agent would be rapidly absorbed into the systemic circulation and brain, and then rapidly redistributed to other body compartments for eventual clearance. Sleep induction is a situation where a rapid onset and reasonably rapid offset are desirable. *Termination of the acute effects of a single dose of a psychotropic is primarily the result of redistribution from brain to other body fat compartments, rather than final elimination* (8, 16, 17, 22, 23).

In other situations, rapidity of onset might be less important than a sustained effect. Examples include maintenance and prophylactic strategies to prevent the recurrence of seizures, panic attacks, psychosis, or manic episodes. A short-lived agent, which requires multiple daily dosing to maintain effective concentrations, increases the likelihood of noncompliance and increases the risk of relapse.

When there is a clear separation between the concentration of drug necessary to obtain a therapeutic effect and higher levels that produce side effects, the clinician can carefully adjust to the former while avoiding the latter. This strategy is particularly true for earlier psychotropics (e.g., TCAs), which have a plethora of effects, each predominating at different concentrations (24). This circumstance is the basis for therapeutic drug monitoring (TDM), which aids the rational adjustment of dose to obtain the desired effect (e.g., antidepressant effect), while avoiding concentrations associated with undesirable effects (e.g., anticholinergic effect). This issue is discussed in more detail later in this chapter.

Alterations in Pharmacokinetics

DRUG-DRUG INTERACTIONS

Knowledge about pharmacokinetic interactions (i.e., the effects of one drug on the absorption, distribution, metabolism, or elimination of another coadministered drug) is critical for the safe and effective use of drug combinations. For example, certain anticonvulsants (e.g., CBZ, phenobarbital) potently *induce* hepatic P-450 enzymes, causing plasma levels of antipsychotics to fall because of an acceleration in their metabolism. Thus, the addition of carbamazepine to control mood swings in a psychotic patient previously stabilized may precipitate an antipsychotic exacerbation relapse unless the medication is adjusted to compensate (25, 26). Conversely, fluoxetine and paroxetine, for example, potently *inhibit* the P-450 isoenzyme IID6, important in the oxidative metabolism of drugs such as the TCAs (27). This effect can result in a quadrupling of a TCA's plasma concentration and can cause serious toxicity unless the TCA dose is reduced (28, 29).

EFFECTS OF AGING AND DISEASE

The pharmacokinetics of a drug can change with aging and/or disease (30–43).

There are several factors that can alter the pharmacokinetic phases in the elderly, making them more prone to psychotropics' effects, including:

- A decrease in *intracellular water*
- A decrease in *protein binding*
- A decrease in *tissue mass*
- An increase in *total body fat.*

These changes act synergistically to increase the effect of most psychotropic drugs in the elderly. A decrease or increase in the total body fat constitutes an enlarged reservoir for drug accumulation. The end result is that drugs tend to persist longer in the elderly. There is also a general *decrease in intestinal absorption* of drugs due to diminished GI tract blood flow and motility, as well as an *increase in gastric pH*. These two changes can reduce the effectiveness of some drugs in the elderly.

There is also an *increase in the free-drug fraction,* so that for every milligram given, as well as for every drug concentration, there is a greater amount of this fraction. In addition, *drug metabolism tends to decrease* in the elderly (related to diminished hepatic blood flow, liver mass, and P-450 enzyme content and activity). *A decrease in renal excretion* also means that potentially active metabolites tend to accumulate more, and may be active in an undesirable way.

In summary, for drugs that undergo extensive biotransformation prior to elimination, aging often produces a substantial lengthening of the required time to eliminate the drug (i.e., its half-life). Thus, older patients frequently clear these agents much more slowly than their younger counterparts, making the elderly more susceptible to toxicity on the same dose of the same drug (44–58).

This phenomenon can also occur with diseases that alter the physiological mechanisms subserving the various pharmacokinetic phases.

The Four Primary Pharmacokinetic Phases

ABSORPTION

> **Case Example.** A 37-year-old schizoaffective patient was treated with *thioridazine* (100 mg by mouth qid), *phenytoin* (100 mg by mouth qid), and *amitriptyline* (50 mg by mouth qid). The patient had been stabilized on this regimen for several weeks but then complained of daytime sedation. The treating physician then combined all three into a single bedtime regimen. The patient expired that night from an acute cardiac arrest.

This case illustrates the possibility of an additive pharmacodynamic impact, as well as the interactive effects of these drugs that could substantially elevate peak plasma concentrations when they are given at the same time.

The principal route of administration for psychoactive drugs is *oral*, with absorption generally occurring *in the small bowel*. The drug is then absorbed into the *portal circulation* and enters *the liver*, where it can undergo extensive metabolism before reaching the *systemic circulation* (i.e., first-pass effect). Most psychotropics are highly lipophilic, so that they readily pass the *blood-brain barrier* (BBB) and enter the central nervous system (CNS) (16, 17). In addition, because of this property, they share several other features:

- *Availability* to the brain
- *Rapid* absorption
- *Complete* absorption

- High *first-pass effect*
- Large *volume of distribution.*

Bioavailability refers to the portion of a drug absorbed from the site of administration. The reference site of administration is intravenous, because this presumably produces 100% *absorption.* Figure 3.2 illustrates three sample drug concentration curves in plasma as a function of time. The area under the curve is the total amount of drug in the systemic circulation available for distribution to the site(s) of action. The dark curve represents the *oral;* medium curve the *intramuscular;* and light curve the *intravenous* concentration. The same dose completely absorbed from any of these routes would produce an identical area under the curve (i.e., 100% bioavailability).

Any decrease in the area under the curve for intramuscular or oral versus intravenous administration would represent a decrease in bioavailability based on that

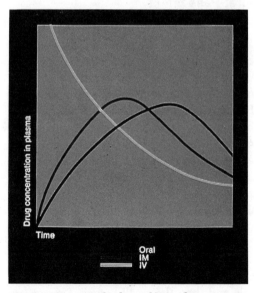

Figure 3.2. Single-dose plasma drug concentration versus time curves for the same dose of the same drug given to the same individual by three different routes: oral (dark); i.m. (medium); and i.v. (light).

route of administration (5). Common factors that influence bioavailability include:

- *Physicochemical properties* of the drug
- *Formulation* of the product
- *Disease states* that influence gastrointestinal function, or first pass effect
- *Precipitation* of a drug at the injection site.

There are other clinically important parameters beyond the extent of absorption that are apparent on the single-dose plasma curve. These include:

- *Peak concentration* (C_{max})
- *Time to the peak concentration* (T_{max}).

Generally C_{max} will be inversely correlated to T_{max} (i.e., the shorter the time for a drug to be absorbed, the higher the peak concentration). A higher C_{max} and shorter T_{max} typically mean a more rapid appearance of clinical activity following administration. These parameters can also determine whether a drug should be developed for a specific indication, since T_{max} and C_{max} are generally a function of a compound's physicochemical properties.

In terms of physicochemical properties, the more polar a compound the slower the absorption from the gastrointestinal tract and the slower the penetration into the brain from the systemic circulation. These two phases (i.e., into the systemic circulation and into the brain) are usually correlated. Oxazepam, the most polar BZD, is slowly absorbed into the systemic circulation as well as into the brain, making it a poor sedative (8, 9). By contrast, lorazepam rapidly penetrates both compartments, inducing sleep in a reasonable time frame (17). While rate of penetration into the brain generally parallels rate of penetration into the systemic circulation, this is not always true. An example is the original formulation of temazepam, which came in a hard gelatin capsule, resistant to gastric breakdown (8). This formulation led to a slow absorption rate, diminishing its effectiveness as a sedative even though it penetrated the brain rapidly from the systemic circulation. A change in the formulation led to more rapid absorption, increasing its usefulness as a sedative-hypnotic.

Fast absorption may not always be desirable, since drug toxicity may be a function of C_{max}. In the case example that began the discussion on absorption, failure to appreciate this fact led to a fatal outcome. **Cardiac toxicity, due to the stabilization of excitable membranes, is as much a function of the peak plasma concentration as it is the steady state tissue concentration.** Thus, changing a formulation to delay T_{max} and reduce C_{max} may significantly increase safety. Dividing the dose into smaller amounts and administering it more frequently can also accomplish the same result. In such a case, the average plasma concentration over the dosing interval and the amount absorbed will remain the same but the peak concentration will be lower and the trough concentration higher.

Differences in bioavailability, particularly as they affect the rate of absorption, can vary significantly among formulations (i.e., products) of the same drug. The Food and Drug Administration considers a generic product to be comparable to a brand name if there is no more than a $\pm 20\%$ difference (more or less) in bioavailability (i.e., T_{max} and C_{max}) (59). Hence, theoretically, there could be as much as a 40% difference between two generic preparations of the same drug. This possibility may explain why a patient who previously tolerated and benefitted from a medication begins to develop side effects or suffers a relapse when another formulation is substituted.

Route of Administration

Different routes of administration can affect the rate of absorption, as well as the ratio of parent compound to its various metabolites. For example, the concentration-time curve is usually shifted to the left with the i.m. route, due to more rapid absorption. Hence, T_{max} is shifted to the left (i.e., shortened) and C_{max} is higher, contracting the curve, even though the area under the curve (AUC) is unchanged.

This pattern is not true for all drugs, however. For example, diazepam and chlordiazepoxide are unstable at a pH of 7.4 and tend to crystallize in tissue when given intramuscularly (8, 9, 17). Therefore, they are less bioavailable when given i.m. versus orally. Their absorption also tends to be erratic and variable, depending on where the injection was given (i.e., near blood vessels, in fat, or muscle), as well as slower and less complete.

First-Pass Effect

When drugs are administered orally, they typically are absorbed in the small bowel, enter the portal circulation, and pass through the liver, where a certain fraction undergoes metabolism in the hepatocytes (i.e., first-pass metabolism or first-pass effect). The extent of this effect can be broadly altered by diseases (e.g., cirrhosis, portacaval shunting, persistent hepatitis, congestive heart failure), and by some drugs (e.g., alcohol, cimetidine, fluoxetine) influencing the peak concentrations achieved and the ratio of the parent compound to metabolites (56, 57).

Once first-pass metabolism has occurred, metabolites are excreted into the bile and then the small bowel. Those that are lipid soluble are reabsorbed into the portal circulation, eventually entering the systemic circulation. These metabolites may have a similar or substantially different pharmacological profile from their parent drug. For example, chlorpromazine undergoes extensive hepatic biotransformation and has 168 theoretical metabolites, of which 70 have been identified in plasma and tissue. Some have dopamine receptor-blocking activity, although they are weaker than the parent compound, making it difficult to separate the effects (good or bad) of the parent compound from its numerous active metabolites.

In contrast to oral administration, drugs administered intravenously or intramuscularly directly enter the systemic circulation, avoiding the first-pass effect. This is why many drugs (e.g., fluphenazine) are more potent when administered intramuscularly and why the i.m. dose must be adjusted to compensate for this difference. Medical conditions such as cirrhosis can cause portacaval shunting, allowing drugs to avoid the first-pass effect and directly enter the systemic circulation, enhancing a psychotropic's effect. Coadministered drugs can affect first-pass metabolism (60–62). For example, acute alcohol intoxication can substantially reduce the first-pass effect on TCAs, leading to a doubling of the C_{max} after the same dose (63). This effect contributes to the increased toxicity that occurs when an overdose of TCAs is taken with alcohol.

DISTRIBUTION

Case Example. A 44-year-old chronic, alcoholic male presented in the emergency room with disorientation and combativeness after 2 days of abstinence. He complained of visual and tactile hallucinations and was found to have an elevated heart rate, blood pressure, and temperature. *Lorazepam* was slowly administered intravenously and after 15 minutes the patient was mildly sedated. He was then transferred to an inpatient unit. During this 30-minute interval, he received no addi-

tional lorazepam, and when he arrived on the floor, his symptoms had returned. He became agitated, struck one of the nursing staff, and had to be physically restrained.

In this case, failure to account for the phenomenon of drug redistribution resulted in a potentially avoidable adverse outcome, as explained in the following discussion. Once in the systemic circulation, the drug distributes to organs in direct proportion to their fat and protein content (64). The rate of accumulation is a function of an organ's vascularity. While highly lipid-soluble drugs accumulate in adipose tissue to the same extent that they accumulate in brain, *the rate of accumulation is much faster in brain than in adipose tissue.*

Figure 3.3 illustrates single and multiple dose pharmacokinetics, with the Y axis representing plasma drug concentration and the X axis the time elapsed since drug administration. When a single oral dose is administered, the drug reaches C_{max} and then undergoes a relatively rapid decline. **This initial decline is due primarily to drug distribution, rather than to elimination. Thus, the initial drug concentration drop is a function of the rate of uptake into other bodily compartments rather than elimination from the body.** This fact is particularly important with the first dose of an i.v.-administered psychotropic since:

- They are quite *lipophilic*
- They have *large volumes of distribution*
- Their *tissue concentrations are typically 10 to 100 times greater than their plasma concentrations.*

The acute effects of a single dose of most psychotropics are terminated by redistribution. An example would be the acute sedative effects of intravenously administered lorazepam, which rapidly pen-

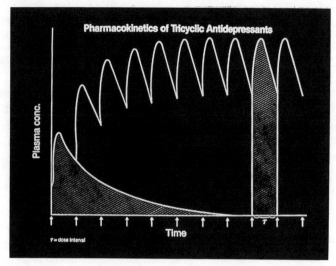

Figure 3.3.   Plasma drug concentration versus time curve following administration of a single oral dose and following repeated administrations of the same oral dose.

etrates the brain. A disproportionate amount of the dose enters the CNS because of its greater vascularity in comparison to peripheral adipose tissue. When plasma concentration falls, however, the drug re-equilibrates out of the brain and into the systemic circulation, from where it is distributed to adipose sites. This fall in brain concentration terminates lorazepam's acute psychoactive effects.

Distribution of the drug is conceptualized as accumulation into various body compartments (e.g., fat; aqueous; bone; brain; etc.). The extent to which drugs differ in their rate and degree of accumulation into various organs is related to the number of compartments into which they equilibrate. Even within a given compartment, such as blood, there may be more than one subcomponent for distribution, including:

• Plasma *water*
• Plasma *protein*
• Circulating *cells* (particularly red blood cells).

Most psychotropics are highly protein-bound (65–68). Such bound drug often account for more than 90% of the total plasma concentration. The clinical significance is that even though the free-drug fraction is the smallest absolute amount, it is the most important, since its concentration determines the final equilibration with the site of action. While a 5% change in the bound amount seems small, the free fraction could have now gone from 5% to 10%, doubling the effective drug concentration in equilibrium with the site of action. Thus, any condition that shifts the ratio of bound to free drug can affect its pharmacodynamics. Conditions that lead to a functional decrease in the amount of circulating protein include:

• *Malnutrition,* as with severe anorexia
• *Wasting,* as in the nephrotic syndrome
• *Aging*
• *Concomitant drugs* that compete for protein binding sites (69, 70).

Increasing the relative amount of the free fraction can increase toxicity. Since most assays do not distinguish between bound and free-drug fractions, therapeutic drug monitoring may not be helpful unless specialized techniques are used.

Acute and chronic inflammatory processes can increase the amount of circulating α_1-acid glycoprotein (which avidly binds a variety of psychotropics), increasing the absolute amount of bound drug, while the free fraction remains unchanged. The result is that the circulating total concentrations may seem excessive but actually represent simply an increase in the bound (but biologically inert) fraction.

The absolute and relative size of the body's fat compartment can change with normal aging and morbid obesity (30, 32, 40, 41). As noted earlier, the percentage of total body water and protein content decreases in the elderly, while their percentage of fat content increases, leaving a relatively larger reservoir to store psychotropics. These changes explain why many psychotropic drugs have a longer, more persistent effect in the elderly. The morbidly obese patient also has an increased reservoir, and a drug's effect will persist, consistent with the size of the adipose compartment.

Under steady state conditions, there is a proportional relationship between the tissue and the plasma compartments (5, 71, 72). This fact underlies the usefulness of therapeutic drug monitoring. While psychotropics do not exert their psychoactive effects in plasma, their plasma concentration is, nonetheless, in equilibrium with tissue levels. **Although tissue concentrations (depending upon the organ) are 10 to 100 times greater than plasma concentrations, the latter provide an indirect measurement of the former.**

METABOLISM

Case Example. A 62-year-old male presented to his internist with a major depressive disorder. His past medical history was significant for two previous myocardial infarctions and related congestive heart failure, well-controlled by digoxin. There was also a past history of significant alcohol abuse, in remission for the past 4 years. The internist prescribed amitriptyline 75 mg p.o. at bedtime. One week later the patient returned with a worsening of his depressive state, and the internist increased the dose to 100 mg. The patient continued to deteriorate, and was referred to a psychiatrist, who hospitalized him. The patient was now suspicious, guarded, and irritable and was given the diagnosis of a psychotic depression. Haloperidol (10 mg p.o.) at bedtime was added. Five days later the patient was found unconscious in his room after complaining of faintness and heart palpitations. He was rushed to the coronary intensive care, where a 2:1 atrioventricular block and periodic runs of premature ventricular contractions (PVCs) were found on the electrocardiogram (ECG). Drug level monitoring revealed a total TCA plasma level of 950 ng/ml. All psychoactive drugs were stopped. As the plasma level fell, the cardiac and psychotic symptoms resolved.

This patient had several risk factors for the development of toxic TCA concentrations even while on a relatively low dose of amitriptyline. The following discussion will elaborate on these.

Biotransformation

Most psychotropics undergo extensive *hepatic biotransformation* leading to the formation of more polar metabolites, which are then excreted in the urine. The necessary *biotransformation* steps may involve one or several of the following steps by way of example:

- Hydroxylation
- Demethylation
- Oxidation
- Sulfoxide formation.

While most drugs undergo extensive biotransformation prior to elimination, some undergo simple conjugation with glucuronic acid, and others are excreted unmetabolized (e.g., lithium) (8, 9, 73). Since conjugation can occur in most organs, this step is not dependent upon liver function. Thus, drugs that undergo only glucuronidation do not have their rate of clearance affected by liver disorders. These include all of the 3-hydroxybenzodiazepines (e.g., lorazepam, oxazepam, temazepam), which are as readily cleared by the old as the young, as long as their renal function is normal. The same is true for patients with severely compromised liver function, which is another reason to use these agents early in the treatment of delirium tremens. Should such patients subsequently develop hepatic failure, they can still readily clear the drug and thus avoid having it persist in the body to worsen cognitive function and level of arousal. By contrast, a drug like diazepam, which requires extensive biotransformation, can be more problematic if the patient develops hepatic failure (74). Further, the metabolites of diazepam have similar pharmacological properties, accumulate in the body, and ultimately contribute to the pharmacological effect.

Hepatic biotransformation results in the formation of metabolites whose pharmacological effects may be similar or dissimilar to the parent compound. Either way they also determine the final behavioral effect(s). For example, norfluoxetine has essentially the same activity as fluoxetine in terms of both serotonin reuptake blockade and inhibition of the hepatic isoenzyme IID6, but is cleared more slowly (27, 28, 75). As a result, norfluoxetine accumulates extensively in the body following chronic administration of fluoxetine, making it, rather than the parent compound, the principal determinant of the clinical effect.

Clomipramine's major metabolite, desmethylclomipramine, has a markedly different pharmacological profile (76). Thus, while clomipramine is a potent inhibitor of serotonin reuptake, desmethylclomipramine is a more potent inhibitor of norepinephrine reuptake. If clomipramine's value in obsessive compulsive disorder depends on its ability to block 5-HT reuptake (and not norepinephrine), then this effect should be a function of the relative ratio between clomipramine and desmethylclomipramine. Thus, this agent could lose its effectiveness for obsessive-compulsive disorder (OCD) if a patient were an efficient convertor to the active metabolite, or became such as a result of enzyme induction or inhibition.

Another important situation is the less efficacious but more toxic metabolite. For example, if the concentration of the hydroxylated metabolite of imipramine (2-hydroxyimipramine) were increased, this TCA could lose its effectiveness while simultaneously increasing its toxicity (77).

Hepatic Enzyme Induction

Alcohol, nicotine, and most anticonvulsants induce liver enzymes (25, 78–83). Barbiturates and carbamazepine induce the metabolism of other drugs as well as their own (i.e., **autoinduction**). Blood levels obtained after 3 or 4 days reflect what the rate of elimination is at that time; however, levels will subsequently fall on the same dose because autoinduction alters the half-life as a function of continued drug administration. Therefore, early therapeutic drug monitoring of carbamazepine cannot assure the eventual concentration reached after several weeks on the drug (see Alternate Treatment Strategies in Chapter 10).

Alcohol has a triphasic effect on the elimination rates of drugs like TCAs that

require extensive biotransformation (63). *Acute* alcohol ingestion in combination with a TCA in a teetotaller who attempts suicide will block first-pass metabolism significantly. This chemical inhibition can triple the peak concentration of a TCA by increasing the rate of absorption and by reducing the extent of first-pass hepatic metabolism. This is why the consumption of alcohol in association with a TCA overdose increases their lethality.

Drinking on a regular basis for several weeks to months can induce liver enzymes, resulting in a lower TCA plasma concentration. Thus, *subacute and subchronic* alcohol consumption induces liver enzymes and causes lower plasma levels of drugs that undergo hepatic biotransformation as a necessary step in their elimination.

Chronic alcohol ingestion can cause cirrhosis, reducing liver enzyme concentration as well as liver mass. This may cause portacaval shunting and plasma drug levels to rise.

Hepatic Enzyme Inhibition

In contrast to anticonvulsants and alcohol, drugs such as quinidine, flecainide, β-blockers, fluoxetine, paroxetine, and antipsychotics can inhibit specific oxidative enzymes in the liver (27, 28, 75, 84–97). TCAs, certain BZDs, bupropion, some steroids, and antipsychotics can all have their metabolism inhibited by fluoxetine. For example, fluoxetine can produce a twofold to tenfold increase in the concentration of a TCA, like amitriptyline, leading to serious or even life-threatening toxicity on a dose that was previously well-tolerated (28, 29, 75).

Hepatic Arterial Flow

After a drug enters the systemic circulation, the delivery back to the liver depends on left ventricular function (LVF). Further, drugs may also affect the biotransformation of other drugs indirectly, through an *effect on hepatic arterial blood flow* (60, 98). The rate of drug conversion is dependent on the rate of delivery to the liver, which is determined by arterial flow. *Cimetidine and β-blockers, such as propranolol, decrease arterial flow*, slowing the metabolism of various drugs that undergo extensive hepatic biotransformation.

Effects of Disease on Hepatic Function

Diseases that *directly affect* hepatic integrity include cirrhosis, viral infections, and collagen vascular diseases. Diseases that *indirectly affect* function include metabolic disorders (e.g., azotemia secondary to renal insufficiency) and cardiac disease. While decreased left ventricular output can result in a decrease in hepatic arterial flow, right ventricular failure causes hepatic congestion, reducing both the first-pass effect and delaying biotransformation.

Thus, the patient with a toxic TCA concentration (case at start of Metabolism section) may have developed excessively high amitriptyline plasma levels due to the additive effects of congestive heart failure (CHF); diminished left ventricular function (LVF) leading to decreased hepatic arterial blood flow; alcohol- and age-related decline in liver function; and, finally, haloperidol inhibition of amitriptyline's metabolism.

ELIMINATION

Case Example. A 48-year-old bipolar female, stabilized on 1200 mg/day of lithium for the past 6 months, had a plasma level that varied between 0.8 to 1.0 mEq/liter.

She developed a recurrence of her rheumatoid arthritis, for which her internist prescribed ibuprofen (800 mg tid). A week later she was brought to the emergency room in a confused, disoriented, and lethargic state. She was also ataxic and had periodic generalized myoclonic jerks. TDM revealed a lithium level of 4.0 mEq/liter, and despite a rapid fall to under 0.5 mEq/liter with plasma dialysis, her neurological status continued to deteriorate. After 5 days, she died.

Failure to account for a critical drug interaction, affecting the renal clearance of lithium, resulted in an otherwise avoidable fatality (99).

The last step in a drug's clearance from the body is elimination, which for most psychotropics occurs via the kidneys. At this point, most compounds have been converted into their polar metabolites, which are more water- and less lipid-soluble than the parent compound, thus facilitating their clearance in urine. On the single-dose concentration-time curve, this step is reflected by the terminal elimination phase, which is typically a gradual and steady decline in the plasma level over time. The slope of this clearance curve is a function of the rates of biotransformation and elimination. Thus, the slope (the K_e or kinetic constant of elimination) represents a summation of the hepatic enzymatic activity required for biotransformation necessary for subsequent elimination and the glomerular filtration rate that clears polar metabolites from the blood (Fig. 3.2).

Obviously, *renal insufficiency* can delay clearance (101, 102). More specifically, it will result in the accumulation of higher concentrations of polar metabolites. Depending on the pharmacological profile of these metabolites, patients may accumulate compounds that are less efficacious

and/or more toxic than the parent compound. *Dehydration* can result in the same outcome since it diminishes glomerular filtration rate. Changing the *plasma pH* (e.g., cranberry juice to acidify, sodium bicarbonate to make more basic) can also hasten or retard the clearance of certain drugs (e.g., amphetamines) via the kidneys. *Drugs* may also affect the ability of the renal tubules to excrete a drug. Two examples are the effect of loop diuretics and nonsteroidal anti-inflammatory agents on lithium renal clearance (99, 103).

Single Dose Prediction Test

The slope of this line can also be used to predict the steady state concentration that will be achieved on a given drug dose (100). This strategy usually involves measuring a blood level 24–36 hours after a test dose. That value is a function of an individual's ability to eliminate the drug and hence is a measure of the individual's K_e. Since the K_e that determines the 24-hour single dose level is the same K_e that determines the steady state concentration (C_{SS}), it can be used to predict the eventual C_{SS} on a given dose. Assuming linear pharmacokinetics, a change in dose will produce a proportional change in blood level, allowing the clinician to predict the dose required to achieve a desired concentration (see Pharmacokinetics/Plasma Levels in Chapter 5).

With repeated administration there is an ascending concentration until steady state is reached. At that point, the concentration remains in a narrow range with continued drug administration, assuming that it does not influence its own metabolism (e.g., carbamazepine can accelerate its own metabolism over several weeks).

Therapeutic Drug Monitoring

Therapeutic drug monitoring has four major clinical applications:

- To monitor *compliance*
- To increase *efficacy*
- To increase *safety*
- To protect against *medical-legal* actions.

The characteristics of a drug that make TDM useful are listed in Table 3.2.

TDM can eliminate or control interindividual variability in pharmacokinetics that can determine clinical outcome (24, 28, 104, 105). It is essentially a refinement of the approach to dose adjustment based upon clinical response. Using this strategy, the clinician titrates the dose in terms of improvement as well as the development of nuisance or toxic effects. The discussion in this chapter has enumerated those pharmacokinetic factors that may produce variable clinical outcomes in different patients taking the same medication.

There are several intervening variables between drug dose and blood levels, blood levels and brain levels, concentration at the site of action, and finally, treatment outcome. Those variables can be grouped into three categories:

I. Pharmacokinetics involves:

- Absorption
- Distribution
- Metabolism
- Elimination.

II. The relationship between plasma concentration and the concentration achieved at the site of action involves:

- The percent of the drug that is actually *tissue-bound versus* the percent of the drug that is in the *free form*
- The ability of the drug to cross the *blood-brain barrier*
- *Disease states* that would alter the blood-brain barrier or regional cerebral blood flow.

III. The relationship between a drug's concentration and its effect at the site of action involves:

- *Receptor* function
- *Enzyme* content
- *Reuptake* mechanisms
- *Feedback* systems.

ROLE OF TDM

One role for TDM is to guard against toxicity. This fact is particularly true for drugs that have narrow therapeutic indices, serious toxic effects, and substantial interindividual variability in metabolism. Such drugs include: lithium, the tricyclic

Table 3.2.
Pharmacodynamic and Pharmacokinetic Characteristics of a Drug that Predict the Clinical Usefulness of Therapeutic Drug Monitoring

Multiple mechanisms of action
Large interindividual variability in metabolism
Narrow therapeutic index
Delayed onset of action
Difficulty detecting early development of
  toxicity

antidepressants, and some anticonvulsants. This is especially crucial when early signs of toxicity are difficult to detect (105–107). For example, the early phases of a delirium due to toxic TCA concentrations may mimic the worsening of a depression. Without guidance from TDM, the clinician might increase the TCA dose due to presumed worsening of the mood disorder and inadvertently cause more toxicity.

TDM may provide objective data when there is a paucity of hard information. For example, while antipsychotic TDM is still controversial, it can provide additional information to determine the optimal dose for a given patient. In this instance, the patient is his own control, with an antipsychotic plasma level obtained after the dose has been stabilized. Then, TDM can be repeated when relapses occur to clarify whether noncompliance or drug refractoriness was responsible. Finally, this issue can be further clarified by repeating TDM when the patient is again stable. This approach avoids the initial impulse to increase the dose or to switch drugs, if the problem was at least partially attributable to noncompliance. It can also avoid a vicious cycle of increasing noncompliance due to adverse effects resulting from higher than necessary doses (and blood levels).

On occasion, TDM may also be used to aid in determining whether:

- There has been an *adequate trial.*
- A patient responded to the active drug or had a *placebo response.*
- The *benefit outweighs* the potential for *adverse effects.*

A sufficient dose for a sufficient interval constitutes an adequate trial. In particularly resistant cases, TDM can define dose adequacy by guiding its adjustment to eliminate differences introduced by pharmacokinetic variations among patients.

Many clinicians assume a patient has experienced a placebo response if improvement occurs more rapidly than the typical time course. This assumption can be further substantiated by documenting a concentration well below that which is typically effective. Effective and safe levels in a patient responding to unusually low doses can help the clinician determine that the patient is likely to be a true drug, rather than a placebo, responder. This information can guide decisions about duration of drug therapy and whether other interventions may be indicated.

Occasionally, some patients respond only to unusually high doses that nonetheless produce safe plasma concentrations. This type of information can alleviate concerns by providing a pharmacokinetic explanation for the necessity to use such high doses. Alternatively, some patients who only respond to high doses may also have high plasma drug levels and thus be at increased risk for serious toxicity. In such instances, prudence may dictate an alternative therapy, or at least following the patient's status more closely. An example would be a depressed patient requiring TCA plasma levels above 450 ng/ml (108). If an alternative antidepressant therapy is not practical, it would be prudent to obtain an ECG and an electroencephalogram (EEG) to assess for physiological evidence of toxicity even though not clinically evident.

TIMING OF SAMPLES FOR TDM

Blood samples for TDM should be obtained in the elimination phase of drug dosing, since these levels are more reproducible than those drawn during the absorption or distribution phases. Determining the elimination phase requires knowing when the C_{max} occurs as well as the rapid fall off due to redistribution.

Errors in the timing of samples (e.g., before steady state has been reached or too early in a dosing interval) can produce misleading results and inappropriate dosing decisions.

FREQUENCY OF TDM

The pharmacokinetics of a drug can also determine the frequency of monitoring. Many believe that TDM requires frequent blood drawings, primarily based on the experience with lithium. This drug is relatively unique, however, in that its levels are determined by different factors. Thus, the plasma level of lithium is not solely a function of the dose and renal status but also of fluid and salt intake and output, which can vary independent of dose, rapidly altering electrolyte balance.

For most drugs, their concentration is a function of dose as well as an individual's rate of metabolism and elimination, which are relatively stable unless a moderating variable intervenes. Examples of such moderating variables include diseases that affect organs important for metabolism or elimination (e.g., liver or heart); or a concurrent agent that induces or inhibits the metabolism or elimination of the target drug. Some clinicians feel that for such drugs, TDM needs to be done only once, early in treatment, but after sufficient time has passed to insure C_{ss} has been achieved. Many clinicians only obtain plasma levels if a problem occurs.

Another instance in which TDM would be repeated is for unexpected events, such as relapse or the development of a new side effect. Except in these situations, TDM does not need to be repeated, since it is a measurement of the patient's ability to metabolize and eliminate a drug, which is generally a reproducible and stable biological phenomenon. This is also why TDM can be used to detect noncompli-

ance. We note that for many agents plasma levels are not useful since assays are not available or there is insufficient pharmacokinetic data to interpret plasma level results.

CONCLUSION

This chapter has reviewed the important pharmacokinetic principles associated with most psychotropics. Further, it has distinguished its phases from the issue of pharmacodynamics. Understanding a drug's pharmacokinetics can enhance safety and efficacy, while helping to correct less than optimal outcomes. Since these principles are an indispensable part of treatment planning and monitoring, they will be considered in the following chapters on specific drug therapies.

REFERENCES

1. Drayer DE. Pharmacologically active drug metabolites: therapeutic and toxic activities, plasma and urine data in man, accumulation in renal failure. Clin Pharmacokinet 1976;1:426–443.
2. Ross EM, Gilman AG. Pharmacodynamics: mechanisms of drug action and the relationship between drug concentration and effect. In: Gilman AG, Goodman LS, Rall TW, Murad F, eds. Goodman and Gilman's the pharmacological basis of therapeutics. 7th ed. New York: Macmillan, 1985:35–48.
3. Weisman A, Koe BK. Contributions of industrial research to basic neuro psychopharmacology: preclinical screening and discovery. In: HV Metzler ed. Psychopharmacology: the third generation of progress. New York: Raven Press, 1987:1649–1658.
4. Preskorn S. The future and psychopharmacology: needs and potentials. Psychiatr Ann, 1990;20(11):625–633.
5. Holford NHG, Sheiner LB. Understanding the dose-effect relationship: clinical application of pharmacokinetic-pharmacodynamic models. Clin Pharmacokinet 1981; 6:429–453.
6. Kenakin TP. Pharmacologic analysis of

drug-receptor interaction. New York: Raven Press, 1987.

7. Meyer UA. Molecular genetics and the future of pharmacogenetics. Pharmacol Ther 1990b;46:349–355.

8. Greenblatt DJ, Shader RI. Clinical pharmacokinetics of the benzodiazepines. In: (Smith DE, Wesson DR, eds.) The benzodiazepines: current standards for medical practice. Lancaster, UK: MTP Press, 1985:43–50.

9. Bellantuono C, Reggi V, Tognoni G, Garattini S. Benzodiazepines: clinical pharmacology and therapeutic use. Drugs 1980; 19:195–219.

10. Ladewig D. Dependence liability of the benzodiazepines. Drug Alcohol Depend 1984;13:139–149.

11. Kitanaka I, Ross RJ, Cutler NR, Zavadil AP III, Potter WZ. Altered hydroxydesipramine concentration in elderly depressed patients. Clin Pharmacol Ther 1982;31:51–55.

12. Nelson JC, Jatlow P. Nonlinear desipramine kinetics: prevalence and importance. Clin Pharmacol Ther 1987;41:666–670.

13. Brosen K. Recent developments in hepatic drug oxidation. Clin Pharmacokinet 1990; 18:220–239.

14. Benfield P, Heel RC, Lewis SP. Fluoxetine: a review of its pharmacodynamic and pharmacokinetic properties, and therapeutic efficacy in depressive illness. Drugs 1986;32:481–508.

15. Tasker T, Kaye C, Zussman D, et al. Paroxetine plasma levels: lack of correlation with efficacy or adverse effects. Acta Psychiatr Scand 1990;80(Suppl 350):152–155.

16. Greenblatt DJ, Ehrenberg BL, Gunderman JS, Locniskar A, Scavone JM, Harmatz JS, Shader RI. Pharmacokinetic and electroencephalographic study of intravenous diazepam, midazolam, and placebo. Clin Pharmacol Ther 1989;45:356–365.

17. Hegarty JE, Dundee JW. Sequelae after the intravenous injection of three benzodiazepines—diazepam, lorazepam and flunitrazepam. Br Med J 1977;2:1384–1385.

18. Hollister LE, Motzenbecker FP, Degan RO. Withdrawal reactions from chlordiazepoxide ("Librium"). Psychopharmacology 1961;2:63–68.

19. Harrison M, Gusto U, Naranjo CA, Kaplan HL, Sellers EM. Diazepam tapering in detoxification of high-dose benzodiazepine abuse. Clin Pharmacol Ther., 1984; 36:527–532.

20. Miller LG, Greenblatt DJ, Barnhill JG, Shader RI. Chronic benzodiazepine administrations: I. Tolerance is associated with benzodiazepine receptor downregulation and decreased aminobutyric acid receptor complex binding and function. J Pharmacol Exp Ther 1987a;246:170–176.

21. Miller LG, Greenblatt DJ, Roy RB, Summer WR, Shader RI. Chronic benzodiazepine administration: II. Discontinuation syndrome is associated with upregulation of aminobutyric acid receptor complex binding and function. J Pharmacol Exp Ther 1987b;246:177–182.

22. Reidenberg MM, Levy M, Warner H, Coutinho CB, Schwartz MA, Yu G, Cheripko J. Relationship between diazepam dose, plasma level, age, and central nervous system depression. Clin Pharmacol Ther 1978;23:371–374.

23. Shader RI, Greenblatt DJ, Harmatz JS, Franke K, Koch-Weser J. Absorption and disposition of chlordiazepoxide in young and elderly male volunteers. J Clin Pharmacol 1977;17:709–718.

24. Preskorn S. Tricyclic antidepressants: whys and hows of therapeutic drug monitoring. J Clin Psychiatry 1989;50(Suppl): 34–42.

25. Pippenger CE. Clinically significant carbamazepine drug interactions: an overview. Epilepsia 1987;28:571–576.

26. Crowley JJ, Cusack BJ, Jue SG, Koup JR, Park BK, Vestal RE. Aging and drug interactions: II. Effect of phenytoin and smoking on the oxidation of theophylline and cortisol in healthy men. J Pharmacol Exp Ther 1988;345:513–523.

27. Crewe HK, Lennard MS, Tucker GT, et al. The effect of paroxetine and other specific serotonin reuptake inhibitors on cytochrome P450 IID6 activity in human liver microsomes. Br J Clin Pharmacol 1991; 32:658p–659p.

28. Preskorn SH, Burke M. Somatic therapy for major depressive disorder: Selection of an antidepressant J Clin Psychiatry 1992; 53(9):5–18.

29. Preskorn SH, Beber JH, Faul JC, Hirschfeld R. Serious adverse effects of combining fluoxetine and tricyclic antidepressants. Am J Psychiatry, 1990;147:4: 532.

30. Edelman, JS, Leibman J. Anatomy of body water and electrolytes. Am J Med 1959; 27:256–277.

31. Abernethy DR, Kertzner L. Age effects on

alpha-1-acid glycoprotein concentration and imipramine plasma protein binding. J Am Geriatr Soc 1984;32:705–708.

32. Cusack B, O'Malley K, Lavan J, Noel J, Kelly JG. Protein binding and disposition of lidocaine in the elderly. Eur J Clin Pharmacol 1985;29:232–329.

33. Campion EW, deLabry LO, Glynn RJ. The effect of age on serum albumin in healthy males: report from the normative aging study. J Gerontol 1988;43:M18–M20.

34. Bhanthumnavin K, Schuster MM. Aging and gastrointestinal function. In: Finch CE, Hayflick L, eds. Handbook of the biology of aging. New York: Van Nostrand Reinhold, 1977:709–723.

35. Evans MA, Triggs EJ, Cheung M, Broe GA, Creasey H. Gastric emptying rate in the elderly: implications for drug therapy. J Am Geriatr Soc 1981;29:201–205.

36. Wallace SM, Verbeek RK. Plasma protein binding of drugs in the elderly. Clin Pharmacokinet 1987;12:41–72.

37. Shock NW, Watkin DM, Yiengst BS, Norris AH, Gaffney GW, Gregerman RE, Falzone JA. Age differences in the water content of the body as related to basal oxygen consumption in males. J Gerontol 1963;18:1–8.

38. Vestal RE, Cusack BJ. Pharmacology and ageing. In: Schneider EL, Rowe JW, eds. Handbook of the biology of aging. 3rd ed. San Diego: Academic Press, 1990:349–383.

39. Bupp SJ, Preskorn SH. The effect of age on plasma levels of nortriptyline. Ann Clin Psychiatry 1991;3(1):61–65.

40. Abernethy DR, Greenblatt DJ, Shader RI. Imipramine and desipramine disposition in the elderly. J Pharmacol Exp Ther 1985; 232:183–188.

41. Salem SAM, Rajjayabun P, Shepherd AMM, Stevenson IH. Reduced induction of drug metabolism in the elderly. Age Ageing. 1978;7:68–73.

42. Schmucker DL. Aging and drug disposition: an update. Pharmacol Rev 1979; 30:445–456.

43. Klotz U, Avant GR, Hoyumpa A, Schenker S, Wilkenson GR. The effects of age and liver disease on the disposition and elimination of diazepam in adult man. J Clin Invest 1975;55:347–359.

44. Berlinger WJ, Goldberg MJ, Spector R, Chiang CK, Ghoneim MM. Diphenhydramine: kinetics and psychomotor effects in elderly women. Clin Pharmacol Ther 1982;32:387–391.

45. Cusack B, Kelly J, O'Malley K, Noel J, Lavan J, Horgan J. Digoxin in the elderly: pharmacokinetic consequences of old age. Clin Pharmacol Ther 1979;25:772–776.

46. Castleden CM, George CF. The effect of ageing on the hepatic clearance of propranolol. Br J Clin Pharmacol 1979;7:49–54.

47. Chandler MH, Scott SR, Blouin RA. Age-associated stereoselective alterations in hexobarbital metabolism. Clin Pharmacol Ther 1988;43:436–441.

48. Christensen JH, Andreasen F, Jansen JA. Influence of age and sex on the pharmacokinetics of thiopentone. Br J Anaesth 1981; 53:1189–1195.

49. Feely J, Crooks J, Stevenson IH. The influence of age, smoking and hyperthyroidism on plasma propranolol steady state concentration. Br J Clin Pharmacol 1981; 12:73–78.

50. Greenblatt DJ, Divoll M, Abernethy DR, Harmatz JS, Shader RI. Antipyrine kinetics in the elderly: prediction of age-related changes in benzodiazepine oxidizing capacity. J Pharmacol Exp Ther 1982;220:120–126.

51. Hayes MJ, Langman MJS, Short AH. Changes in drug metabolism with increasing age: 2. Phenytoin clearance and protein binding. Br J Clin Pharmacol 1975;2:73–79.

52. Mucklow JC, Fraser HS. The effects of age and smoking upon antipyrine metabolism. Br J Clin Pharmacol 1980;9:612–614.

53. Woodhouse KW, Mutch E, Williams FM, Rawlins MD, James OFW. The effect of age on pathways of drug metabolism in human liver. Age Ageing 1984;13:328–334.

54. Woodhouse KW, Wynne HA. Age-related changes in liver size and hepatic blood flow: the influence of drug metabolism in the elderly. Clin Pharmacokinet 1988; 15:287–294.

55. Wynne HA, Cope LH, Mutch E, Rawlins MD, Woodhouse KW, James OFW. The effect of age upon liver volume and apparent liver blood flow in healthy man. Hepatology 1989;9:297–301.

56. Lindeman RD, Tobin J, Shock NW. Longitudinal studies on the rate of decline in renal function with age. J Am Geriatr Soc 1985;33:278–285.

57. Rowe JW, Andres R, Tobin JD, Norris AH, Shock NW. The effect of age on creatinine clearance in man: a cross-sectional and longitudinal study. J Gerontol 1976;31:155–163.

58. Beers MH, Ouslander JG. Risk factors in geriatric drug prescribing: a practical guide to avoiding problems. Drugs 1989;37:105–112.

59. Schwartz LL. The debate over substitution policy. Its evolution and scientific bases. Am J Med 1985;79(suppl. 2B):38–44.

60. Divoll M, Greenblatt DJ, Abernethy DR, Shader RI. Cimetidine impairs clearance of antipyrine and desmethyldiazepam in the elderly. J Am Geriatr Soc 1982c;30:684–689.

61. Vestal RE, Cusack BJ, Mercer GD, Dawson GW, Park BK. Aging and drug interactions: I. Effect of cimetidine and smoking on the oxidation of theophyline and cortisol in healthy men. J Pharmacol Exp Ther 1987;241:488–500.

62. Greenblatt DJ, Preskorn SH, Cotreau MM, Horst WD, Harmatz JS. Fluoxetine impairs clearance of alprazolam but not of clonazepam. Clin Pharmacol Ther 1992; 52:479–486.

63. Weller R, Preskorn S. Psychotropic drugs and alcohol: pharmacokinetic and pharmacodynamic interactions. Psychosomatics 1984;25:301–309.

64. Klotz U. Pathophysiological and disease-induced changes in drug distribution volume: Pharmacokinetic implications. Clin Pharmacokinet 1976;1:204–218.

65. Jusko WJ, Gretch M. Plasma and tissue protein binding of drugs in pharmacokinetics. Drug Metab Rev 1976;5:43–140.

66. MacKichan JJ. Protein binding drug displacement interactions. Fact or fiction? Clin Pharmacokinet 1989;16:65–73.

67. Vallner JJ. Binding of drugs by albumin and plasma protein. J Pharm Sci 1977; 66:447–465.

68. Routledge PA. The plasma protein binding of basic drugs. Br J Clin Pharmacol 1986; 22:499–506.

69. Goulden KJ, Dooley JM, Camfield PR, Fraser AD. Clinical valproate toxicity induced by acetylsalicylic acid. Neurology 1987;37:1392–1394.

70. Paxton JW. Effects of aspirin on salivary and serum phenytoin kinetics in healthy subjects. Clin Pharmacol Ther 1980; 27:170–178.

71. Glotzbach R, Preskorn S. Brain concentrations of tricyclic antidepressants: Single-dose kinetics and relationship to plasma concentration in chronically dosed rats. Psychopharmacology 1982;78:25–27.

72. Frade L, Wiesel FA, Halldin C, Sedvall G. Central D2-dopamine receptor occupancy in schizophrenic patients treated with antipsychotic drugs. Arch Gen Psychiatry 1988;45:71–76.

73. Wilkinson GR, Shand DG. Commentary: a physiological approach to hepatic clearance. Clin Pharmacol Ther 1975;18:377–390.

74. Bertilsson L, Henthorn TK, Sanch E, Tybring G, Sawe J, Villen T. Importance of genetic factors in the regulation of diazepam metabolism: relationship to S-mephenytoin, but not debrisoquine: a case report supporting a coregulation of certain phase I and II metabolic reaction. Ther Drug Monit 1988;10:242–244.

75. Preskorn S, Alderman J, Harris S, Chung M, Harrison W. Desipramine levels after sertraline or fluoxetine. Presented at the 145th annual meeting of the American Psychiatric Association, May 2–7, 1992, Washington D.C.

76. Rudorfer MV, Potter WZ. Pharmacokinetics of antidepressants. In: HV Metzler, ed. Psychopharmacology: the third generation of progress. New York: Raven Press, 1987: 1353–1363.

77. Jandhyala B, Steenberg M, Perel J, et al. Effects of several tricyclic antidepressants on the hemodynamics and myocardial contractility of the anesthetized dogs. Eur J Pharmacol 1977;42:403–410.

78. Altafullah I, Talwar D, Loewenson R, Olson K, Lockman LA. Factors influencing serum levels of carbamazepine and carbamazepine-10, 11-epoxide in children. Epilepsy Res 1989;4:72–80.

79. Bourgeois BFD. Pharmacologic interactions between valproate and other drugs. Am J Med 1988;84:29–33.

80. Patel IH, Levy RH, Trager WF. Pharmacokinetics of carbamazepine-10, 11-epoxide before and after autoinduction in the rhesus monkey. J Pharmacol Exp Ther 1978;206:607–613.

81. Jusko WJ. Smoking effects in pharmacokinetics. In: Benet, L.Z.;Massoud, N.; Gambertoglio, J.G., eds. Pharmacokinetic basis for drug treatment. New York: Raven Press, 1984:311–320.

82. Jusko WJ. Role of tobacco smoking in pharmacokinetics. J Pharmacokinet Biopharm 1980;6:7–39.

83. Vestal RE, Wood AJJ. Influence of age and smoking on drug kinetics in man: studies using model compounds. Clin Pharmacokinet 1980;5:309–319.

84. Balant-Gorgia AE, Balant LP, Genet C, Dayer P, Aeschlimann JM, Garonne G. Importance of oxidative polymorphism and levopromazine treatment on the steady-state blood concentration of clomipramine and its major metabolites. Eur J Clin Pharmacol 1986;31:449–455.

85. Brosen K, Gram LF, Haghfelt T, Bertilsson L. Extensive metabolizers of debrisoquine become poor metabolizers during quinidine treatment. Pharmacol Toxicol 1987;60:312–314.

86. Fonne-Pfister R, Meyer UA. Xenobiotic and endobiotic inhibitors of cytochrome P450dbl function, the target of the debrisoquine/sparteine type polymorphism. Biochem Pharmacol 1988;37:3829–3835.

87. Gram LF, Debruyne D, Caillard V, Boulenger JP, Lacotte J, Moulin M, Zarifian E. Substantial rise in sparteine metabolic ratio during haloperidol treatment. Br J Clin Pharmacol 1989;27:272–275.

88. Haefely WE, Bargetzi MJ, Follath F, Meyer UA. Potent inhibition of cytochrome P450IID6 by flecainide in vitro and in vivo. J Cardiovasc Pharmacol 1990;15:776–779.

89. Hirschowitz J, Bennet JA, Semian FP, Garber D. Thioridazine effect of desipramine plasma levels. J Clin Psychopharmacol 1983;3:376–379.

90. Leeman T, Dayer P, Meyer UA. Single-dose quinidine treatment inhibits metropolol oxidation in extensive metabolizers. Eur J Clin Pharmacol 1986;29:739–741.

91. Gram LF, Overo KF. Drug interaction: Inhibitory effect of neuroleptics on metabolism of tricyclic antidepressants in man. Br Med J 1972;1:463–465.

92. Otton SV, Inaba T, Kalow W. Competitive inhibition of sparteine oxidation in human liver by beta-adrenoceptor antagonists and other cardiovascular drugs. Life Sci 1984;34:73–80.

93. Siris SG, Cooper TB, Rifbain AE, Brenner R, Liebermann JA. Plasma imipramine concentration in patients receiving concomitant fluphenazine decanoate. Am J Psychiatry 1982;139:104–106.

94. Steiner E, Dumont E, Spina E, Dahlqvist R. Inhibition of desipramine 2-hydroxylation by quinidine and quinine. Clin Pharmacol Ther 1988;43:577–581.

95. Syvahlahti EKG, Lindberg R, Kallio J, de Vocht M. Inhibitory effects of neuroleptics on debrisoquine oxidation in man. Br J Clin Pharmacol 1986;22:89–92.

96. Vestal RE. Kornhauser DM, Hollifield JW, Shand DG. Inhibition of propranolol metabolism by chlorpromazine. Clin Pharmacol Ther 1979;25:19–24.

97. Wright JM, Stokes EF, Sweeney VP. Isoniazid-induced carbamazepine toxicity and vice versa. A double drug interaction. N Engl J Med 1982;307:1325–1327.

98. Feely J, Pereira L, Guy E, Hockings N. Factors affecting the response to inhibition of drug metabolism by cimetidine—dose response and sensitivity of elderly and induced subjects. Br J Clin Pharmacol 1984; 17:77–81.

99. Ragheb M, Ban TA, Buchanan D, Frolich JC. Interaction of indomethacin and ibuprofen with lithium in manic patients under a steady-state lithium level. J Clin Psychiatry 1980;41:11:397–398.

100. Madakasira S, Preskorn S, Weller R, Pardo M. Single dose prediction of steady state plasma levels of amitriptyline. J Clin Psychopharmacol 1982;2:136–139.

101. Simard M, Gumbiner B, Lee A, Lewis H, Norman D. Lithium carbonate intoxication. A case report and review of the literature. Arch Intern Med 1989;149:36–46.

102. Sansome ME, Ziegler DK. Lithium toxicity: a review of neurologic complications. Clin Neuropharmacol 1985;8:242–248.

103. Mehta BR, Robinson BHB. Lithium toxicity induced by triamterene-hydrochlorothiazide. Postgrad Med J 1980;56:783–784.

104. Preskorn S, Mac D. The implication of concentration-response studies of tricyclic antidepressants for psychiatric research and practice. Psychiatr Dev 1984; 3:201–222.

105. Preskorn SH, Fast GA. Therapeutic drug monitoring for antidepressants: efficacy, safety, and cost effectiveness. J Clin Psychiatry 1991;52(6):23–33.

106. Preskorn SH, Jerkovich GS. Central nervous system toxicity of tricyclic antidepressants: Phenomenology, course, risk factors, and role of therapeutic drug monitoring. J Clin Psychiatry 1990;2:223–224.

107. Preskorn SH, Fast G. Tricyclic antidepressant-induced seizures and plasma drug concentration. J Clin Psychiatry 1992;53(5):160–162.

108. Goldman DL, Katz SE, Preskorn SH. What to do about extremely high plasma levels of tricyclics. Am J Psychiatry 1989; 146:3:401–402.

CHAPTER 4

Indications for Antipsychotics

The primary indication for antipsychotics is the presence of psychosis in such disparate conditions as:

- *Schizophrenia*
- *Schizophreniform* disorder
- *Schizoaffective* disorder
- *Brief reactive* psychosis
- *Delusional* (paranoid) disorder
- *Affective* disorders with mood congruent or incongruent psychotic symptoms
- *Organic* psychoses.

Since the most common psychotic condition is schizophrenia, this will be the primary disorder discussed. We will also consider those conditions characterized as "schizophrenic spectrum" (e.g., delusional, schizophreniform, schizoaffective); affective illness with psychotic features; and various nonpsychotic conditions (e.g., in the developmentally disabled) for which this class of drugs has been employed. (See Appendices A, C, E, F, G, and H.)

Schizophrenia

HISTORY OF THE CONCEPT

The identification of this illness in modern psychiatry begins with Kahlbaum, who described catatonia; Hecker, who described hebephrenia; and finally, Emil Kraepelin, who described dementia praecox (1–4).

The syndrome identified by Kraepelin is similar to the Diagnostic and Statistical Manual, 3rd edition, revised (DSM-III-R) diagnosis of schizophrenia and the Research Diagnostic Criteria (RDC) definition of chronic schizophrenia. It usually begins in adolescence or young adulthood, and frequently follows a progressively deteriorating course, with few patients ever making a complete recovery.

In contrast to Kraepelin, who emphasized the progressive course and poor outcome, the Swiss psychiatrist Eugen Bleuler employed a much broader concept of schizophrenia (5). Focusing on the thought disorder and the inconsistent, inappropriate, and disorganized affect, he identified four fundamental symptoms:

- Autism
- Ambivalence
- Abnormal thoughts
- Abnormal affect.

He also emphasized the incongruent relationships among thought, emotions, and behavior. Unlike his predecessors, he did not believe hallucinations and delusions were fundamental to the schizophrenic process, considering them accessory symptoms.

Historically, the diagnosis of schizophrenia in the United States has been based on bleulerian and psychoanalytic theory, partly due to the greater influence of the latter group in the fifties and sixties. By contrast, European psychiatry used a narrower set of diagnostic criteria, similar to Kraepelin's approach.

Psychoanalytic theory conceptualized schizophrenia as the use of primitive defenses (e.g., denial) against anxiety in the presence of a weakened ego. Since these patients are unable to employ more mature defenses against id-derived impulses, they regress to a more primitive level of functioning, with the intrusion of primary process thinking into consciousness. Since this condition was seen as a severe regression, almost any significantly ill patient could be diagnosed as schizophrenic. If this hypothesis were true, anxiolytics should have an antipsychotic effect, but that is typically not the case. Further, antipsychotics have a different biochemical action (i.e., dopamine receptor blockade) than the antianxiety agents (modulation of GABA receptor-chloride ion channels), constituting both a mechanistic and a clinical difference between these two drug classes. More importantly, the lack of efficacy with anxiolytics displaces the role of anxiety as critical to the pathogenesis of schizophrenia.

Another perspective comes from *family systems theory*. Here, the family is characterized as having disordered communication, with various members playing unusual or aberrant roles. Thus, patients experience "double binds," when contradictory expectations are placed on them (6). Initial controversial hypotheses held that the "schizophrenogenic" mother was the critical factor and then later that the

schizophrenic's father also played a significant role (7–9). Intensive therapy, in the context of in-hospital separation from the family, was considered the treatment of choice. In contrast to classical psychodynamic therapy, which focuses on the individual patient, family therapy attempts to resolve conflicts in the system, as well as in the patient's psyche. Typically this involves sessions that include all or as many members as possible. Thus, even though one member is identified as the patient, it is the disturbed communication and interactions among all members that is the focus of therapy.

DESCRIPTIVE/PHENOMENOLOGICAL APPROACH

At one time, because schizophrenia was then a much broader concept, almost all patients with moderate to severe psychotic symptoms were given this diagnosis. By contrast, bipolar disorder was defined very narrowly and only diagnosed in classic cases. Indeed, hospitalized patients diagnosed as schizophrenic in the United States were almost double those in Great Britain. Conversely, mood disorders were diagnosed five times more frequently in Great Britain than in the United States. To explore these differences, the United States and the United Kingdom conducted a systematic, structured interview research study of patients in Brooklyn, New York, and London (10, 11). The Present State Examination was used to standardize the diagnostic process, and as a result, many schizophrenic patients in New York were rediagnosed as having mood disorders, usually psychotic depression or mania. This project demonstrated that many United States patients diagnosed as schizophrenic would have received a diagnosis of mania or depression in the United Kingdom.

American psychiatry's approach to diagnosis began to change substantially with the development of specific diagnostic criteria, (as well as effective treatments such as lithium). These criteria were initially formulated by Feighner and Robins (The Feighner criteria), and later expanded by Spitzer, Endicott, and Robins into the RDC, which were the basis of the DSM-III, DSM-III-R, and upcoming DSM-IV (12, 13). In addition to being more descriptive in orientation, this approach recognized the importance of empirical data to develop explicit inclusion and exclusion criteria, which can then be scrutinized for reliability and validity.

EPIDEMIOLOGY

Throughout the world the lifetime prevalence of schizophrenia is about 1%. While the prevalence is slightly higher in the lower classes, data from a number of countries indicates that the social class distribution of the parents of schizophrenic probands is similar to the general population (14–16). This supports the "social drift" hypothesis, that the concentration of schizophrenics in the lower socioeconomic stratum is the result of their impaired functioning.

Schizophrenic patients tend to be born during the late winter or early spring in the Western hemisphere, an observation that suggests the possibility of a viral infectious process in the mother and the fetus, most probably during the first trimester (17, 18). Both sexes are equally affected, but females have a somewhat later onset of illness (i.e., approximately 6 years) than males and somewhat milder course.

SYMPTOMS

Schizophrenia is best characterized by delusions and hallucinations occurring in a clear sensorium, and in the absence of a significant mood disturbance. It is also associated with a variety of bizarre behaviors; illogical and/or tangential thinking; and shallow, blunted, or inappropriate affect.

Delusions are false beliefs that the patient maintains in the face of incontrovertible, contradictory evidence. The schizophrenic patient usually has no insight that these beliefs are not real, but rather maintains a firm conviction in them. Schizophrenia is characterized by a variety of delusions, of which the persecutory type predominates. Other delusions often involve bizarre bodily changes.

Hallucinations are false perceptions in the absence of a real sensory stimulus. They are typically auditory, consisting of voices that arise from both within and outside the body. They may be threatening, can ridicule, or urge patients to objectionable acts (i.e., command hallucinations). Visual hallucinations are also relatively frequent, but olfactory (e.g., unpleasant smells arising from the patient's own body) or tactile hallucinations (e.g., animals crawling inside one's body, or insects crawling over the skin) are uncommon.

Catatonia (withdrawn type), is characterized by prolonged immobility, waxy flexibility, posturing, and grimacing. Since catatonic symptoms can also occur in affective and organic psychosis, they are not specific to schizophrenia.

Schneiderian, first-rank symptoms describe hallucinations and delusions thought to be typical of schizophrenics (19, 20). Examples include:

- *Audible thoughts* (i.e., voices speak the patient's thoughts out loud)
- *Voices arguing* (two or more voices can argue or discuss issues, sometimes referring to the patient in the third person)

- *Voices commenting* on the patient's behavior
- *Somatic passivity* imposed by outside forces
- *Thought withdrawal* by outside forces, leaving the patient feeling as if his mind is empty
- *Thought insertions* by outside forces
- *Thought broadcasting* (i.e., thoughts escape from the patient's mind and are overheard by others)
- *Impulses, volitional acts, or feelings* that are not one's own but are imposed by outside forces
- *Delusional perceptions* (i.e., the patient attributes delusional meaning to normal perceptions).

COURSE OF ILLNESS

Several studies investigated the outcome in schizophrenic patients before antipsychotics were available (21–23). They generally found that an early onset of insidious symptoms, most characterized by negativity and a gradual deterioration into psychosis without clear precipitating events, was predictive of a poor outcome. These patients typically never married and often demonstrated asocial and bizarre behavior during childhood (24–27).

Longitudinal follow-up of narrowly defined schizophrenics shows that approximately 95% have a lifetime illness, with these patients rarely rediagnosed as having a mood disorder later (28, 29). They also often had:

- Poor performance in school
- Slightly lower IQs
- Abnormalities in cognitive and motor development
- Visual-motor incoordination
- Proprioceptive and vestibular difficulties.

By contrast, patients with good premorbid personalities and more typical functioning during childhood who later developed schizophrenic symptoms, especially in the face of massive precipitating events, had better outcomes. They also tended to have family histories of mood disorders, as well as affective features as part of their own illness. This led to the concept of process versus reactive schizophrenia (e.g., poor prognosis versus good prognosis) (30, 31).

BIOLOGICAL CORRELATES

In 1976, Johnstone, Crow, and coworkers applied the then newly developed computed tomography (CT) scan technology to study schizophrenic patients, and reported slightly larger ventricles as compared to matched controls (32). Indeed, these abnormalities were first noted in 1927, when Jacoby and Winkley reported enlarged ventricles using pneumoencephalography, with a number of open studies subsequently confirming this result in the 1930s (33). Furthermore, those with larger ventricles were usually more cognitively impaired and had fewer positive and more negative symptoms. Crow's suggestion of enlarged ventricles in association with negative symptoms spurred even more interest in this distinction. Subsequent studies with CT scans, and later magnetic resonance imaging, have verified that many schizophrenics have enlarged ventricles and associated cortical atrophy, especially in the temporal lobe and hippocampal nuclei (34–37). While schizophrenics do not show a specific abnormality like hydrocephalus, blind measurements over many studies have replicated these changes with several different radiographic techniques. It is important to note that the ventricular enlargement and cortical atrophy are statistical phenomena. Thus, although the abnormality is present in 30–40% of schizophrenics, there is significant overlap with normal controls, as well as a wide variety of other psychiatric conditions.

There is also evidence that the mothers of schizophrenics have a higher incidence of obstetrical complications. Furthermore, schizophrenics have more soft neurological signs and developmental anomalies associated with fetal damage. All these complications occur more frequently in schizophrenics with enlarged ventricles.

Enlarged ventricles and cortical atrophy are positively correlated with:

- *Negative* symptoms
- *Poor performance* on some neuropsychological tests
- The presence of *soft neurological signs*
- *Poor response* to treatment
- A *worse prognosis.*

Finally, there is evidence that blood flow is reduced in schizophrenics, particularly to the frontal lobes, and that glucose metabolism, as measured by positron emission tomography, is reduced in the same area. This is particularly evident when a patient is stimulated with a mental task that induces frontal lobe activity, such as the Wisconsin Card Sort Test.

The implication of these findings for nomenclature is that these patients tend to present clinically as the kraepelinian, poor prognosis type.

FAMILIAL AND GENETIC ISSUES

There is a large literature showing that this disorder has a familial and hereditary pattern (38–41). Therefore, the genetic relatives of schizophrenic patients have an increased risk of developing this disorder. Studies on identical and fraternal twins

from different countries find that 50–60% of monozygotic twins are concordant for schizophrenia, in contrast to only 15% of dizygotic twins (42–47).

There are also several cross-fostering studies of children of schizophrenic parents, adopted away by nonschizophrenic foster parents, who were compared to adopted children of normal parents raised by schizophrenic foster parents (48, 49). Invariably, those children whose biological parents had schizophrenia developed this disorder more frequently than the offspring of nonschizophrenic parents. This was true even when the latter were reared by schizophrenic foster families. In addition, the concordance rate for the illness in schizophrenic monozygotic twins reared apart was comparable to monozygotic twins reared together. These findings leave little doubt of a hereditary factor in schizophrenia. The advent of molecular genetics has provided powerful techniques for chromosomal localization of these disorders, and there is intense investigation to localize the responsible gene (or genes) associated with schizophrenia.

COST OF SCHIZOPHRENIA

Schizophrenia is a devastating illness crippling virtually every aspect of an individual's identity. Thus, it interferes with the ability to correctly interpret perceptions; to relate appropriately to others on both a cognitive and emotional basis; and to articulate one's thoughts clearly. Schizophrenics rarely achieve as much in life as their nonaffected age cohort. Prior to the discovery of antipsychotics, about 50% of hospital beds were occupied by these patients, and even now, they still occupy 25%. The disorder begins relatively early in life, (i.e., late teens and early twenties) and rarely remits. It produces severe social deficits and at times continuous hospitalization. A substantial number of the homeless are schizophrenics, as well as many who live isolated, unproductive lives in facilities such as halfway houses. In sum, it represents a major burden to society and a tragedy for both patients and their families.

ROLE OF ANTIPSYCHOTICS IN SCHIZOPHRENIA

An important question is whether or not these agents are indicated for all patients with active schizophrenia. While there is general agreement that they are beneficial, a small group of therapists emphasize the role of psychotherapy, even though their patients often require medication as well. Thus, although the majority benefit from these drugs, it is possible that a small subgroup may do well without medication. For example, "reactive" schizophrenics have recovered from an episode without drug treatment.

A classic, double-blind, random assignment investigation by Cole, Klerman, and Goldberg (1964), compared the response of schizophrenics treated with antipsychotics or placebo (50, 51). In a re-examination of the data, we compared the fate of the 10–20% who had the best outcome. A small percentage completely recovered without residual symptoms in 6 weeks, representing about 16% of those on drugs; but only about 1% on placebo. This is a remarkable difference; and, while some did relatively well without medication, it is likely that they would have done even better with active drug therapy.

Further, in the drug-treated group, only 2% deteriorated, in contrast to 33% in the placebo group. It is true that some patients show little improvement with drugs, but if they had been given only placebo, they most likely would have deteriorated even more. Thus, at both ends of the prognostic spectrum, there appears to be a substantial benefit from drugs.

Other Psychotic Disorders

SCHIZOPHRENIFORM DISORDER

Patients with this condition manifest the symptoms of an acute exacerbation of schizophrenia, but they make a complete recovery, with the prodromal, active, and residual phases lasting no more than 6 months.

SCHIZOAFFECTIVE DISORDER

This category is characterized by both psychotic and affective symptoms, with patients not clearly meeting the diagnosis of schizophrenia or of a major mood disorder. While this category is not well understood, the possibilities include:

- It is a *variant of schizophrenia*
- It is a *variant of a mood disorder*
- It represents patients who have *both disorders simultaneously*
- It is a *separate entity*
- There is a *continuum between schizophrenia and mood disorders* without any sharp division between them, with schizoaffective disorder representing the middle portion of this continuum.

A number of studies on the heredity of schizoaffective disorder (SA) have found that these patients have more relatives with both affective and schizophrenic conditions, when compared to normals controls (52–55). While they also had some relatives with schizoaffective disorder, the predominant familial illnesses were schizophrenic or affective. The course of illness and prognosis appear to fall somewhere between that of mood and schizophrenic disorders. Thus, a greater percentage of SA patients recover, with better functioning than schizophrenics, but do not improve as much as those with pure mood disorders (56–58). The number of SA patients who have a progressively deteriorating course also falls somewhere between schizophrenic and mood disorders. Finally, some SA patients respond to lithium during an acute episode, which then also appears to prevent future relapses.

BRIEF REACTIVE PSYCHOSIS

This is an acute response to a severe stressor that generally subsides in a day or two. This phenomenon is frequently seen in adolescence and young adulthood without prodromal symptoms or lasting impairment. There is little information available about such factors as prevalence and heredity, other than that which is inherent in the diagnosis.

DELUSIONAL (PARANOID) DISORDER

This category is attributed to Kahlbaum and Kraepelin, who both saw paranoia as a chronic, unremitting system of delusions distinguished by both the absence of hallucinations and the deterioration seen in schizophrenia.

Paranoia is a stable, delusional system of at least 6 months' duration, while by definition *acute paranoia* lasts less than 6 months. In *shared paranoia*, a close friend or relative passively accepts the delusional belief system of the more dominant member, thus, the symptoms may not necessarily be truly delusional. DSM-III-R criteria distinguishes between paranoia, which incorporates systematized delusions without hallucinations, and *paraphrenia*, which also includes hallucinations.

Delusional disorder is relatively uncommon, with an incidence 25 times less than that of schizophrenia, and both sexes are involved equally. The term *late paraphrenia* refers to the development of delusions (often with hallucinations) in elderly patients (i.e., patients over 55 without preexisting major psychiatric disease). Interestingly, deafness is present in a substantial number of this group.

Delusions can be held throughout life despite considerable contradictory evidence, which is usually reinterpreted to coincide with one's false beliefs. They are usually highly systematized; interrelated by a common theme; and often encapsulated, (i.e., a person's thinking remains unimpaired except for the systematized delusions, which markedly depart from reality).

Subtypes of Delusional Disorders

Examples of delusional subtypes include:

- Erotomanic
- Grandiose
- Jealous
- Persecutory
- Monosymptomatic hypochondriacal
- Megalomanic.

Erotomanic Type

The central core of this delusional variant is that one is loved in a highly idealized, romantic, or spiritual manner. Sometimes the delusion is kept secret, but frequently efforts (i.e., telephone calls, letters, gifts, visits) are made to contact the person who is the object of the delusion, often a famous person, or a superior at work. While female patients are usually seen clinically, many males are often seen in a forensic context because they come into contact with the law when they stalk or try to inappropriately contact the individual who is the focus of their delusion.

Grandiose Type

These delusions often take the form of a false belief that the patient possesses some great, unrecognized talent; is the son or daughter of a famous person; or actually is the famous person, while the true celebrity is an imposter.

Jealous Type

Here, the patient is convinced, despite overwhelmingly contrary evidence, that a spouse or a lover is unfaithful. As evidence of infidelity, these patients may use seemingly unrelated events to support their delusional system. Often they will confront their spouse or lover, take steps to intervene, or initiate investigations into the perceived infidelity.

Persecutory Type

Here, patients believe that they are being conspired against, poisoned, or drugged by someone. They may even take action against their perceived persecutors, on occasion resorting to violence.

Somatic Type

Patients may feel that they emit a foul odor from some part of their body; that they have insects on their skin or suffer from internal parasites; or feel certain parts of the body are misshapen or ugly. They have no insight and will persistently seek treatment from the appropriate medical specialist.

Course of Illness

Lifetime prevalence is about 0.03–0.5%. While delusional disorders can occur at any age, onset is generally after the age of 40 years. The course is highly variable, with some patients holding their false beliefs all their lives; others may have episodes that can remit within a few months or follow a waxing and waning course. While these patients are generally intellectually and occupationally intact, frequently their delusional system interferes with social functioning.

While large-scale studies have not been done, anecdotal case reports indicate that these disorders are helped by antipsychotics, with some patients, such as late paraphrenics, quite responsive. Unfortunately, since many of these patients are paranoid, they may not seek medical help or cooperate with treatment recommendations.

PSYCHOTIC MOOD DISORDERS

It is well established that monotherapy with various antidepressants, (e.g., tricyclic antidepressants (TCAs), monoamine oxidase inhibitors (MAOIs)), is relatively ineffective (i.e., they are necessary but not sufficient) for treating depression or mania with associated delusions and/or hallucinations. Thus, psychotically depressed patients are best managed with a combination of antipsychotic-antidepressant or with electroconvulsive therapy (ECT).

While there is no doubt that antipsychotics have a more rapid onset of action than lithium in an acute manic episode, we are unaware of clinical trials that examine the differential effect of antipsychotics or lithium for nonpsychotic versus psychotic mania. This topic is discussed further in Chapter 10.

ORGANIC PSYCHOSES

There are few controlled studies of antipsychotics used in a wide variety of organic psychoses; instead, most of the literature consists of anecdotal case reports (single cases, or series of cases).

Agitation in the Demented Elderly

For agitated and demented elderly patients, the use of low-dose, high-potency antipsychotics is considered the treatment of choice. There is some controversy about the use of these agents (see The Elderly Patient in Chapter 14), and recently, the federal authorities have attempted to curtail the use of these agents in the elderly population. This may be misguided, however, since the only studies addressing this question found that antipsychotics had a clear calming effect in a demented, nursing home population (59, 60). Indeed, the Finkle study found that after the federal regulations went into effect there was a decrease in the use of antipsychotics and an increase in nursing home deaths. They also found a greater death rate in the placebo group. Thus, it is possible that unchecked agitation may increase mortality in a frail, elderly person.

There are four small studies on the use of antipsychotics in agitated patients treated on geriatric units of state hospitals (61–64). These patients had a wide variety of organic psychoses, and probably constitute a different population from the chronically demented group, since many were admitted because of an acute exacerbation of their psychosis. Our meta-analysis of these data found a statistically significant benefit favoring the use of antipsychotics in this population (see The Elderly Patient in Chapter 14).

Steroid Psychosis

Davis et al. (1992) recently reviewed the literature on steroid psychosis, locating 29 cases where low doses of antipsychotics alone were used to treat this condition and found a remission rate of 82% (65). The response was remarkably rapid, with a third of the patients remitting in a few days, 60% by 1 week, and 80% by 2 weeks. Parenthetically, ECT also benefits steroid psychosis, tricyclics make the psychosis worse, and prophylactic lithium can prevent its occurrence.

Nonpsychotic Disorders

Anxiolytics are the treatment of choice for *anxiety disorders,* and antipsychotics should not be used for this purpose. Previously, psychotropics were classified as major and minor tranquilizers, a categorization we now know to be conceptually incorrect. There is evidence however that adding benzodiazepines (BZDs) to antipsychotics might improve the treatment of various acute psychotic episodes complicated by agitation, although this has not been well studied. (See Chapters 5 and 10).

Antipsychotics are widely used to treat behavioral disturbances in the *developmentally disabled.* While there is a large body of anecdotal evidence to support their efficacy, there are little data from well-controlled clinical trials. These agents are also effective in treating a wide variety of *secondary psychoses,* including those resulting from various diseases that can affect brain function (e.g., primary degenerative dementia, delirium, etc.).

CONCLUSION

Knowing (or at least suspecting) certain empirical facts, one can use these as the basis for specific diagnostic criteria. If diagnosis is then made by these criteria, the diagnostic scheme will subsequently predict the original, empirical observation. Since the very same facts were used to create the diagnostic criteria, a circularity in thinking about categories is established (albeit inadvertently).

One of the more bizarre theories of schizophrenia is the "labelling" theory. Proponents feel that schizophrenia does not exist, and what is called schizophrenia is merely the result of labelling individuals with social dysfunction. There is a wealth of empirical information that the various mental disorders are not "sociopathologic," but instead have different:

- *Symptom* clusters
- Clinical *outcomes*
- Brain *imaging* findings
- Autopsy *brain structural* findings
- Responses to various *endocrine challenges*
- *Genetic* patterns.

Confirmation should not be sought from factors implicit in the diagnostic criteria, but rather through independent lines of evidence. Perhaps the most convincing is the response of schizophrenia and other psychotic disorders to the antipsychotics.

REFERENCES

1. Kahlbaum K. Die Gruppirung der Psychischen Krankheiten. Danzig: Kafemann, 1863.
2. Kahlbaum K. Die Katatonie oder das Spannungsirresein. Berlin: Hirschwald, 1874.
3. Hecker E. Die Hebephrenie. Arch Pathol Ant Physiol Klin Med, 1871;52:394–429.
4. Kraepelin E. Dementia praecox and paraphrenia. Huntington, New York: Robert Krieger, 1971 (facsimile of 1919 edition. Barclay RM, trans).
5. Bleuler E. Dementia praecox or the group of schizophrenias. Zinkin J, trans. New York: International Universities Press, 1950.
6. Bateson G, Jackson DD, Haley J, Wakland JH. Toward a theory of schizophrenia. Behav Sci 1956;1:251–264.
7. Lidz R, Lidz T. The family environment of schizophrenic patients. Am J Psychiatry 1949;106:332–345.
8. Lidz T. Intrafamilial environment of the schizophrenic patient: VI. The transmission of irrationality. Arch Neurol Psychiat 1958;79:305–316.
9. Wynne LC, Ryckoff IM, Day J, Hirsch S. Pseudomutuality in the family relations of schizophrenics. Psychiatry 1958;21:205–220.
10. Cooper B. Epidemiology. In: Wing JK, ed. Schizophrenia: toward a new synthesis. New York: Grune & Stratton, 1978.
11. Cooper JE, Kendell RE, Gurland BJ, Sharpe L, Copeland JRM, Simon R. Psychiatric diagnosis in New York and London: a comparative study of mental hospital admissions. London: Oxford University Press, 1972. (Institute of Psychiatry, Maudsley Monographs, no. 20).
12. Feighner JP, Robins E, Guze SB, Woodruff RA, Winokur G, Munoz R. Diagnostic criteria for use in psychiatric research. Arch Gen Psychiatry 1972;26:57–63.
13. Spitzer RL, Endicott J, Robins E. Research diagnostic criteria: rationale and reliability. Arch Gen Psychiatry 1978;35:773–786.
14. Dunham HW. Community and schizophrenia. Detroit: Wayne State University Press, 1965.
15. Faris REL, Dunham HW. Mental disorders in urban areas. Chicago: University of Chicago Press, 1939.
16. Goldberg EM, Morrison SL. Schizophrenia and social class. Br J Psychiatry 1963;109:785–802.
17. Watson CG, Kucala T, Tilleskjor C, Jacobs L. Schizophrenic birth seasonality in relation to the incidence of infectious diseases and temperature extremes. Arch Gen Psychiatry 1984;41:85–90.
18. Hare EH. Season of birth in schizophrenia

and neurosis. Am J Psychiatry 1975;132: 1168–1171.

19. Mellor CS. First rank symptoms of schizophrenia. Br J Psychiatry 1970;117:15–23.

20. Taylor MA. Schneiderian first-rank symptoms and clinical prognostic features in schizophrenia. Arch Gen Psychiatry 1972;26:64–67.

21. Astrup C, Fossum A, Holmboe R. Prognosis in functional psychoses. Springfield, Illinois: CC Thomas, 1962.

22. Astrup C, Noreik K. Functional psychoses: diagnostic and prognostic models. Springfield, Illinois: CC Thomas, 1966.

23. Belmaker R, Pollin W, Wyatt RJ, Cohen SA. Follow-up of monozygotic twins discordant for schizophrenia. Arch Gen Psychiatry 1974;30:219–222.

24. Albee G, Lane E, Reuter JM. Childhood intelligence of future schizophrenics and neighborhood peers. J Psychol 1964;58: 141–144.

25. Offord DR. School performance of adult schizophrenics, their siblings and age mates. Br J Psychiatry 1974;125:12–19.

26. Jones MB, Offord DR. Independent transmission of IQ and schizophrenia. Br J Psychiatry 1975;126:185–190.

27. Pfohl B, Winokur G. Schizophrenia: course and outcome. In: Henn FA, Nasrallah HA, eds. Schizophrenia as a brain disease. New York: Oxford University Press, 1982.

28. Guze SB, Cloninger R, Martin RL, Clayton PJ. A follow-up and family study of schizophrenia. Arch Gen Psychiatry 1983; 40:1273–1276.

29. Tsuang MT, Woolson RF, Winokur G, Crowe RR. Stability of psychiatric diagnosis: schizophrenia and affective disorders followed up over a 30- to 40-year period. Arch Gen Psychiatry 1981;38:535–539.

30. Stephens JH. Long-term course and prognosis of schizophrenia. Seminars in Psychiatry 1970;2:464–485.

31. Stephens JH, Astrup C. Prognosis in "process" and "non-process" schizophrenia. Am J Psychiatry 1963;119:945–953.

32. Johnstone EC, Crow TJ, Frith CD, Husband J, Kreel L. Cerebral ventricular size and cognitive impairment in chronic schizophrenia. Lancet 1976;2:924–926.

33. Weinberger DR, Wyatt RJ. Brain morphology in schizophrenia: in vivo studies. In: Henn FA, Nasrallah HA, eds. Schizophrenia as a brain disease. New York: Oxford University Press, 1982.

34. Weinberger DR, Bigelow LB, Kleinman JE, Klein ST, Rosenblatt JE, Wyatt RJ. Cerebral ventricular enlargement in chronic schizophrenia: an association with poor response to treatment. Arch Gen Psychiatry 1980;37:11–13.

35. Luchins DJ. Computed tomography in schizophrenia: disparities in the prevalence of abnormalities. Arch Gen Psychiatry 1982;39:859–860.

36. Nasrallah HA, McCalley-Whitters M, Jacoby CG. Cerebral ventricular enlargement in young manic males: a controlled CT study. J Affective Disord 1982;4:15–19.

37. Rieder RO, Mann LS, Weinberger DR, van Kammen DP, Post RM. Computed tomographic scans in patients with schizophrenia, schizoaffective, and bipolar affective disorder. Arch Gen Psychiatry 1983;40:735–739.

38. Tsuang MT, Vandermey R. Genes and the mind: inheritance of mental illness. London: Oxford University Press, 1980.

39. Tsuang MT, Winokur G, Crowe RR. Morbidity risks of schizophrenia and affective disorders among first degree relatives of patients with schizophrenia, mania, depression, and surgical conditions. Br J Psychiatry 1980;137:497–504.

40. Fowler RC, Tsuang MT, Cadoret RJ. Parental psychiatric illness associated with schizophrenia in the siblings of schizophrenics. Compr Psychiatry 1977;18:271–275.

41. Fowler RC, Tsuang MT, Cadoret RJ. Psychiatric illness in the offspring of schizophrenics. Compr Psychiatry 1977;18:127–134.

42. Karlsson JL. Genealogic studies of schizophrenia. In: Rosenthal D, Kety SS, eds. The transmission of schizophrenia. Oxford; Pergamon Press, 1968:85–94.

43. Kendler KS. Overview. A current perspective on twin studies of schizophrenia. Am J Psychiatry 1983;140:1413–1425.

44. Fischer M. Psychoses in the offspring of schizophrenic twins and their normal cotwins. Br J Psychiatry 1971;118:43–52.

45. Fischer M, Harvald B, Hauge M. A Danish twin study of schizophrenia. Br J Psychiatry 1969;115:981–990.

46. Kallmann FJ. The genetic theory of schizophrenia. An analysis of 691 twin index families. Am J Psychiatry 1946;103:309–322.

47. Gottesman II, Shields J. Contributions of twin studies to perspectives in schizophre-

nia. In: Maher BA, ed. Progress in experimental personality research. Vol 3. New York: Academic Press, 1966:1–84.

48. Kety SS, Rosenthal D, Wender PH, Schulsinger F, Jacobsen B. The biologic and adoptive families of adopted individuals who became schizophrenic: prevalence of mental illness and other characteristics. In: Wynne LC, Cromwell RL, Matthysse S, eds. The nature of schizophrenia: new approaches to research and treatment. New York: John Wiley & Sons, 1978:25–37.

49. Heston LL. Psychiatric disorders in foster home-reared children of schizophrenic mothers. Br J Psychiatry 1966;112:819–825.

50. Cole JO, Goldberg SC, Klerman GL. Phenothiazine treatment in acute schizophrenia. Arch Gen Psychiatry 1964;10:246–261.

51. Cole JO, Goldberg SC, Davis JM. Drugs in the treatment of psychosis: controlled studies. In: Solomon P, ed. Psychiatric drugs. New York: Grune & Stratton, 1965:153–180.

52. Tsuang MT, Dempsey M, Rauscher F. A study of "atypical schizophrenia": comparison with schizophrenia and affective disorder by sex, age of admission, precipitant, outcome, and family history. Arch Gen Psychiatry 1976;33:1157–1160.

53. Tsuang MT, Woolson RF. Mortality in patients with schizophrenia, mania, depression, and surgical conditions. Br J Psychiatry 1977;130:162–166.

54. Coryell WH, Tsuang MT. DSM-III schizophreniform disorder: comparisons with schizophrenia and affective disorder. Arch Gen Psychiatry 1982;39:66–69.

55. Pope HG, Lipinski JF, Cohen BM, Axelrod DT. "Schizoaffective disorder": an invalid diagnosis? A comparison of schizoaffective disorder, schizophrenia and affective disorder. Am J Psychiatry 1980;137:921–927.

56. Tsuang MT, Woolson RF, Fleming JA. Long-term outcome of major psychoses. I. Schizophrenia and affective disorders compared with psychiatrically symptom-free surgical conditions. Arch Gen Psychiatry 1979;36:1295–1301.

57. Bleuler M. The schizophrenic disorders: long-term patient and family studies. New Haven Connecticut: Yale University Press, 1978 (originally published in 1972, Clemens S. trans).

58. Ciompi L. Catamnestic long-term study on the course of life and aging in schizophrenics. Schizophr Bull 1980;6:606–618.

59. Barnes R, Veith R, Okimoto J, Raskind M, Gumbrecht G. Efficacy of antipsychotic medications in behaviorally disturbed dementia patients. Am J Psychiatry 1982;139:1170–1174.

60. Finkle SI, Lyons JS, Anderson RL, Sherrell K, Davis JM, Cohen-Mansfield J, et al. A double blind study of thiothixene in agitated nursing home elderly (in press).

61. Sugerman AA, Williams BH, Adlerstein AM. Haloperidol in the psychiatric disorders of old age. Am J Psychiatry 1964;120:1190–1192.

62. Rada RT, Kellner R. Thiothixene in the treatment of geriatric patients with chronic organic brain syndrome. J Am Geriatr Soc 1976;24:105–107.

63. Petrie WM, Ban TA, Berney S, Fujimori M, Guy W, Ragheb M, Wilson WH, Schaffer JD. Loxapine in psychogeriatrics: a placebo- and standard-controlled clinical investigation. J Clin Psychopharmacol 1982;2(2):122–126.

64. Stotsky B. Multi-center study comparing thioridazine with diazepam and placebo in elderly, non-psychotic patients with emotional and behavioral disorders. Clin Ther 1984;6:546–559

65. Davis JM, Leach A, Merk B, Janicak PG. Treatment of steroid psychoses. Psychiatric Annals 1992;22:487–491.

CHAPTER 5

Treatment with Antipsychotics

History

As in other areas of clinical science, serendipity, as well as careful scientific investigation, have contributed to our knowledge about antipsychotics, including their:

- *Discovery*
- *Potential mechanism(s) of action*
- Range of *complications*.

Chlorpromazine's (CPZ) efficacy was recognized partially by chance, when it was initially synthesized as an antihistamine and chosen for human investigation because it was a relatively mild sedative. The concept of an antipsychotic, however, was unknown at that time. CPZ's sedating properties then led the French anesthesiologist, surgeon Henri Leborit, to use CPZ in a lytic cocktail to reduce autonomic response with surgical stress (1). He also recommended its use for treatment of a wide variety of other disorders, encouraging John Delay and Pierre Deniker (1952), who then administered CPZ to schizophrenic patients; the rest is history (2, 3).

Even though CPZ did not produce a permanent cure for schizophrenia or for any other psychotic disorder, it had a dramatic impact, benefitting many as no other treatment had before. News of its effectiveness spread rapidly, and within a year or two, CPZ was employed worldwide, altering the lives of millions of psychotic patients in a positive manner.

The relocation of treatment from chronic inhospital settings to outpatient community mental health centers is, in part, due to the efficacy of antipsychotics. Naturalistic studies before the era of psychotropics revealed that two of three psychotic patients (primarily schizophrenic) spent most of their lives in state asylums. Before the mid-1950s, there had been a steady increase in state hospital populations, which paralleled the general population growth; but antipsychotics contributed to a marked reduction in those hospitalized for various psychoses. Presently, more than 95% of these patients live outside of the hospital, even though many continue to relapse and/or demonstrate residual symptoms. Thus, while the antipsychotics have not been a panacea, they make community-based care a reality for many who would otherwise have remained chronically institutionalized.

Reserpine, used as a folk medicine in

India, was also discovered to have antipsychotic properties at about the same time as CPZ. Both agents affected the dopaminergic system, albeit in different ways, but the functional results were similar (i.e., lowering dopamine activity). This phenomenon has continued to be the basis for hypotheses about the mechanism of action of these drugs and for biological theories about the pathophysiology of psychotic disorders.

The revolutionary idea that drugs could exert a specific antipsychotic effect, coupled with a growing recognition of their significant adverse effects, led to the search for other substances with similar properties. Some compounds, such as rauwolfia, came from traditional folk medicine; some were discovered empirically; whereas others were the result of systematic clinical investigations with chemically or structurally related compounds. This has led to a variety of effective drugs for schizophrenia and for other major psychotic disorders. Among these drugs are:

- The phenothiazines
- The thioxanthenes
- The dibenzoxazepines
- The dibenzodiazepines
- The butyrophenones
- The dihydroindolones
- The diphenylbutyrylpiperidines
- The rauwolfian alkaloids
- Experimental agents.

Table 5.1 presents the classes, names, and typical doses for the most commonly used antipsychotics.

Figure 5.1 presents the basic chemical structure of most agents with antipsychotic effects.

REFERENCES

1. Laborit H, Huguenard P, Alluaume R. Un nouveau stabilisateur végétatif, le 4560 RP. Presse Med 1952;60:206–208.
2. Delay J, Deniker P. Le traitement des psychoses par une methode neurolytique derivee de l'hibermotherapie. Congres des medecins alienistes et neurologistes de France, Luxembourg, July, 1952:497–502.
3. Delay J, Deniker P. Trente-hit cas de psychoses traitees par la cure-prolongee et continue de 4560 RP. Le Congres de AL et Neurologie de Langue Francaise, in Compte Rendue Congress. Paris: Marson et Cie, 1952.

Mechanism of Action

The common denominator underlying the efficacy of the neuroleptic antipsychotics is the blockade of central dopamine (DA) receptors. The extrapyramidal reactions, particularly parkinsonian symptoms, are a major adverse effect of these drugs, as well as an important clue to their mechanism of action. True Parkinson's disease is caused by a DA deficiency in the nigrostriatal system. Further, crystallographic data have demonstrated that CPZ's molecular configuration is similar to that of DA, which could explain its ability to block this neurotransmitter's receptors. Drugs with similar structures that do not block DA receptors (e.g., promethazine, imipramine) do not have antipsychotic activity. The isomer of flupenthixol that blocks DA receptors is an effective antipsychotic, but the isomer that does not is ineffective (1).

Interestingly, the atypical antipsy-

Table 5.1.
Antipsychotic Agents

Types		Dosage (average range, orally, per day)
Phenothiazines		
Aliphatics		
• Thorazine	(Chlorpromazine)	100–1000 mg
• Sparine	(Promazine)	25–1000 mg
• Vesprin	(Triflupromazine)	20–150 mg
Piperidines		
• Mellaril	(Thioridazine)	30–800 mg
• Serentil	(Mesoridazine)	20–200 mg
• Quide	(Piperacetazine)	20–160 mg
Piperazines		
• Stelazine	(Trifluoperazine)	2–60 mg
• Prolixin	(Fluphenazine)	5–40 mg
• Trilafon	(Perphenazine)	2–60 mg
• Tindal	(Acetophenazine)	40–80 mg
• Compazine	(Prochlorperazine)	15–125 mg
Thioxanthenes		
Navane	(Thiothixene)	6–60 mg
Taractan	(Chlorprothixene)	10–600 mg
Dibenzoxazepines		
Loxitane	(Loxapine)	20–250 mg
Dibenzodiazepines		
Clozaril	(Clozapine)	100–900 mg
Butyrophenones		
Haldol	(Haloperidol)	3–50 mg
Dihydroindolenes		
Moban	(Molindone)	15–225 mg
Diphenylbutyrylpiperidines		
Semap	(Penfluridol)	100 mg/wk
• long acting oral medicine		
• not yet approved in United States		
Orap	(Pimozide)	1–10 mg
Rauwolfian Alkaloids		
Serpasil	(Reserpine)	0.1–1 mg
Experimental Agents		
Propranolol		
Naloxone		
Apomorphine		
Lithium		
α-methyl-p-tyrosine		

Adapted from Davis JM, Janicak PG, Lindon R, et al. Neuroleptics and psychotic disorders. In: Coyle JT, Enna SJ, eds. Neuroleptics: neurochemical, behavioral and clinical perspectives. New York: Raven Press, 1983.

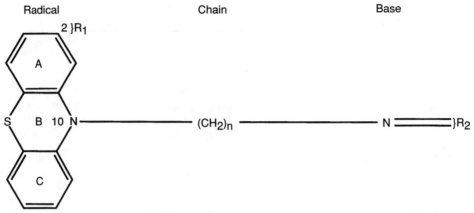

Figure 5.1.   Basic requirements for antipsychotic activity: distance between N_{10} of radical and the base N atom must equal at least three carbons (n = 3), with a suitable substituent R_2 mainly determining the qualitative properties of the group; the A_2 substituent R_1 mainly determines the quantitative properties of the individual compounds.

chotic clozapine does not produce extrapyramidal side effects. This is an important observation, because it offers the hope that these two effects can be dissociated. Generally, the term "neuroleptic" is applied to all drugs that produce both extrapyramidal and antipsychotic effects, but clozapine may be an antipsychotic without being a neuroleptic, perhaps making the interchangable use of the terms neuroleptic and antipsychotic passé.

The evidence that antidopaminergic agents ameliorate psychosis and that DA agonists can produce psychosis or worsen pre-existing disorders, supports a central role for DA in any theory about pathophysiology. Further, there is a high correlation among directly measured *DA receptor binding*, the clinical potency of these agents, animal behavioral models, and data about DA blockade.

Other drug effects that decrease DA activity also support this position. Thus, when DA synthesis is blocked by α-methyl-*p*-tyrosine (AMPT), the dose necessary for an antipsychotic effect is reduced (i.e., the dose-response curve is shifted to the left by the interaction between dopamine and AMPT). Finally, a drug such as reserpine that can deplete DA stores also has relatively mild antipsychotic properties.

DOPAMINERGIC PATHWAYS OF THE CENTRAL NERVOUS SYSTEM

Because the existing evidence strongly implicates the DA system in psychosis, it is pertinent to discuss this neurotransmitter's central dopaminergic pathways. There are five tracts:

- The *striatal* system (A-9)
- The *mesolimbic* system (A-10)
- The *mesocortical* system
- The *retinal* system
- The *neurohypophyseal* system

The last system is of interest in regard to the elevation in prolactin, which is closely associated with drug efficacy.

Postmortem studies of patients with idiopathic Parkinson's disease demonstrate cell loss in the striatal system (A-9), directly implicating this tract vis-à-vis the neuroleptic-induced pseudoparkinsonian side effects. The assumption that psychosis is related to the A-10 system is made by exclusion. There is also evidence that clozapine may differentially block DA pathways. Specifically, it seems to act on the mesolimbic dopaminergic system (A-10), while being relatively inactive in the striatal system (A-9); however, this remains controversial. Since clozapine may block specific DA receptors, its antipsychotic activity could be consistent with an antidopaminergic mechanism of action. Conversely, clozapine does not typically induce extrapyramidal symptoms, which are presumably subserved by the A-9 system. Thus, while clozapine is known to block striatal DA receptors in positron emission tomography (PET) studies, resolution is not sufficient to clarify effects on other tracts. Furthermore, low doses of metoclopramide, which significantly decreases the number of DA neurons spontaneously active in A-9, do not have antipsychotic effects (except at high doses) but can induce tardive dyskinesia (TD), as well as acute extrapyramidal side effects (EPS).

NEUROPHYSIOLOGICAL STUDIES

Another way to measure striatal (A-9) or mesolimbic (A-10) activity is through neurophysiological studies involving the firing rate of these neurons. The acute administration of antipsychotics will cause DA neurons to initiate a burst pattern of firing, with the opposite occurring when a DA agonist is administered. Eventually, some degree of tolerance develops and the enhanced DA synthesis decreases with time on drug, as demonstrated in both human cerebrospinal fluid (CSF) studies and rat brain slices. On a more chronic basis, repeated drug administration results in a dramatic decrease in the proportion of spontaneously active dopaminergic neurons (i.e., excitation-induced depolarization blockade of the DA neuron spike-generating region). Both the depolarization blockade and the antipsychotic effects of these drugs develop slowly. Classic antipsychotics induce nigrostriatal and mesolimbic DA neurons into depolarization blockade, while atypical antipsychotics, such as clozapine, only induce depolarization in the mesolimbic-mesocortical DA neurons.

The working assumption that the striatal system is only involved with extrapyramidal function (e.g., parkinsonian side effects, dystonias, and tardive dyskinesia) and that the mesolimbic or mesocortical systems are only involved with psychosis may be an oversimplification. Many of the neuroanatomical studies on the identified dopaminergic tracts are done with rats. In the monkey, by contrast, there are many more DA tracts that are either absent in the rat, or, at least, markedly different; and human systems could well be different from the rat's or monkey's. Understanding the neuropharmacology of the antipsychotics is further complicated, given that neither the mesolimbic-mesocortical nor the striatal systems are homogeneous, but may also include various subsystems.

DOPAMINE RECEPTOR SUBTYPES

D_1 through D_5

There are several different types of dopaminergic receptors, and antipsychotics most likely produce their effects by blocking the D_2 subtype, but some also block D_1 receptors. The D_1 and the D_2 subtypes of postsynaptic receptors can be differentiated by their specific antagonists and agonists. These receptors, in turn, alter the adenyl cyclase and other second messenger systems in a variety of ways. The assumption that antipsychotics produce their effect only via the D_2 receptors is not a certainty, inasmuch as it is possible that D_3, D_4, or D_5 could also be involved. For example, the specific role of D_1 and D_5 receptor subtypes has yet to be clarified.

Dopamine Autoreceptors

There are also dopaminergic presynaptic receptors (or autoreceptors) that generally play a negative feedback role. These autoreceptors sense the level of neurotransmitter and produce a negative feedback influence on DA synthesis and release. Thus, high DA release results in high intrasynaptic concentrations, which stimulate the autoreceptors, ultimately inducing a slowing of DA's synthesis and release. Conversely, blockade of the postsynaptic receptors may lead to positive feedback loops, which can:

- activate *tyrosine hydroxylase* in the presynaptic dopaminergic neuron
- increase DA *synthesis*
- increase the *firing rate*
- increase the levels of DA metabolites, such as *homovanillic acid (HVA)*.

Further complicating the picture is the induction of autoreceptor supersensitivity with chronic neuroleptic administration, as well as the fact that at least one tract—the mesocortical, which projects to the prefrontal cortex—may lack such autoreceptors. The authors have conducted preliminary, single-dose studies with apomorphine, which at a dose that stimulated presynaptic DA autoreceptors, thus reducing synthesis and release, also had a measurable acute antipsychotic effect (2, 3).

DECREASING DOPAMINERGIC ACTIVITY

Given the typical time course of adaptation to the biochemical and electrophysiological effects induced by antipsychotics in most dopaminergic systems, it is important to consider the time course for their efficacy. While an apparent clinical benefit can be seen within a few hours after treatment is initiated, there is usually a lag period of 1–2 weeks.

Time-dependent changes in plasma HVA (a major metabolite of DA) during neuroleptic treatment are consistent with the hypothesis that these agents' mechanism involves a slowly developing decrease in presynaptic DA synthesis and release. Whereas decreases in plasma HVA appear to parallel the time course of antipsychotic efficacy, peripheral DA systems may also contribute to plasma or urine HVA levels. Further, because different brain areas may or may not develop tolerance, it is quite possible that CSF HVA levels reflect those areas producing most of the HVA, but are not relevant to the psychotic process. With these caveats in mind, human CSF and plasma data are generally consistent with the animal studies, both of which have contributed considerable evidence implicating DA blockade and its aftermath. The relevance of these findings to the biological mechanisms subserving psychosis, however, has yet to be determined.

TOLERANCE

It is relevant to examine whether tolerance develops to the antipsychotic effect of these agents. For example, Sharma et al. (1993) found that "nontolerant" psychotic patients had a significantly inferior clinical response to antipsychotics, in contrast to their "tolerant" counterparts (4). Further, they found an earlier age of illness onset and a more refractory course in the "nontolerant" group. Although biochemical and electrophysiological tolerance (i.e., return of HVA to more normal levels and depolarization inactivation, respectively) develop in most DA systems, they do not occur in all.

For example, prefrontal and cingulate cortices may be spared, perhaps because of the absence of autoreceptors in these tracts. There is also evidence that many areas in nonhuman, primate brains develop biochemical tolerance to the neuroleptic-induced HVA rise, but other areas do not. Thus, with chronic neuroleptic treatment, certain areas (cingulate, dorsal frontal, and orbital frontal cortex) maintain their HVA increases. Patients who were examined postmortem after chronic antipsychotic therapy were found to have increased HVA levels in certain areas, such as the cingulate and perifalciform cortex. It is also interesting that stress and/or benzodiazepine receptor agonists can selectively stimulate DA neurons in the mesoprefrontal area, but not in other dopaminergic tracts.

By using D_2-blocking isotopes in a PET scanner, it is possible to image the striatum in psychotic patients. There is preliminary evidence from one PET scan study that some drug-free schizophrenics manifested an increase in D_2 dopamine receptors, but another study failed to find such an alteration (5, 6). These studies used different receptor ligands, different assumptions, and both had a small sample size, so that definitive conclusions are not possible. Finally, when PET scans were done on patients receiving clinically effective doses of neuroleptics, all of these agents (including clozapine and sulpiride) produced D_2 receptor blockade in the striatum (7). Furthermore, they do so at the typical doses used to treat schizophrenic patients.

INCREASING DOPAMINERGIC ACTIVITY

If decreasing dopaminergic activity benefits psychosis, what is the effect of increasing dopaminergic activity? **Potentiation of DA by a variety of mechanisms is a common denominator for inducing para-noia, hallucinations, and other manifestations of psychosis.** For example:

- *L-Dopa* (3, 4-dihydroxyphenylalanine), which is converted to DA in the body, can produce psychosis as a side effect
- *Amantadine,* another dopaminergic drug, can also induce psychotic symptoms
- *Stimulants,* such as amphetamine and methylphenidate, are potent releasers of DA, while cocaine also interferes with its reuptake, increasing DA concentrations at synaptic sites and producing paranoid reactions in some abusers.
- Bromocriptine, apomorphine, lisoride, and other *direct-acting DA agonists* all benefit Parkinson's disease, and can cause psychotic reactions at high doses.

Large doses of amphetamine, cocaine, and other sympathomimetics can cause acute paranoid reactions, either spontaneously in abusers or experimentally in normal volunteers. For example, an injection of a large amphetamine dose often produces a paranoid psychosis within hours. Frequent smaller doses over several days can also produce a paranoid psychotic reaction. An episode's duration usually parallels the length of time the drug remains in the body.

Additional evidence comes from studies of increasing dopaminergic activity in patients with active psychosis. For example, small intravenous (i.v.) doses of methylphenidate (e.g., 0.5 mg/kg) can result in a marked exacerbation of an acute schizophrenic episode (8). By contrast, such doses usually do not produce psychotic symptoms in normal controls or in remitted patients. The phenomenon of worsening a pre-existing psychosis may be different from that of producing a paranoid reaction in normal subjects. Thus, specific pre-existing psychotic symptoms worsen (e.g., catatonic patients become more catatonic), but patients without paranoia do not demonstrate such "new" symptoms. Methylphenidate is more potent in this regard than dextroamphetamine, consistent with the hypothesis that it intensifies psychotic symptoms by releasing central intraneuronal stores of norepinephrine and DA from the reserpine-sensitive pool (9).

Finally, sensitivity to an amphetamine test dose in recovered patients seems to predict an impending relapse (10). Interestingly, when physostigmine, a drug that increases brain acetylcholine, is administered before methylphenidate, it prevents the exacerbation, indicating that the worsening is mediated by a dopaminergic-cholinergic imbalance (11). Physostigmine itself, however, does not reduce psychosis, suggesting that the underlying process is not amenable simply to altering cholinergic tone.

CONCLUSION

All clinically effective neuroleptic-antipsychotics block DA receptor activity. Further, stimulation of this neurotransmitter can induce psychotic symptoms "de novo" or exacerbate an existing psychotic disorder. Atypical agents such as clozapine offer the promise of selectively targeting specific DA tracts that mediate the pathological condition, while sparing those tracts that mediate the unwanted adverse effects (e.g., extrapyramidal side effects, tardive dyskinesia).

REFERENCES

1. Johnstone EC, Crowe TJ, Frith CD, Carney MWP, Price JS. Mechanism of the antipsychotic effect in the treatment of acute schizophrenia. Lancet 1978;1:848.
2. Smith RC, Tamminga C, Davis JM. Effect of apomorphine on schizophrenic symptoms. J Neural Transm 1977;40(2):171–176.
3. Schaffer MG, Davis JM, Tamminga CA. Apomorphine's antipsychotic activity. Arch Gen Psychiatry 1985;42:927.
4. Sharma RP, Javaid JI, Janicak PG, Faull K, Davis JM. Homovanillic acid in the cerebrospinal fluid: patterns of response after four weeks of neuroleptic treatment. Biol Psychiatry 1993, in press.
5. Sedvall GC, Farde L, Persson A, Wiesel F. Imaging of neurotransmitter receptors in the living brain. Arch Gen Psychiatry 1986;43:995–1005.
6. Wong DF, Wagner HN, Tune LE, Dannals RF, Pearlson GD, Links JM, et al. Positron emission tomography reveals elevated D-2 dopamine receptors in drug naive schizophrenia. Science 1986;234:1558–1563.
7. Farde L, Wiesel FA, Holldin C, Sedvall G. Central D2-dopamine receptor occupancy in schizophrenic patients treated with antipsychotic drugs. Arch Gen Psychiatry 1988;45:71–76.
8. Sharma RP, Javaid JL, Pandey GN, Janicak PG, Davis JM. Behavioral and biochemical effects of methylphenidate in schizophrenic and non-schizophrenic patients. Biol Psychiatry 1991;30:459–466.
9. Lieberman JA, Kane JM, Gadaleta D, Brenner R, Lesser MS, Kinon B. Methylphenidate challenge as a predictor of relapse in schizophrenia. Am J Psychiatry 1984;141:633–638.
10. Angrist B, Preselow E, Rubinstein M, Wolkin A, Rotrosen J. Amphetamine response and relapse risk after depot neuroleptic discontinuation. Psychopharmacology 1985;85:277–283.
11. Janowsky DS, El-Yousef MK, Davis JM. Antagonistic effects of physostigmine and methylphenidate in man. Am J Psychiatry 1973:130:1370–1376.

Effects on Cognition and Behavior

Investigators have attempted to assess the impact of antipsychotics on the cognitive and the behavioral disturbances characteristic of schizophrenia. The antipsychotics decrease typical but nonspecific symptoms such as hallucinations and delusions (Table 5.2). Thus, labelling them as antischizophrenic agents is too restrictive inasmuch as they also benefit such disparate disorders as psychotic depression or mania; late onset paraphrenia; and organic-induced psychosis. As the symptoms reduced by neuroleptics are typical of psychosis in general, these agents are best conceptualized as a type of antipsychotic.

Serious mental disorders fundamentally alter one's personality, and evidence from controlled studies demonstrates that antipsychotics "normalize" thought processes. Some claim that the involuntary administration of these drugs violates a patient's freedom of speech. In fact, with the onset of a psychotic episode, patients' "normal" mental processes become loose, rambling, illogical, circumstantial, inco-

herent, inappropriately concrete, and are often manifested by bizarre thought and speech patterns. Delusional ideas may dominate, with or without visual or auditory hallucinations.

There are several studies measuring cognitive performance before (drug-free) and after treatment that find a marked improvement on medication. Whereas it is true that some drugs have sedative properties, this is more than counteracted by their ability to correct disturbances of thought. The net effect is that a patient's cognitive functions are much improved, often approaching premorbid status.

Antipsychotics can activate retardation or diminish excitation; therefore, the term "tranquilizer" is a misnomer. These agents do not, in any real sense, produce a state of

Table 5.2.
Effect of Antipsychotics on Symptoms of Schizophrenia[a]

Bleuler's Classification of Schizophrenic Symptoms	VA Study No. 1	VA Study No. 3	Kurland, 1962	NIMH-PSC No. 1	Gorham and Pokorny, 1964 vs. Group Psychotherapy
Fundamental Symptoms					
Thought disorder	+ +	+ +	+ +	+ +	+ +
Blunted affect-indifference				+ +	+
Withdrawal-retardation	+ +	+ +	0	+ +	+ +
Autistic behavior-mannerisms	+ +	+ +	0	+ +	+
Accessory symptoms					
Hallucinations	+ +	+ +	+	+	0
Paranoid ideation	0	+ +	0	+	+
Grandiosity	0	0	0	0	+
Hostility-belligerence	+ +	+ +	H.R.	+	+
Resistiveness-uncooperativeness	+ +	+ +	H.R.	+ +	+ +
Nonschizophrenic symptoms					
Anxiety-tension-agitation	0	0	H.R.	+	0
Guilt-depression	+ +	0	0	0	0
Disorientation				0	
Somatization					0

[a] + +, symptom areas showing marked drug-control group differences; +, those showing significant but less striking differences; 0, areas not showing differential drug superiority; H.R., heterogeneity of regression found on analysis of covariance of the measures indicated. (This invalidates this particular statistical procedure but does not mean that there was *no* drug effect.)
Adapted from Klein D, Davis JM. Diagnosis and drug treatment of psychiatric disorders. In: Review of antipsychotic drug literature, Baltimore: Williams & Wilkins, 1969:90.

tranquility in normal or psychotic individuals; in fact, normal controls often find their effects unpleasant. An appropriate analogy may be aspirin, which reduces an elevated temperature, but typically does not alter normal temperature. Another example is insulin, which replaces the absent endogenous supply and restores a diabetic to normal glucostasis. So too, APs normalize cognition and behavior, presumably through their DA-blocking effects.

In 1977, Spohn and coworkers studied the effect of these agents in 40 chronic patients, who underwent a 6-week, placebo washout phase and were then randomly assigned to CPZ or placebo (1). In contrast to placebo, CPZ was found to:

- Enhance *concentration*
- Reduce *overestimation and fixation time* on a perceptual task
- Increase the *accuracy of perceptual judgment*.

The common denominator was the patients' ability to attend appropriately to a given task. Further, attentional dysfunction, information-processing impairment, and autonomic dysfunction were improved more in the drug-treated group.

In another study drug-induced improvement in schizophrenic symptoms was also measured using the Brief Psychiatric Rating Scale (BPRS) and the Holtzman-Johnstone Thought Disorder Index, which elicits responses to standardized stimuli (i.e., the Rorschach test and the Wechsler Adult Intelligence Scale) (2). Each response was blindly categorized to quantify the level of thought disorder, which although substantial before treatment, showed a marked reduction with adequate drug therapy. Further, thought disorder improved during the same period and to the same degree as the other symptoms (Fig. 5.2).

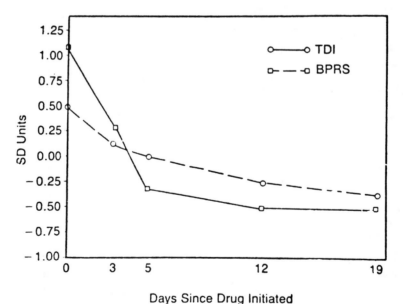

Days Since Drug Initiated

Figure 5.2. Effects of antipsychotics on thought disorder and behavioral symptoms of schizophrenia. BPRS, Brief Psychiatric Rating Scale; TDI, Thought Disorder Index. From Davis JM, Baxter JT, Kane JM. Antipsychotic drugs. In: Kaplan and Sadock, eds. Comprehensive textbook of psychiatry. 5th ed. Baltimore: Williams & Wilkins, 1989:1604.

CONCLUSION

Assuming antipsychotics work by blocking DA receptors, it is not known why such blockade leads to a lessening of psychosis, but they clearly do more than control agitation. Terminology should reflect available data, particularly since the cause of schizophrenia is not known, nor how an antidopamine action benefits psychotic disorders in general. PET studies of obsessive-compulsive disorder (OCD) find increased activity in the basal ganglia, which may prolong the "on-line" time of obsessive ideation. It is tempting to speculate that antipsychotics also working through their effects on the basal ganglia, allow thought patterns to stay "on line" for longer periods, thus approximating a more normal pattern. The practical consequence of drug treatment is that patients become less psychotic, as manifested by an improvement in all aspects of the syndrome, including thought disorder, attention deficits, and behavior.

REFERENCES

1. Spohn HE, Lacousiere R, Thompson K, Coyne L. Phenothiazine effects on psychological and psychophysiological dysfunction in chronic schizophrenics. Arch Gen Psychiatry 1977;34:633.
2. Hurt SW, Holzman PS, Davis JM. Thought disorder. Arch Gen Psychiatry 1983;40: 1281–1285.

Management of Acute Psychosis

EFFICACY FOR ACUTE TREATMENT

Most double-blind studies evaluating the efficacy of antipsychotics find them superior to placebo for the treatment of acute and chronic psychotic disorders (primarily schizophrenia). In some of the studies the dosage was too low to produce an effect, but when adequate, these agents were consistently superior to placebo. The magnitude of improvement in the drug-treated group was considerable whether evaluated by the degree of change (e.g., worse, no change, slight improvement, marked improvement) or degree of remission (e.g., full remission, only minimal symptoms, still mildly ill, moderately ill, or severely ill). Results from a National Institute of Mental Health (NIMH) Collaborative Study, combining both types of evaluation, are presented in Table 5.3 (1, 2). These results can be summarized as follows:

- 16% of the drug-treated versus only 1% of the placebo-treated groups were in *complete remission* or *very much improved*
- 29% of the drug-treated and 11% of the placebo group were evaluated as *improved, with only borderline symptoms*
- 16% of the drug-treated and 10% of the placebo group were evaluated as *improved, with mild symptoms* remaining
- 8% of patients *did poorly* on active drug (i.e., rated as not improved or still ill), compared with 48% on placebo
- One-third of the placebo patients *deteriorated* during 6 weeks of treatment, in contrast to only 2% of those on an antipsychotic
- The *largest differences* between the drug- and the placebo-treated patients are *seen at both ends of the outcome spectrum.*

This study also found that new schizophrenic symptoms often emerged during the 6 weeks of placebo treatment, whereas worsening of symptoms was prevented by antipsychotics. **Heinz Lehmann coined the term "psychostatic" to describe the ability of phenothiazines to prevent the re-emergence of psychotic symptoms (3).**

Table 5.3.
Efficacy of Antipsychotics[a]

Degree of Remission	Degree of Change	Drug (%)	Placebo (%)
Remitted	Very much improved	16	1
Only borderline symptoms remain	Improved	29	11
Mild symptoms still present	Improved	16	10
Moderately ill	Slightly improved	31	31
Moderately ill	Not improved	6	15
Severely ill	Worse	2	33

[a]From Cole JO, Davis JM. Antipsychotic drugs. In: The schizophrenic syndrome. New York: Grune & Stratton, 1969:478–568.

The time course of improvement for most acutely psychotic patients on these agents (Fig. 5.3) demonstrates that most therapeutic gain occurs during the first 6 weeks, although further progress can be realized much later. Thus, some patients improve rapidly within a few days, while others show gradual changes over several months. There is no evidence for clinical tolerance, for if there were, one would have to increase the dose over time. Fixed dose studies, however, show that the initial effective amount of drug does not lose efficacy. In addition, patients do not require higher doses after several weeks of treatment, but instead the reverse appears to be true. It is also clear that antipsychotics do not produce dependency of the barbiturate, stimulant, or narcotic type.

Comparative Efficacy

In the hope of developing either a more effective agent or one with fewer adverse effects, medicinal chemists have synthe-

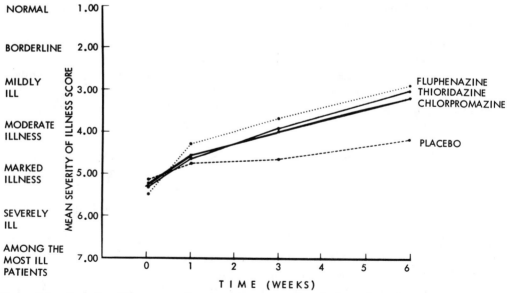

Figure 5.3. Severity of illness over time in patients treated with phenothiazines. From Davis JM, Baxter JT, Kane JM. Antipsychotic drugs. In: Kaplan and Sadock, eds. Comprehensive textbook of psychiatry. 5th ed. Baltimore: Williams & Wilkins, 1989:1595.

sized a number of new compounds. Preclinical animal model studies are used to select potentially useful drugs, utilizing a profile of pharmacological properties that reflect dopamine blockade. This research has led to the development of several new classes, as noted earlier in this chapter.

The question immediately arises as to whether any of the drugs in these various classes are superior to CPZ for the typical patient, for particular symptom(s), or for subgroups of patients.

With the exception of promazine and mepazine, all are clearly superior to placebo or nonspecific sedatives (e.g., phenobarbital (Tables 5.4, 5.5, 5.6, and 5.7). Comparisons with CPZ in controlled trials found mepazine and promazine inferior to CPZ, but all other agents were equal to CPZ in therapeutic efficacy (Table 5.8). Other controlled trials using thioridazine or trifluoperazine as standards also found all other antipsychotics to be comparable to these agents (Table 5.8). Whereas there were trends at times favoring one agent over another, they were usually not statis-

Table 5.4.
Drug versus *Placebo* in Controlled Studies of Schizophrenia[a]

	Number of Studies in Which Drug Was	
Drug	More Effective than Placebo	Equal to Placebo
Chlorpromazine	55	11
Reserpine	20	9
Triflupromazine	9	1
Perphenazine	5	0
Prochlorperazine	7	2
Trifluoperazine	16	2
Fluphenazine	15	0
Butaperazine	4	0
Thioridazine	7	0
Mesoridazine	3	0
Carphenazine	2	0
Chlorprothixene	4	0
Thiothixene	2	0
Haloperidol	9	0
Pimozide	2	2
Molindone	1	0
Loxapine	5	1
Phenobarbital	0	3

[a]Adapted from Klein D, Davis JM. Diagnosis and drug treatment of psychiatric disorders. In: Review of antipsychotic drug literature. Baltimore: Williams & Wilkins, 1969:54.

Table 5.5.
Recent Antipsychotics versus *Placebo* for Schizophrenia: Acute Treatment

		Responders (%)				
Number of Studies	Number of Subjects	Drug (%)	Placebo (%)	Difference (%)	Chi Square	*p* Value
		Loxapine versus Placebo				
5	197	61	34	27	16.8	4×10^{-5}
		Molindone versus Placebo				
1	29	20	0	20	3.12	0.08
		Risperidone versus Placebo				
1	40	62	22	39	11.0	9×10^{-4}

Table 5.6.
Standard Antipsychotics (used in comparison studies with Loxapine, Molindone, Risperidone, Table 5.5) versus *Placebo* for Schizophrenia: Acute Treatment

		Responders (%)				
Number of Studies	Number of Subjects	Drug (%)	Placebo (%)	Difference (%)	Chi Square	*p* Value
7	266	56	29	27	25.0	6×10^{-7}

Table 5.7.
Antipsychotics versus *Phenobarbital* for Schizophrenia: Acute Treatment

Number of Studies	Number of Subjects	Responders (%)		Difference (%)	Chi Square	*p* Value
		Antipsychotics (%)	Phenobarbital (%)			
2	153	50	14	36	17.4	3×10^{-5}

Table 5.8.
Effectiveness of Antipsychotics Compared with Chlorpromazine, Thioridazine, and Trifluoperazine[a]

Drug	Number of Studies in Which Drug Was		
	More Effective than *Chlorpromazine*	As Effective	Less Effective
Mepazine	0	0	4
Promazine	0	2	4
Triflupromazine	0	10	0
Perphenazine	0	6	0
Prochlorperazine	0	10	0
Trifluoperazine	0	11	0
Butaperazine	0	2	0
Thioridazine	0	12	0
Mesoridazine	0	7	0
Fluphenazine	0	9	0
Carphenazine	0	2	0
Acetophenazine	0	1	0
Thiopropazate	0	1	0
Chlorpromazine	0	6	0
Thiothixene	0	4	0
Haloperidol	0	4	0
Molindone	0	6	0
Loxapine	0	14	1
Phenobarbital	0	0	6

	More Effective than *Thioridazine*	As Effective	Less Effective
Mesoridazine	0	2	0
Carphenazine	0	1	0
Haloperidol	0	2	0
Piperacetazine	0	3	0

	More Effective than *Trifluoperazine*	As Effective	Less Effective
Mesoridazine	0	1	0
Carphenazine	0	3	0
Acetophenazine	0	1	0
Butaperazine	0	3	0
Chlorprothixene	0	1	0
Haloperidol	0	4	0

[a]Adapted from Klein D, Davis JM. Diagnosis and drug treatment of psychiatric disorders. In: Review of antipsychotic drug literature. Baltimore: Williams & Wilkins, 1969:59.

tically significant, and an inspection of the data finds no agent to be consistently superior to any other. Furthermore, all these drugs produced consistent changes in the same symptoms. These similarities are quite striking and support the theory that they work through a common mechanism of action (i.e., dopamine blockade). Furthermore relevant differences are primarily related to their side-effect profiles.

Pimozide is Food and Drug Administration (FDA)-labelled for Tourette's disorder and is particularly interesting in that it is a highly specific DA antagonist that may produce fewer adverse effects than haloperidol. In open studies with adequate doses, this agent has demonstrated efficacy for acute schizophrenia. Several double-blind trials comparing pimozide to standard antipsychotics also found it to be an equally effective maintenance therapy (4–9). We consider this agent to be as effective as the other standard agents, with the same but perhaps less severe side effects.

An Atypical Antipsychotic

Clozapine is the first clinically effective antipsychotic with an atypical profile (10, 11). Compared to classic (or standard) neuroleptics it:

- Has a lower affinity for D_2 *receptors*
- Binds proportionately more to D_1 *receptors*
- Appears to act selectively on *cortical and mesolimbic DA* neuronal systems (in preference to the nigrostriatal and tuberoinfundibular areas)
- Blocks 5-HT_2 receptors
- Probably has no *EPS* effects (e.g., no known cases of TD)
- Has broad effects on *other neurotransmitter systems* (e.g., norepinephrine (NE), acetylcholine (Ach))
- Has a decreased rate of *sexual and reproductive* dysfunction.

Evidence supporting its efficacy comes from one double-blind, placebo-controlled study and six other antipsychotic-controlled, random-assignment studies (12–16, Sandoz, unpublished data). When compared to standard antipsychotics such as CPZ and haloperidol, it was found to be more effective (i.e., three studies found clozapine significantly superior and two others found a trend favoring clozapine ($p = 0.10$)). When the results of these studies were combined, the probability that clozapine is superior to antipsychotics was highly statistically significant ($p = 1 \times 10^{-10}$) (see Tables 5.9 and 5.10).

Remembering that when a large num-

Table 5.9.
Clozapine versus *Standard Antipsychotics* for Schizophrenia: Acute Treatment— Individual Studies

Number of Studies	Number of Subjects	Responders (%)		Difference (%)	Chi Square	*p* Value
		Clozapine (%)	Std Drug (%)			
1	25	85	75	10		
1	102	92	80	12		
1	216	70	57	13		
1	79	31	10	21		
1	267[a]	30	4	26		
1	50	92	60	32		
6	739	57%	36%	21%	41.7	1×10^{-10}

[a]Kane et al. (1988)

Table 5.10.
Clozapine versus *Standard Antipsychotics* for Schizophrenia: Acute Treatment—Summations

Number of Studies	Number of Subjects	Responders (%)		Difference (%)	Chi Square	p Value
		Clozapine (%)	Std Drug (%)			
		Low Difference Groups				
4	422	31	45	15	10.4	0.001[a]
		High Difference Groups				
2	317	40	12	28	39.6	3×10^{-10a}

[a]Homogeneity chi square = not significant

ber of patients are studied, a relatively small effect can become statistically significant, this evidence seems to establish that clozapine is more effective than standard antipsychotics. Since clozapine is marketed in over 20 countries, there has been wide clinical experience and several open trials supporting its efficacy as well.

Even though this agent has been found to be superior to standard antipsychotics, as well as to placebo, and beneficial in about 30% of nonresponders, its side-effect profile has been a major obstacle to its widespread utilization. Specifically, agranulocytosis (approximately 1% incidence) and seizures (usually with higher doses (>500–600 mg) are the most serious.

Given clozapine's significant adverse effects, Lieberman and Kane recommend its use only in psychotic patients who are clear nonresponders to standard agents, in that they:

- Failed three trials of different agents from at least two chemical classes
- Were treated for at least 6 weeks
- Received doses in excess of 1000 mg CPZ equivalents
- Had therapeutic drug monitoring (TDM) and/or parenteral administration to control for rapid metabolism and/or a large first-pass effect.

Starting doses should be in the range of 25–50 mg/day and titrated up slowly to minimize EPS and hypotension. The usual therapeutic range is 300–500 mg/day (the maximum allowable dose is 900 mg/day). This dose is typically achieved in 2–5 weeks and should be maintained for several more before considering an increase. In this context, Perry and colleagues found a therapeutic threshold clozapine plasma level of 350 ng/ml (i.e., 64% with levels above this responded, versus only 22% with levels below this point), which required an average dose of 380 mg/day (17).

Dosing Strategies

The goal of drug therapy is to achieve maximum improvement by treating the underlying disease process, rather than a given symptom. For example, retarded schizophrenic patients may respond dramatically, even in the absence of more obvious target symptoms such as agitation and aggression. Although the goal is to treat the underlying process, the monitoring of more typical psychotic symptoms serves as a barometer for assessing a drug's effect.

In general, low doses (e.g., haloperidol, 2–10 mg/day) are preferable when possible, usually sufficient, and help avoid toxicity. This is especially important with long-term treatment since the cumulative effects may predispose to TD.

Because the onset of improvement is approximately 1–2 weeks with the antipsychotics many clinicians prefer to start with a moderate dose (i.e., haloperidol, 10–15 mg/day; thioridazine, 300–400 mg/day) and maintain the dose for that period. Whereas dosage can be adjusted more frequently to control adverse effects, it should not be adjusted daily on the basis of therapeutic effect because of the length of these agents' half-lives.

Some clinicians employ a loading dose (e.g., 60 mg haloperidol) for quick control of psychotic symptoms, and then taper off slowly to a lower maintenance regimen. Others prefer to start with a low dose and gradually increase it as needed. There is no strong evidence as to which approach produces a quicker or better long-term result. Under either regimen, the reduction of overt psychotic symptoms and a gradual cognitive reorganization are the goals. Initially, the clinician often administers a drug several times a day, but later phases of treatment usually require only once-a-day dosing because of these agents' longer half-lives (20–24 hours). A single bedtime dose is convenient and practical inasmuch as the peak sedative effect occurs shortly thereafter.

Although the studies previously discussed failed to find that "megadoses" (e.g., haloperidol, 100–150 mg/day) produced a better response than standard dosages, there is anecdotal information that an occasional patient will benefit from this approach. Some recover slowly, however, and improvement might be erroneously attributed to the later, high-dose strategy (i.e., in time, they might have responded equally well to a lower dose). Although nonresponders can be tried on moderately high doses, in view of the dose-response curve, there is no reason to treat most patients with heroically high doses.

Toxicity

The dose-response curve for toxicity is similar to the therapeutic dose-response curve. There are slightly more adverse effects at higher doses, but massive doses fail to produce appreciably greater toxicity. Thus, patients who received high-dose treatment for several months (e.g., 1200 mg fluphenazine or 700 mg trifluoperazine) had the same incidence of adverse effects as those on standard doses, and no significant increase in toxicity (18, 19). Even though serious complications may not occur with high doses, this does not mean it is a good idea. Although there is only a weak correlation between dose and TD, assuming it is at least partially dose and time-on-drug related, lifetime drug exposure is an important consideration. Whereas TD may also be associated with short-term, high doses, there is no definitive evidence to support this hypothesis. Although long-term, high-dose treatment might produce more TD, it is unlikely to occur during short-term higher dosing if clinically necessary. In fact, length of time on treatment is probably more important than dose.

CHOICE OF ANTIPSYCHOTIC

If all antipsychotics are equally effective, how does one choose the best drug for a given patient? Because their action is related to structural similarities shared by most compounds in this class, there is no reason to expect a given patient to respond differentially to a particular agent. So the critical consideration usually involves differences in adverse effects. For example, thioridazine has fewer extrapyramidal complications, whereas haloperidol has fewer sedative and cardiovascular effects. Thus, a patient who requires a high activity level to maintain his/her psychological well-being may do better on a less sedating agent.

The clinical myth exists that agitated patients respond best to a sedating agent (such as CPZ) and that withdrawn patients respond best to a less sedating agent (such as trifluoperazine, fluphenazine, or haloperidol). This has never been proven, and indeed, evidence from early NIMH collaborative studies indicated that a second-order factor, labelled "apathetic and retarded," predicted a differentially good response to CPZ (20). This finding was not replicated in another large clinical trial (21). Several schema have been developed to predict which patients would respond to which antipsychotics, but validation studies uniformly failed to support these initial findings.

Determining whether a particular subtype of patient responds differentially to a given drug is an empirical question. Despite the lack of clear differential indications, clinicians continue to encounter patients who respond to one AP but not another. It is also possible that patients maintained on the original agent may have done equally well. Some patients may preferentially improve on a particular drug due to differences in:

- Absorption
- Distribution
- Accumulation at receptor sites
- Pharmacodynamic actions
- Metabolism of its derivatives
- Adverse cognitive effects, such as sedation.

It is also important to consider that improvement in some patients too quickly switched to another agent may be falsely attributed to the latter drug, rather than a delayed response to the first medication. Thus, it is unwise to change too rapidly or too frequently. The optimal dose of a single agent should be ascertained empiri-

cally and then allowed a reasonable time to exert its effects. At some point (i.e., several days or weeks in a severely disturbed patient; or several weeks or months in a less dramatically impaired patient), however, a trial with a second drug (preferably with as different a side-effect profile as possible) is warranted. We emphasize that the effectiveness of this strategy has not been demonstrated in controlled clinical trials.

Cost of Treatment

We have analyzed all available double-blind studies comparing various antipsychotics and used these data to calculate the equivalent daily dosages, as well as the cost of different agents (22). The pharmaceutical industry generally markets a drug so that a three-times-a-day dosage is much more expensive than once-a-day dosing. Thus, cost is primarily determined by the number of tablets rather than the milligram dose in each tablet. For example, 25 mg of CPZ costs almost as much as a 100-mg tablet, and four 25-mg tablets cost nearly three times as much as one 100-mg tablet. Therefore, giving the largest available dose in a once-a-day regimen will save considerable expense, while also substantially reducing nursing time and other related hospital costs. Further, for outpatients, a bedtime dose may be easier to remember and monitor, thus improving compliance. Usually, once-a-day dosing can be achieved with standard tablets. Delayed-release, oral forms are available for some agents, but there is no evidence that these more expensive formulations have any advantage over standard preparations.

The clinician needs to know a patient's financial status when considering a dosing regimen. In a patient with limited financial means, the cost of medication may be a deterrent to compliance, and arrangements should be made to minimize any economic obstacles. From a societal point of view, the cost of medication is small in comparison to an outpatient visit, and both of these are negligible in comparison to the expense of hospitalization.

TREATMENT OF PSYCHOTIC AGITATION

Rapid control of acutely disruptive behavior, often associated with an exacerbation of various types of psychotic disorders, is desirable to:

- *Lessen* the propensity toward *violence*
- *Avoid* physical *restraints*
- *Expedite* diagnostic *assessment*
- Facilitate *more definitive treatment.*

Violent behavior may have numerous causes, yet in most cases treatment must be initiated before an accurate diagnosis can be made. Nevertheless, a tentative diagnosis should be attempted. The most common causes of such behavior in emergency room settings include psychosis, personality disorder, and alcohol or drug intoxication or withdrawal. In medical or surgical wards, delirium is the more likely cause.

Psychosis. Schizophrenia or mania should be suspected when there is a history of psychiatric illness; onset of symptoms has been gradual; there is evidence of hallucinations, delusions, and/or disorganized thought; and orientation is intact.

Drugs. Cocaine and amphetamine intoxication may cause an agitated paranoid psychotic episode. Physical signs include dilated pupils, slurred speech, ataxia, hyperreflexia, and nystagmus, as well as evidence of drug use (e.g., needle "tracks", nasal septum erosion). Vital signs, if obtainable, include elevated blood pressure, pulse rate, and temperature (see also The Alcoholic Patient in Chapter 14).

Delirium. Characteristics include the sudden onset of symptoms, disorientation, visual hallucinations, and transient, often paranoid, delusions. The intensity of symptoms often fluctuates, and the patient may have a known medical illness but no psychiatric history.

Standard Drug Therapies

Antipsychotics and benzodiazepines, used alone or in combination, are the treatment of choice for achieving rapid control of acute agitation. While aggressively administered high-dose antipsychotics can control extremely disruptive behavior, their adverse effects may be quite severe (23–27). At times, anxiolytics may be effective when used alone or in combination for prompt control, while lessening the chance for adverse events. If both are used, lower dosages of each are required. Intramuscular paraldehyde has also been used, although it must be given by deep injection to avoid painful lesions. Barbiturates are not recommended.

Route of administration depends on a variety of factors, including the degree of patient agitation and the availability of the various formulations of given drugs (see Table 5.11). While oral medication is preferable whenever possible, when a patient refuses or is unable to cooperate, parenteral administration may be required. Although i.v. administration produces the most rapid effect, it may not be feasible in extremely agitated, uncooperative patients.

Parenteral Antipsychotics

The primary indication for standard intramuscular (i.m.) administration is when a patient is too disturbed to take oral

Table 5.11.
Route of Administration of Psychotropics

Liquid	Tablet	Intramuscular	Intravenous
Thiothixene	Lorazepam	Droperidol	Droperidol
Haloperidol	Diazepam	Haloperidol	Haloperidol
Loxapine	Chlordiazepoxide	Lorazepam	Diazepam
			Lorazepam

medication. Because drugs are more rapidly absorbed when given parenterally, and their effect occurs about 60 minutes faster than with oral administration (i.e., 30 versus 90 minutes), violent or otherwise dangerously disturbed patients should initially receive i.m. injections. Further, since orally administered drugs are metabolized in the gut, as well as during their first pass through the liver, less than 50% may reach the systemic circulation for ultimate availability at the intended brain sites.

Extremely psychotic, explosive patients usually respond (at least partially) to i.m. treatment in 15–30 minutes, often avoiding any serious incidents that might occur with oral administration's slower onset of action. Although orally administered drugs take longer to act, they may still be used for emergency titration after one (or several) i.m. injections have produced a rapid onset of action.

Intravenous adminstration of low-dose, high-potency agents is also an option in certain clinical situations. For example, i.v. haloperidol, alone or in combination with i.v. lorazepam, has been safe and effective in managing delirium in critically ill, medical patients (28, 29). At times, effective doses of haloperidol may be as low as 0.5–1 mg when given by this route.

Dosing Strategies for Antipsychotics

Some clinicians prefer a sedating agent, such as CPZ, while others prefer a high-potency agent, such as haloperidol, fluphenazine, or thiothixene because their side-effect profiles may allow for more aggressive dosing (e.g., low sedation, low anticholinergic, low hypotension). The authors conducted a controlled trial in acute, psychotically manic patients who required concomitant antipsychotics (30). In addition to lithium, they were randomly assigned to oral CPZ or thiothixene. The results between the two drug treatments over a 2-week period were very similar, with no clinically or statistically significant differences. The experimental design of this study dictated that the need for an additional dose of antipsychotic be reassessed every 2 hours during the day. While such highly excited, manic patients are often treated with augmenting agents, they are not usually monitored as frequently. By having their status re-evaluated every 2 hours (according to the study design), most patients improved with relatively low doses of either agent, and as a result, none experienced intolerable adverse effects. Had they not been monitored as frequently, higher than necessary doses may have been given (see also Chapter 10).

Although some rapidly escalate the dose of antipsychotic to high levels (a strategy referred to as rapid tranquilization or a loading dose approach), we encourage flexibility in the:

- *Route* of administration
- *Dose* required to meet the patient's clinical state

- *Frequency of re-evaluations* assessing drug response and adverse effects.

Repeated high i.m. doses over several days are inadvisable inasmuch as most patients do not require such aggressive intervention, and this strategy may increase the risk for severe EPS and/or the neuroleptic malignant syndrome (NMS). Finally, it is preferable to switch patients to oral treatment as quickly as possible to manage the remainder of an acute episode.

Benzodiazepines

Benzodiazepines (BZDs) may be given to patients with moderate agitation due to drug intoxication. These agents also are the treatment of choice in alcohol withdrawal states, characterized by agitation, tremors, or change in vital signs (See also The Alcoholic Patient in Chapter 14) (31).

Lorazepam. Recently, there has been an increased use of lorazepam to control psychotic aggressivity (32–42). One reason is that, of all the BZDs available in parenteral form, lorazepam has a pharmacokinetic profile (quick, reliable absorption) that makes it particularly suitable for this type of use. Open, retrospective, and controlled studies indicate that oral or parenteral lorazepam added to an antipsychotic controls disruptive behavior safely and effectively for most patients. The combination may also permit an overall reduction of the antipsychotic dose, although this assumption requires further study (37, 39, 41).

An open, comparative study of 14 acutely psychotic patients treated with lorazepam alone (N = 8, mean dose = 20.9 mg/day) or lorazepam plus haloperidol (mean dose = 15 mg/day; mean dose = 5.2 mg/day; respectively) demonstrated a significant decrease in psychotic symptoms over 48 hours (36). Although the

improvement in both groups was equal, the doses of haloperidol were low, and there was no comparative placebo group.

Another *retrospective chart review* reported on patients treated in a 24-hour psychiatric emergency unit during two separate 6-month periods (37). During the first period (1982), patients usually received standard i.m. haloperidol for behavioral control; during the second period (1984), they received either i.m. haloperidol or a combination of i.m. haloperidol plus i.m. lorazepam. Further, the doses used during the second period (with or without lorazepam) were significantly lower, compared with the 1982 period. Although the authors concluded that the BZD allowed for lower doses of antipsychotics, it is difficult to determine its influence because all patients received lower doses of APs during the second period.

In another *open study*, agitated patients were randomly assigned to receive i.m. alprazolam (4 mg), i.m. haloperidol (5 mg), or a combination of the two (41). Agitation, assessed every 30 minutes, was better managed with the combination than either treatment alone.

Lorazepam (2 mg i.m.) was found to be equivalent to haloperidol (5 mg i.m.) either alone or when added to ongoing antipsychotic treatment, and significantly reduced the likelihood of akathisia and dystonia (42). In the treatment of acute mania, lorazepam has also been reported useful as an adjunct to lithium as well as antipsychotics (32, 38, 40, 43, 44).

Clonazepam. Case reports and one small double-blind study indicate that oral clonazepam may be useful for psychotic agitation when combined with lithium or an antipsychotic (see also Management of an Acute Manic Episode in Chapter 10) (45–50).

Midazolam. Intramuscular midazolam, another BZD with reliable parenteral absorption, has produced rapid sedation in acutely psychotic patients with marked agitation (51).

Alprazolam. In a review of high-potency BZDs for psychotic disorders, Bodkin recommended avoidance of alprazolam for psychotic agitation because it may be activating and may induce belligerence or mania (57–61).

Complications of Benzodiazepines

Sedation, ataxia, and cognitive impairment may occur frequently with high BZD dosages. Other adverse effects reported in the treatment of schizophrenia include:

- Behavioral *disinhibition*
- *Increase in anxiety* and *depression* (38, 62–70).

Concomitant use of a BZD and the atypical antipsychotic clozapine may increase the risk of sedation, dizziness, collapse with loss of consciousness, respiratory distress, and fluctuating blood pressure (71).

Other Strategies

Barbiturates

Prior to the discovery of the neuroleptics/antipsychotics, episodes of psychotic excitement were usually managed with i.v. amobarbital in doses sufficient to heav-

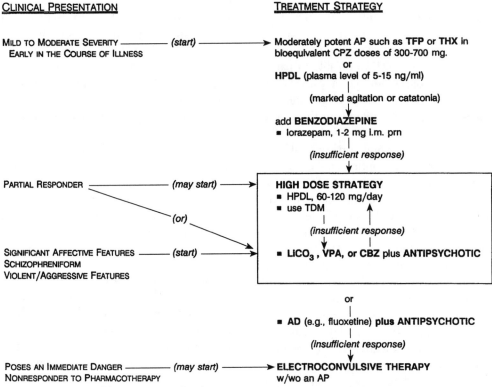

Figure 5.4.   Strategy for the treatment of an acute psychotic episode.

ily sedate or actually put patients to sleep. Upon awakening, they were often much less excited. The role that sleep deprivation plays in the onset of psychotic symptoms may be a partial explanation for this beneficial effect. Although sedatives have no specific effect on the underlying psychosis, they can calm psychotic excitement. Because the extreme excitement, rage, and explosivity often associated with a psychotic exacerbation are amenable to intervention with sedatives, this raises the possiblity that these symptoms may have a different underlying mechanism than that subserving the psychosis itself.

Finally, *lithium*, *β-blockers*, and *carbamazepine* may be effective for the management of chronic, but not acute, intermittent assaultiveness and agitation (72–79).

CONCLUSION

The authors have developed a treatment strategy to manage an acute psychotic exacerbation, and it is outlined in Figure 5.4. When possible, the judicious, time-limited use of sedatives in combination with an antipsychotic may bring about a more rapid and qualitatively better effect than aggressively pushing the dose of antipsychotic. Parenteral administration is frequently required during the earliest phases of treatment and may avoid serious sequelae in the explosive, assaultive, or violence-prone patient. There is also a distinction between the use of augmenting sedatives for the acutely agitated and/or violent patient versus the chronically agitated or assaultive patient. In the former situation, sedatives might be added initially, and in the latter, after several weeks of antipsychotic therapy to improve the final result. Alternatively, β-blockers, anticonvulsants (e.g., CBZ), or lithium may also be beneficial with or without a concur-

rent antipsychotic to manage the chronically aggressive patient.

REFERENCES

1. Cole JO. Phenothiazine treatment in acute schizophrenia. Arch Gen Psychiatry 1964; 10:246–261.
2. Cole JO, Goldberg SC. Davis JM. Drugs in the treatment of psychosis: controlled studies. In: Solomon P, ed. Psychiatric drugs. New York: Grune and Stratton, 1966:153–180.
3. Lehman HE. Drug treatment of schizophrenia. In: Kline NS, Lehmann ME, eds. International psychiatry clinics. Vol. 2, No. 4. Boston: Little, Brown, 1965:717–751.
4. Falloon I, Watt DC, Sheperd M. A comparative controlled trial of pimozide and fluphenazine decanoate in the continuation therapy of schizophrenia. Psycol Med 1978;8:59–70.
5. Janssen P, Brugmans J, Dony J, Schuermans V. An international double-blind clinical evaluation of pimozide. J Clin Pharmacol 1972;12:26–34.
6. Gross H. A double-blind comparison of once-a-day pimozide, trifluoperazine, and placebo in the maintenance care of chronic schizophrenic outpatients. Curr Ther Res 1974;16:696-705.
7. Clark ML, Huber W, Hill D, Wood F, Costiloe JP. Pimozide (and thioridazine) in chronic schizophrenic outpatients. Dis Nerv Syst 1975;36:137–141.
8. Clark ML, Huber W, Serafetinides EA, Colmore JP. Pimozide (Orap): a tolerance study. Clin Trials Journal 1971;8 (suppl 2):25–32.
9. Janssen P, Brugmans J, Dony J, Schuermans V. An international double-blind clinical evaluation of pimozide. J Clin Pharmacol 1972;12:26–34.
10. Lieberman JA, Kane JM, Johns CA. Clozapine: guidelines for clinical management. J Clin Psychiatry 1989;50:329–338.
11. Baldessarini R, Frankenburg FR. Clozapine: a novel antipsychotic agent. N Engl J Med 1991;324:746–754.
12. Kane J, Honigfeld G, Singer J, Meltzer H. Clozaril collaborative study group: clozapine for the treatment-resistant schizophrenic: a double-blind comparison with chlopromazine. Arch Gen Psychiatry 1988; 45:789–796.
13. Fischer-Cornelssen KA, Ferner UJ. An

example of European multi-center trials: multispectral analysis of clozapine. Psychopharmacol Bull 1976;12:34–39.

14. Honigfeld G, Patin J, Singer J. Clozapine: antipsychotic activity in treatment-resistant schizophrenics. Adv Ther 1984;1: 77–97.

15. Shopsin B, Klein H, Aaronson M, Collora M. Clozapine, chlorpromazine, and placebo in newly hospitalized, acutely schizophrenic patients: a controlled, double-blind comparison. Arch Gen Psychiatry 1979;36:657–664.

16. Claghorn J, Honigfeld G, Abuzzahab FS, Wang R, Steinbook R, Tuason V, Klerman G. The risks and benefits of clozapine versus chlorpromazine. J Clin Psychopharmacol 1987;7:377–384.

17. Perry P, Miller D, Arndt SV, Cadoret RJ. Clozapine and norclozapine concentrations and clinical response in treatment refractory schizophrenic patients. Am J Psychiatry 1991;148:231–235.

18. Quitkin F, Rifkin A, Klein DF. Very high dosage vs standard dosage fluphenazine in schizophrenia: a double-blind study of nonchronic treatment-refractory patients. Arch Gen Psychiatry 1975;32:1276–1281.

19. Wijsenbeek H, Steiner M, Goldberg SC. Trifluoperazine: a comparison between regular and high doses. Psychopharmacologia (Berlin) 1974;36:147–150.

20. Goldberg SC, Mattison N, Cole JO, Klerman GL. Prediction of improvement in schizophrenia under four phenothiazines. Arch Gen Psychiatry 1967;16:107–117.

21. Goldberg SC, Frosch WA, Drossman AK, Schooler NR, Johnson GFS. Prediction of response to phenothiazines in schizophrenia: a cross-validation study. Arch Gen Psychiatry 1972;26:367–373.

22. Jurman RJ, Davis JM. Comparison of the costs of psychotropic medications: an update. In: Janicak PG, Davis JM, eds. Psychiatric Med 1991;2:349–359.

23. Reschke RW. Parenteral haloperidol for rapid control of severe, disruptive symptoms of acute schizophrenia. Dis Nerv Sys 1974;35:112–115.

24. Anderson WH, Kuehnle JC, Catanzano RM. Rapid treatment of acute psychosis. Am J Psychiatry 1976;133:1076–1078.

25. Salzman C, Hoffman SA. Rapid tranquilization. Hosp Comm Psychiatry 1982;33: 346.

26. Huyse F, Van Schijndel RS. Haloperidol and cardiac arrest. Lancet 1988;2:568–569.

27. Modestin J, Krapf R, Boker W. A fatality during haloperidol treatment: mechanism of sudden death. Am J Psychiatry 1981; 138:1616–1617.

28. Tesar GE, Murray GB, Cassem NH. Use of high-dose intravenous haloperidol in the treatment of agitated cardiac patients. J Clin Psychopharmacol 1985;5:344–347.

29. Adams F. Emergency intravenous sedation of the delirious, medically ill patient. J Clin Psychiatry 1988;49(suppl 12):22–27.

30. Janicak PG, Bresnahan DB, Sharma R, Davis JM, Comaty JE, Malinick C. A comparison of thiothixene with chlorpromazine in the treatment of mania. J Clin Psychopharmacol 1988;8:33–37.

31. Dubin WR, Weiss KJ. Handbook of psychiatric emergencies. Springhouse, PA: Springhouse Corporation, 1991.

32. Modell JG, Lenox RH, Weiner S. Inpatient clinical trial of lorazepam for the management of manic agitation. J Clin Psychopharmacol 1985;5:109–113.

33. Bick PA, Hannah AL. Intramuscular lorazepam to restrain violent patients. Lancet 1986;1:206.

34. Ward ME, Saklad SR, Ereshefsky L. Lorazepam for the treatment of psychotic agitation. Am J Psychiatry 1986;143:1195–1196.

35. Dever A, Schweizer E. Rapid remission of organic mania after treatment with lorazepam. J Clin Psychopharmacol 1988;8:227–228.

36. Modell JG. Further experience and observations with lorazepam in the management of behavioral agitation. J Clin Psychopharmacol 1986;6:385–387.

37. Salzman C, Green AI, Rodriguez-Villa F, Jaskiw G. Benzodiazepines combined with neuroleptics for management of severe disruptive behavior. Psychosomatics 1986;27 (suppl):17–23.

38. Arana GW, Ornsteen ML, Kanter F, Friedman HL, Greenblatt DJ, Shader RI. The use of benzodiazepines for psychotic disorders: a literature review and preliminary clinical findings. Psychopharmacol Bull 1986;22:77–87.

39. Campbell R, Simpson GM. Alternative approaches in the treatment of psychotic agitation. Psychosomatics 1986;27 (suppl):23–26.

40. Lennox RH. Newhouse PA, Creelman WL, Whitaker TM. Adjunctive treatment of manic agitation with lorazepam versus haloperidol: a double-blind study. J Clin Psychiatry, 1992;52(2):47–52.

41. Garza-Trevino ES, Hollister LE, Overall JE, Alexander WF. Efficacy of combinations of intramuscular antipsychotics and sedative-hypnotics for control of psychotic agitation. Am J Psychiatry 1989;146:1598–1601.

42. Salzman C, Solomon D, Miyawaki E, Glassman R, Rood L, Flowers E, Thayer S. Parenteral lorazepam versus parenteral haloperidol for the control of psychotic disruptive behavior. J Clin Psychiatry 1991; 52(4):177–180.

43. Cohen S, Khan A, Johnson S. Pharmacological management of manic psychosis in an unlocked setting. J Clin Psychopharmacol 1987;7:261–264.

44. Busch FN, Miller FT, Weiden PJ. A comparison of two adjunctive strategies in acute mania. J Clin Psychiatry 1989;50:453–455.

45. Freinhar JP. Clonazepam in the treatment of mentally retarded persons. Am J Psychiatry 1986;143:1324.

46. Freinhar JP, Alvarez WH. Clonazepam: a novel therapeutic adjunct. Int Psychiatry Med 1985–1986;15:321–328.

47. Altamura AC, Mauri MC, Mantero M, Brunetti M. Clonazepam/haloperidol combination therapy in schizophrenia: a double-blind study. Acta Psychiatr Scand 1987;76:702–706.

48. Freinhar JP, Alvarez WH. Use of clonazepam in two cases of acute mania. J Clin Psychiatry 1985;46:29–30.

49. Chouinard G, Young SN, Annable L. Antimanic effect of clonazepam. Biol Psychiatry 1983;18:451–466.

50. Chouinard G. The use of benzodiazepines in the treatment of manic depressive illness. J Clin Psychiatry 1988;49 (suppl):15–19.

51. Mendoza AR, Djenderedjian AH, Adams J, Ananth J. Midazolam in acute psychotic patients with hyperarousal. J Clin Psychiatry 1987;48:291–292.

52. Bodkin JA. Emerging uses for high-potency benzodiazepines in psychotic disorder. J Clin Psychiatry 1990;5 (suppl):41–46.

53. Feighner JP, Aden GC, Fabre LF, Rickels K, Smith WT. Comparison of alprazolam, imipramine and placebo in the treatment of depression. JAMA 1984;249:3057–3064.

54. Fawcett J, Edwards JH, Kravitz HM. Alprazolam: an antidepressant? J Clin Psychopharmacol 1987;7:295–310.

55. Gardner DL, Cowdry RW. Alprazolam-induced dyscontrol in borderline personality disorder. Am J Psychiatry 1985;142:98–100.

56. Rosenbaum JF, Woods SW, Groves JE, Klerman GL. Emergence of hostility during alprazolam treatment. Am J Psychiatry 1984;141:792–793.

57. Arana GW, Pearlman C, Shader RI. Alprazolam-induced dyscontrol in borderline personality disorder. Am J Psychiatry 1985; 142:369.

58. Goodman WK, Charney DS. A case of alprazolam, but not lorazepam, inducing manic symptoms. J Clin Psychiatry 1987; 48:117–118.

59. France RD, Krishnan KRR. Alprazolam-induced manic reaction. Am J Psychiatry 1984;141:1127–1128.

60. Pecknold JC, Fleury D. Alprazolam-induced manic episodes in two patients with panic disorder. Am J Psychiatry 1986; 143:652–653.

61. Strahan A, Rosenthal J, Kaswan M, Winston A. Three cases of acute paroxysmal excitement associated with alprazolam treatment. Am J Psychiatry 1985;142(7): 859–861.

62. Michaux MH, Kurland AA, Agallianos DD. Chlorpromazine-chlordiazepoxide and chlorpromazine-imipramine treatment of newly hospitalized, acutely ill psychiatric patients. Curr Ther Res 1966;8 (suppl):117–152.

63. Hanlon TE, Ota KY, Agallianos DD, Berman SA, Bethon GD, Kobler F, Kurland AA. Combined drug treatment of newly hospitalized, acutely ill psychiatric patients. Dis Nerv Syst 1969;30:104–116.

64. Hanlon TE, Ota KY, Kurland AA. Comparative effects of fluphenazine, fluphenazine-chlordiazepoxide and fluphenazine-imipramine. Dis Nerv Syst 1970;31:171–177.

65. Jimerson DC, van Kammen DP, Post RM, Docherty JP, Bunney Jr WE. Diazepam in schizophrenia: a preliminary double-blind trial. Am J Psychiatry 1982;139(4):489–491.

66. Lingjaerde O. Effect of the benzodiazepine derivative estazolam in patients with auditory hallucinations: a multi-centre double-blind, crossover study. Acta Psychiatr Scand 1982;65:339–354.

67. Karson CN, Weinberger DR, Bigelow L, Wyatt RJ. Clonazepam treatment of chronic schizophrenia: negative results in a double-blind, placebo-controlled trial. Am J Psychiatry 1982;139:1627–1628.

68. Pato CN, Wolkowitz OM, Rapaport M, Schulz SC, Pickar D. Benzodiazepine aug-

mentation of neuroleptic treatment in patients with schizophrenia. Psychopharmacol Bull 1989;25(2):263–266.

69. Bacher NM, Lewis HA, Field PB. Combined alprazolam and neuroleptic drug in treating schizophrenia. Am J Psychiatry 1986;143:1311–1312.

70. Dixon L, Weiden PJ, Frances AJ, Sweeney J. Alprazolam intolerance in stable schizophrenic outpatients. Psychopharmacol Bull 1989;25(2):213–214.

71. Sassim N, Grohmann R. Adverse drug reactions with clozapine and simultaneous application of benzodiazepines. Pharmacopsychiatry 1988;21:306–307.

72. Shader RI, Jackson AH, Dodes LM. The antiaggressive effects of lithium in man. Psychopharmacologia 1974;40:17–24.

73. Sheard MH, Marini JL, Bridges CI, Wagner E. The effect of lithium on impulsive aggressive behavior in man. Am J Psychiatry 1976;133(12):1409–1413.

74. Williams DT, Mehl R, Yudofsky S, Adams D, Roseman B. The effect of propranolol on uncontrolled rage outbursts in children and adolescents with organic brain dysfunction. J Am Acad Child Psychiatry 1982; 21:129–135.

75. Ratey JJ, Morrill R, Oxenkrug G. Use of propranolol for provoked and unprovoked episodes of rage. Am J Psychiatry 1983;140: 1356–1357.

76. Yudofsky SC, Stevens L, Silver J, Barsa J, Williams D. Propranolol in the treatment of rage and violent behavior associated with Korsakoff's psychosis. Am J Psychiatry 1984;141(1):114–115.

77. Greendyke RM, Kanter DR, Schuster DB, Verstreate S, Wootton J. Propranolol treatment of assaultive patients with organic brain disease. J Nerv Ment Dis 1986; 174(5):290–294.

78. Sorgi PJ, Ratey JJ, Polakoff S. Beta-adrenergic blockers for the control of aggressive behaviors in patients with chronic schizophrenia. Am J Psychiatry 1986;143: 775–776.

79. Hyman SE, Arana GW. Handbook of psychiatric drug therapy. Boston: Little, Brown, 1988.

Maintenance/Prophylaxis

Since the majority of schizophrenic patients have a chronic disorder, the issue of maintenance therapy becomes critical. Shortly after the introduction of antipsychotics, it became apparent that many patients quickly relapsed when their medications were withdrawn; conversely, maintainance pharmacotherapy prevented such relapses.

There may be exceptions, however, to this general rule. For example, a brief reactive psychosis in response to a severe stressor may occur only once, making long-term maintenance unnecessary. Before the era of antipsychotics there were many naturalistic investigations that identified acute onset, floridly psychotic episodes in patients who had a good premorbid history and subsequently made a full recovery. Because there are no systematic data on maintenance medication in such patients, it is hard to determine the optimal course of action after a first episode. Given the likelihood that psychotic episodes in reaction to an overwhelmingly stressful event will not recur, delaying maintenance medication may be the most prudent course to avoid adverse effects such as TD. Under certain circumstances, it may also be reasonable to use short-term treatment for 6–12 months to ensure a solid recovery without resorting to longer-term treatment.

EFFICACY OF MAINTENANCE ANTIPSYCHOTICS

The efficacy of antipsychotics in preventing relapse is supported by at least 35 random-assignment, double-blind studies, which reported the number who relapsed on placebo versus maintenance medication (Table 5.12, Davis, 1975; results initially summarized are updated here). A total of 3720 patients were randomly assigned to either placebo or an AP (at least 6 weeks with oral therapy or 2 months with i.m. depot treatment), with 55% on placebo relapsing, compared with only 21% on maintenance medication. On the basis of the Mantel-Haenszel test, the combined studies indicated a highly significant difference (chi square = 483, df = 1, $p < 10^{-107}$). **This finding represents overwhelming statistical evidence that in schizophrenia, antipsychotics prevent relapse.**

Some of these studies included remit-

Table 5.12.
Efficacy of Antipsychotics in Preventing Relapse[a]

Study	Year of Study	Number of Subjects	Relapsed (%) Placebo (%)	Relapsed (%) Drug (%)	Difference (%) (Placebo − Drug)
Schauver et al.	1959	80	18	5	13
Diamond and Marks	1960	40	70	25	45
Blackburn and Allen	1961	53	54	24	30
Gross and Reeves	1961	109	58	14	44
Adelson and Epstein	1962	281	90	49	41
Freeman and Alson	1962	94	28	13	15
Troshinsky et al.	1962	43	63	4	59
Whitaker and Hoy	1963	39	65	8	57
Caffey et al.	1964	259	45	5	40
Kinross-Wright and Charalampous	1965	40	70	5	65
Garfield et al.	1966	27	31	11	20
Melnyk et al.	1966	40	50	0	50
Englehardt et al.	1967	294	30	15	15
Morton	1968	40	70	25	45
Prien and Cole	1968	762	42	16	26
Prien et al.	1969	325	56	20	36
Baro et al.	1970	26	100	0	100
Rassidakis et al.	1970	84	58	34	24
Clark et al.	1971	19	70	43	27
Leff and Wing	1971	30	83	33	50
Hershon et al.	1972	62	28	7	21
Hirsch et al.	1973	74	66	8	58
Hogarty et al.	1973	361	67	31	36
Gross	1974	61	65	34	31
Chien and Cole	1975	31	87	12	75
Clark et al.	1975	35	78	27	51
Schiele	1975	80	60	3	57
Andrews et al.	1976	31	35	7	28
Rifkin et al.	1977	62	68	7	61
Levine et al. (p.o.)	1980	33	59	33	26
Levine et al. (i.m.)	1980	34	30	18	12
Cheung	1981	28	62	13	49
Wistedt	1981	38	63	38	25
Nishikawa et al.	1982	55	100	85	15
Ruskin and Nyman	1991	18	50%	13%	37%

[a]Summary statistics, p less than 10^{-107}
Adapted from Davis JM, Andriukaitis S. The natural course of schizophrenia and effective maintenance drug treatment. J. Clin Psychopharmacol 1986;6:2s–10s.

ted patients studied in outpatient trials, while others were still symptomatic inpatients or outpatients. In those fully remitted for several years, the APs could be characterized as having a clear prophylactic effect. In those partially remitted, this effect could be characterized as continued maintenance treatment. In the latter case, symptomatology worsened substantially with drug discontinuation. In each study, the placebo group is compared with the drug group, thus randomizing all of the above-mentioned factors. Even though many populations in several countries were used, the drug-placebo difference was still evident.

To illustrate the effectiveness of long-term medication, we will summarize two critical studies. Hogarty and Goldberg (1973) reported on 361 schizophrenic outpatients who, after discharge and a stabilization period on phenothiazines, were randomly assigned to CPZ or placebo (1). Half of each group also received psychotherapy from an individual caseworker plus vocational rehabilitation counseling. After 1 year, relapse had occurred in 73% of those receiving placebo without psychotherapy and in 63% of those given placebo plus psychotherapy. In contrast, only 33% of the CPZ-only and 26% of the CPZ-plus-psychotherapy group suffered a relapse. Overall, 31% of the drug-treated group relapsed, compared with 67% on placebo. Furthermore, the relapse rate with CPZ dropped to 16% when those who abruptly stopped their medication were excluded. Thus, almost half of the drug-treated relapses may have been secondary to medication noncompliance. While the psychotherapy groups had only slightly fewer relapses than patients not receiving psychotherapy, those who received drug plus psychotherapy functioned better than those on drug alone. Psychotherapy may take more time to work, because its effect

was more apparent after 18 months of treatment. **It appears that these two treatments complement each other, with psychotherapy improving psychosocial functioning and drugs preventing relapses.**

The second study was a Veterans Administration (VA) collaborative project (Caffey et al., 1964) which included 171 patients who received a placebo and 88 on either CPZ or thioridazine (total N = 259) (2). In this study, compliance was assured, for it included only inpatients, with nurses administering the medication. Relapse occurred in 45% of the placebo group, in contrast to only 5% of the drug-treated group.

Time Course of Relapse

An important issue in maintenance treatment is the rate of relapse upon discontinuation of therapy, which differs markedly from study to study, perhaps due to their varying durations. In addition, the definition of relapse varied, so that the rate was higher when defined as a modest re-emergence of psychotic symptoms rather than an exacerbation sufficient to cause rehospitalization. Using the former criteria, the relapse rate may be as high as 5–20% per month, whereas the more conservative criteria might yield a 1–10% rate.

The number of patients not yet relapsed versus time was plotted in Figure 5.5 to address the question of whether recurrence occurred at a constant or varying rate. When the data for long-term placebo treatment were analyzed, relapses tended to occur along an exponential function analogous to that seen with the half-life of drugs in plasma (3). This indicates that relapse occurs at a constant rate.

Beginning with a fixed number of patients in a study group, the number relapsing at fixed time points will always be a constant percentage of the overall number

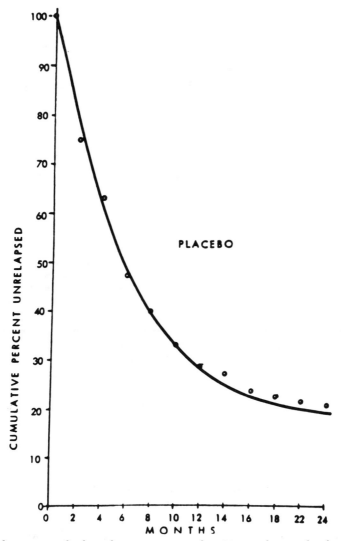

Figure 5.5. Relapse rate of schizophrenic patients after 24 months on placebo. Adapted from Davis JM et al. Important issues in the drug treatment of schizophrenia. Schizophr Bull 1980;6(1):82.

remaining in the study. Thus, over time, the actual number of patients relapsing will decrease because of a diminishing pool, but the rate does not change. For example, if we begin with 100 patients and a constant relapse rate of 10% per month, 10 will relapse at the end of the first month, leaving 90 in the trial. In the second month, 10% of 90, or 9, will relapse, leaving 81 patients, and so on.

Data from several large collaborative studies were plotted, with results fitting the exponential model (for constant relapse rate) more accurately than a linear model. The relapse rates for these studies included:

- A *constant relapse rate of 15.7%* per month in a VA hospital collaborative study (Caffey et al., 1964) (see Fig. 5.6)

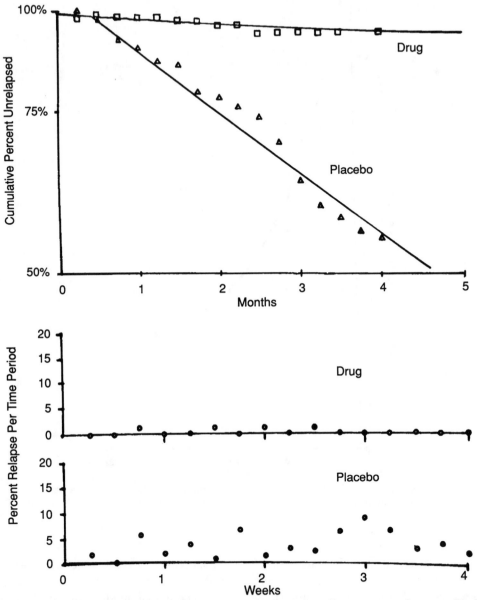

Figure 5.6. Relapse rate of schizophrenic patients after 4 months on active drug or placebo. Bottom panels present hazard rate per week. Adapted from Davis JM, Janicak PG, Chang S, Klerman K. Recent advances in the pharmacologic treatment of the schizophrenic disorders. In: Grinspoon L, ed. Psychiatry 1982 annual review. Washington DC: APPI Press, 1982:192.

- A *constant relapse rate of 10.7%* for those on placebo in the NIMH Hogarty and Goldberg study (1973) (see Fig. 5.7)
- A *constant relapse rate of 8%* per month in the collaborative NIMH study (Prien and Cole, 1969) (see Fig. 5.8).

The least-squares analysis of these data provided an excellent fit, with r^2 approaching 0.95.

In a long trial, it is expected that all at risk will have relapsed. Those not at risk will not, leaving a constant number of

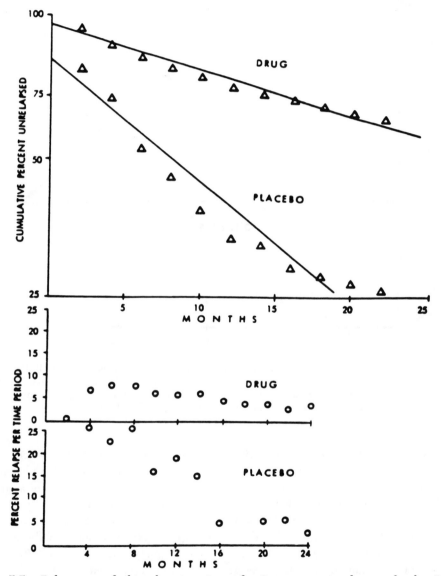

Figure 5.7. Relapse rate of schizophrenic patients after 2 years on active drug or placebo. Bottom panels present hazard rate per 2 month period. Adapted from Davis JM, Janicak PG, Chang S, Klerman K. Recent advances in the pharmacologic treatment of schizophrenic disorders. In: Grinspoon L, ed. Psychiatry 1982 annual review. Washington DC: APPI Press, 1982:193.

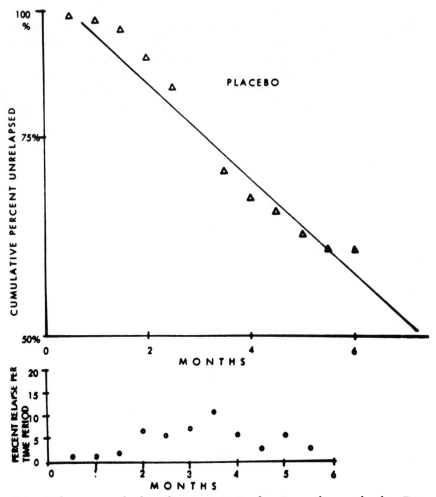

Figure 5.8. Relapse rate of schizophrenic patients after 6 months on placebo. Bottom panel presents hazard rate per month. Adapted from Davis JM, Janicak PG, Chang S, Klerman K. Recent advances in the pharmacologic treatment of schizophrenic disorders. In: Grinspoon L, ed. Psychiatry 1982 annual review. Washington DC: APPI Press, 1982:194.

"5-year survivors." In an attempt to clarify this point, Hogarty et al. (1976) followed their placebo group for 2 or more years after the initial study and found that almost all had relapsed or were lost to follow-up (4). Indeed, after 18 months, the data hinted that the relapse rate was decreasing, but so few remained that the placebo group did not yield a sufficient number of unrelapsed patients for reasonable conclusions.

If one prevents an exacerbation for 2–3

years, are patients less likely to relapse or will the rate remain about 10% per month? (i.e., does maintenance of remission for a sustained interval fundamentally alter the course of illness?). In the drug-treated groups of Hogarty and Goldberg (1974) and Hogarty and Ulrich (1976, 1979), there were ample subjects for this type of assessment (5). **When the APs were withdrawn after 2–3 years of successful treatment, the relapse rates were similar to those when maintenance medications** were stopped after only 2 months of therapy.

There is also evidence that patients with inadequate plasma levels are more likely to relapse, with the most frequent reason being inadequate compliance. A drop in a plasma level that was previously constant usually indicates poor compliance. Ironically, the act of drawing blood levels often encourages patient compliance.

A false conclusion frequently states that 50% of patients relapse without drugs whereas 50% do not and, therefore, may not need medication; however, the follow-up period in most studies was only 4–6 months, at which time a rate of 10% per month yields about a 50% relapse rate per year. If the period had been extended to 1 year, the rate would have increased to 75% (3). If the observation of a constant rate is true, the great majority of patients will relapse when active medication is discontinued, if followed long enough. Given the existing evidence, the majority of chronic patients should receive indefinite maintenance medication.

After several recurrences there is substantial evidence that maintenance treatment is necessary. Patients who have had many episodes but make a good recovery from the acute exacerbation benefit most from maintenance medication. Those who have the least drug/psychotherapy versus no treatment difference tend to benefit least from maintenance pharmacotherapy (6). For example, Prien and his colleagues (1971) found that chronically hospitalized patients maintained on low-dose antipsychotics had fewer relapses than those who needed more medication (see Table 5.13, relapse percentages by categories of medication dose and chronicity) (7–9).

It is also possible that in some chronic patients their illness "burns out" and they no longer require medication. To test this possibility, Morgan and Cheadle (1974) selected 74 of 475 patients who were clinically judged to be appropriately suitable for nondrug management, but only five remained stable after several years (10). Relapse occurred an average of 4.5 months after cessation of therapy, indicating that even better-functioning psychotic patients are at high risk if not maintained on active drug therapy. In conclusion, while maintenance therapy may not always be appropriate, especially after a single acute reactive episode, its discontinuation poses a complicated clinical decision (11).

Effects on Natural Course of Illness

In addition to the prevention of relapse or recurrence is the related, and critical, question of whether relapses or untreated episodes affect the natural course of a psychotic disorder. Two studies by May and collaborators, who investigated the outcome of 228 hospitalized schizophrenic patients randomly assigned to five treatment plans, provide data on the long-term effects of treating or not treating an acute episode (12, 13). These patients were initially assigned to one of the following regimens: electroconvulsive therapy (ECT); a phenothiazine alone; psychotherapy alone; a phenothiazine in combination with psychotherapy; or no specific treatment (control group).

Table 5.13.
Percent Clinically Deteriorated or Relapsed by Current Medication Dose and Length of Hospitalization in Chronic Schizophrenia[a]

Chronicity	CPZ eq.[b] (mg)	Number of Subjects	Relapsed (%)
Very chronic[c]	< 300	45	22
Chronic[d]	< 300	54	53
Very chronic[c]	> 300	108	70
Chronic[d]	> 300	64	73

[a]From Prien RF, Levine J, Switalski RW. Discontinuation of chemotherapy in chronic schizophrenia. Hospital & Community Psychiatry 1971:22:4–7.
[b]CPZ eq. = chlorpromazine equivalents
[c]Very chronic = 15 years or over
[d]Chronic = less than 15 years

Following stabilization, they were discharged into the community. Those with poor responses were generally in the groups not receiving drug or ECT. After 6–12 months, the remaining 48 nonresponding, hospitalized patients from all treatment groups then received pharmacotherapy and psychotherapy. Only two did not respond to the combination, and all were eventually discharged. **The principal difference among the groups at this point was that those initially assigned to the no drug or no ECT groups had their episode prolonged for 6 or more months until a drug was started.**

The patients were then followed for 3–5 years after the index admission. When the total number of days rehospitalized were compared, those who received only psychotherapy spent about twice as much time in the hospital as those who received pharmacotherapy plus psychotherapy. This was despite the fact that poststudy treatment was similar in both groups (i.e., current treatment was then an uncontrolled, clinically determined variable). Those who received no drug/no psychotherapy also did substantially poorer than the drug/no psychotherapy group. It is of particular interest that the patients who initially received ECT, and were then maintained on APs as needed, did as well as those who received drug treatment throughout. A critical aspect of May's study was the random assignment to an initial drug-free period (6–12 months), because it is presently impossible to have patients go unmedicated for such a long period due to ethical concerns.

This study provides significant evidence that antipsychotics and ECT positively alter the natural course of illness and that experiencing a psychotic episode without early definitive therapy is harmful. The precise mechanism involved in producing this harm is unknown, but we would assume that:

- A psychotic episode may induce some *lasting damage*, making future episodes more likely
- The *disruptive psychotic behavior plus the long hospital stay* may have irreparable effects on social or family functioning
- Or *both scenarios may contribute* to the prognosis.

In another study, Greenblatt et al. (1965) compared four variations of drug and social therapies in chronic schizophrenics continuously hospitalized and randomly divided into drug and nondrug groups. They were also subdivided into those receiving intensive or minimal social therapy (14). Because they had been continuously hospitalized for many years, the outcome of the two nondrug groups is critical in evaluating the effect of a long drug-free period on ultimate status. At the 6-month point the greatest improvement occurred in the two medication groups (drugs with and without social therapy). After 6 months, there was a trend toward greater symptomatic improvement in the drug plus intensive social therapy group (33%) when compared with the drug plus minimal social therapy group (23%). Those receiving intensive social therapy and no drugs fared poorly during this 6-month period, and then received 6 more months of psychosocial treatment plus drugs. In the final evaluation, intensive social therapy without drugs impeded improvement; and when finally placed on medication, this group never gained the same benefit achieved by those initially treated with drugs plus intensive social therapy. By contrast, the therapy plus drug intervention combination was helpful, with intensive social therapy facilitating discharge into the community. As in the May studies, the 6 month drug-free period seemed to produce a carry-over negative effect.

METHODS OF DRUG ADMINISTRATION

Targeted Treatment Strategy

Prophylaxis may act not by preventing episodes but rather by treating them as they occur, thus attenuating a major exacerbation. In this light, an alternate drug maintenance approach may be to carefully follow patients longitudinally, and only medicate to abort an episode when there are early warnings of a relapse. Unfortunately, many relapses occur abruptly, and it is doubtful that an episode can be halted once the process has started. Yet, some episodes may be preceded by a week or two of prodromal signs.

In targeted treatment, pharmacotherapy is only used when prodromal symptoms become manifest, in the few days or weeks preceding a recurrence. Such nonspecific symptoms may include:

- Increased anxiety; dysphoria; lability of mood
- Loss of interest; reduced energy; discouragement about the future
- Reduced attention; increased preoccupation; increased illusions; racing thoughts
- Vague digressive speech; eccentric behavior
- Nightmares.

A targeted treatment strategy utilizes these symptoms as cues to initiate drug therapy, thus avoiding continual antipsychotic therapy. The problem with this approach is that the organ needed to do the monitoring (i.e., the brain) is the organ that is dysfunctional.

There are four double-blind studies targeting treatment to an impending relapse as an alternate strategy to continuous maintenance medication. Jolley et al. (1989, 1990) reported that of 25 patients in a continuous-medication control group, only three relapsed, with two requiring hospitalization (15, 16). By contrast, of 24 patients in a targeted treatment group, 12 relapsed, and eight required hospitalization. Herz et al. (1990) compared over 100 patients on continuous or targeted therapy and observed more relapses in the targeted group (17). Using a survival analysis, they found a significant superiority for continuous medication. Herz and his coworkers (1991) then studied another group of 101 finding 15 of 50 targeted patients relapsed, with 12 rehospitalized. By contrast, only 8 of 51 maintenance-treatment patients relapsed, with three hospitalized (18).

Gaebel and his coworkers (1991) reported in an abstract a 2-year multicenter study in Germany using random assignment to early intervention, crisis intervention, or maintenance therapy (19). Out of 364 patients, 159 completed the trial and 23% of the maintenance-medication group relapsed, contrasted to 63% of the crisis intervention and 45% of the early intervention groups. It should be noted that the early intervention group also received substantially more drug than the crisis intervention group. Their targeted treatment was a variant of low-dose therapy, with patients on antipsychotics much of the time when they were manifesting prodromal symptoms.

Based on the published abstract of their work, we multiplied the 23% who did not relapse with maintenance medication times the assumed 121 in each arm of the trial; averaged the 63% and 45% for the two nonmedication strategies; and then multiplied this mean (i.e., 53.5%) by the 242 in these two arms of the trial. The results indicated that 25% of continuously medicated patients relapsed, in contrast to 50% in the targeted treatment groups, a highly statistically significant difference.

Carpenter et al. (1990) performed a similar unblinded comparison study (20). Of the 57 targeted patients, 53% relapsed, compared to only 36% of the 59 continuous-therapy patients. Survival analysis demonstrated again that a continuous regimen was clearly more effective than targeted therapy (i.e., relapse rate with continuous therapy was 1.6, versus 3.18 for the targeted therapy).

Analyzing only the three published studies with explicit data, 23% of the continuous group and 38% of the targeted group required hospitalization. The Mantel-Haenszel test also found this difference statistically significant (chi square = 6.7; df = 1; p = .01). In summary, the four controlled studies of targeted versus continuous treatment found that outcome was poorer with the targeted strategy.

Low-Dose Strategy

An alternate strategy would be to maintain patients on a continuous lower dose of APs (either i.m. or oral) that is then increased only when prodromal signs occur. Studies have shown that standard doses are more effective than lower doses, but again, many factors should be considered before embarking on a given approach.

There have been four dose-response studies of maintenance depot medication (see also Long-Acting Antipsychotics later in this chapter). Generally, most groups used a standard dose of 25 mg fluphenazine decanoate given i.m. every 2 weeks, although some compared standard with lower doses. The lowest doses were used by Kane and his coworkers (1983), who chose 1.25–5 mg (21). In their study, three patients in the standard dose group relapsed and 61 patients remained well, while 26 patients in the low-dose group relapsed and 36 remained well. Marder et al. (1987) used doses of 25 mg in comparison with 5 mg, but patients who showed very early signs of relapse could have their dose slightly increased (22). For purposes of our discussion, we consider the 5 or 25 mg their fixed starting dose. Of those on the standard dose of 25 mg, 10 relapsed and 21 remained well, while 22 relapsed and 13 remained well on the lower dose. When the patients had early signs of relapse, their dose was increased, and as a result, the dose-response relationship began to level out to no difference. Hogarty et al. (1988) used doses of 25 mg, versus an average of 3.8 mg, and found a nonsignificant difference between the two groups (23). Thus, in the standard dose group, 19 did not relapse, and six did; whereas in the low-dose group, 21 did not relapse and nine did. Johnson et al. (1987) used flupenthixol decanoate, so there is the question of exact equivalence, but their low-dose group was roughly equivalent to the Hogarty and Marder groups (24). Of those on the regular dose, four of 31 relapsed in 18 months, and of those who received half of the usual dose, 12 of 28 relapsed in this time period. Kane et al. (unpublished data) studied the 6-month relapse rate in patients randomly assigned to 25, 50, 100, or 200 mg of haloperidol decanoate on a monthly schedule. The relapse rate was lowest for those on 200 mg monthly. **If all studies are considered collectively, we see an increased relapse rate at the lower dose levels, with the threshold for a minimally effective dose probably slightly higher than the lowest utilized.**

When patients are randomly assigned

to a lower than standard dose, the relapse rate rises slightly, but there are substantially fewer adverse effects. With a greater decrease in dose, however, there is a substantial increase in the relapse rate. The question is further complicated, in that different patients may require different doses. Given these tradeoffs, clinicians must often rely on trial and error. In studies demonstrating a slight increase in the relapse rate with slightly lower doses, an increase in dose almost always aborted a relapse, without the need for rehospitalization.

To supplement depot medication, oral preparations can be used when early warning signals of an impending relapse occur because the pharmacokinetics of depot preparations require months to reach steady state (see also Pharmacokinetics/Plasma Levels later in this chapter). By contrast, oral administration brings about an altered steady state in several days. **We recommend treating most patients with the minimally effective dose to avoid more serious adverse effects, even at the cost of a few more relapses, provided this strategy does not lead to rehospitalization or produce serious impairment in functioning.**

In conclusion, clinicians must balance several factors when choosing the proper therapy, including the:

- Problem of *dysphoric adverse effects*
- Disruption of a *minor relapse*
- Likelihood of a *severe relapse*
- Long-term risk of *tardive dyskinesia*
- Likelihood of *suicide* during a relapse.

Choice of Maintenance Medication

As in the treatment of an acute episode, all antipsychotics are theoretically equieffective, so the choice of agent is made on the basis of adverse effects and half-life.

Pimozide is a specific DA antagonist that may have merit as a maintenance medication because of its long oral half-life and minimal side-effect profile (25, 26).

Clozapine has recently been approved for more severe forms of schizophrenia in patients who have failed to respond to adequate trials of standard agents or cannot tolerate their adverse effects. Data from long-term open evaluations of clozapine demonstrate that improvement is maintained over time, even when the dose is reduced. Further, patients did not develop tolerance to its antipsychotic effect. Naturalistic reports indicate that an adequate trial for acute response in some patients may be at least 6 months. Further, a small number (8 of 14) of previously refractory patients were successfully maintained on clozapine for up to 2 years (27). To date, however, no controlled trials have addressed the question of its usefulness as a maintenance strategy.

Complications

Post-Psychotic Depression

There is a significant difference between unremitted or partially remitted patients with pronounced negative symptoms and those in remission who experience a depressive episode. Siris et al. (1987) selected candidates with a history of schizophrenia who recovered and then experienced a major depression that resolved with antidepressant (AD) therapy (28). Thirty-three patients receiving both maintenance APs and ADs were studied in a double-blind design that included an AP plus random administration of either an AD or placebo. The group receiving both types of psychotropic had a statistically superior outcome ($p = 0.020$, two-tailed Fisher's test) on their global scores for each of the subscales in the depression ratings, but there was no difference in the measure of psychosis or adverse effects between the two groups. Siris et al. (1990) also conducted a follow-up study on the previous AD-treated group, maintaining them on fluphenazine decanoate and benztropine, as well as adjunctive imipramine (29). After 6 months, their imipramine was tapered to a placebo or they continued on the same medication regimen for 1 more year. All six who were tapered off active drug relapsed into a depressive state, in contrast to only two of the eight remaining on imipramine ($p = 0.009$). Of note is that those who relapsed again improved once adjunctive imipramine was reinstituted. Johnson (1981) studied 50 schizophrenics in remission who were randomly assigned to receive nortriptyline or placebo for a 5-week trial (30). More subjects in the nortriptyline group (i.e., 28%) were free of depression at the end of the trial than in the placebo group (i.e., 8%). Prusoff et al. (1979) studied 40 schizophrenic outpatients with depressive episodes treated with amitriptyline or placebo in addition to their maintenance perphenazine (31). In general, improvement in depression was modest, not statistically impressive, and there was a suggestion of worsening in psychosis.

In summary, episodes of superimposed depression benefit from intervention with concurrent AD therapy, but these agents do not appear to help patients who suffer from a more chronic, negative symptom presentation.

Supersensitivity Psychosis

Supersensitivity psychosis (SSP) has been described as the rapid re-emergence of psychotic symptoms upon discontinuation of long-term neuroleptic treatment. Chouinard and Steinberg's (1984) criteria for the diagnosis are presented in an abbreviated form in Table 5.14, and descriptions of patients who meet these criteria can be found in Hunt et al. (1988) (32, 33). This phenomenon is thought to be secondary to an up-regulation of DA receptors in the neural circuit(s) subserving psychosis. This concept is analogous to the hypothesis regarding TD, which postulates a DA receptor supersensitivity secondary to striatal neuroleptic blockade (i.e., dopaminergic receptor up-regulation in the neural tract relevant to movement). Thus, withdrawal of these drugs may induce a rebound psychosis, just as it may cause TD.

Peet (1991), in a chart review study of 55 outpatients, found seven who met the criteria for SSP (34). Singh et al. (1990) compared five patients with a history of SSP to five without, predicting that those with SSP would relapse more rapidly upon discontinuation (35). In the study design, antipsychotic medication was abruptly replaced by placebo without any tapering, and the emergence of psychosis or TD was evaluated. The authors found no evidence of relapse into psychosis over a 2-week period. As the relapse rate of untreated schizophrenics is about 10% per month,

---

Table 5.14.
Criteria for Supersensitivity Psychosis

History of receiving neuroleptics or antipsychotics for at least 6 months
    Patient has had a decrease or discontinuation of medication with appearance of psychosis
       or
    Patient has had no decrease or discontinuation of medication during treatment but has more relapses or increased tolerance to antipsychotic effects
Exclusion Criteria:
    Patients in the acute phase of the illness
    Patients with continued psychotic illness that did not respond to neuroleptic treatment

we might expect some relapses during this time, but the sample size of this study was too small for definitive conclusions (i.e., 10 patients). To prove the existence of SSP one would have to show that there is an *increased relapse rate* or at least a worsening of symptoms greater than would otherwise be expected. Although the clinician must remain alert to this possibility, we would give this hypothesis the "Scotch verdict" of not proven, with the burden of proof resting with those who have proposed this syndrome.

CONCLUSION

Continuous, moderate-dose maintenance APs afford the best chance of avoiding relapse in psychotic patients. Low doses should theoretically diminish the possibility of TD, but in fact, are only weakly correlated. Further, with too low a dose, patients are at risk of developing more frequent exacerbations, which usually require in-creased doses, and/or may contribute to higher levels of psychopathology not amenable to future drug intervention.

The utilization of maintenance strategies must always be considered in the context of the long-term consequences to minimize more serious adverse effects (i.e., TD and perhaps SSP). There is a trade-off between the risk of TD using adequate dose long-term medication and the higher risk of relapse with lower dose strategies. Because a recurrence of psychotic behavior may interfere with vocational and social functioning and, at the extreme, result in violence or suicide, the cost of an episode to patients, their families, and society must be carefully considered. Finally, psychosocial therapies can enhance the beneficial effects of medication, improving the overall quality of life.

Figure 5.9 outlines a recommended strategy for managing the chronic, relapsing psychotic patient.

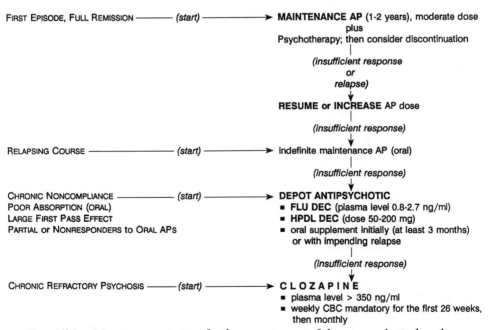

Figure 5.9.   Maintenance strategy for the management of chronic psychotic disorders.

REFERENCES

1. Hogarty GE, Goldberg SC. Collaborative study group. Drug and sociotherapy in the aftercare of schizophrenic patients. One-year relapse rates. Arch Gen Psychiatry 1973;28:54–64.
2. Caffey EM, Diamond LS, Frank TV, Grasberger JC, Herman L, Klett CJ, et al. Discontinuation or reduction of chemotherapy in chronic schizophrenics. J Chronic Dis 1964;17:347–358.
3. Davis JM, Dysken MW, Haberman SJ, Javaid J, Chang S, Killian G. Use of survival curves in analysis of antipsychotic relapse studies. In: Cattabeni F, Racogni G, Spano P, ed. Long-term effects of neuroleptics (Adv Biochem Psychopharmacol, Vol. 2) New York: Raven Press, 1980:471–481.
4. Hogarty GE, Ulrich RF, Mussare F, Aristigueta H. Drug discontinuation among long-term successfully maintained schizophrenic outpatients. Dis Nerv Sys 1976; 37:494–500.
5. Hogarty GE, Ulrich RF. Temporal effects of drug and placebo in delaying relapse in schizophrenic outpatients. Arch Gen Psychiatry 1977;34:297–301.
6. Goldberg SC, Schooler NR, Hogarty GE, Roper M. Prediction of relapse in schizophrenic outpatients treated by drug and sociotherapy. Arch Gen Psychiatry 1977; 34:171–184.
7. Prien RF, Cole JO. High dose chlorpromazine therapy in chronic schizophrenia. Report of National Institute of Mental Health Psychopharmacology Research Branch Collaborative Study Group. Arch Gen Psychiatry 1968;18:482–95.
8. Prien RF, Cole JO, Belkin NF. Relapse in chronic schizophrenics following abrupt withdrawal of tranquilizing medication. Br J Psychiatry 1969;115:679–686.
9. Prien RF, Levine J, Switalski RW. Discontinuation of chemotherapy for chronic schizophrenics. Hosp Community Psychiatry 1971;22:4–7.
10. Morgan R, Cheadle J. Maintenance treatment of chronic schizophrenia with neuroleptic drugs. Acta Psychiatr Scand 1974; 50:78–85.
11. Davis JM, Marter JT, Kane JM. Antipsychotic drugs. In: Kaplan HI, Saddock BJ, eds. Comprehensive textbook of psychiatry. 5th ed., V.2. Baltimore: Williams & Wilkins, 1989:1591–1626.
12. May PRA, Tuma AH, Dixon WJ. Schizophrenia. A follow-up study of results of treatment. I. Design and other problems. Arch Gen Psychiatry 1976a;33:474–478.
13. May PRA, Tuma AH, Yale C, Potepan P, Dixon WJ. Schizophrenia—A follow-up study of results of treatment. II. Hospital stay over two to five years. Arch Gen Psychiatry 1976;33:481–486.
14. Greenblatt M, Solomon MH, Evans AS, Brooks GW, eds. Drug and social therapy in chronic schizophrenia. Springfield, IL: Charles C Thomas, 1965.
15. Jolley AG, Hirsch SR, McRink A, Manchanda R. Trial of brief intermittent neuroleptic prophylaxis for selected schizophrenic outpatients: clinical outcome at one year. Br Med J 1989;298:985–990.
16. Jolley AG, Hirsch SR, Morrison E, McRink A, Wilson L. Trial of brief intermittent neuroleptic prophylaxis for selected schizophrenic outpatients: clinical and social outcome at two years. Br Med J 1990;301(6756):837–842.
17. Herz MI, Glazer WM, Mostert MA, Sheard MA, Szymanski HV. Intermittent vs maintenance medication in schizophrenia. Two year results. Clin Neuropharmacol 1990;13 (suppl 2):426–427.
18. Herz MI, Glazer WM, Mostert MA, Sheard MA, Szymanski HV, Hafez H, Mirza M, Vana J. Intermittent vs. maintenance medication in schizophrenia. Arch Gen Psychiatry 1991;48:333–339.
19. Gaebel W, Kopcke W, Linden M, Muller P, Muller-spahn F, Pietzcker A, Tegeler J. 2-Year outcome of intermittent vs. maintenance neuroleptic treatment in schizophrenia. Schiz Res 1991;4:288.
20. Carpenter WT, Hanlon TE, Heinrichs DW, Summerfelt AT, Kirkpatrick B, Levine J, Buchanan RW. Continuous versus targeted medication in schizophrenic outpatients: outcome results. Am J Psychiatry 1990;147(9):1138–1148.
21. Kane JM, Rifkin A, Woerner M, Reardon G, Sarantakos S, Schiebel D, et al. Low-dose neuroleptic treatment of outpatient schizophrenics. I. Preliminary results for relapse rates. Arch Gen Psychiatry 1983; 40:893–896.
22. Marder SR, Van Putten T, Mintz J, Lebell M, McKenzie J, May PRA. Low- and conventional-dose maintenance therapy with fluphenazine decanoate. Two-year outcome. Arch Gen Psychiatry 1987;44:518–521.

23. Hogarty GE, McEvoy JP, Munetz M, Di-Barry AL, Bartone P, Cather R, Cooley SJ, Ulrich RF, Carter M, Madonia MJ, the EPICS Research Group. Dose of fluphenazine, familial expressed emotion, and outcome in schizophrenia. Results of a two-year controlled study. Arch Gen Psychiatry 1988;45:797–805.

24. Johnson DAW, Ludlow JM, Street K, Taylor RDW. Double-blind comparison of half-dose and standard-dose flupenthixol decanoate in the maintenance treatment of stabilized outpatients with schizophrenia. Br J Psychiatry 1987;151:634–638.

25. Clark ML, Huber W, Serafetinides EA, Colmore JP. Pimozide (Orap). A tolerance study. Clin Trial J 1971;2 (suppl):25–32.

26. Clark ML, Huber W, Hill D, et al. Pimozide in chronic outpatients. Dis Nerv Sys 1975;36:137–141.

27. Mattes JA. Clozapine for refractory schizophrenia: an open study of 14 patients treated up to 2 years. J Clin Psychiatry 1989;50:389–391.

28. Siris SG, Morgan V, Fagerstrom R, Rifkin A, Cooper TB. Adjunctive imipramine in the treatment of postpsychotic depression: a controlled trial. Arch Gen Psychiatry 1987;42:533–539.

29. Siris SG, Mason SE, Beranzohn PC, Alvir JM, McCorry TA. Adjunctive imipramine maintenance in post-psychotic depression/negative symptoms. Psychopharmacol Bull 1990;26:91–94.

30. Johnson DAW. Studies of depressive symptoms in schizophrenia. J Psychiatr 1981;139:89–101.

31. Prusoff BA, Williams DH, Weissman MM, Astrachan BM. Treatment of secondary depression in schizophrenia. A double-blind, placebo-controlled trials of amitriptyline added to perphenazine. Arch Gen Psychiatry 1979;36:569–575.

32. Chouinard G, Steinberg S. New clinical concept on neuroleptic-induced supersensitivity disorders. In: Stancer HC, Garfinkel PE, Rakoff VM, eds. Guidelines for use of psychotropic drugs. New York: Spectrum Publications, 1984:205–227.

33. Hunt JI, Singh H, Simpson GM. Neuroleptic-induced supersensitivity psychosis: retrospective study of schizophrenic inpatients. J Clin Psychiatry 1988;49:258–261.

34. Peet M. Supersensitivity psychosis (Letter to the Editor). J Clin Psychiatry 1991;52:90.

35. Singh H, Hunt JL, Vitiello B, Simpson GM. Neuroleptic withdrawal in patients meeting criteria for supersensitivity psychosis. J Clin Psychiatry 1990;51:319–321.

Long-Acting Antipsychotics

A depot antipsychotic is one that can be administered in such a way that, after a single dose, a therapeutically efficient tissue concentration of at least 1 week's duration is achieved (1, 2). Slow release of the active drug is produced by combining the base antipsychotic with a fatty acid (decanoic acid). The alcohol group of the antipsychotic is esterified by the acid, producing a lipophilic compound whose solubility in oil increases. An oil, usually sesame, is then used as a vehicle for intramuscular injection, where the ester, which is not pharmacologically active, is hydrolyzed by tissue esterases, slowly releasing the active compound.

Depot preparations should be the first line of treatment in patients with several relapses, as well as in those who have clear problems with noncompliance. Because many patients stop their oral drugs, often precipitating a relapse, long-acting, depot fluphenazine and haloperidol (HPDL) represent a major tactical advantage in chemoprophylaxis (3). In open trials, many who fared poorly on oral management were greatly benefited by i.m. depot medication. This improvement was presumably because of previous noncompliance with their oral regimens, but it is also possible that some patients rapidly metabolize oral preparations (e.g., a large first-pass effect), never achieving adequate plasma levels by this route of administration.

While these preparations are an important addition to the therapeutic armamentarium, particularly for outpatients, they may also occasionally benefit inpatients. It is important to appreciate the different pharmacokinetic properties of long-acting injectable drugs, especially the longer time period (i.e., 3–4 months) required to achieve steady state concentrations, which must be taken into account when titrating dose.

LITERATURE REVIEW

Table 5.15 shows the difference in the percentage of patients who relapsed while on oral or depot antipsychotics from six random-assignment, double-blind studies (3–8). Although the outcome is mixed, three of the studies found an appreciable difference between the two regimens. For example, one study found a 3% relapse rate per month on oral versus a 1% rate on depot fluphenazine. The three other studies, however, found little difference, but they also may have had more compliant patients. Combining these data with the Mantel-Haenszel test reveals a significantly lower relapse percentage on depot

versus oral medication (chi square = 13.5, $p = 0.0002$). The usefulness of depot medication is also supported by Johnson et al. (1979, 1983, 1990), who used matched controls; as well as Marriott and Hiep (1976); Tegeler and Lehmann (1981); and Freeman (1980), who used mirror image controls (i.e., relapse in patients on oral medication and later on depot medication) (9–14).

Several longitudinal studies have also found that patients stabilized on depot fluphenazine relapsed when switched to an oral antipsychotic preparation (15). Mirror-image studies also found depot fluphenazine (decanoate or enanthate) reduced the incidence of relapse, as well as the number of days hospitalized, when compared with oral therapy. These open, crossover studies switched patients from oral to depot forms, and the outcome with each approach was evaluated.

Complicated research protocols make significant demands on patients; therefore, only those who can give informed consent, and are thus more likely to be compliant, enter such trials. Further, the *Hawthorne effect* may be operative, in that the interest of the investigator may effectively communicate to patients the importance of taking their medication. The increased quality of clinical care, which is often a

Table 5.15.
Percent Difference in Relapse between Depot and Oral Preparations[a]

Study	Number of Subjects	Study Duration	Relapsed (%) Oral (%)	Relapsed (%) Depot (%)	Difference (Oral minus Depot) (%)
Crawford and Forest (1974)	29	40 weeks	27	0	27
del Guidice et al. (1975)	82	1 year	91	43	48
Rifkin et al. (1977)	51	1 year	11	9	2
Falloon et al. (1978)	41	1 year	24	40	− 16
Hogarty et al. (1979)	105	2 years	65	40	25
Schooler et al. (1979)	214	1 year	33	24	9

Mantel-Haenszel: $p < 0.0002$
[a]Adapted from Davis JM, Andriukaitis S. The natural course of schizophrenia and effective maintenance drug treatment. J Clin Psychopharmacol 1986;6:2s–10s.

byproduct of research, may inspire some to become better educated about their disorder and its treatment and more highly motivated to take medication. Such factors could cloud any differences in efficacy between oral and depot forms.

STANDARD DEPOT PREPARATIONS

Fluphenazine

Whereas the fluphenazine depot preparations are superior to placebo in preventing relapse in groups of remitted schizophrenic patients, their advantage over oral fluphenazine is less clear. Rifkin et al. followed remitted schizophrenics for 1 year and found that 63% treated with placebo relapsed, whereas only 5% on depot and 4% on oral fluphenazine relapsed during that period (5). Schooler et al. treated schizophrenic patients with either fluphenazine decanote or oral fluphenazine for 1 year and again found no significant difference in relapse rates between these two groups (i.e., 24 versus 33%, respectively) during that time (16). By contrast, at least two other controlled studies conducted in a *typical clinical setting* found a clear difference favoring depot over oral preparations (Table 5.15).

For example, Kane, Woerner, and Sarantakos, point out that some studies may not have effectively evaluated the potential benefit of depot fluphenazine (17). For example, patients volunteering for such studies are those who would be compliant whether they took oral or depot medications; therefore, these studies may underrepresent the noncompliant population. Second, inasmuch as relapse may not occur for 3–7 months after medications have been completely discontinued, a 1-year study period may not be long enough to evaluate the relative effectiveness of a depot versus oral antipsychotic.

In this context, Hogarty et al. followed patients who were treated with either i.m. fluphenazine hydrochloride or i.m. fluphenazine decanoate for 2 years (7). After the first year, the relapse rate did not differ between the two groups (i.e., 40% for hydrochloride and 35% for decanoate). During the second year, however, 42% of those remaining in the hydrochloride group relapsed, as compared with only 8% of those remaining in the decanoate group. Although the difference was not statistically significant, the figures suggest an advantage favoring the decanoate preparation in minimizing relapse during the second year of treatment.

Fluphenazine enanthate and decanoate are similar in potency, efficacy, and adverse effects. They differ only in that the decanoate preparation is slightly more potent and slightly longer acting, requiring lower doses and less frequent administrations. Because the decanoate form manifests marginally fewer adverse effects, it is probably preferable.

Dose

When initiating depot fluphenazine, a conservative dose should be chosen, realizing that it may take several months to establish steady state levels. It may also be necessary to supplement treatment with oral fluphenazine during this early phase until the required maintenance level is ascertained. If psychotic symptoms should re-emerge, oral fluphenazine can also be used to establish control and the depot dosage can be increased accordingly at the next scheduled injection. If the depot dose is too high, as evidenced by the appearance of persistent adverse effects, then appropriate symptomatic treatment should be initiated and the dose reduced or injection intervals extended until adverse effects are controlled. The goal is to establish the lowest effective maintenance dose, mindful that too low a dose may increase the risk of relapse and rehospitalization (see Kane (18)). Conversely, too high a dose may expose the patient to unnecessary adverse effects and noncompliance.

Haloperidol

Haloperidol decanoate is an effective depot agent comparable to standard oral preparations (19–22). It can be given monthly, and has a marginally lower incidence of EPS compared with the fluphenazine formulations.

Clinically, haloperidol decanote has been administered to hundreds of chronic shizophrenic patients in several open studies to determine its efficacy, pharmacokinetics, safety, and adverse effects. The trials ranged from 4 months to 2 years, with dosages ranging from 25 to 500 mg given once every 4 weeks. The results of these studies have consistently shown that depot haloperidol:

- Is as effective in controlling psychotic symptoms in chronic schizophrenic patients as oral haloperidol, other oral antipsychotics, or depot fluphenazine
- Has not produced any clinically significant changes in hematological or biochemical values
- Produces a steady plasma level that declines slowly by one-half during the interinjection interval
- Does not increase and may even decrease the incidence of extrapyramidal and other adverse effects when compared to those produced by oral preparations (22–28).

Dose

The calculation of an appropriate dosage for the depot form requires converting from a given oral dose of haloperidol. Earlier observations found the bioavailability of oral haloperidol to be 60 –70%, indicating that this would correspond to a monthly dose of haloperidol decanoate of about 20 times the daily oral dose (see Deberdt et al. (23)). For example, if a patient is stabilized on a daily oral dose of 10 mg, then a corresponding monthly dose of the decanoate formulation would be 200 mg. Kane and others, however, suggest a lower starting ratio of 10–15:1 (29). Doses will usually need to be adjusted individually, however, based on a given patient's response and the emergence of adverse effects.

Fluphenazine Depot versus Haloperidol Depot

In general, double-blind comparisons have found the two depot formulations to be equieffective in the maintenance treatment of schizophrenic patients. Kissling et al. evaluated both fluphenazine and haloperidol decanoate in a 6-month double-blind study involving 31 schizophrenic patients (30). They found both were equally effective in preventing relapse, with a slight advantage with haloperidol decanoate, which produced fewer and less severe adverse effects, as reflected by fewer adverse effect-related dropouts and a decreased need for antiparkinsonian medications. Wistedt compared fluphenazine decanoate and haloperidol decanoate in a double-blind study involving 51 schizophrenic patients over a 20-week treatment period. He found no difference between the drug groups on ratings of global clinical changes, with both showing a significant improvement over the course of the study (31). The haloperiodol-treated group, however, did show a greater degree of improvement in ratings on a clinical psychopathology scale, and less depressive symptomatology compared with the fluphenazine group. Although there was no difference in EPS between groups, the patients on fluphenazine required higher doses of antiparkinsonian medication during the study, perhaps indicating a greater severity of EPS. Chouinard et al. randomly assigned 12 schizophrenic outpatients to receive either haloperidol decanoate or fluphenazine decanoate in a dose ratio of 3:1. This was a double-blind study over an 8-month period, and it found no significant differences between the drug groups on any of the psychopathology ratings, parkinsonian symptoms, or the need for antiparkinsonian medication (32).

Fluphenazine decanoate may cause more acute EPS than haloperidol decanote due to a phenomenon known as "dose dumping." Here, a small amount of depot formulation is released into the systemic circulation shortly after an injection. There may be a tendency for haloperidol to be more effective on a subset of schizophrenic symptoms, less depressogenic, and slightly less likely to exacerbate extrapyramidal symptoms. These effects are not large, however; may not be clinically significant; and are not consistently evident in all studies.

REFERENCES

1. Comaty JE, Janicak PG. Depot neuroleptics. Psychiatric Ann 1987;17:491–496.
2. Knudsen P. Chemotherapy with neuroleptics. Clinical and pharmacokinetic aspects with a particular view to depot preparations. Acta Psychiatr Scand 1985;322 (72, suppl):51–75.
3. del Guidice J, Clark WG, Gocka EF. Prevention of recidivism of schizophrenics treated with fluphenazine enanthate. Psychosomatics 1975;16:32–36.
4. Crawford R, Forrest A. Controlled trial of depot fluphenazine in out-patient schizophrenics. Br J Psychiatry 1974;124:385–391.
5. Rifkin A, Quitkin F, Rabiner CJ, Klein DF. Fluphenazine decanoate, fluphenazine hydrochloride given orally, and placebo in remitted schizophrenics. I. Relapse rates after one year. Arch Gen Psychiatry 1977;34:43–47.
6. Falloon I, Watt DC, Shepherd M. A comparative controlled trial of pimozide and fluphenazine decanoate in the continuation therapy of schizophrenia. Psychol Med 1978;8:59–70.
7. Hogarty GE, Schooler NR, Ulrich R, Mussare F, Ferro P, Herron E. Fluphenazine and social therapy in the aftercare of schizophrenic patients. Relapse analyses of a two-year controlled study of fluphenazine decanoate and fluphenazine hydrochloride. Arch Gen Psychiatry 1979;36:1283–1294.
8. Schooler NR, Levine J, Severe JB. NIMH-PRB collaborative fluphenazine study group. Depot fluphenazine in the prevention of relapse in schizophrenia: evaluation of a treatment regimen. Psychopharmacol Bull 1979;15:44–47.
9. Johnson DAW. Further observations on the duration of depot neuroleptic maintenance therapy in schizophrenia. Br J Psychiatry 1979;135:524–530.
10. Johnson DAW, Pasterski JM, Ludlow JM, Street K, Taylor RDW. The discontinuance of maintenance neuroleptic therapy in chronic schizophrenic patients: drug and social consequences. Acta Psychiatr Scand 1983;67:339–352.
11. Johnson DAW, Wright NF. Drug prescribing for schizophrenic outpatients on depot injections: repeat surveys over 18 years. Br J Psychiatry 1990;156:827–834.
12. Marriott P, Hiep A. A mirror image outpatient study at a depot phenothiazine clinic. Aust N Z J Psychiatry 1976;10:163.
13. Tegeler J, Lehmann E. A follow-up study of schizophrenic outpatients treated with depot neuroleptics. Prog NeuroPsychopharm 1981;5:79–90.
14. Freeman H. Twelve years' experience with the total use of depot neuroleptics in a defined population. In: Cattabeni F et al., eds. Long-term effects of neuroleptics (Adv. Biochem. Psychopharmacol.) New York: Raven Press, 1980;559–564.
15. Davis JM, Andriukaitis S. The natural course of schizophrenia and effective maintenance drug treatment. J Clin Psychopharmacol 1986;6 (1, suppl):2S–10S.
16. Schooler NR, Levine J, Severe JB, Brauzer B, Di Mascio A, Klerman GL, Tuason VB. Prevention of relapse in schizophrenia. An

evaluation of fluphenazine decanoate. Arch Gen Psychiatry 1980;37:16–24.

17. Kane JM, Woerner M, Sarantakos S. Depot neuroleptics: a comparative review of standard, intermediate, and low-dose regimens. J Clin Psychiatry 1986;47 (suppl):30–33.

18. Kane JM. The use of depot neuroleptics: clinical experience in the United States. J Clin Psychiatry 1984;45:5–12.

19. Zissis NP, Psaras M, Lyketsos G. Haloperidol decanoate, a new long-acting antipsychotic, in chronic schizophrenics: double-blind comparison with placebo. Curr Ther Res 1982;31:650–655.

20. Viukari M, Salo H, Lamminsivu U, Gordin A. Tolerance and serum levels of haloperidol during parenteral and oral haloperidol treatment in geriatric patients. Acta Psychiatr Scand 1982;65:301–308.

21. Zuardi AW, Giampietro AC, Grassi ER, et al. Double-blind comparison between two forms of haloperidol. An oral preparation and a new depot decanoate in the maintenance of schizophrenic patients. Curr Ther Res 1983;34 (2, sec 1):253–261.

22. Nair NPV, Suranyi-Cadotte B, Schwartz G, Thavundayil JX, Achim A, Lizondo E, Nayak R. A clinical trial comparing intramuscular haloperidol decanoate and oral haloperidol in chronic schizophrenic patients: efficacy, safety, and dosage equivalence. J Clin Psychopharmacol 1986;6(1, suppl):30S–37S.

23. Deberdt R, Elens P, Berghmans W, Heykants J, Woestenborghs R, Driesens F, Reyntjens A, van Wijngaarden I. Intramuscular haloperidol decanoate for neuroleptic maintenance therapy. Efficacy, dosage schedule and plasma levels. An open multicenter study. Acta Psychiatr Scand 1980;62(4):356–363.

24. Reyntjens AJM, Heykants JJP, Woestenborghs RJH, Gelders YG, Aerts TJ. Pharmacokinetics of haloperidol decanoate. A 2-year follow-up. International Pharmacopsychiatry 1982;17(4):238-246.

25. Gelders YG, Reyntjens AJM, Ash CW, Aerts TJ. 12-month study of haloperidol decanoate in chronic schizophrenic patients. International Pharmacopsychiatry 1982;17(4):247–254.

26. Suy E, Woestenborghs R, Heykants J. Bioavailability and clinical effect of two different concentrations of haloperidol decanoate. Current Therapeutic Research 1982;31:982–991.

27. Youssef HA. A one-year study of haloperidol decanoate in schizophrenic patients. Curr Ther Res 1982;31:976–981.

28. Bucci L, Marini S. Haloperidol decanoate in chronic schizophrenic patients. Curr Ther Res 1985;37:1091–1097.

29. Kane JM. Dosage strategies with long-acting injectable neuroleptics, including haloperidol decanoate. J Clin Psychopharmacol 1986;6 (suppl):20S–23S.

30. Kissling W, Moller HJ, Walter K, Wittmann B, Krueger R, Trenk D. Double-blind comparison of haloperidol decanoate and fluphenazine decanoate effectiveness, adverse effects, dosage and serum levels during a six months' treatment for relapse prevention. Pharmacopsychiatry 1985; 18:240–245.

31. Wistedt B, Persson T, Hellbom E. A clinical double-blind comparison between haloperidol decanoate and fluphenazine decanoate. Curr Ther Res 1984;35:804–814.

32. Chouinard G, Annable L, Campbell W, Boisvert D, Bradwejn J. A double-blind, controlled clinical trial of haloperidol decanoate and fluphenazine decanoate in the maintenance treatment of schizophrenia. Psychopharmacol Bull 1984;20(1):108–109.

Pharmacokinetics/Plasma Levels

Clinically relevant pharmacokinetic factors involving the antipsychotics include:

• Good *absorption* from the gastrointestinal tract
• An extensive *"first-pass"* hepatic effect

• *Subsequent high systemic clearance* due to this large hepatic extraction ratio each time the plasma recirculates through the liver
• *Extensive distribution* (V_D) due to highly lipophilic character

- *Plasma half-life* ($t_{1/2}$) of about 20 hours
- Primary *route of elimination* is hepatic metabolism
- The presence of *metabolites* with varying pharmacological profiles (e.g., some may be more effective than their parent compound (e.g., mesoridazine); some may not reach the brain (e.g., sulfoxides); and some may have greater toxicity than the parent compound).

Antipsychotics are a chemically diverse group of drugs having in common the ability to ameliorate psychotic symptoms. Unfortunately, a significant percentage of patients fail to respond adequately or may develop adverse effects such as acute EPS; various tardive syndromes (e.g., TD, dystonia, etc.); and less commonly, even more life-threatening adverse events such as NMS.

The utilization of drug plasma levels to effect optimal clinical response and to minimize adverse or toxic effects is standard practice in general medicine (e.g., phenytoin, digoxin), as well as in psychiatry (e.g., lithium, TCAs, and carbamazepine) (see Chapter 3). The theoretical basis for plasma level monitoring rests on several factors, including:

- The existence of a *long interval* between drug administration and clinical response
- *Large interindividual differences* in response to the same dose for the same diagnosis
- It may help establish the *minimally effective dose*
- It may help *estimate the average dose* required to achieve a certain concentration when a positive correlation exists between a given steady state concentration (C_{SS}) and the dose required.

Unfortunately, for a number of methodological and clinical reasons, similar success (as with the TCAs) has not been achieved with the monitoring of antipsychotic steady state plasma concentrations. The major difficulties are:

- *Insufficient sample sizes*
- The inclusion of *refractory, nonhomogeneous, noncompliant* patients
- *Nonrandom adjustment of the dose* based on response, adverse effects, or initial presentation
- *Concurrent treatments*
- Too brief an *observation period* for clinical effects to occur
- Variable time of *blood sampling*
- *Inadequate evaluation* of clinical response
- Presence of numerous active *metabolites*
- Inadequate *assay methods*, such as radioreceptor assays (RRA).

FIXED DOSE DESIGNS

Literature Review

While large interindividual variability in the steady state plasma concentrations among patients treated with similar doses of a given antipsychotic is well established, the existence of a critical range of plasma concentration for therapeutic response or significant adverse effects remains controversial. However, there is a growing body of data from a number of fixed-dose studies, some of which indicate a possible linear or curvilinear (inverted U-shaped) relationship between plasma levels and clinical response for such agents as:

- Chlorpromazine (1)
- Fluphenazine (2, 3)
- Trifluoperazine (4)
- Thiothixene (5)
- Haloperidol (6–13).

Prospective studies targeting large numbers of acutely ill patients to certain plasma levels to test a putative therapeutic threshold or range are also being conducted for agents such as haloperidol.

Chlorpromazine

Curry et al. found a wide range of effective plasma drug levels in schizophrenics treated with comparable doses of CPZ, establishing that an upward or downward shift of 50% in dose usually produced adverse effects or an exacerbation, respectively (14, 15). In one patient who had not responded to 1900 mg of orally administered CPZ daily, a one-third reduction resulted in a corresponding decrease in the plasma level as well as a satisfactory clinical response. Wode-Helgodt et al. studied CPZ plasma concentrations in 44 schizophrenics on different doses in a constant dose design (1). They found a positive correlation between plasma levels and clinical response, suggesting a lower threshold level of 40 ng/ml. By contrast, May et al. found no relationship between plasma levels and response in 48 patients on fixed doses of CPZ (6.6 mg/kg/day) (16). It is important to note that this agent is particularly problematic because of its many, potentially confounding, metabolites, which are typically not measured.

Fluphenazine

Several groups have investigated fluphenazine plasma levels with either the oral or the intramuscular, depot form. In one study, clinical response as a function of the mean C_{SS} of oral fluphenazine suggested an upper therapeutic end based on three nonresponding patients who had mean C_{SS} above 2.8 ng/ml (3). Further, a lower end was suggested by two nonresponders and one partial responder whose levels were below 0.2 ng/ml. More recently, Van Putten et al. found that higher fluphenazine plasma levels (up to 4.23 ng/ml) were significantly associated with a higher rate of improvement; however, 90% (65 of 72 patients) experienced disabling adverse effects with levels greater than 2.7 ng/ml (17). In a 2-year, double-blind comparison of 5 mg or 25 mg of fluphenazine decanoate, Marder et al. found a significant relationship between fluphenazine plasma levels and psychotic exacerbations after 6–9 months of maintenance therapy (18). Thus, those with levels less than 0.5 ng/ml did much worse than those with levels above 1.0 ng/ml. Therefore, levels between 1.0 and 2.8 ng/ml may be the ideal range for most patients.

Trifluoperazine

Recently, we reported on a potential therapeutic window with the commonly used phenothiazine trifluoperazine (4). An acutely psychotic group of patients (N = 36) was treated with a relatively low, fixed dose (5 mg twice a day) for 2 weeks. Clinical improvement was correlated with plasma levels at the end of this treatment phase. As with previous studies, there was a wide interindividual difference in steady state levels (i.e., range = 0.20–3.50 ng/ml; or an 18-fold difference). There was also evidence for a lower therapeutic threshold, around 1 ng/ml, and a suggestion of an upper end around 2.3 ng/ml (see Fig. 5.10). While trifluoperazine is known to have active metabolites in plasma, it is unknown whether they pass the blood-brain barrier, and because this study only measured the parent compound, their potential impact is unknown. While there was some heterogeneity in the diagnostic categories (i.e., 30 patients were diagnosed as schizophrenic, five as schizoaffective, and one as unspecified functional psychosis), the design was such that a drug response was fully expected, because all patients had experienced a recent, florid, clearly ratable, psy-

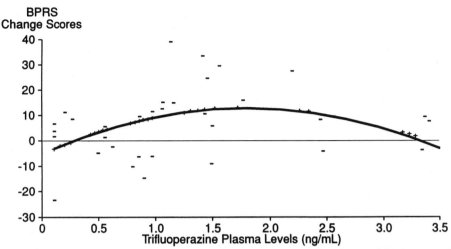

Figure 5.10.   Brief Psychiatric Rating Scale change scores in relationship to trifluoperazine plasma levels. Janicak PG, Javaid JI, Sharma RP, et al. Trifluoperazine plasma levels and clinical response. J Clin Psychopharmacol 1989; 9:340–346.

chotic exacerbation (i.e., delusions and/or hallucinations) requiring acute hospitalization. Further, when the results were analyzed using only those 30 patients diagnosed as schizophrenic, the outcome was virtually identical. All patients improved sufficiently during the index admission (average hospital stay approximately 2 months) and were discharged to outpatient care.

Based on our review of dose-response studies, 9–15 mg of trifluoperazine would be almost equivalent to 300 mg of CPZ and should fall near the lower part of the linear portion of the dose-response curve. Indeed, with a 10 mg dose, there appeared to be a lower end (1 ng/ml plasma) to a postulated therapeutic window in the present patient sample that is consistent with the previous predicted dose-response calculations. There were also preliminary data defining a potential upper end (i.e., 2.3 ng/ml plasma) of the therapeutic window for this drug.

Thiothixene

Yesavage et al. treated 48 acute schizophrenics with thiothixene (80 mg/day),

measuring serum and RBC concentrations 2 hours after the morning dose (19). Serum levels ranged from 3–45 ng/ml, with a linear relation between clinical response during the first week of treatment and serum (r = 0.5) as well as red blood cell (RBC) levels (r = 0.64). By contrast, Mavroidis et al. found a curvilinear relationship between thiothixene plasma levels and clinical response (5). Thus, levels ranging between 2.0 and 15 ng/ml, measured 10 to 12 hours after the dose, were associated with clinical improvement; however, of 19 patients, only 1 had plasma levels greater than 15 ng/ml.

Haloperidol

Haloperidol (HPDL) is the most commonly prescribed antipsychotic, and unlike most others, it has only one pharmacologically active metabolite (i.e., reduced haloperidol). We recently reviewed the literature on HPDL plasma levels and summarized the outcome (20). Although there are several studies examining the relationship between HPDL steady state plasma levels and clinical response, they have used varying methodologies in terms of patient selection, symptom profile, diagnostic criteria, assay techniques, and the use of variable or fixed dose schedules. Hence, the results of these studies are difficult to interpret collectively. As with other agents, the results with the fixed dose studies of HPDL have also been conflicting, although at least six have demonstrated a curvilinear relationship (i.e., therapeutic window) between its plasma levels and clinical response. Whereas optimal levels differed slightly among these studies, the mean low end was 4.2 ng/ml, and the mean high end was 16.8 ng/ml (6–11, 13) (see Table 5.16).

Positive Studies.   Mavroidis et al. studied 14 DSM-III schizophrenics for 2 weeks (7). After a 2-day washout, patients were randomly assigned to fixed doses of 6 mg/day, 12 mg/day, or 24 mg/day for 14 days. Patients were rated with the New Haven Schizophrenic Index (NHSI), and plasma HPDL was measured by gas liquid chromatographic assay (GLC). Their study suggested that a curvilinear relationship existed between HPDL plasma levels and NHSI ratings (i.e., at least a 40% improvement) with a therapeutic window between 4.2 and 11.0 ng/ml over the 2-week treatment course. In a study of RBC and plasma HPDL levels (also measured by GLC in the same patient population), Garver et al. found, in a further analysis, evidence for a plasma therapeutic range (3.4–11 ng/ml) by day 14 of treatment using the same fixed doses (6, 12, or 24 mg/day) (8). Seventeen patients who met DSM III criteria for schizophrenia in acute exacerbation were assessed for changes in baseline pathology with the serial modified NHSI. Of the 14 patients who completed the 2-week trial, those whose levels were within this range (N = 6) showed a significantly better response than those who were outside this range (N = 8).

Smith et al. studied 27 Research Diagnostic Criteria (RDC)-diagnosed schizophrenic or schizoaffective patients over 24 days (6). They excluded patients with a history of nonresponse to antipsychotics, long inpatient hospitalizations, or lack of predominance of positive symptoms from the study. Patients were kept drug-free from 1–3 weeks and then randomly assigned to 10 mg/day or 25 mg/day of HPDL, and blood was drawn 11½ hours after the last dose and plasma levels mea-

Table 5.16.
Fixed-Dose Studies Finding a Curvilinear Relationship between Haloperidol Plasma Levels and Clinical Response[a]

Study	Assay Method[b]	Therapeutic Range	Rating Scale	Study Duration
Garver (1984) Mavroidis (1983)	GLC	4–11 ng/ml	NHSI	14 Days
Smith (1984)	GLC (RRA)	7–17 ng/ml	BPRS Psychosis Factor	24 Days
Potkin (1985)	RIA	4–26 ng/ml	CGI	6 Weeks
Van Putten (1985)	RIA	5–16 ng/ml	BPRS	7 Days
Van Putten (1988)	RIA	2–12 ng/ml	BPRS Psychosis Factor	4 Weeks
Santos (1989)	RIA	12–35.5 ng/ml (7.4–24.9 in subchronic group)	BPRS Total Score	21 Days

[a]Adapted from Janicak PG, Javaid JI, Davis JM. Neuroleptic plasma levels: methodological issues, study design, and clinical applicability. In: Marder SR, Davis JM, Janicak PG, eds. Clinical use of neuroleptic plasma levels. Washington DC: APPI Press, pp. 17–44, in press.
[b]See Table 1.8.

sured by both GLC and RRA. They reported a curvilinear relationship between the GLC-measured plasma levels and the BPRS psychosis factor, with maximum efficacy related to plasma levels between 7 and 17 ng/ml. Even though a subsequent letter by Smith reported an inability to replicate their original results, when the data was combined (i.e., the old and the new samples, excluding the presumed chronic nonresponders), a significant relationship persisted (21).

Potkin et al. studied 43 DSM-III diagnosed schizophrenic and schizophreniform patients (17–45 years old) with an illness duration less than 5 years (9). Patients were drug free for 1 week and randomly assigned to a fixed-dose schedule of either 0.4 mg/kg body weight or 0.15 mg/kg body weight of haloperidol for 45 days. The Clinical Global Index (CGI) and the Brief Psychiatric Rating Scale (BPRS) were used on days 7, 14, 28, and 42, and plasma levels were obtained 12 hours after the last dose and were measured by radioimmunoassay (RIA). This study again suggested a curvilinear relationship between blood levels and clinical ratings, with a therapeutic window between 4.0 and 26.0 ng/ml.

Van Putten et al. studied 47 schizophrenic patients who were drug free up to 3 weeks and then randomly assigned to fixed doses of 5 mg/day, 10 mg/day, or 20 mg/day of HPDL (10). After 4 weeks, the dose for nonresponders was increased up to 30 mg/day for another 4 weeks. Patients were evaluated with the BPRS, Nurses' Observation Scale for Inpatient Evaluation (NOSIE), and CGI rating scales; blood was drawn 12 hours after the last dose; and HPDL was measured by RIA. They reported a curvilinear relationship between the BPRS/CGI and plasma levels only during the first week of treatment, with a therapeutic range of 5–16 ng/ml. They also noted that the daily dose positively corre-

lated with plasma levels. A second study by Van Putten et al. (1988) included 76 male schizophrenic patients, used an RIA assay, and found a curvilinear relationship (i.e., 2–12 ng/ml) between HPDL plasma levels and the BPRS psychosis factor after 4 weeks of treatment (11).

Santos et al. (1989) treated 30 schizophrenic patients with three randomly assigned doses of haloperidol (15, 20, and 30 mg/day) for 21 days, after at least 10 days washout from oral and 4 months from depot medication (13). Ten patients each were assigned to one of the three fixed-dose groups, and plasma levels were determined on treatment days 4, 7, 14, and 21 with RIA. They found evidence for an inverted U-shaped relationship between the percent improvement from baseline on the total BPRS and the C_{SS} of haloperidol, with an overall effective concentration range of 12.0–35.5 ng/ml. When patients were classified as subchronic or chronic, however, the therapeutic ranges were 7.4–24.9 ng/ml and 14.8–38.5 ng/ml, respectively. They postulated that, possibly due to the development of tolerance in the DA system(s), the effective concentration interval may vary with chronicity of illness.

Two other studies with more complicated methodologies had similar findings. Magliozzi et al. reported a fixed-dose study on 17 patients (16 outpatients) over a period of 3–12 weeks (22). The fixed doses ranged from 2 mg/day to 120 mg/day, with plasma levels ranging from undetectable to 96 ng/ml. Of the 17 individuals, two had their doses changed during the study. Magliozzi used an "index of improvement" to determine response and showed that improvement was significantly greater for patients who had a mean HPDL serum concentration between 8 and 18 ng/ml. Davis et al. conducted a 3-week fixed-dose study in 25 acutely decompensated schizophrenics (12). This was a comparison study of high-dose haloperidol (60 mg/day, i.m., for 5 days, followed by p.o. 45 mg/day for 2 days, 30 mg/day for 2 days, 20 mg/day for 3 days, and then 15 mg/day for the final week of the study); and standard dose HPDL (15 mg/day, p.o., for 3 weeks). They found that 43% of the responders had plasma levels between 5 and 21 ng/ml, in contrast to only 10% of the nonresponders.

Negative Studies. There have also been a number of studies that show a linear relationship or no correlation at all between plasma HPDL and clinical response.

Volavka and Cooper reviewed seven HPDL fixed-dose studies and found that two demonstrated a linear relationship and five demonstrated no relationship (23). The studies with a linear relationship had used low doses (6 mg/day and 0.2 mg/kg/day, respectively); hence, it may be that they were only reaching the lower limits of a possible therapeutic window. Of the five studies that showed no relationship at all, two used chronically ill patients and one used a heterogeneous group of psychotic disorders.

Perry et al. reviewed five studies that included only schizophrenics who were on fixed-dose schedules, were treated for 2 or more weeks, and demonstrated at least a 30% improvement on the BPRS (24). Using a logistic regression analysis, they found that these studies together demonstrated a linear rather than a curvilinear relationship between HPDL plasma levels and clinical response.

TARGETED PLASMA LEVEL DESIGNS

Thus far, the most valid experimental design for examining the relationship between blood levels and clinical response has employed fixed doses and analyzed the relationship retrospectively. In many of these studies, however, the number of patients who did not respond at higher plasma levels was very small. Further, because the data were analyzed after the completion of the study, we do not know if these patients would have responded had there been a reduction in their plasma levels. There are also statistical problems with a post hoc assignment to a given plasma level category using data from a single study. Because the plasma level-clinical response relationship may be non-linear, it would be useful to characterize this relationship with the initial data so that subsequent validation studies can be conducted. To confirm such a categorization one could pool data from several studies to achieve an adequate sample size that would clearly define the optimal cutoff point for a lower end and possibly for an upper end as well, and then use these data to design a targeted plasma level study.

Since such data are available for HPDL, various investigators are presently conducting "targeted" plasma level studies to prospectively test the hypothesis of a curvilinear relationship with HPDL.

Volavka et al. failed to find evidence for a therapeutic window after randomly assigning 111 schizophrenic or schizoaffective patients to one of three HPDL plasma levels (i.e., 2–13; 13.1–24; or 24.1–35 ng/ml) for 6 weeks (25). Patients who did not respond were then reassigned to another level for an additional 6 weeks. Interpretation of their results, however, may be complicated by too high a level for the low and perhaps middle ranges and a prolonged period of time to titrate to the middle and high HPDL plasma levels.

An ongoing study at the Illinois State Psychiatric Institute includes patients hospitalized with an acute exacerbation of their psychosis who are first randomly assigned in a double-blind design to one of three empirical doses (2, 5, or 10 mg bid) to achieve a "targeted" HPDL C_{SS} range of >5 ng/ml (low), 6–18 ng/ml (middle), or ≥25 ng/ml (high). If a patient does not achieve the assigned range after 5 days, the dose is adjusted using the following formula:

$$D_2 = D_1 \times C_{SS2} \div C_{SS1}$$

where D_1 is the original dose; D_2 is the new dose required for the "targeted" C_{SS2}; and, C_{SS1} is the observed steady state concentration with the original dose.

As part of this study a dose prediction formula was developed to more rapidly achieve the desired HPDL C_{SS}. For this purpose the first 28 patients, prior to receiving the initial assigned dose for achieving their targeted level, received a 15 mg "test" dose (PO) of HPDL, and blood samples were drawn 24 and 48 hours afterwards. Data analysis indicated a strong linear relationship between the targeted log C_{SS} achieved and the dose required when the 24 hour log transformed plasma level was included in a linear regression model (r = 0.933) (26). This formula is now being prospectively tested for its validity in determining the dose required to achieve the desired HPDL C_{SS}. Figure 5.11 demonstrates the range and mean HPDL plasma level C_{SS} achieved thus far during the first treatment phase.

Once the "targeted" C_{SS} range is achieved a patient is maintained on the same dose for 2 weeks. If there is a 30% or greater improvement from the baseline BPRS score, patients are classified as responders and remain in their assigned plasma level range for 2 more weeks. Half of the initial nonresponders in the low and the high ranges are reassigned to the middle range, and half of the middle level initial nonresponders are assigned to the high plasma level to ascertain whether

they then convert to a responder status. The other half of the nonresponders remain in their originally assigned plasma level to control for the effect of time on treatment response.

Results on the first 55 patients revealed the following qualitative outcomes:

- *Low Group*
  - 40% (2 of 5) of the initial nonresponders reassigned to the middle group converted to responders.
  - 20% (1 of 5) of the initial nonresponders assigned to remain in the low group converted to responders.
  - 17% (1 of 6) of the initial responders assigned to remain in the low group worsened (i.e., their total BPRS scores increased).
- *Middle Group*
  - 50% (2 of 4) of the initial nonresponders assigned to remain in the middle group converted to responders.
- *High Group*
  - 75% (3 of 4) of the initial nonresponders reassigned to the middle group converted to responders.
  - 60% (3 of 5) of the initial responders assigned to remain in the high group worsened.

After an adequate sample size has been obtained, the results of this study should help to establish or refute the existence of a plasma level-clinical response relationship for HPDL in acute psychotic exacerbations.

Case Example. A 29-year-old female was admitted to our research unit due to an exacerbation of her schizoaffective disorder. After giving informed consent, the patient participated in the targeted HPDL plasma level study. She was randomly assigned initially to the high plasma level and began treatment with 60 mg/day of HPDL for 3 weeks. She scored a 40 on the BPRS at baseline (after an 11-day medication-free period). Her mean HPDL plasma level was 38.4 ng/ml for the first 3

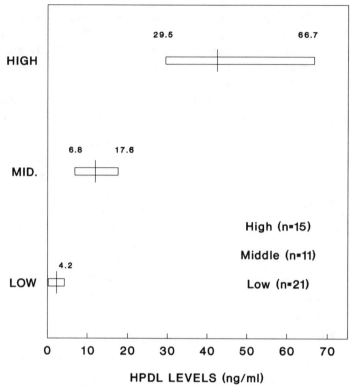

Figure 5.11.   Haloperidol (HPDL) plasma level ranges and means by targeted groups.

weeks, and her BPRS score was 39 at the end of that period. She was then randomly reassigned to a middle plasma level, with a reduction of HPDL to 16 mg/day. At the end of this phase (24 days later), the patient's BPRS score was 22, with an average plasma level of 14.2 ng/ml. After no improvement in the first phase, the patient experienced a 45% decrease from her total baseline BPRS score during the second phase. Keeping in mind the lowest score on the BPRS is 18, this was an 82% drop in ratable symptoms.

Case Example. A 29-year-old male schizophrenic patient was admitted to our research unit due to a worsening in his paranoid delusions and auditory hallucinations. After giving informed consent and undergoing a 12-day medication washout, he scored a 48 on the BPRS. He was randomly assigned initially to a low plasma level and received haloperidol, 2 mg/day, with an average plasma level of 1.29 ng/ml over 3 weeks. He demonstrated a slight

improvement, scoring a 37 on the BPRS at that point (i.e., a 23% change). He was then randomly reassigned to a middle plasma level, and the dose of haloperidol was increased to 18 mg/day. After 27 days, he had an average plasma level of 12.0 ng/ml, and rated a 21 on the BPRS, or a 55% improvement from his baseline symptoms. Again, considering 18 is the lowest total BPRS score possible, this was an 84% drop in rateable symptoms.

Both patients demonstrated clinically relevant and statistically significant decreases in psychotic symptoms after their plasma HPDL concentrations were targeted within the 10–15 ng/ml range. While it is possible they improved during the second phase solely due to time on treatment, their scores on the BPRS dropped rapidly, once switched into the middle range. In addition, they demonstrated little to minimal improvement during the first 3 weeks.

Scores on the Simpson Angus side-effect scale were in the mild range for both patients, and did not change during either phase. Thus, this would not support decrease in toxicity as the reason for improvement, especially when the dose, and blood levels, were reduced in the first patient.

CONCLUSION

In summary, the value of routine plasma level monitoring remains uncertain; however, TDM can be useful in the following situations:

- To determine patient *compliance*
- To establish *adequacy* of the pharmaco-therapy in nonresponders
- To *avoid toxicity* due to unnecessarily high plasma levels
- To monitor patients with other *medical disorders* and/or on *concurrent psychotropics or other medical drugs*
- To *maximize the clinical response* where the drug plasma level-response relationship is elucidated
- To help define the *dose-response relationship*
- To safeguard clinicians in potential *medical-legal situations.*

REFERENCES

1. Wode-Helgodt B, Borg S, Fyro B, Sedvall G. Clinical effects and drug concentrations in plasma and cerebrospinal fluid in psychotic patients treated with fixed doses of chlorpromazine. Acta Psychiatr Scand 1978;58:149–173.
2. Chang SS, Javaid JI, Dysken MW, Casper RC, Janicak PG, Davis, JM. Plasma levels of fluphenazine during fluphenazine decanoate treatment in schizophrenia. Psychopharmacology 1985;87:55–58.
3. Dysken MW, Javaid JI, Chang SS, Schaffer C, Shahid A, Davis, JM. Fluphenazine

pharmacokinetics and therapeutic response. Psychopharmacology 1981;73:205–210.
4. Janicak PG, Javaid JI, Sharma RP, Comaty JE, Peterson J, Davis JM. Trifluoperazine plasma levels and clinical response. J Clin Psychopharmacol 1989;9(5):340–346.
5. Mavroidis ML, Kanter DR, Hirschowitz J, Garver, DL. Clinical relevance of thiothixene plasma levels. J Clin Psychopharmacol 1984;4(3):155–157.
6. Smith RC, Baumgartner R, Misra CH, Mauldin M, Shvartsburd A, Ho BT, De John C. Haloperidol. Plasma levels and prolactin response as predictors of clinical improvement in schizophrenia. Chemical versus radioreceptor plasma level assays. Arch Gen Psychiatry 1984;41:1044–1049.
7. Mavroidis ML, Garver L. Plasma haloperidol levels and clinical response: confounding variables. Psychopharmacol Bull 1985; 21:62–65.
8. Garver DL, Hirschowitz J, Glicksteen GA, Kanter DR, Mavroidis ML. Haloperidol plasma and red blood cell levels and clinical antipsychotic response. J Clin Psychopharmacol 1984;4:133–137.
9. Potkin SG, Shen Y, Zhou D, Pardes H, Shu L, Phelps B, Poland R. Does a therapeutic window for plasma haloperidol exist? Preliminary Chinese data. Psychopharmacol Bull 1985;21(1):59–61.
10. Van Putten T, Marder SR, May PRA, Poland RE, O'Brien RP. Plasma levels of haloperidol and clinical response. Psychopharmacol Bull 1985;21:69–72.
11. Van Putten T, Marder SR, Mintz J, Poland RE. Haloperidol plasma levels and clinical response: a therapeutic window relationship. Psychopharmacol Bull 1988;24:172–175.
12. Davis JM, Ericksen SE, Hurt S, Chang SS, Javaid JI, Dekirmenjian H, Casper R. Haloperidol plasma levels and clinical response: basic concepts and clinical data. Psychopharmacol Bull 1985;21:48–51.
13. Santos JL, Cabranes JA, Vasquez FF, Almoguera I, Ramos JA. Clinical response and plasma haloperidol levels in chronic and subchronic schizophrenia. Biol Psychiatry 1989;26:381–388.
14. Curry SH. Determination of nanogram quantities of chlorpromazine or its metabolites in plasma using gas liquid chromatography with an electron capture detector. Anal Chem 1968;40:1251–1255.
15. Curry SH, Marshall JHL, Davis JM, Janowsky DS. Chlorpromazine plasma levels

and effects. Arch Gen Psychiatry 1970; 22:289–296.

16. May PRA, Van Putten T, Jenden DJ, Yale C, Dixon WJ. Chlorpromazine levels and the outcome of treatment in schizophrenic patients. Arch Gen Psychiatry 1981;38: 202–207.

17. Van Putten T, Aravagiri M, Marder SR, Wirshing WC, Mintz J, Chabert N. Plasma fluphenazine levels and clinical response in newly admitted schizophrenic patients. Psychopharmacol Bull 1991;27(2):91–96.

18. Marder SR, Van Putten T, Aravagiri M, Hawes EM, Hubbard JW, McKay G, Mintz J, Midha KK. Fluphenazine plasma levels and clinical response. Psychopharmacol Bull 1990;26:256–259.

19. Yesavage JA, Holman CA, Cohn R, Lombrozo L. Correlation of initial serum levels and clinical response. Arch Gen Psychiatry 1983;40:301–304.

20. Janicak PG, Javaid JI, Davis JM. Neuroleptic plasma levels: methodological issues, study design, and clinical applicability. APPI Press (in Press)

21. Smith, RC. Plasma haloperidol levels and clinical response. Arch Gen Psychiatry 1987;44:1110–1112.

22. Magliozzi JR, Hollister LE, Arnold KV, Earle GM. Relationship of serum haloperidol levels to clinical response in schizophrenic patients. Am J Psychiatry 1981; 138(3):365–367.

23. Volavka J, Cooper TB. Review of haloperidol level and clinical response: looking through the window. J Clin Psychopharmacol 1987;7:25–30.

24. Perry PJ, Pfohl BM, Kelly MW. The relationship of haloperidol concentrations to therapeutic response. J Clin Psychopharmacol 1988;8:38–43.

25. Volavka J, Cooper T, Czobor P, Bitter I, Meisner M, Laska E, Gastanaga P, Krakowski M, Chou JC-Y, Crowner M, Douyon R. Haloperidol blood levels and clinical effects. Arch Gen Psychiatry 1992; 49:354–361.

26. Javaid JI, Janicak PG, Hedeker D, Sharma, RP, Davis, JM. Steady-state plasma level prediction for haloperidol from a single test dose. Psychopharmacol Bull 1991;27(1):83–88.

Alternate Treatment Strategies

In partially responsive or nonresponsive patients the first issue is to determine if an individual is truly treatment-resistant, since many receive subtherapeutic doses and are too hastily considered refractory. In such situations, more aggressive treatment (dose increase; augmentation) may be appropriate, if not precluded by adverse effects. In selected cases it may also be helpful to monitor plasma levels to assure that they are in a reasonable range (see Pharmacokinetics/Plasma Levels earlier in this chapter). If a patient continues to demonstrate significant symptoms after a sufficient trial (2–3 weeks) the addition of lithium, an anticonvulsant, or an antidepressant may be helpful, especially if affective symptoms are present.

There is no evidence that combining two APs is superior to comparable amounts of a single agent. For studies to address this question validly, treatment groups must be given bioequivalent amounts of medication. When this is done, increasing the dose of a single agent demonstrated a similar dose-response relationship to the combination of two drugs.

DOSING STRATEGY

Whereas lower doses are desirable and often sufficient, some patients may require short-term, higher dose treatment. Because many clinicians are reluctant to use this approach fearful of severe adverse effects, they may prematurely seek alternative strategies. These concerns may not be entirely warranted, however. For example,

Dubin et al. reviewed 10 papers addressing the prevalence of adverse effects during rapid tranquilization in 676 cases (1). Overall, their prevalence was extremely low (<8%) and consisted mostly of EPS or hypotension (with low potency agents).

Tardive dyskinesia is also frequently mentioned as a reason to minimize exposure, but this condition usually develops following more chronic exposure. **The relationship between TD and prior neuroleptic dosing is uncertain at this time, and the authors are not aware of any studies indicating that an acute, time-limited use of higher neuroleptic doses increases the prevalence of this disorder** (2). Fortunately, the occurrence of the neuroleptic malignant syndrome (NMS) is an infrequent event (less than 1.5%), and no occurrences were noted in the 676 cases reviewed by Dubin. In the discussion on adverse effects, however, we note a higher incidence has been found by others during rapid dose increases.

ANTIPSYCHOTICS PLUS OTHER PSYCHOTROPICS

A second major question is the relative benefit of other concurrent psychotropic agents. Issues that are often raised include:

- Do adjunctive *benzodiazepines* help aggressivity in psychotic patients?
- Do adjunctive *mood stabilizers* help depressed, excited or apathetic schizophrenic patients?
- Do adjunctive *anticonvulsants* help with seizure-related complications, associated aggression, or affective symptoms?

Benzodiazepines Plus Antipsychotics

Despite the advent of new, atypical APs, there are continued efforts to identify other adjunctive medications that may improve response to standard treatments. One such strategy is the addition of benzodiazepines to an antipsychotic regimen. This pharmacological approach is partially based on the evidence that GABA, which is facilitated by BZDs, inhibits certain dopamine tracts and that these medications may attenuate the dopamine system via a different route (3–7).

Literature Review

Most of the literature addressing this issue consists of anecdotal reports; retrospective chart reviews; uncontrolled studies in small patient samples; plus a small number of controlled trials. To our knowledge at least 12 studies (including over 450 patients) have evaluated the efficacy of adjunctive BZDs in nonresponsive schizophrenics (Table 5.17). Two of three open studies showed positive results, as did two controlled, single-blind studies (8–12). In seven double-blind, crossover studies (six with placebo controls) the results are more contradictory, in that five showed no advantage to an adjunctive BZD, and one of the two positive studies had a small sample size (13–19).

A chart review of 380 patients discharged from the Boston Veterans Administration Hospital found one group who were prescribed either an antipsychotic alone (N = 22, mean dose = 560 mg/day CPZ eq.) or with lorazepam (N = 8, mean dose = 265 mg/day CPZ eq.; 2.75 mg/day lorzepam) (20). Although it was concluded that the addition of lorazepam necessitated less antipsychotic, the patient distribution was quite unequal (only eight patients were on AP/BZD treatment), and this trend may have disappeared with a larger, more equalized sample size. A second group of 32 patients, discharged during the same time period, were prescribed an

Table 5.17.
Benzodiazepines (type/dose range) Used in Controlled Treatment Trials of Schizophrenia

As Sole Agent	In Conjunction with Antipsychotics
Chlordiazepoxide (20–700 mg/day)	Alprazolam (0.5 mg/day to highest dose tolerated)
Diazepam (15–400 mg/day)	Camazepam (40 mg/day)
	Chlordiazepoxide (30–300 mg/day)
	Clonazepam (1 mg/day to optimum dose)
	Diazepam (15–200 mg/day)
	Estazolam (6 mg/day)
	Lorazepam (0.75 mg/day to highest dose tolerated)

antipsychotic (mean dose = 771 mg/day CPZ eq.) and benztropine, or an antipsychotic (933 mg/day CPZ eq.), benztropine, and lorazepam. Those treated with the AP/BZD combination plus benztropine were actually on higher doses of an AP in comparison to the antipsychotic-alone group, contradicting the earlier results.

The Spring Grove State Hospital group compared a phenothiazine plus a benzodiazepine to a phenothiazine alone in a double-blind, random-assignment trial and found the combination inferior to the single agent (15, 16). Clinicians could increase the dose of the blinded medication until the patient became sedated. As a result, a much lower dose of phenothiazine was used when combined with the BZD than when given alone, probably because of the excessive sedation. Thus, the lower doses of phenothiazine in the combination group could have contributed to their poorer response.

Catatonia

Recently, a large number of case reports have found that BZDs (mainly lorazepam) are effective in the treatment of catatonia. Lorazepam, clonazepam and diazepam have been reported to induce temporary remission of catatonic symptoms (21–28). BZD treatment of catatonia is usually considered diagnostic, however, because symptoms return as the drug's therapeutic effect wanes. Continuing BZD treatment may produce longer symptom remission, but treatment should be directed to the underlying cause of the catatonia (29). In a review of 30 cases (with various psychiatric diagnoses), only two organic patients failed to demonstrate a significant clinical response (23, 30). Based on these reports, lorazepam appears to be effective in "functional" catatonia. Further, i.v. diazepam (10–20 mg) has also been reported to be effective (27). All these cases are consistent, in that patients tended to demonstrate a marked response to i.m. or i.v. administration of a BZD, and this response persisted when the medication was given on a maintenance basis (usually p.o.). By contrast, patients tended to relapse within 24 hours if the BZD was discontinued prior to initiating treatment for the underlying psychopathology. The motivation to use lorazepam is its safe and rapid onset of action. If adequate results are not seen quickly (i.e., after 4–8 hours of 2 mg i.m. q 2 hours), however, one should then treat aggressively with a high potency antipsychotic. With careful monitoring, antipsychotics have been noted to produce symptom reduction within 24–96 hours. ECT should also be considered if the situation is deteriorating and/or life threatening. Catatonia is an infrequent event, and for obvious ethical reasons controlled studies would be impossible. Thus, while many of these case reports are impressive and indicate the effectiveness of parenteral BZDs, confirmatory controlled trials are unlikely.

Adverse Effects

Although less toxic than antipsychotics, benzodiazepines can produce adverse effects (31–35). Ataxia, sedation, dysarthria, nausea, vomiting, confusion, excitation, disinhibition, and/or assaultiveness have all been reported. In one study, 32% experienced sedation and drowsiness, and 34% demonstrated arousal, excitation, or assaultiveness resembling a manic state (this was higher than reported in most other studies) (20). Thus, although BZDs may benefit some patients, they may be counterproductive in others.

Conclusion

In summarizing the results, there appears to be little or no advantage to an AP/BZD combination in most patients. There was a consistent, although small, group of individuals, however, who demonstrated a rapid, dramatic, and sustained response (e.g., catatonic) when treated with this combination. Some attribute this to a placebo effect, but the quick onset, lasting effect and degree of improvement speak against this. Another possibility is that improvement may actually be secondary to relief from extra-pyramidal side effects, such as akathesia; however, it is unlikely that the dramatic improvement in some patients could be explained by this alone. Finally, there may be a small subpopulation that experiences a true drug effect. Thus, schizophrenia, viewed by many as a heterogeneous disease, may encompass subgroup(s) that benefit from BZDs (36). Definitive controlled studies using adequate doses of antipsychotics in both groups (i.e., antipsychotics alone versus an antipsychotic plus BZD) have yet to be done. In part, this is due to the excessive sedation seen in the combined drug group. To avoid this, low-dose high-potency, less-sedating agents (e.g., HPDL) should be employed.

In clearly nonresponding, nonaffective, psychotic patients, BZDs may be of benefit, but presently there is no way to predict which ones. Although there is no evidence that any particular BZD is more effective than another, we would recommend the use of higher potency agents such as lorazepam or clonazepam.

Antidepressants Plus Antipsychotics

A collaborative VA study (1961) found the addition of imipramine or an MAOI to CPZ did not benefit chronic psychotic patients any more than CPZ alone (37). Further, the addition of an amphetamine was slightly harmful. This finding has since been replicated in several studies on apathetic schizophrenic patients (38). A 1979 study of chronic ambulatory schizophrenics compared amitriptyline plus perphenazine to perphenazine alone (39). They found the combination slightly better in ameliorating depressive symptoms, but at the cost of a slight increase in patients' thought disorder.

Tricyclic antidepressants (TCAs) plus phenothiazines benefited an occasional patient with schizoaffective or catatonic symptoms. Since it is difficult to distinguish a severe, apathetic depression from a patient with catatonic features, an augmenting AD should be tried. TCAs may help a postpsychotic depression in outpatients, suggesting the importance of identifying subgroups that might benefit from this approach. Thus, while ADs do not appear helpful in the apathetic, negative-symptom patient, they may help those with a coexisting major depression. This combination is also much more effective than AD monotherapy in psychotic depression (see also Chapter 6).

More recently, preliminary findings indicate that the addition of fluoxetine may increase response or benefit treatment-resistant schizophrenic patients (40, 41). Further, deficit symptoms seemed to improve in some patients, supporting a possible role for $5\text{-}HT_2$ hypersensitivity as the underlying mechanism (42). Care must be taken to monitor plasma levels of such agents, which may rise when an AP is combined with this SRI.

Mood Stabilizers

Lithium

Because there is some evidence that lithium may help patients with schizoaffective or schizophreniform disorders, this raises the question of whether lithium added to an antipsychotic would produce a better response.

Biederman et al. (1979) compared haloperidol alone to HPDL plus lithium in a group of 36 schizoaffective patients and found four of 18 improved with HPDL, versus 11 of 18 on the combination (43).

Anticonvulsants

There is limited evidence that carbamazepine plus an AP may also benefit some schizophrenic patients—an interesting possibility in view of the similar antimanic properties of lithium and carbamazepine (44). This area requires further research, especially to clarify the indications for combining anticonvulsants with an antipsychotic. For example, mania complicated by psychotic features, may benefit from *lithium, carbamazapine,* or *valproic acid* (or valproate, or divalproex sodium) augmented by APs. Because CBZ induces the metabolism of at least some APs (e.g., haloperidol, thiothixene), dose adjustment based on TDM may be necessary to achieve the optimal effect.

NON-ANTIPSYCHOTIC ALTERNATIVES

Benzodiazepines

Although numerous controlled trials have examined the role of selected BZDs, their effects range from deterioration, to no change in most patients, to striking improvement in a rare patient when using BZDs either as the sole agent or as an adjunct to antipsychotics (15, 16, 18, 31, 36, 45–69). Reported effects include:

- *Amelioration of anxiety and tension* superimposed over chronic schizophrenia in 3 of 6 patients, a finding not replicated by others (58, 59, 71)
- An experimental benzodiazepine (estazolam) in addition to an antipsychotic *reduced auditory hallucinations* in selected chronic schizophrenics (18)
- A few studies find beneficial effects, but most find *no significant benefit or even deterioration* with BZD treatment.

When it occurs, onset of therapeutic activity may be rapid (within hours, days, or 1–2 weeks). Even in those few patients with good initial response, however, therapeutic effects attributable to BZDs may be temporary. Several controlled studies have found that tolerance developed by the fourth week of treatment (15, 16, 45, 55, 56, 67). High doses appear to be associated with more favorable response, but data are limited, contradictory, and inconclusive (11, 29, 31, 33).

There is little evidence available indicating that one BZD is more effective than another. Because the duration of most controlled studies has been 8 weeks or less, data on more prolonged treatment are anecdotal.

Sedation, ataxia and cognitive impairment may occur frequently with use of high BZD dosages. Other adverse effects reported with use of BZDs in the treatment of schizophrenia include behavioral disinhibition, exacerbation of psychosis and increase in anxiety and depression (15, 16, 18, 20, 31, 36, 54, 65, 70, 71). Concomitant use of a BZD and the atypical antipsychotic clozapine may increase the risk of sedation, dizziness and severe collapse with loss of consciousness (72).

Lithium

The role of lithium in treating schizophrenia has not been well delineated. Although it may be useful in certain patients with aggression, agitation, or psychomotor excitement, many believe it has no true antipsychotic properties. Clinical evidence from a small number of controlled trials find lithium alone is not beneficial for process schizophrenia. For example, an earlier double-blind, controlled trial of lithium versus chlorpromazine for chronic schizophrenics found lithium completely ineffective and possibly harmful in the more chronic patients, while the antipsychotic had its expected beneficial effect (73).

For many years, schizophrenia was divided into process (core) and reactive types. More recent investigations indicate

that the reactive psychotic group has many affective, as well as schizophrenic features (e.g., family histories). This distinction is recognized in the DSM-III-R as either schizophreniform, schizoaffective, or brief reactive psychosis.

It is possible that there are three major functional disorders:

- Core schizophrenia
- Reactive schizophreniform disorder
- Mood disorders

but the present nosological system only recognizes two categories:

- Schizophrenia
- Mood disorders.

Schizophreniform disorder is usually classified in the schizophrenic spectrum, but some would categorize it as a mood disorder. For many years, United States patients were diagnosed manic if they met narrowly defined criteria, and schizophrenia was a broader, more inclusive category. Recently, however, the DSM-III-R criteria for schizophrenia have become more restrictive, and the pendulum has swung, with some defining this diagnosis narrowly and mood disorders quite broadly. The picture is further complicated by those with mixed schizophrenic and manic symptoms, who are then classified as having a schizoaffective disorder.

There is a limited body of evidence that lithium helps atypical mania, schizoaffective, or schizophreniform disorder, both as an acute treatment and for prevention of recurrence. There are younger patients who demonstrate both schizophrenic and manic features early in the course of their illness. When in doubt about the diagnosis, lithium may be preferable for an acute episode because, if successful, it will most likely be an effective prophylaxis as well. Clearly, some are so disturbed that the clinician cannot wait until lithium becomes fully effective, and an antipsychotic must be added, but often it can be discontinued after a brief period to determine if lithium alone is sufficient.

Hirschowitz et al. (1980) further explored the range of lithium's efficacy by systematically treating patients with schizophrenic or schizophreniform disorders (74). They found that "poor prognosis" schizophrenia rarely responded to lithium, while good prognosis schizophrenia did benefit. Since there was no control group, it is possible that some were placebo responders.

Because little work has been done on the drug treatment of schizophreniform or brief reactive psychosis, investigations conducted at the Illinois State Psychiatric Institute are important to note. Patients presenting with acute schizophrenic symptoms underwent a drug-free washout period, received lithium only initially, and then APs later (74). Lithium was ineffective for core schizophrenia as defined by the DSM-III, but those meeting criteria for schizophreniform disorder did respond to lithium. Whether schizophreniform illness is a variant of mood disorders (a reasonable hypothesis in view of their lithium response) or a separate entity that is lithium-sensitive is still unclear. It is known that these patients have family histories that include mood disordered as well as schizophrenic relatives. In a small pilot study, physostigmine (a drug with possible antimanic but no antipsychotic properties) benefited schizophreniform patients who responded to lithium, but had no effect in those who did not (Garver DL, personal communication).

Antipsychotics have a broad-spectrum effect, improving psychosis in schizophrenia, schizophreniform disease, mania, and organic psychosis; but response to lithium suggests an affective core. **Whereas al-most all schizophreniform patients are presently treated with antipsychotics, it is possible that lithium may be more specific and safer in their management.**

Propranolol

Propranolol may have specific antiaggressive effects for mentally retarded, organic, and certain schizophrenic patients with episodic violence. High-dose propranolol in patients with episodic aggression has been recommended, but this is based primarily on case reports. These indications should be distinguished from its use with or without an antipsychotic as a specific treatment for schizophrenia. For example, some open studies using high doses of propranolol (i.e., 500 mg to 2 g) reported success in an occasional schizophrenic patient, but not all studies confirmed this outcome (75–82).

In a review of the literature, we found three controlled trials, one demonstrating propranolol to be slightly superior to an antipsychotic, but two others finding it no better than placebo for schizophrenia (83).

When given concurrently, there is limited evidence that this agent may increase an antipsychotic's plasma level, which could explain the enhanced effect. Thus, three controlled studies found propranolol plus an antipsychotic superior to propranolol alone; however, two studies found the combination no more effective than an antipsychotic alone. In view of these negative studies, propranolol's efficacy remains doubtful; but there is sufficient positive evidence to consider it potentially helpful for some patients.

Electroconvulsive Therapy

Antipsychotics have long since replaced insulin shock and ECT for the treatment of schizophrenia. Several studies, however, have found ECT equal in efficacy to these agents, while one large-sample, controlled trial found it less effective than drugs, but more effective than psychotherapy (84). Some clinicians believe that selected patients may benefit when ECT is given concurrently with an antipsychotic. For example, one controlled study found that ECT in combination with a phenothiazine led to a more rapid remission than the phenothiazine alone (85). Clinical experience has clearly documented an important role for ECT in catatonic excitement or withdrawal, as well as for other severe, life-endangering psychotic states.

CONCLUSION

Figure 5.4 demonstrates a strategy to manage an acute psychotic exacerbation, with alternate interventions if response is insufficient or complications, such as aggressivity, catatonia, or mood disturbances, occur.

REFERENCES

1. Dubin WR. Rapid tranquilization: antipsychotic or benzodiazepine. J Clin Psychiatry 1988;49(12):5–11.
2. Casey DE. Tardive dyskinesia. In: Meltzer HY, ed. Psychopharmacology, the third generation of progress. New York: Raven Press, 1987:1411–1419.
3. Fornum F. Biochemistry, anatomy, and pharmacology of GABA neurons. In: Meltzer HY, ed. Psychopharmacology: the third generation of progress. New York: Raven Press, 1987:173–182.
4. Garbutt J, VanKammen DPO. The interactions between GABA and dopamine: implications for schizophrenia. Schizophrenia Bull 1983;9(3):336–353.
5. Lloyd KG, Murselli PL. Psychopharmacology of GABAergic drugs. In: Meltzer HY, ed. Psychopharmacology: the third generation of progress. New York: Raven Press, 1987:183–195.
6. Meldrum B. Pharmacology of GABA. Clin Neuropharmacol 1982;5(3):293–316.
7. Mohler IJ, Evans SJ. γ-aminobutyric acid (GABA), receptors and their association with benzodiazepine recognition sites. In: Meltzer HY, ed. Psychopharmacology: the third generation of progress. New York: Raven Press 1987:265–272.
8. Csernansky JG, Lombrozo L, Gulevich GD, Hollister LE. Treatment of negative schizophrenic symptoms with alprazolam: A preliminary open-label study. J Clin Psychopharmacol 1984;4(6):349–352.
9. Douyon R, Angrist B, Peselow E, Cooper T, Rotrosen J. Neuroleptic augmentation with alprazolam: clinical effects and pharmacokinetic correlates. Am J Psychiatry 1989;146(2):231–234.
10. Nestoros JN, Nair NPV, Pulman JR, Schwartz G, Bloom D. High doses of diazepam improve neuroleptic-resistant chronic schizophrenic patients. Psychopharmacology 1983;81:42–47.
11. Weizman A, Tyano S, Wijsenbeek H, Ben DM. High dose diazepam treatment and its effect on prolactin secretion in adolescent schizophrenic patients. Psychopharmacology 1984;82:382–385.
12. Wolkowitz OM, Breier A, Doran A, Kelsoe J, Lucas P, Paul SM, Pickar D. Alprazolam augmentation of the antipsychotic effects of fluphenazine in schizophrenic patients. Arch Gen Psychiatry 1988;45:664–671.
13. Csernansky JG, Riney SJ, Lombrozo L, Overall JE, Hollister LE. Double-blind comparison of alprazolam, diazepam, and placebo for the treatment of negative schizophrenic symptoms. Arch Gen Psychiatry 1988;45:655–659.
14. Holden JMC, Itil TM, Keskiner A, et al. Thioridazine and chlordiazepoxide, alone and combined, in the treatment of chronic schizophrenia. Compr Psychiatry 1968; 9(6):633–643.
15. Hanlon TE, Ota KY, Kurland AA. Comparative effects of fluphenazine, fluphenazine-chlordiazepoxide and fluphenazine-imipramine. Dis Nerv Syst 1970;31:171–177.
16. Hanlon TE, Ota KY, Agallianos DD, et al. Combined drug treatment of newly hospitalized acutely ill psychiatric patients. Dis Nerv Syst 1969;30:104–116.
17. Kellner R, Wilson RM, Muldawer MD, Pathak D. Anxiety in schizophrenia: the responses to chlordiazepoxide in an intensive design study. Arch Gen Psychiatry 1975;32:1246–1254.
18. Lingjaerde O. Effect of the benzodiazepine derivative estazolam in patients with audi-

tory hallucinations: a multi-centre double-blind, crossover study. Acta Psychiatr Scand 1982;65:339–354.

19. Ruskin P, Averburch I, Buchman RW, et al. Benzodiazepines in chronic schizophrenia. Biol Psychiatry 1979;14(3):557–558.

20. Arana GW, Ornsteen ML, Kanter F, Friedman HL, Greenblatt DJ, Shader RI. The use of benzodiazepines for psychotic disorders. A literature review and preliminary clinical findings. Psychopharmacol Bull 1986;22(1):77–87.

21. Salam SA, Pillai A, Beresford TP. Lorazepam for psychogenic catatonia. Am J Psychiatry 1987;144:1082–1083.

22. Salam SA, Kilzich N. Lorazepam in psychogenic catatonia: an update. J Clin Psychiatry 1988;49(suppl):16–21.

23. Greenfeld D, Conrad C, Kincare P, Bowers Jr MB. Treatment of catatonia with low-dose lorazepam. Am J Psychiatry 1987;144:1224–1225.

24. Walter-Ryan WG. Treatment for catatonic symptoms with intramuscular lorazepam. J Clin Psychopharmacol 1985;5:123–124.

25. Wetzel H, Heuser I, Benker O. Stupor and affective state: alleviation of psychomotor disturbances by lorazepam and recurrence of symptoms with RO 15-1788. J Nerv Ment Dis 1987;175:240–242.

26. Martenyi F, Harangozo J, Laszlo M. Clonazepam for the treatment of catatonic schizophrenia. Am J Psychiatry 1989;146:1230.

27. McEvoy JP, Lohr JB. Diazepam for catatonia. Am J Psychiatry 1984;141:284–285.

28. Menza MA, Harris D. Benzodiazepines and catatonia: an overview. Biol Psychiatry 1989;26:842–846.

29. Bodkin JA. Emerging uses for high-potency benzodiazepines in psychotic disorder. J Clin Psychiatry 1990;5(suppl):41–46.

30. Saltana AS, Kilzieh N. Lorazepam treatment of psychogenic catatonia: an update. J Clin Psychiatry 1988;49(12):16–21.

31. Jimerson DC, Van Kammen DP, Post RM, Docherty JP, Bunney WE Jr. Diazepam in schizophrenia: a preliminary double-blind trial. Am J Psychiatry 1982;139(4):489–491.

32. Cohen S, Khan A, Johnson S. Pharmacological management of manic psychosis in an unlocked setting. J Clin Psychopharmacol 1987;7(4):261–264.

33. Hass S, Emrich HM, Beckmann H. Analgesic and euphoric effects of high dose diazepam in schizophrenia. Neuropsychobiology 1982;8:123–128.

34. Mondell JG. Further experience and observations with lorazepam in the management of behavioral agitation (letter). J Clin Psychopharmacol 1986;6(6):385–387.

35. Salzman C. Use of benzodiazepines to control disruptive behavior in inpatients. J Clin Psychiatry 1988;49(suppl 12):13–15.

36. Pato CN, Wolkowitz OM, Rapaport M, Schulz SC, Pickar D. Benzodiazepine augmentation of neuroleptic treatment in patients with schizophrenia. Psychopharmacol Bull 1989;25(2):263–266.

37. Casey, JF, Hollister LE, Klett CJ, Lasky JJ, Caffey GM. Combined drug therapy of chronic schizophrenics. Controlled evaluation of placebo, dextro-amphetamine, imipramine, isocarboxazid, and trifluoperazine added to maintenance doses of chlorpromazine. Am J Psychiatry 1961;117:997–1003.

38. Davis JM. The treatment of schizophrenia. Curr Opin Psychiatry 1990;3:29–34.

39. Weissman M. The psychological treatment of depression. Evidence for the efficacy of psychotherapy alone, in comparison with, and in combination with pharmacotherapy. Arch Gen Psychiatry 1969;36:1261–1269.

40. Goff DC, Brotman AW, Waites M, McCormick S. Trial of fluoxetine added to neuroleptics for treatment-resistant schizophrenic patients. Am J Psychiatry 1990;147(4):492–494.

41. Goldman MB, Janecek HM. Adjunctive fluoxetine improves global function in schizophrenia. J Neuropsych Clin Neurosci 1990;2:429–431.

42. Bleich A, Brown S, Kann R, et al. The role of serotonin in schizophrenia. Schizophr Bull 1988;14:297–325.

43. Biederman J, Lerner Y, Belmaker RH. Combination of lithium carbonate and haloperidol in schizo-affective disorder. A controlled study. Arch Gen Psychiatry 1979;36:327–333.

44. Okuma T, Yamashita I, Takahashi R, Itoh H, Otsuki S, Watanabe S, Sarai K, Hazama H, Inanaga K. A double-blind study of adjunctive carbamazepine versus placebo on excited states of schizophrenic and schizoaffective disorders. Acta Psychiatr Scand 1989;80:250–259.

45. Altamura AL, Mauri MC, Mantero M, et al. Clonazepam/haloperidol combination therapy in schizophrenia: a double-blind

study. Acta Psychiatr Scand 1987;76:702–706.

46. Smith ME. A clinical study of chlorpromazine and chlordiazepoxide. Conn Med 1961;25:153–157.

47. Hankoff LD, Rudorfer L, Paley HM. A reference study of ataraxics: a two-week double blind outpatient evaluation. J New Drugs 1962;2:173–178.

48. Azima H, Arthurs D, Silver A. The effects of chlordiazepoxide (Librium) in anxiety states. Can Psychiatr Assoc J 1962;7:44–50.

49. Merlis S, Turner WJ, Krumholz W. A double-blind comparison of diazepam, chlordiazepoxide and chlorpromazine in psychotic patients. J Neuropsychiatry 1962;3(suppl):S133–S138.

50. Rao AV. A controlled trial with "Valium" in some psychiatric disorders. Indian J Psychiatry 1964;4:188–192.

51. Maculans GA. Comparison of diazepam, chlorprothixene and chlorpromazine in chronic schizophrenic patients. Dis Nerv Sys 1964;25:164–168.

52. Stonehill E, Lee H, Ban TA. A comparative study with benzodiazepines in chronic psychotic patients. Dis Nerv Sys 1966;27:411–413.

53. Gundlach R, Engelhardt DM, Hankoff L, et al. A double-blind outpatient study of diazepam (Valium) and placebo. Psychopharmacologia 1966;9:81–92.

54. Michaux MH, Kurland AA, Agallianos DD. Chlorpromazine-chlo rdiazepoxide and chlorpromazine-imipramine treatment of newly hospitalized, acutely ill psychiatric patients. Curr Ther Res 1966;8(suppl):117–152.

55. Hekimian LJ, Friedhoff AJ. A controlled study of placebo, chlordiazepoxi de and chlorpromazine with thirty male schizophrenic patients. Dis Nerv Sys 1967;28:675–678.

56. Holden JMC, Itil TM, Keskiner A, et al. Thioridazine and chlordiazepoxide, alone and combined, in the treatment of chronic schizophrenia. Compr Psychiatry 1968;9:633–634.

57. Guz L, Moraea R, Sartoretto JN. The therapeutic effects of lorazepam in psychotic patients treated with haloperidol: a double-blind study. Curr Ther Res 1972;14:767–774.

58. Kellner R, Wilson RM, Muldawer MD, et al. Anxiety in schizophrenia: the responses to chlordiazepoxide in an intensive design study. Arch Gen Psychiatry 1975;32:1246–1254.

59. Ruskin P, Averbukh I, Belmaker RH, et al. Benzodiazepines in chronic schizophrenia. Biol Psychiatry 1979;14:557–558.

60. Marneros A. Anxiolytische zusatzbehandlung bei den affektbetonten schizphrenien. Therapiewoche 1979;29:7533–7538.

61. Lingjaerde O, Engstrand E, Ellingsen P, et al. Antipsychotic effect of diazepam when given in addition to neuroleptics in chronic psychotic patients: a double blind clinical trial. Curr Ther Res 1979;26:505–514.

62. Lerner Y, Lwow E, Levitin A, et al. Acute high-dose parenteral haloperidol treatment of psychosis. Am J Psychiatry 1979;136:1061–1064.

63. Nishikawa T, Tsuda A, Tanaka M, et al. Prophylactic effect of neuroleptics in symptom-free schizophrenics. Psychopharmacology 1982;77:301–304.

64. Nestoros JN, Suranyi-Cadotte BE, Spees RC, et al. Diasepam in high doses is effective in schizophrenia. Prog Neuropsychopharmacol Biol Psychiatry1982;6:513–516.

65. Karson CN, Weinberger DR, Bigelow L, et al. Clonazepam treatment of chronic schizophrenia: negative results in a double-blind, placebo-controlled trial. Am J Psychiatry 1982;139:1627–1628.

66. Nestoros JN, Nair NPV, Pulman JR, et al. High doses of diazepam improve neuroleptic-resistant chronic schizophrenic patients. Psychopharmacology 1983;81:42–47.

67. Csernansky JG, Riney SJ, Lombrozo L, et al. Double-blind comparison of alprazolam, diazepam and placebo in the treatment of negative schizophrenic symptoms. Arch Gen Psychiatry 1988;45:655–659.

68. Wolkowitz OM, Breier A, Doran AR, et al. Alprazolam augmentation of the antipsychotic effects of fluphenazine in schizophrenic patients: preliminary results. Arch Gen Psychiatry 1988;45:664–671.

69. Wolkowitz OM, Pickar D. Benzodiazepines in the treatment of schizophrenia: a review and reappraisal. Am J Psychiatry 1991;148:714–726.

70. Bacher NM, Lewis HA, Field PB. Combined alprazolam and neuroleptic drug in treating schizophrenia. Am J Psychiatry 1986;143:1311–1312.

71. Dixon L, Weiden PJ, Frances AJ, et al. Alprazolam intolerance in stable schizophrenic outpatients. Psychopharmacol Bull 1989;25:213–214.
72. Sassim N, Grohmann R. Adverse drug reactions with clozapine and simultaneous application of benzodiazepines. Pharmacopsychiatry 1988;21:306–307.
73. Shopsin B, Kim SS, Gershon S. A controlled study of lithium vs. chlorpromazine in acute schizophrenics. Br J Psychiatry 1971;119:435–440.
74. Hirschowitz J, Casper R, Garver DL, Chang S. Lithium response in good prognosis schizophrenia. Am J Psychiatry 1980; 137(8):916–920.
75. Atsmon A, Blum I. Treatment of acute porphyria variegata with propranolol. Lancet 1970;24:196–197.
76. Atsmon A, Blum I. The discovery. In: Roberts E, Amacher P, eds. Propranolol and schizophrenia. New York: Alan Liss, Inc., 1978.
77. Atsmon A, Blum I, Steiner M, Latz A, Wijsenbeek H. Further studies with propranolol in psychotic patients. Psychopharmacologia 1972;27:249–254.
78. Atsmon A, Blum I, Wijsenbeek H, Maoz P, Steiner M, Zielgelman G. The short-term effects of adrenergic-blocking agents in a small group of psychotic patients. Psychiatria Neurologia Neurochirurgia 1971; 74:251–258.
79. Yorkston NJ, Zaki SA, Havard CWH. Propranolol in the treatment of schizophrenia: an uncontrolled study with 55 adults. In: Roberts E, Amacher P, eds. Propranolol and schizophrenia. New York: Alan R. Liss, Inc., 1978.
80. Yorkston NJ, Zaki SA, Malik MKU, Morrison RC, Havard CWH. Propranolol in the control of schizophrenic symptoms. Br Med J 1974;4:633–635.
81. Yorkston NJ, Zaki SA, Themen J, Havard CWH. Propranolol to control schizophrenic symptoms. Adv Clin Pharmacol 1976;12:91–104.
82. Yorkston NJ, Zaki SA, Themen J, Havard CWH. Safeguards in the treatment of schizophrenia with propranolol. Postgrad Med J 1976;52(suppl 4):175–180.
83. Davis JM, Janicak PG, Chang S, Klerman K. Recent advances in the pharmacologic treatment of the schizophrenic disorders. In: Grinspoon L, ed. Psychiatry 1982 annual review. Washington D.C.: APPI, 1982.
84. Langsley DG, Enterline JD, Hickerson GX. A comparison of chlorpromazine and EST in treatment of acute schizophrenic and manic reactions. Arch Neurol Psychiat 1959;81:384–391.
85. Smith K, Surphlis WRP, Gynther MD, Shimkunas AM. ECT and chlorpromazine compared in the treatment of schizophrenia. J Nerv Ment Dis 1967;144:284–290.

Role of Psychosocial Therapies

There is virtually unanimous agreement among experienced mental health workers regarding the unique benefit of the antipsychotics. Some with limited patient experience, however, are critical of these agents. Unfortunately, this attitude is based on inaccurate information that schizophrenia is a psychological condition and, as a logical deduction, that drugs are, at best, an ancillary therapy and, at worst, harmful. Another reason for increasing one's knowledge about this issue is that some members of the legal profes-

sion, at times supported by misguided mental health activists, have attempted to make drug therapy illegal, claiming that the definitive treatment is psychotherapy because it addresses the basic cause. This argument is less than compelling, since, while the exact cause of schizophrenia and other psychotic conditions is unknown, they are almost certainly biological disorder(s).

Having established the primary role of antipsychotics, there is evidence that psychosocial therapies, when administered with these agents, improve long-term prognosis. Because chronically psychotic patients have difficulties with social adjustment, reason dictates that they and their families could benefit from such interventions. Regardless of theoretical orientation, it is clear that practitioners should provide psychosocial therapy as part of a comprehensive treatment strategy.

EFFICACY OF PSYCHOSOCIAL THERAPIES

Psychotherapy Only versus Drug Therapy

There is no empirical evidence that long-term, inhospital psychotherapy without drugs is beneficial. Indeed, in any study that compared psychotherapy only to drug therapy under any circumstances, the psychotherapy group always did poorly. The May study found that patients receiving psychotherapy alone did poorly, both initially as well as during follow-up (1, 2). The study found that psychotherapy did not increase improvement scores over that observed in the control group; and indeed, there was a nonsignificant trend in the other direction. Since patients received only 24 hours of psychotherapy by relatively inexperienced counselors, this does not constitute a definitive test of this intervention's potential efficacy (Table 5.18).

Drug Therapy Only versus Drug plus Psychotherapy

At the Massachusetts Mental Health Center (MMHC), a small group of chronically ill, schizophrenic patients who were treated by senior psychoanalysts deteriorated when a placebo was substituted for thioridazine. Further, there was no evidence that the drugs made patients less responsive to psychoanalytically oriented psychotherapy, and in fact, many were more responsive to the psychotherapeutic process when on thioridazine (3–5).

In another MMHC study, chronic state hospital patients were randomly assigned to four variations of drug and *social therapies: high intensity* social therapy *with drugs; high intensity* social therapy *without drugs; low intensity* social therapy *with drugs;* or *low intensity* social therapy *with-*

Table 5.18.
Assessment of Outcome in Patients with Schizophrenia Treated with and without Antipsychotic Drugs and Psychotherapy[a]

	No Drugs		Drug	
	No Psychotherapy	Psychotherapy	No Psychotherapy	Psychotherapy
Percent released	59%	64%	95%	96%
Nurses' rating MACC total	38	38	48	48
Menninger nurses' health-sickness rating	26	23	29	30
Nurses' idiosyncratic symptoms $(125 \times)$[b]	37	29	66	74
Therapists' rating on symptom rating sheet $(50 \times)$[b]	22	21	27	27
Analysis rating of insight	3.4	3.3	3.7	4.1

[a]Adapted from Davis JM, Janicak PG, Chang S, Klerman K. Recent advances in the pharmacologic treatment of the schizophrenic disorders. In: Grinspoon L, ed. Psychiatry 1982 annual review. Washington DC: APPI Press, 1982:221.
[b]A higher number reflects greater improvement. In order to have the two scales fit with this convention, scores were subtracted from an arbitrary constant.

out drugs. High intensity social therapy consisted of a variety of psychotherapies, social work intervention, occupational therapy, psychodrama, and "total push" therapies. The low intensity social therapy consisted of milieu interventions administered in a state hospital. Improvement rates in the drug-treated patients were significantly higher than the rates observed in the nondrug groups, either in the state hospital milieu (10%) or at the MMHC (0%). Further, there was no significant symptomatic improvement in the *drug-plus-high*-intensity-social-therapy group (33%), when compared to the *drug-plus-low*-intensity social-therapy group (23%) (Table 5.19). If anything, the high intensity social therapy without drugs impeded improvement, because this group, even after being placed back on drugs after a 6-month hiatus, never caught up with the continuously drug-treated groups.

The VA performed a double-blind study comparing group therapy alone, group therapy with an AP, and AP therapy alone (6). In most cases, drug treatment with or without group therapy, produced substantially better improvement than group therapy only. Again, as in the earlier studies of social therapy, the antipsychotics proved crucial. The VA also performed a comparable study in chronic, elderly schizophrenic patients with similar results (7).

Three other studies have compared psychotherapy or group therapy plus drug to drug alone in hospital settings and found that those receiving psychotherapy do marginally better (8–10).

In a 2-year, collaborative study of psychotherapy in hospitalized, acute schizophrenic patients, investigators compared *exploratory and insight-oriented psychotherapy* (E-IO) with a control treatment of *reality-adaptive-supportive* (RAS) psychotherapy (i.e., essentially a placebo psychotherapy). All study patients were also placed on APs. One hundred and sixty-four patients entered the study; but 42% dropped out before the required minimum participation of 6 months, and only one-third of the initial sample remained at the end of 2 years. Seventy-two patients (35 E-IO and 37 RAS) at 12 months and 47 (22 E-IO and 25 RAS) at 24 months were available for analyses. Although the differences between the E-IO and RAS groups were small, the RAS patients, over a 2-year follow-up period, spent more time functioning independently, spent less time in the hospital, and were more likely to be employed. The results indicated only a minimum outcome difference between the two types of psychotherapy, regardless of the outcome measure examined. These results are consistent with several other small studies of psychotherapy plus drugs versus drugs alone.

John Rosen claimed that *direct analysis* (a psychoanalytic-like technique) produced improvement in 37 cases of deteriorated schizophrenia (11, 12). He defined improvement as the ability to live comfort-

Table 5.19.
Results of Four Treatments in Chronic Schizophrenia[a]

	High Social Therapy[b]	Low Social Therapy[c]
Percentage showing high improvement at 6 months' evaluation		
Drug therapy	33%	23%
No drug therapy	0%	10%
Percentage showing high improvement after 36 months		
Drug therapy	35%	19%
No drug therapy for 6 months, then drug therapy	26%	6%

[a]Adapted from Klein D, Davis JM. Diagnosis and drug treatment of psychiatric disorders. In: Review of antipsychotic drug literature. Baltimore: Williams & Wilkins, 1969:92.
[b]Patients transferred to Massachusetts Mental Health Center.
[c]Patients remaining in state hospitals.

ably outside of an institution, with the achievement of psychological integrity, emotional stability, and character structure such that a patient could withstand as much environmental stress as one who never experienced a psychotic episode. The credibility of this claim, however, was shattered by an independent evaluation of these patients' outcome. Five years later, a follow-up of Rosen's group found that 37% had not been initially diagnosed as schizophrenic, but rather as psychoneurotic, manic-depressive, or possibly hyperthyroid (e.g., one patient recovered after her thyroid was removed). The remainder met criteria for schizophrenia, and during the next 10 years, 75% had between two and five subsequent readmissions. Thus, Rosen's initial claims were not substantiated because many did not have schizophrenia, and most of those who did were not able to sustain their improvement.

In another study, psychotherapy with and without drugs was compared with a *"no formal psychotherapy"* control group (13–15). No valid conclusions can be drawn from this study, however, because there was no adequate control group with respect to medication. Further, the majority of the psychotherapy group received medication and the control group was treated in an entirely different milieu, with many apparently transferred to a chronic facility.

Another study evaluating two types of *behaviorally oriented therapy* is open to the same criticism because it did not include adequate information about the drug treatment of those remaining in the state hospital (16, 17). It is known that at the beginning of the trial most patients were not on adequate doses of appropriate drugs and some were not even receiving an antipsychotic. At various times during the study, a variable percentage (at times as great as 50%) of the psychological treatment groups also received medication. Thus, no valid conclu-

sions can be drawn because the psychological treatment groups received drug therapy and many in the control group may not have received adequate drug therapy. This study is important in supporting the usefulness of specific behavioral interventions in comparison to milieu treatment, but any conclusion concerning the role of drugs is clearly invalid.

R.D. Laing employed *family-oriented therapy* with schizophrenic patients, reporting that 25% received no "tranquilizers" at all (implying that 75% did receive medication!) (18). Further, he and his coworkers used a broad definition of schizophrenia, much less restrictive than that which was common in Great Britain at the time, so it is possible that all core schizophrenic patients received medication (Laing, in a personal communication to JMD acknowledged that he did refer his patients to a competent psychiatrist for drug treatment.)

Four controlled, random-assignment studies comparing brief hospital treatment with relatively longer periods of hospital-based psychological intervention found that the brief hospital stays produced comparable results to the longer stay regimen (19–24).

Patients from families with high expressed emotion (demanding, critical, high expectations) have a higher relapse rate than those from families with low expressed emotion (25–28). These findings suggested that certain patients may be vulnerable to emotional confrontations and led to the use of family therapy to reduce high expressed emotion. Families are taught techniques for coping with the patient and, perhaps more importantly, are educated about the disorder and the need for medication compliance.

Table 5.20 shows the effect of psychosocial treatment on relapse rates in seven studies (29–35). All patients received

Table 5.20.
Outcome of Patients Treated with Antipsychotic Drugs with and without Psychosocial Treatment[a]

Study	Evaluation Interval	Drug Alone (number of subjects)		Drug and Psychosocial Therapy (number of subjects)	
		Well	Relapsed	Well	Relapsed
Hogarty et al. (1974)	2 years	73	22	80	15
Goldstein et al. (1978)	6 weeks	42	8	44	2
Hogarty et al. (1979)	2 years	25	27	30	23
Falloon et al. (1982)	9 months	9	9	16	2
Tarrier et al. (1988)	9 months	8	8	29	3
Leff et al. (1990)	2 years	3	9	6	6
Hogarty et al. (1991)	2 years	11	10	39	15
TOTAL		171	93	244	66
% Well/Relapsed		65%	35%	79%	21%

[a]MH chi square = 16.5; df = 1; p = 0.00005
Adapted from Davis JM, Andriukaitis S. The natural course of schizophrenia and effective maintenance drug treatment. J Clin Psychopharmacol 1986;6:2s–10s.

maintenance APs, and the experimental variable was the presence or absence of some form of psychosocial therapy. Thus, these studies assessed whether psychoeducation/family intervention has any additional benefit beyond that produced by medication. The number who relapsed in each treatment group was reported, so we combined the data from all seven studies and found a consistently better outcome for those with psychoeducation/family therapy intervention in comparison with those on maintenance drug therapy only (chi square = 16.5; df = 1; p = 0.00005). Whereas the psychosocial treatments used in these seven studies employed similar techniques, not all were focused exclusively on lowering the family's expressed emotion toward the patient. Nevertheless, the consistently better outcome for those receiving some type of social therapy, in addition to APs, is a promising finding. Since these cannot be truly "blind," we would emphasize that these trials have been conducted by proponents of psychotherapy. Therefore, until they are replicated by others, we need to interpret the results cautiously. **These results underscore the importance of a careful transition from an inpatient to outpatient environment in preventing relapse.**

CONCLUSION

In the hospital setting, several groups failed to find psychotherapy without drugs effective, and the addition of psychotherapy to drug treatment produced marginal and inconsistent gains. In general, psychotherapeutic interventions are more appropriate in the outpatient setting. The role of these therapies can be analogized to the treatment of a broken leg, with medication comparable to casting the fracture and psychosocial therapies to the physical therapy that then facilitates the healing process.

Clinicians must be thoughtful in choosing the appropriate psychosocial treatment for specific patients. Any such intervention should be proven helpful, rather than chosen solely on the basis of a theoretical model. Finally, more complicated psychological strategies, often costlier in terms of time and expense, appear to offer no advantage over more economical sociotherapeutic models.

REFERENCES

1. May PRA, Tuma AH, Dixon WJ. Schizophrenia—A follow-up study of results of treatment. I. Design and other problems. Arch Gen Psychiatry 1976;33;474–478.
2. May PRA, Tuma AH, Yale C, Potepan P, Dixon WJ. Schizophrenia—A follow-up study of results of treatment. II. Hospital stay over two to five years. Arch Gen Psychiatry 1976;33:481–486.
3. Grinspoon L, Ewalt JR, Shader RI. Schizophrenia: pharmacotherapy and psychotherapy. Baltimore: Williams & Wilkins, 1968: 67–74.
4. Grinspoon L, Ewalt JR, Shader RI. Schizophrenia: pharmacotherapy and psychotherapy. Baltimore: Williams & Wilkins, 1972.
5. Messier J, Finnerty R, Botvin C, Grinspoon L. A follow-up study of intensively treated chronic schizophrenic patients. Am J Psychiatry 1969;125:1123–1127.
6. Gorham DR, Pokorny AD. Effects of a phenothiazine and/or group psychotherapy with schizophrenics. Dis Nerv Sys 1964; 25:77–86.
7. Honigfeld G, Rosenbaum MP, Blumenthal IJ, Lambert HL, Roberts AJ. Behavioral improvement in the older schizophrenic patient: drug and social therapies. J Am Geriatr Soc 1965;8:57–72.
8. Dvangelakis MG. De-institutionalization of patients. Dis Nerv Sys 1961;22:26–32.
9. Rogers CR, Gendlin EG, Kiesler DJ, Traux CB, eds. The therapeutic relationship and its impact: a study of psychotherapy with schizophrenics. Madison: University of Wisconsin Press, 1967.
10. Gunderson JG, Frank AF, Katz HM, Vannicelli ML, Frosch JP, Knapp PH. Effects of psychotherapy in schizophrenia: II. Comparative outcome of two forms of treatment. Schizophr Bull 1984;10:564–598.
11. Rosen JN. The treatment of schizophrenic psychoses by direct analytic therapy. Psychiatr Q 1947;21:117–119.
12. Rosen JN. Direct analysis: selected papers. New York: Grune & Stratton, 1953.
13. Karon B, O'Grady P. Intellectual test changes in schizophrenic patients in the first six months of treatment. Psychotherapy theory, research and practice 1969;6: 88–96.
14. Karon BP, Vandenbos GR. Experience, medication and the effectiveness of psychotherapy with schizophrenics. Br J Psychiatry 1970;116:427–428.
15. Karon BP, Vandenbos GR. The consequences of psychotherapy to schizophrenic patients. Psychotherapy theory, research and practice 1972;9;111–119.
16. Paul GL, Lentz RJ. Psychosocial treatment of chronic mental patients: milieu vs social learning programs. Cambridge: Harvard University Press, 1977.
17. Paul GL, Tobias LL, Holly, BL. Maintenance psychotropic drugs in the presence of active treatment programs: a "triple-blind" withdrawal study with long-term mental patients. Arch Gen Psychiatry 1972;27:106–115.
18. Esterson A, Cooper DG, Laing RD. Results of family-oriented therapy with hospitalized schizophrenics. Br Med J 1965;2: 1462–1465.
19. Knight A, Hirsch S, Platt SD. Clinical change as a function of brief admission to a hospital in a controlled study using the present state examination. Br J Psychiatry 1980;137:170–180.
20. Herz MI, Endicott J, Spitzer RL. Mesnikoff A. Day vs. inpatient hospitalization: a controlled study. Am J Psychiatry 1971; 127:1371–1382.
21. Herz MI, Endicott J, Spitzer RL. Brief hospitalization: a two year follow-up. Am J Psychiatry 1977;134:502–507.
22. Glick ID, Hargreaves WA, Drues J, Showstack JA. Short vs long hospitalization: a prospective controlled study. IV. One-year follow-up results for schizophrenic patients. Am J Psychiatry 1976;133:509–514.
23. Glick ID, Hargreaves WA, Raskin M, Kutner J. Short vs long hospitalization: a prospective controlled study. I. The preliminary results of a one year follow-up of schizophrenics. Arch Gen Psychiatry 1974; 30:363–369.
24. Caffey EM, Jones RB, Diamond LS, Burton E, Bowen WT. Brief hospital treatment of schizophrenia: early results of a multiple hospital study. Hosp Community Psychiatry 1968;19:282–287.
25. Brown GW, Birley JLT, Wing JK. Influence of family life on the course of schizophrenic disorders: a replication. Br J Psychiatry 1972;121:241–258.
26. Leff JP, Wing JK. Trial of maintenance therapy in schizophrenics. Br Med J 1971; 2:599–604.
27. Vaughn CE, Leff JP. The influence of family and social factors on the course of psychiatric illness. A comparison of schizophrenic and depressed neurotic patients. Br J Psychiatry 1976;129:125–137.

28. Vaughn CE, Snyder KS, Jones S, Freeman WB, Falloon IRH. Family factors in schizophrenic relapse. Replication in California of British research on expressed emotion. Arch Gen Psychiatry 1984;41:1169–1177.
29. Falloon IRH, Boyd JL, McGill CW, Razani J, Moss HB, Gilderman AM. Family management in the prevention of exacerbations of schizophrenia. A controlled study. N Engl J Med 1982;306:1437–1440.
30. Goldstein MJ, Rodnick EH, Evans JR, May PRA, Steinberg MR. Drug and family therapy in the aftercare of acute schizophrenics. Arch Gen Psychiatry 1978;35:1169–1177.
31. Hogarty GE, Goldberg SC, Schooler NR, Ulrich RF. Collaborative Study Group. Drug and sociotherapy in the aftercare of schizophrenic patients. II. Two-year relapse rates. Arch Gen Psychiatry 1974;31:603–608.
32. Hogarty GE, Schooler NR, Ulrich R, Mussare F, Ferro P, Herron E. Fluphenazine and social therapy in the aftercare of schizophrenic patients. Relapse analyses of a two-year controlled study of fluphenazine decanoate and fluphenazine hydrochloride. Arch Gen Psychiatry 1979;36:1283–1294.
33. Hogarty GE, Anderson CM, Reiss DJ, Kornblith SJ, Greenwald DP, Ulrich RF, Carter M, the EPICS Research Group. Family psychoeducation, social skills training, and maintenance chemotherapy in the aftercare treatment of schizophrenia. II. Two-year effects of a controlled study on relapse and adjustment. Arch Gen Psychiatry 1991;48:340–347.
34. Leff J, Berkowitz R, Shavit N, Strachan A, Glass I, Vaughn C. A trial of family therapy versus a relatives' group for schizophrenia. Two-year follow-up. Br J Psychiatry 1990;157:571–577.
35. Tarrier N, Barrowclough C, Vaughn C, Bamrah JS, Porceddu K, Watts S, Freeman H. The community management of schizophrenia. A controlled trial of a behavioural intervention with families to reduce relapse. Br J Psychiatry 1988;153:532–542.

Adverse Effects

A long list of adverse effects may imply that many patients have most adverse effects, to a significant degree. In fact, while almost all patients will experience some mild effects with these drugs, such as dry mouth or tremor, they are usually transitory and disappear with time, medication reduction, or discontinuation. Fortunately, these effects are rarely serious or irreversible, and on the average, the typical complications with antipsychotics are no worse than with medications prescribed for other medical disorders.

CENTRAL NERVOUS SYSTEM

Acute Extrapyramidal Side Effects

Acute EPS effects can be classified into three categories:

• Parkinsonian syndrome
• Acute dystonias
• Akathisia.

Lower potency agents, such as thioridazine and CPZ, have a decreased incidence of EPS when compared to higher potency agents, such as haloperidol or fluphenazine.

The *parkinsonian syndrome* is characterized by a mask-like facies, resting tremor, cogwheel rigidity, shuffling gait, and psychomotor retardation. A more subtle form may present as emotional blunting (e.g., an apathetic appearance lacking in spontaneity) and a relative inability to engage in social activities, which can be confused with the emotional withdrawal, apathy, and retardation that are part of a schizophrenic disorder or a postpsychotic depression. The syndrome is symptomatically identical to idiopathic parkinsonism and responds to antiparkinsonian medications (e.g., benztropine). Parkinsonian rigidity and akinesia may also respond to amantadine. Rarely, neuroleptics have been reported to produce a catatonic-like state, similar to akinetic mutism, which may also be responsive to amantadine.

The *dystonias* consist of torticollis, retrocollis, oculogyric crisis, and opisthotonos.

Akathisia is a motor restlessness manifested by the urge to move about and an inability to sit still. This can be confused with psychotic agitation because patients are driven by a restlessness which is primarily motor and cannot be controlled by their own volition. Unlike psychotic agitation, however, akathisia is accompanied by subjective distress, worsened by increasing the antipsychotic dose, and often benefited by a decrease.

The parkinsonian syndrome and akathisia often occur early in therapy and tend to persist if not treated. They can also appear years later, frequently coexisting with TD. EPS, in general, occur equally in both sexes and all ages, with the elderly at greatest risk for TD. However, there are age- and sex-related differences in the incidence of various types of EPS (e.g., akathisia, acute dystonia, etc.).

Although these adverse effects have fairly characteristic presentations, their diagnosis can occasionally be missed. For example:

- Dystonia can be confused with bizarre mannerisms
- Akathisia can be confused with agitation
- Parkinsonian akinesia can be confused with schizophrenic apathy or a retarded depression.

Treatment: Acute

An accurate diagnosis is important because these manifestations may be mis-taken for an exacerbation of the psychosis, prompting an escalation in dose when a decrease or an antiparkinsonian drug should be considered. A therapeutic trial with an agent such as procyclidine, benztropine, or diphenhydramine can be diagnostic, because acute dystonic reactions usually respond in minutes to parenteral administration of these agents.

EPS often present a clinical quandary because options can include: blocking them with an antiparkinsonian drug; reducing the dose; changing to another agent; or some combination of these three. The decision should be based partly on clinical improvement, so if a patient's psychosis is stabilized, a decrease in the dose would be reasonable. If the patient is still quite psychotic, however, adding an antiparkinsonian drug or switching to another antipsychotic may be more appropriate. If adverse effects limit a clinically appropriate dose increase, switching to another agent is recommended.

Acute dystonias are typically seen in the first few days to weeks of treatment and can occur with even limited exposure (e.g., children treated with a single dose of prochlorperazine for nausea). Although dystonias may disappear spontaneously, they should be treated aggressively, as they are often painful and upsetting to the patient. Occasionally, an acute dystonic reaction is resistant to standard treatment but may respond to parenteral diazepam, caffeine sodium benzoate, or barbiturate-induced sleep.

Akathisia may respond to propranolol, BZDs, amantadine, anticholinergics, or by simply switching to a different antipsychotic. The fact that β-blockers benefit akathisia is an important observation, suggesting that it is mediated by noradrenergic mechanisms. The observation that propranolol is beneficial is supported by several double-blind studies, suggesting that this agent may be the treatment of choice (1–4). While akathisia is generally thought of as an extrapyramidal reaction, the beneficial effects of propranolol may suggest a more complex etiology.

Although propranolol is often considered the treatment of choice for akathisia, low doses of clonazepam, diazepam, or lorazepam may also reduce its severity (5–11). These BZDs may be a useful alternative when propranolol is contraindicated (e.g., in patients with asthma, insulindependent diabetes mellitus, cardiac conduction abnormalities) or as an adjunct when akathisia persists despite stepwise escalation of propranolol (12).

Treatment: Prophylaxis

Prophylactic antiparkinsonian medication for all patients on neuroleptics is controversial. Arguments against this approach include:

- Many patients *never manifest EPS*
- There are *side effects associated with these medications,* such as dry mouth, blurred vision, confusion, urinary retention, and, very rarely, paralytic ileus
- *Dental caries* and *diverticuli* may occur with chronic use
- Patients can develop *behavioral toxicity,* which, in its severe form may be characterized by disorientation, loss of immediate memory, and florid hallucinations
- The *expense* of treatment is increased
- Anticholinergics can produce a feeling of euphoria and *can be abused.*

Arguments in favor of their prophylactic use include:

- *EPS are often distressing,* particularly when they occur outside the hospital; and on rare occasions can be life-threatening (e.g., oculogyric crisis or opisthotonus when alone or while driving)
- Diagnosis can be difficult because *EPS may be subtle and easily confused with psychotic symptoms*
- *Serious adverse effects are uncommon* with the addition of antiparkinsonian drugs.

Studies in which antiparkinsonian medications were discontinued have significant methodological problems. One specific issue is that patients placed on prophylactic therapy, who then fail to develop symptoms when their antiparkinsonian medication is withdrawn, may never have developed EPS at all. Still, 10 to 70% of patients have been noted to exhibit EPS after discontinuation of their antiparkinsonian drug, indicating that these agents indeed have prophylactic efficacy.

The appropriate study design to address their prophylactic efficacy is the random assignment of patients to active drug or placebo. The Spring Grove study, using this design, found that 27% of patients on perphenazine without antiparkinsonian drug developed an EPS, in contrast to only 10% of those on an antiparkinsonian drug (13). Further, those on the perphenazine/benztropine combination had comparable therapeutic improvement to those on perphenazine-placebo.

The authors conducted a prospective double-blind, placebo-controlled trial of low-dose benztropine (i.e., 2 mg/day) maintenance therapy (14). After an acute EPS had been stabilized with 2 days of active antiparkinsonian medication, the recurrence of EPS did not differ significantly between those maintained on active drug or those switched to placebo over the next 8 days. While there was a trend favoring the active drug group, low-dose maintenance benztropine (i.e., 2 mg/day) afforded little benefit in comparison to placebo.

A classic study by Chien et al. (1974) randomly assigned chronic schizophrenics to three groups: fluphenazine enanthate plus daily antiparkinsonian drugs; antiparkinsonian drugs for 5 days after each fluphenazine injection; or no prophylactic antiparkinsonian drug after fluphenazine enanthate (15).

In all groups EPS were treated when they occurred. Neither the daily-antiparkinsonian-drug group nor the 5-days-after-fluphenazine-injection group showed complete abolition of EPS, with 8 to 20% experiencing symptoms. Nevertheless, the rates were substantially less than the 54% EPS incidence in those on no prophylactic drugs.

There is also evidence of the prophylactic effect of antiparkinsonian drugs from a chart review study showing that they substantially prevented EPS (16).

Patients who have been on antiparkinsonian drugs for more than 3 months should have them slowly tapered and, if possible, stopped. Those who redevelop symptoms should have their antiparkinsonian drug therapy resumed, with periodic attempts to reduce the dosage, subsequently. Again, an alternate strategy is to switch agents. Thioridazine and clozapine produce the fewest EPS; haloperidol, thiothixene, perphenazine, trifluoperazine, and fluphenazine produce the most, with CPZ, chlorprothixene, and acetophenazine occupying an intermediate position.

Late-Onset (Tardive) EPS

Tardive dyskinesia presents with abnormal involuntary movements, usually associated with chronic (i.e., longer than 2 years) therapy (17). Although there is some debate whether the antipsychotics are either necessary or sufficient to produce this syndrome in psychiatric patients, the consensus is that they at least play an important role. TD is characterized by:

- Buccolinguomasticatory movements:
  - Sucking, smacking of *lips*
  - Choreoathetoid movements of the *tongue*
  - Lateral *jaw* movements
- Choreiform or athetoid movements of the *extremities and/or truncal areas*
- *Any combination* of these symptoms.

TD varies in presentation, and should always be considered in the differential diagnosis of any abnormal involuntary movements in patients exposed to neuroleptics or DA-receptor blocking agents used for other medical conditions (e.g., prochlorperazine or metoclopramide).

While TD usually occurs after several years of drug therapy, some patients can develop symptoms within less than 1 year of cumulative drug exposure. In Kane's study of younger adult patients (mean age 29 years) the incidence of TD was about 4% per year of cumulative drug exposure, for at least the first 5 years (18). The incidence is higher in older persons treated for similar lengths of time and lower in younger age groups. Longitudinal studies find that the incidence of TD may decrease and the prevalence remain constant at steady state drug levels. Thus, the number of new cases is balanced by those who spontaneously remit. Frequently, TD first becomes evident with dose reduction or withdrawal, but also can appear on stable doses. Symptoms disappear during sleep, while varying in intensity during the waking hours. Movements may be more pronounced in stressful or emotional situations, but can also be apparent in relaxed states.

Although many cases are relatively mild and nonprogressive, a small percentage are so severe that they result in significant disability. Because reliable predictors to identify patients who will develop the more severe forms have not been established, antipsychotic therapy should always be cautiously employed in every patient. Recent data suggest that TD may improve in some patients despite continued drug treatment, particularly if the doses are lowered (18). Clearly, a comprehensive assessment of the relative, long-term risks and benefits must be an integral part of the treatment plan for any patient on maintenance therapy.

Associated Risk Factors

Several variables appear to increase the chance of developing TD, with advancing age being the single most important risk factor in terms of incidence, severity, and persistence. Older females appear to be at greater risk, as do older patients with mood disorders. This last category (i.e., mood disorders) emphasizes the importance of an accurate diagnosis and consideration of alternate treatments when the diagnosis is unclear (e.g., mood stabilizer rather than an antipsychotic).

Treatment Issues

For vulnerable patients, dose and duration of neuroleptic treatment are important variables, underscoring the preventative benefit of using the minimum effective dose for long-term treatment. Antiparkinsonian medications may aggravate tardive dyskinesia, while reserpine-like drugs and those that raise brain acetylcholine levels (e.g., physostigmine, choline, lecithin) may help (19). Caution is required in interpreting the results of such treatments, however, since many patients recover spontaneously when the neuroleptic is discontinued. TD is infrequent in those not exposed to long-term, high-dose

therapy. Further, spontaneous development of TD has been reported and can be as high as 50% (20). For example, dyskinesias in schizophrenic patients were also described by Kraepelin almost a century before the discovery of the neuroleptics.

TD and the Atypical Antipsychotic Clozapine

It is thought that neuroleptic-induced DA-receptor blockade produces a denervation supersensitivity, ultimately increasing the number of receptor sites. As noted earlier, clozapine does not typically induce EPS. For example, we are not aware of any documented, unequivocal report of clozapine-induced dystonia or parkinsonian rigidity or tremor. In blind studies, a small number of patients are rated as having a mild degree of parkinsonian symptoms (i.e., hypokinesis, rigidity, tremor, akathisia), but this incidence is comparable to that seen with placebo and should be considered "background noise." Since it is difficult to distinguish akathisia from psychotic agitation, or withdrawal and apathy from hypokinesis, these symptoms may actually have been misidentified as EPS. If clozapine produces EPS, then unequivocal reactions such as dystonia should occur. It is remotely possible, however, that clozapine produces very mild EPS, at a much lower rate than observed with typical neuroleptics. A placebo/clozapine comparison with blind ratings would be required to clarify this question, but to date there have been no such large-scale studies with sufficient statistical power (e.g., several thousand patients on clozapine for at least 5 years).

A relatively small number of patients (about 300) have been on clozapine for a few years, and TD has not developed. A number of studies have investigated patients with TD who were switched to clozapine for periods of 3 weeks to 6 months (21–24). Some appeared to improve, but these findings are difficult to interpret because control groups would be needed to demonstrate conclusively that clozapine does not cause TD. **Theoretically, if clozapine does not cause acute EPS, then it should not cause TD.**

Other Tardive Syndromes

Late-onset or tardive dystonia, akathisia, and possibly other types of EPS have also been described as separate disorders from classic TD. Tardive dystonia is characterized by the late appearance of dystonias that persist even though neuroleptics are discontinued. It is rare, with a prevalence of about 1.5%. It is probably a separate diagnostic entity since anticholinergics benefit tardive dystonia whereas these drugs worsen tardive dyskinesia. The onset of tardive dystonia occurs after a shorter exposure time to neuroleptics than generally seen with tardive dyskinesia. Treatments include cessation of the neuroleptic (if possible); anticholinergic agents; and dopamine depleting drugs, such as reserpine or tetrabenazine.

Other CNS Side Effects

Seizures

Most antipsychotics lower the seizure threshold in animals, but this complication rarely occurs in humans, even on high doses of these compounds. They are usually not contraindicated in those with seizure disorders, but should be used cautiously. In the absence of controlled data, it is our clinical opinion that epileptic patients who also require these agents generally show improvement in both their psychosis and seizure disorder. When seizures do occur, it is generally on higher doses and they consist of a single, isolated

episode. A slightly lower dose or the addition of an anticonvulsant can bring about control of both disorders. Investigation into other possible medical conditions as the cause of a seizure episode should also be done.

Clozapine produces seizures, especially in the dose range of 600–900 mg/day. Fortunately, these levels are substantially above the usual therapeutic range of 300–400 mg/day. Rarely, seizures can occur on lower doses, as well. According to the drug's manufacturer, the reported incidence of seizures, based on daily dosage, is:

- 1 to 2% on less than 300 mg
- 3 to 4% on 300 to 599 mg
- 5% on 600 to 900 mg.

Withdrawal Syndrome

The antipsychotics do not produce a classic withdrawal syndrome of the type seen with barbiturates or opioids; nor do they produce psychological dependency, as seen with psychostimulants (e.g., cocaine, amphetamine). Addicts and patients both dislike these drugs and do not spontaneously increase their dose. Indeed, they are more likely to discontinue them without medical advice.

Abrupt discontinuation, however, is associated with certain symptoms, usually within 2–7 days, including:

- *Nausea* and *vomiting*
- Increased *sweating*
- Sensations of *heat or cold*
- *Insomnia*
- *Irritability*
- *Headache.*

Patients abruptly withdrawn from an antipsychotic/antiparkinsonian drug combination generally experience one or two of these symptoms, usually to a mild degree, and rarely develop all of them. One study that randomly assigned patients to abrupt discontinuation of both drugs, or to abrupt discontinuation of the antipsychotic only, found that symptoms occurred almost entirely in the group withdrawn from both drugs. When the antipsychotic alone was discontinued, no withdrawal symptoms were experienced, presumably due to the continuation of the antiparkinsonian drugs. Patients who had their antiparkinsonian drugs abruptly discontinued 4 weeks later also experienced withdrawal symptoms, again suggesting that this syndrome results from the antiparkinsonian drug withdrawal. Because withdrawal phenomena have also been reported in patients on antipsychotics alone, we cannot exclude the possibility that their discontinuation (possibly because of their anticholinergic properties) can also produce these symptoms. We note that parkinsonian patients who discontinue their anticholinergic, antiparkinsonian drugs, experience a marked rebound in their symptoms. Although this syndrome is mild, we recommend tapering both drugs gradually, perhaps at a slightly slower rate for the antiparkinsonian agent.

Sedation

Sedation is a common adverse behavioral change that usually occurs during the first few days after starting an antipsychotic, with some rapidly developing tolerance. While patients should be warned about driving or operating machinery, the drowsiness is generally not troublesome. In general, sedative side effects are inversely proportional to the milligram potency of these drugs. Thus, chlorpromazine and thioridazine produce more sedation than fluphenazine, haloperidol, thiothixene, or trifluoperazine. When necessary it can be controlled by reducing the dose, switching to a less-sedating agent, or giving the entire dose at bedtime. These agents typically produce sedation in normal subjects, but paradoxically enhance the mental functioning of patients due to the reduction in their psychosis. Remoxipride, a novel antipsychotic in development, apparently does not produce sedation.

Cognitive Effects

It is difficult to evaluate cognitive changes in psychotic patients because deficits caused by the disorder must be separated from drug-induced cognitive impairment. Symptoms such as insomnia, bizarre dreams, impaired psychomotor activity, aggravation of psychosis, confusional states, and somnambulism can be seen on or off drug treatment. An apparent worsening of psychosis, which is thought to be an ideational analogue or variant of akathisia, may also occur. Some confusional states, particularly in the elderly, are due to the anticholinergic properties of these drugs, which are often compounded when anticholinergics are given to manage EPS, at times resulting in a central anticholinergic syndrome.

Temperature Dysregulation

The neuroleptic malignant syndrome is an acute disorder of thermoregulation and neuromotor control carrying a mortality rate of about 21% when untreated. **The term neuroleptic malignant syndrome is probably a misnomer, and a better name might be the "hypodopaminergic, hyperpyrexia syndrome."**

The most frequent symptoms of NMS include:

- *Fever,* often greater than 40°C or 104°F
- Severe *muscle rigidity,* typically "lead pipe" or "plastic"

- *Altered consciousness,* usually with clouding of the sensorium, at times progressing to stupor or coma
- *Autonomic changes* characterized by fluctuating blood pressure, tachypnea, diaphoresis, etc.

NMS can occur with a wide variety of agents, including atypical antipsychotics such as tiapride, sulpiride, and clozapine. In addition, it occurs with DA-blocking agents used for other purposes, such as phenothiazine antiemetics (e.g., Prochlorperazine); antipsychotics as adjuncts to anesthesia (e.g., droperidol); or amoxapine, an antidepressant with a neuroleptic-like metabolite. Fluoxetine has also been reported to cause NMS, perhaps indirectly through the effect of increased 5-HT activity on DA neurons in the substantia nigra. DA-depleting agents (e.g., reserpine) and combined antagonist/depleting agents (e.g., tetrabenazine) also may cause NMS. It can also occur when antiparkinsonian agents (e.g., amantadine) are decreased or discontinued. This suggests that NMS is caused by a decrease in dopaminergic tone, and supports the therapeutic benefit of dopaminergic agonists. Paradoxically, NMS has also been reported with amphetamine or cocaine use.

More recently, Keck et al. in 1991 reported an incidence of NMS ranging from 0.02 to 2.4% in a large number of neuroleptic-treated patients and found there was a 0.67% pooled mean estimate (25). Such studies probably overestimate the incidence, since cohorts without NMS are usually not reported. Large-scale epidemiological studies are required to obtain a more precise figure. Further, a significant proportion (i.e., 40%) of these patients were diagnosed as having mood disorders. The ratio of males to females who developed NMS was 3:2, and the mean reported age was about 40 years old.

Other possible risk factors include:

- Presence of an organic mental disorder
- Agitation
- Dehydration
- The rate, route, and dose of neuroleptic administration
- The use of concurrent psychotropics (e.g., lithium).

While 80% of NMS cases occur within the first 2 weeks of initiation or an increase in the dose, it must be emphasized that NMS can occur at any time. Typically, the syndrome progresses rapidly, fully developing in 24–48 hours, and lasts for an average of 7–14 days, but up to 30 days is not unusual. The duration is usually twice as long when depot agents are involved.

Patients with NMS almost always have elevated creatine phosphokinase (CPK) levels. Increases are usually in the 2000–15,000 v/L range and rarely above 100,000 v/L. The absence of an elevation in CPK would speak against the diagnosis of NMS; however, it is nonspecific and can also be markedly increased with agitation; many forms of strenuous physical exercise; dystonic reactions; or intramuscular injections (i.e., CPK is a high sensitivity, low specificity test). Often agitated psychotic patients are given intramuscular injections, further increasing CPK levels. SGOT, SGPT, lactate dehydrogenase (LDH) are usually elevated, indicating liver involvement. White cell elevations range from 15,000 to 30,000/L, with a shift to the left occurring in about 40% of cases. The EEG is usually normal but may show diffuse slowing or other nonspecific abnormalities.

Differential Diagnosis

In *malignant hyperthermia* (MH), muscle rigidity and fever develop rapidly, following exposure to inhalation anesthetic agents and/or succinylcholine. The gene for this disorder has recently been described. Other differential diagnostic considerations include:

- Lethal catatonia
- Heat stroke
- Viral encephalitis
- Tetanus
- Other infections

Treatment

The most important step to effective treatment of NMS is early recognition and prompt withdrawal of the offending agent. In addition, supportive measures should be instituted as quickly as possible. If the patient is receiving an antiparkinsonian agent, it probably should be continued; however, data are lacking to support their usefulness, and care must be taken to avoid an anticholinergically induced worsening of mental status and perhaps further temperature increase. If there is reasonable certainty that the syndrome is NMS, the patient should be transferred to a medical setting in which intensive observation and treatment can be provided.

A variety of supportive measures can be used, including cooling blankets, ice packs or an ice-water enema. The goal should be to return the temperature as close to normal as possible. One should also be ready to treat complications and give supplemental oxygen with or without mechanical ventilation (the amount of oxygen and the method of delivery will depend on the patient's needs).

Drug Treatment. Because of the nature of the disorder, there are no controlled studies; however, most investigators suggest a trial with one or more of the following agents:

- Dantrolene
- Bromocriptine
- Amantadine
- Some combination of these agents.

The initial dose of *dantrolene* should be 2–3 mg/kg over 10–15 minutes. The total dosage should not exceed 10 mg/kg/day, because of the increased risk of hepatotoxicity. The dosage range reported as effective is 0.8–10 mg/kg/day. The typical oral dosage of *bromocriptine* is 2.5–10 mg three times daily; with increases up to 60 mg/day. Some have used bromocriptine in conjunction with dantrolene, with similar dosage patterns. The oral dose of *amantadine* is 200–400 mg/day in divided doses. *Levodopa plus carbidopa* has been infrequently used, and efficacy is not well documented. Dosage of carbidopa is 25 mg plus levodopa 100 mg (three to eight times daily). The *calcium channel blocker* nifedipine has also been used to treat NMS, and further data on this drug would be important, given its beneficial effect in a single case report (26).

The authors found that the specific drug treatment with dantrolene and/or dopaminergic agonists significantly reduced the mortality rate from NMS (i.e., 10% versus 21%), and did so uniformly in mild, moderate and severe cases (27). To test the significance of this finding, we performed case-controlled analyses using as a control the mortality rate of NMS patients who had not received any specific treatment. Thus, by definition the control group consisted of patients who had not received bromocriptine, amantadine, other DA agonists, dantrolene, any form of dopa or ECT.

Electroconvulsive Therapy. ECT is an effective treatment for psychotic and/or severe mania, depression, catatonia, schizophrenic excitement, and schizoaffective disorder. However, its use for the treatment of NMS is controversial because some patients have died or developed cardiac arrest during ECT, whereas others benefited when it was given during or shortly after an episode had resolved (28). The authors reviewed the world literature and found a mortality rate of 11% when ECT was employed during an episode of NMS (29). This compares to a 10% rate in patients treated with specific drug therapy (e.g., dantrolene, DA agonists) and a 21% rate in patients who received only nonspecific treatment for their episode. Further, in the three deaths with ECT, high potency APs were continued before, during and after ECT. Thus, the failure of the NMS to improve may have been due to the continued administration of the offending drug. There were also other cases when antipsychotics were continued with ECT throughout the episode of NMS, and the outcomes were not favorable, though the patients survived. Again, these drugs should be discontinued whenever the possibility of NMS is suspected. While there is insufficient case report data to prove ECT helps NMS, it is clear that this therapy does not worsen the condition. Since some acutely psychotic patients require immediate intervention, ECT may be lifesaving, whereas premature re-introduction of an antipsychotic may worsen an NMS episode.

Retreatment after an NMS Episode. *Retreatment strategies* after an episode of NMS include:

- *ECT* for psychotic depression or other emergencies (30)
- *Lithium* or alternate treatments such as divalproex sodium or carbamazepine for bipolar, manic; schizoaffective; and schizophreniform disorders. Alternate *non-neuroleptic interventions*, may be better in light of reports that affectively disordered patients with psychotic features may be more susceptible to tardive dyskinesia and NMS.
- In psychotic manic episodes *lower doses* in combination with lithium may be as effective as higher doses and perhaps diminish the possibility of an NMS recurrence (31)

If an antipsychotic is necessary, treatment should be instituted as long as possible after an episode (i.e., at least 2 weeks). Because as many as 50% of patients re-exposed to an antipsychotic again develop the syndrome, an antipsychotic from a different family, and preferably a lower potency agent such as thioridazine should be administered. The recommendation to use thioridazine and/or an agent from a different family is based on common sense and not empirical data.

Further, it is best to *start with a very low dose and titrate up slowly* in a hospital setting to carefully monitor clinical response, temperature, and neurological and mental status as well. Using low doses will not necessarily jeopardize chances for an adequate clinical response. For example, we have recently found evidence for a therapeutic effect with low-dose trifluoperazine (32). This finding is consistent with a growing body of literature indicating that "less may indeed be more" when it comes to the dose of antipsychotic.

An alternate agent that has been considered is *clozapine;* however, three recent case reports indicate that this agent used alone may also induce NMS (33–35). We know of a fourth unpublished case and two cases with clozapine-other drug combinations. An unusual adverse effect of clozapine is *hyperthermia* in 10–15% of patients (usually 0.5 to 1°C, but virtually never above 40°C (104°F)). This symptom usually occurs between the fifth and the 15th days of treatment, after which, temperature returns to normal. *Benzodiazepines* (e.g., lorazepam) have also been recommended to either avoid or at least minimize the dose of neuroleptic.

We would also suggest *prophylactic concomitant bromocriptine* for several weeks, with gradual tapering after that time period. Such prophylactic approaches during the retreatment phase have been attempted in a few patients, but there are no controlled studies. Nevertheless, it seems like a sensible strategy and poses little additional risk.

AUTONOMIC ADVERSE EFFECTS

Anticholinergic Effects

Neuroleptics and antidepressants block central and peripheral muscarinic cholinergic receptors, producing many anticholinergic adverse effects, such as:

- Blurred vision
- Dry mouth
- Constipation
- Urinary retention (36).

Patients may develop some tolerance to these effects, which tend to be most troublesome during the early stages of treatment. Dry mouth is one of the most frequent complaints, and patients should be advised to rinse their mouths frequently, and to use *sugarless* gum or candy (sugar products provide a good cultural medium for fungal infection, such as moniliasis, and may also increase the incidence of dental cavities). Further, dry mouth in general can predispose to infections, because saliva is bacteriostatic. Urecholine can alleviate urinary retention.

Approximately one-third of patients on clozapine experience *hypersalivation*, both during the day and at night (e.g., patients often complain of waking up with a wet pillow). While generally mild to moderate in intensity, it can be more se-

vere, even warranting discontinuation of the drug. The increased salivation may disappear with time or with a reduction in dose, but can also persist. Anticholinergics or amitriptyline may help.

CARDIOVASCULAR EFFECTS

Orthostatic Hypotension

Lower potency agents (e.g., CPZ) with α-adrenergic blocking effects and clozapine produce a dose-related postural hypotension and related tachycardia, most pronounced with moderate to higher doses. This can occur after the first dose, worsen on the second or third day, but then subside due to tolerance. It also tends to be more problematic in the elderly and those on higher doses of parenteral medication. It is prudent to monitor blood pressure (lying and standing) after the first dose and during the first few days of treatment. Effective management of this effect begins with a gradual increase in a drug like clozapine (e.g., 25 mg bid or tid for 2 days, then 50 mg tid for several days), with a slower escalation over the next week to 10 days until the minimal therapeutic level (e.g., 300–450 mg/day in divided doses) is achieved. Such a schedule produces significant hypotension in only 3–5% of patients on clozapine, although many will experience milder degrees.

The chief danger with this adverse effect is fainting or falling, although such occurrences are rare. This is an important complication since injuries related to such falls can produce significant morbidity. The α-adrenergic blocking properties are the most likely basis (37).

Treatment

Patients should be instructed to:

- Rise from bed gradually
- Sit with legs dangling for a brief period

- Wait at least 1 minute before standing
- Sit or lie down if feeling faint
- Use support hose, if hypotension persists.

Rarely is it necessary to keep a patient in bed for prolonged periods. Those with serious cardiovascular disease, should have their doses increased very slowly, with blood pressure frequently monitored. Acute orthostasis can usually be managed by having the patient lie down with feet elevated. On rare occasions, volume expanders or vasopressors may be required.

Cardiac Rhythm Disturbances

Patients with known or suspected cardiac disease should have a pretreatment electrocardiogram (ECG). An abnormality consisting of broadened, flattened, or clove T-waves, with increased Q-R intervals has been described with thioridazine at doses as low as 300 mg/day, but does not seem to be associated with any significant clinical consequences. "Torsade des pointes" has been described with several antipsychotics and is characterized by a peculiar type of ventricular tachycardia in which the amplitude of successive beats fluctuates in a sine wave pattern (37).

Clozapine also produces nonspecific inverted T-waves, but again, this is not considered clinically relevant. As far as is known, abrupt discontinuation of antipsychotics, including clozapine, does not produce serious adverse effects, although common sense dictates a gradual reduction over several days (38).

Sudden death is a rare phenomenon with the antipsychotic. An accurate assessment as to whether these drugs are causally or coincidentally involved cannot be made, because sudden death can occur in young, apparently healthy persons on no medication. For example, every year in

the United States some 600,000 people die suddenly. Although the most commonly postulated cause of sudden death is ventricular fibrillation, it can also result from:

- *Asphyxia* caused by regurgitated food
- An endobronchial *mucous plug in asthmatics*
- *Shock* in patients with acquired *megacolon*
- As a complication of *seizures*
- Slowed *intracardiac conduction* (similar to Type II antiarrhythmics and TCAs)

In the past, sudden death was thought to be the result of myocardial infarction, but with more patients surviving such episodes, it appears that many had ventricular arrhythmias without evidence of cardiac muscle damage.

Statistically, the incidence of sudden death in mental patients has not increased since the introduction of antipsychotics, and no one type is more implicated, with deaths occurring on high- and low-potency agents. Medical examiners should refrain from attributing sudden death to these drugs, or to any other cause for that matter, until research clearly establishes a causal, not coincidental, link.

DERMATOLOGIC AND OCULAR EFFECTS

A variety of *dermatological effects*—including urticarial, maculopapular, petechial, and edematous eruptions—occurs infrequently and usually early (in the first few weeks) in treatment. A contact dermatitis can even occur in personnel who handle CPZ. Because sunlight plays a role, difference in incidence may relate to variations in sun exposure. Photosensitivity of the phototoxic type resembles severe sunburn and most often occurs with CPZ;

therefore, patients should be encouraged to avoid excessive sunlight and/or use sunscreens (36).

Chloropromazine—Specific Skin and Eye Changes

Both the dermatological and ocular changes are a reaction to high levels of sunlight and chronic CPZ use. Dermatological effects specific to CPZ include a blue-gray, metallic discoloration in areas exposed to sunlight (face, neck, and the dorsum of hands), beginning with a tan or golden brown color and progressing to slate gray, metallic blue or purple. Histological studies of skin biopsies reveal pigmentary granules similar, but not identical to melanin.

Eye changes have been noticed after chronic, high-dose chlorpromazine and are described as whitish brown granular deposits concentrated in the anterior lens and posterior cornea, visible only by slit lamp examination (these are quite different from, and in no way related to, senile cataracts). Statistically, opacities occur more frequently with skin discoloration, but retinal damage does not occur and vision is virtually never impaired. The occurrence and severity of both effects are related to the duration and total lifetime dose of CPZ (e.g., usually greater than a total dose of 1–3 kg). In the past 2 decades, with the increased use of high-potency agents, these adverse effects have virtually disappeared; but it is not clear that they are totally absent, because this complication is only apparent under a slit lamp. Treatments consist of minimizing exposure to the sun and switching from chlorpromazine to a nonphenothiazine.

Thioridazine—Specific Eye Effects

Thioridazine poses a potentially greater danger to the eyes than CPZ. At doses greater than 800 mg/day, a *retinitis pigmentosa* may appear, leading to substantial visual impairment or even blindness. In some cases, the condition does not fully remit when the drug is stopped; therefore, thioridazine doses of more than 800 mg/day are never recommended to allow for a reasonable margin of safety (36).

ENDOCRINE EFFECTS

There is a large body of preclinical research on the neuroendocrine effects of antipsychotics in a variety of species. Clinical studies find that they induce small, inconsistent effects on sex, adrenocortical, thyroid, and pituitary hormone-related activity. Although much of this literature is not directly relevant to humans, two important effects are *increased lactation* and *possible sexual impotence*. These agents presumably induce their effects by blocking DA receptors in the pituitary, producing a marked increase in prolactin (particularly in females, but also in males). This increase causes breast engorgement and lactation in female patients. If every patient were checked for lactation by manual pressure on the breast, the incidence could be as high as 20–40%, but complaints of overt lactation are relatively rare (i.e., less than 5%). *Gynecomastia* in male patients is also described. There is no evidence that elevated prolactin levels produce any serious consequences, and treatment involves dose reduction or switching to another antipsychotic.

Delayed ejaculation occurs with thioridazine, perhaps due to its greater autonomic effects. Clinicians must be sensitive to these effects because many patients are embarrassed to talk about them.

Glucose-tolerance curves may be shifted in a fashion consistent with diabetes, and false-positive pregnancy tests have been reported.

The marked *weight gain* sometimes associated with drug therapy has not been explained on any endocrine basis. If problematic, one can switch to molindone, which may not cause as much weight gain.

GASTROINTESTINAL EFFECTS

Hepatic

Shortly after the introduction of CPZ, *jaundice* was noted to occur in about one out of every 200 patients. More recently, its incidence has inexplicably decreased to one in 1000, although accurate data are lacking. Jaundice is most often seen about 1–5 weeks after the initiation of therapy and is usually preceded by a flu-like syndrome (malaise, abdominal pain, fever, nausea, vomiting, and diarrhea), resembling mild gastroenteritis or infectious hepatitis. Important clinical factors include:

- *Temporal association* between jaundice and the recent initiation of drug therapy
- Lack of an enlarged or tender *liver*
- Chemical evidence of *choleostasis*, such as an increase in direct relative to indirect bilirubin
- Increased *alkaline phosphatase*
- A reduction of *esterified cholesterol*
- Moderately increased *aminotransferases*
- Peripheral blood smears demonstrating *eosinophilia*
- Liver biopsies showing *bile plugs in the caniliculi*, with eosinophilic infiltration in the periportal space.

This disorder usually disappears after several weeks, with a complete return to normal liver function expected. Rarely, a longer-lasting exanthematous biliary cirrhosis occurs, characterized by a more chronic course of 6 months to 1 year, but also eventually clears. This may be an allergic phenomenon, as evidenced by:

- *Onset* in the first few weeks of treatment
- Frequent association with *other allergic reactions*
- Association with peripheral *eosinophilia* and eosinophilic infiltrations in the liver
- *Prolonged retention of sensitivity* on the challenge test
- Development of a *second episode* as long as 10 years after the first.

The majority of cases reported in the literature have occurred with chlorpromazine and rarely with other agents such as promazine, thioridazine, mepazine, prochlorperazine, fluphenazine, and triflupromazine. There is no convincing evidence that haloperidol or other nonphenothiazine agents produce this type of jaundice. It is occasionally useful to obtain baseline liver function tests on patients with increased susceptibility (e.g., prior history of hepatitis) in the unlikely event that jaundice may develop. Routine serial liver function tests have never proven useful or necessary. The offending drug should be discontinued if a patient develops jaundice, but the value of this practice is also unproven, because many patients have been maintained on CPZ throughout an episode of jaundice without adverse consequences (39).

Hematologic Effects

Leukopenia is a reduction in the white blood cell count (WBC) to less than 3500/mm^3 and a granulocyte count of at least 1500. *Granulocytopenia* is a reduction in the granulocyte count below 1500, whereas *agranulocytosis* is defined as a reduction below 500. Standard antipsychotics induce leukopenia or granulocytopenia in about 5–15% of patients, but this phenomenon has no clinical significance. In comparative studies, the incidence of clopazine-induced leukopenia and granulocytopenia was less than that with chlorpromazine or haloperidol (19). Patients on any of these drugs may experience a WBC drop below 5000, which shortly returns to a normal range, or a drop below 5000, which then remains between 3500 and 5000, with some fluctuation. This drop in WBC does not typically progress to agranulocytosis.

Agranulocytosis occurs rarely with CPZ, and to a lesser extent with promazine, prochlorperazine, mepazine, and thioridazine. It can be assumed to arise with any phenothiazine. It is usually seen in older females with other complicating systemic diseases, and is considerably rarer in young, healthy adults. It generally occurs in the first 6–8 weeks of treatment, with an abrupt onset consisting of a sore throat, ulcerations, and fever. The mortality rate is high, often exceeding 30%.

The offending drug should be discontinued immediately, the patient transferred to a setting with reverse isolation facilities, and aggressive treatment of any infection must be instituted. Cross-sensitivity to other phenothiazines is assumed to be possible, but supporting data are lacking. The value of routine, weekly CBCs is highly questionable because agranulocytosis develops so rapidly. On occasion, phenothiazines may temporarily reduce the total WBC by as much as 30–60%, but this is a different and more benign hematological phenomenon, requiring neither special treatment nor discontinuation of drug therapy. Rarely, thrombocytopenic or nonthrombocytopenic purpura, hemolytic anemias, and pancytopenia are precipitated by phenothiazines, necessitating a switch to another antipsychotic in a different chemical class.

Clozapine-Related Agranulocytosis

About 115 cases of agranulocytosis have been reported worldwide with clozapine,

36 of which occurred during 1975. Many other drugs also cause agranulocytosis, and in some cases patients were receiving such agents in addition to clozapine. A number of patients were not on any other potential offending drug, however, implicating clozapine as the cause (38, 40).

The WBC of patients on clozapine must be followed closely (i.e., with weekly or even twice weekly complete blood counts), especially during the period of greatest risk (i.e., weeks 5–25). If a patient's WBC count drops below:

- 5000, counts should be repeated three times a week
- 3500 and/or the granulocyte count falls below 1500, clozapine should be immediately discontinued
- 1000 or granulocytes below 500, the patient should be placed in reverse isolation.

Risk factors. Two of three patients suffering from agranulocytosis are female, but there is no apparent relationship to age or dose of clozapine. Agranulocytosis is rare in the first 4 weeks of treatment, peaking in incidence during the period between the fifth and 25th weeks of treatment. This observation is important because some patients may be given clozapine on a trial basis for approximately 4 weeks without an appreciable risk of agranulocytosis; and the drug can be discontinued in clear nonresponders before the period of greatest liability. Patients with early, clinically significant response would be the best candidates to continue beyond the period of risk.

Initially, the mortality rate from clozapine-induced agranulocytosis was about 40%, but more recently it has decreased by more than half. Now, while the mortality rate of agranulocytosis complicated by infection is still 40%, without infection it is approximately 15%. In United States clini-

Table 5.21.
Adverse Effects of Antipsychotics

Adverse Effects	Clinical Alerts	Treatment Approaches	Most Common Offenders
I. *Central nervous system*			
A. Acute EPS			
• Pseudoparkinsonism	• Rigidity, bradykinesia, tremor, masked facies	• Decrease dose • Add antiparkinson agent • Switch to another agent	All agents, especially: Haloperidol Fluphenazine Thiothixene
• Dystonias	• Retrocollis, oculogyric crisis, opisthotonus, torticollis • Rarely, laryngeal spasm	• Parenteral antiparkinsonian agent	Loxapine Molindone Perphenazine Trifluoperazine
• Acute dyskinesias	• Rapid, involuntary, coordinated stereotypical movements, usually of mouth, tongue, face		
• Akathisia	• Restlessness, inability to sit still, pacing	• β-blockers; diazepam	
B. Late-onset (tardive) syndromes	• Dyskinesias (usually of tongue, mouth, lips) • Dystonic symptoms	• Stop drugs, if possible • Reserpine may help temporarily	All agents
C. Decrease in seizure threshold	• Convulsion(s)	• Minimize dose • Slowly increase, if necessary • Add anticonvulsants (CBZ, VPA)	Chlorpromazine Promazine
D. Withdrawal syndrome	• GI symptoms, irritability, headaches	• Slowly taper AP drug	
E. Drowsiness, oversedation		• Give as bedtime dose • Increase caffeine intake • Decrease dose • Change to less-sedating agent (e.g., fluphenazine)	Chlorpromazine Thioridazine
F. Cognitive effects	• Toxic psychosis	• Stop or decrease anticholinergic agents e.g.,	Thioridazine
• Central anticholinergic syndrome	Delirium	• Antiparkinsonian • Antidepressant • Antipsychotic • i.v. physostigmine (?)	Chlorpromazine

Table 5.21.—continued
Adverse Effects of Antipsychotics

Adverse Effects	Clinical Alerts	Treatment Approaches	Most Common Offenders
G. Temperature dysregulation • Neuroleptic malignant syndrome	• Hypothermia • Hyperthermia, rigidity, autonomic instability	• Stop drug • Cooling techniques, antipyretics, other supportive treatment • Dantrolene, bromocriptine, other DA agonists, ECT	All agents
2. Autonomic A. Anticholinergic • Difficulty in accommodation; increased intraocular pressure • Dry mouth • Constipation • Hesitancy, urinary retention • Nasal congestion	• Pupillary changes, blurred vision • May develop oral fungal infection • Absent bowel sounds, can progress to paralytic ileus • Delayed or inhibited ejaculation	• Eyeglasses needed (rare) • Decrease dose • Decrease or stop concomitant anticholinergic agent • Frequent, small sips of water • Sugarless candy or gum • Bulk laxatives • Increase fluids • Switch to agent with less anticholinergic effect	Thioridazine Mesoridazine Chlorpromazine
B. Secondary to α-receptor blockade • Hypotension • Tachycardia • Pallor	• Dizziness, syncope • Postural hypotension	• Decrease dose • Change to higher potency agent • Support hose N.B. epinephrine should be avoided	Chlorpromazine Thioridazine
3. Cardiovascular A. ECG changes B. Torsade des pointes C. Sudden death	• Flattening of T wave • Ventricular tachycardia • Probable lethal arrhythmia (uncertain if neuroleptics are associated causally or coincidentally)	• No clinical significance • Stop drug • Avoid lower potency agents, if possible	Thioridazine

	Manifestation	Treatment	Drug
4. Dermatologic-Ocular			
A. Dermatoses			
• Contact	• Urticarial, maculopapular, petechial, edematous eruptions	• Stop drug	Phenothiazines (especially chlorpromazine)
• Systemic			
• Photosensitivity	• Severe sunburn	• Prevent by using sunscreens	
B. Discoloration of skin and corneal or lens opacities	• Blue-gray metallic discoloration of skin • Whitish deposits on ocular exam (do not interfere with vision)	• Decrease dose • Switch drug • Avoid sunlight	Chlorpromazine Thiothixene
C. Pigmentary retinopathy	• Brownish discoloration of vision • Decrease in visual acuity • Pigmentation of fundi	• Do not exceed 800 mg/day thioridazine • Stop drug if symptoms appear	Thioridazine
5. Endocrine system			
A. Galactorrhea, gynecomastia	• Lactation • Breast enlargement	• Decrease or change agent	Especially phenothiazines
B. Amenorrhea	• Menstrual irregularities	• Check for pregnancy • Decrease or change agent • Decrease or change agent	
C. Disturbances in sex drive			
D. Disturbances in glucose metabolism	• Unexplained elevated blood sugar or abnormal G.T.T.		
E. Weight gain, edema (?)		• Restrict caloric intake • Increase exercise • Perhaps switch to molindone if gain is excessive	
6. Gastrointestinal	• Decreased bowel motility and associated constipation		
Hepatic	• Jaundice, followed in 1–7 days by fever, nausea, RUQ pain, malaise	• Stop drug, switch to a non-phenothiazine	Chlorpromazine

Table 5.21.—continued
Adverse Effects of Antipsychotics

Adverse Effects	Clinical Alerts	Treatment Approaches	Most Common Offenders
7. *Hematological* A. Agranulocytosis B. Leukopenia	• Unexplained sore throat, fever, petechiae, malaise	• Weekly CBC with clozapine • Stop drug • Reverse isolation • Antibiotics, supportive care	Clozapine Chlorpromazine (rare with other phenothiazines—never proven to occur in nonphenothiazines)
8. *Drug–drug interactions* e.g.: • Antacids • Barbiturates • Lithium	• Unexplained decrease in efficacy or increase in toxicity	• Avoid concommitant use of agents known to have synergistic or antagonistic effects	All agents (especially chlorpromazine)
9. *Overdose*	• Signs and symptoms: effects maximum w/in 4–6 hours • CNS: agitation, confusion, delirium, twitching, dystonic movements, EPS, convulsions, hyperthermia • C-V: increased HR, decreased BP, arrhythmias, C-V collapse	• Supportive, gastric lavage (H$_2$O soluble) • Antiparkinsonian drugs (diphenhydramine) • Forced diuresis and hemodialysis not helpful • Lipoid dialysis may be beneficial	All antipsychotics

Adapted from Davis JM, Janicak PG, Lindon R, et al. Neuroleptics and psychotic disorders. In: Coyle JT, Enna SJ, eds. Neuroleptics: neurochemical, behavioral and clinical perspectives. New York: Raven Press, 1983.

cal trials the incidence is about 1 per 100, but because this outcome is based on only 1000 patients, it may not be an accurate estimate. It is notable that some who developed clozapine-induced agranulocytosis were later able to tolerate phenothiazines without a recurrence, again implying a different underlying mechanism. When clozapine is discontinued, the WBC gradually returns to normal levels over 2–4 weeks. Treatment requires reverse isolation and management of intercurrent infections with appropriate antibiotics.

CONCLUSION

Although it is difficult to quantify discomfort, the adverse effects of APs most often experienced are less severe than symptoms associated with the common cold. Serious adverse events are much less common. There is a risk to every treatment, but it is erroneous to suggest that because a serious event may occur, it is likely to occur. For example, one of the most dangerous activities we engage in is driving or riding in an automobile; yet that does not mean that every time we drive to work there is a high probability that we will experience a serious injury or death.

We have summarized our recommended clinical strategy for psychotic disorders in Figures 5.4 and 5.9 as well as the important adverse events seen with antipsychotics in Table 5.21. We emphasize the chronic nature of these disorders and, in that light, the necessity of developing treatment plans with the optimal risk/benefit balance.

REFERENCES

1. Adler LA, Rieter S, Corwin J, Hemdal P, Angrist B, Rotrosen J. Differential effects of propranolol and benzotropine in patients with neuroleptic-induced akathisia. Psychopharmacol Bull 1987;23(3):519–521.

2. Kramer MS, Gorkin RA, Johnson C, Sheves P. Propranolol in the treatment of neuroleptic-induced akathisia(nia) in schizophrenics: a double-blind, placebo-controlled study. Biopsychiatry 1988;24:823–827.

3. Lipinski JF, Zubenko GS, Cohen BM, Barriera PJ. Propranolol in the treatment of neuroleptic-induced akathisia. Am J Psychiatry 1984;141:412–415.

4. Adler L, Angrist B, Peselow E, Corwin J, Maslansky R, Rotrosen J. A controlled assessment of propranolol in the treatment of neuroleptic-induced akathisia. Br J Psychiatry 1986;149:42–45.

5. Altamura AC, Mauri MC, Mantero M, Brunetti M. Clonazepam/haloperidol combination therapy in schizophrenia: a double-blind study. Acta Psychiatr Scand 1987;76:702–706.

6. Marneros A. Anxiolytische zusatzbehandlung bei den affektbetonten schizphrenien. Therapiewoche 1979;29:7533–7538.

7. Adler L, Angrist B, Peselow E, Corwin J, Rotrosen J. Efficacy of propranolol in neuroleptic-induced akathesia. J Clin Psychopharmacol 1985;5:164–166.

8. Lipinski JF, Zubenko GS, Cohen BM, Barreira PJ. Propranolol in the treatment of neuroleptic-induced akathisia. Am J Psychiatry 1984;141:412–415.

9. Donlan PT. The therapeutic use of diazepam for akathisia. Psychosomatics 1973;14:222–225.

10. Kutcher S, Williamson P, MacKenzie S, Marton P, Ehrlich M. Successful clonazepam treatment of neuroleptic-induced akathisia in older adolescents and young adults: a double-blind, placebo-controlled study. J Clin Psychopharmacol 1989;9(6):403–406.

11. Gagrat D, Hamilton J, Belmaker RH. Intravenous diazepam in the treatment of neuroleptic-induced acute dystonia and akathisia. Am J Psychiatry 1978;135:1232–1233.

12. Bodkin JA. Emerging uses for high-potency benzodiazepines in psychotic disorder. J Clin Psychiatry 1990;5(suppl):41–46.

13. Hanlon TE, Schoenrich C, Frenck W, Turek I, Kurland AA. Perphenazine benzotropine mesylate treatment of newly admitted psychiatric patients. Psychopharmacologia 1966;9:328–339.

14. Comaty JE, Janicak PG, Rajaratnam J, Sharma RP, Baker D, Davis JM. Is mainte-

nance antiparkinsonian treatment necessary? Psychopharmacol Bull 1980;26:267–271.

15. Chien CP, DiMascio A, Cole JO. Antiparkinsonian agents and depot phenothiazine. Am J Psychiatry 1974;131:86–90.

16. Lapolla A, Nash LR. Treatment of phenothiazine-induced parkinsonism with biperiden. Curr Ther Res 1965;7:536–541.

17. Crane GE. Dyskinesia and neuroleptics. Arch Gen Psychiatry 1968;19:700–703.

18. Tardive Dyskinesia. A task force report of the American Psychiatric Association. Washington, D.C.: American Psychiatric Association, 1992.

19. Davis JM, Barter JT, Kane JM. Antipsychotic drugs. In: Kaplan HI, Sadock BJ, eds. Comprehensive textbook of psychiatry. 5th ed. Vol 2. Baltimore: Williams & Wilkins, 1989:1591–1626.

20. Owens DG, Johnstone EC, Frith CD. Spontaneous involuntary disorders of movement. Arch Gen Psychiatry 1982:39:452–461.

21. Caine ED, Polinsky RJ, Kartzinel R, Ebert MH. The trial use of clozapine for abnormal involuntary movement disorders. Am J Psychiatry 1979;136(3):317–320.

22. Cole JO, Gardos G, Tarsay D, et al. Drug trials in persistent dyskinesia. In: Fann WE, Davis JM, Domino E, Smith RC, eds. Tardive dyskinesia: research and treatment. New York: Spectrum Medical, 1980.

23. Gerbino L, Shopsin B, Collora M. Clozapine in the treatment of tardive dyskinesia: an interim report. In: Fann WE, Davis JM, Domino E, Smith RG, eds. Tardive dyskinesia: research and treatment. New York: Spectrum Medical, 1980.

24. Lieberman JA, Saltz BL, Johns CA, Pollack S, Kane JM. Clozapine effects on tardive dyskinesia. Psychopharmacol Bull, 1989;25(1);57–62.

25. Keck PE, McElroy SL, Pope HG: Epidemiology of NMS. J Clin Psychiatry 1991; 21:148–151.

26. Hermesh H, Molcho A, Aizenberg D, Munitz H. The calcium antagonist nifedipine in recurrent neuroleptic malignant syndrome. Clin Neuropharmacol 1988;II:552–555.

27. Sakkas P, Davis JM, Hau J, Wang Z. Pharmacotherapy of NMS. Psychiatr Ann 1991;21:157–164.

28. Addonizio G, Susman VL. ECT as a treatment alternative for patients with symptoms of neuroleptic malignant syndrome. J Clin Psychiatry 1987;48:102–105.

29. Davis JM, Janicak PG, Sakkas P, Gilmore C, Wang Z. Electroconvulsive therapy in the treatment of the neuroleptic malignant syndrome. Convulsive Therapy 1991;7(2): 111–120.

30. Janicak PG, Easton MS, Comaty JE, Dowd S, Davis JM. Efficacy of ECT in psychotic and nonpsychotic depression. Convulsive Ther 1989;5(4):314–320.

31. Janicak PG, Bresnahan DB, Sharma R, Davis JM, Comaty JE, Malinick C. A comparison of thiothixene with chlorpromazine in the treatment of mania. J Clin Psychopharmacol 1988;8(1):33–37.

32. Janicak PG, Javaid JI, Sharma RP, Comaty JE, Peterson J, Davis JM. Trifluoperazine plasma levels and clinical response. J Clin Psychopharmacol 1989;9(5):340–346.

33. Miller DD, Sharafuddin MJA, Kathol RG: A case of clozapine-induced NMS. J Clin Psychiatry 1991;52:99–101.

34. Anderson ES, Powers PS. NMS associated with clozapine use. J Clin Psychiatry 1991;52:102–104.

35. DasGupta K, Young A. Clozapine-induced NMS. J Clin Psychiatry 1991;52:105–107.

36. Cole JO, Davis JM. Antipsychotic drugs. In: Bellak L, ed. The schizophrenic syndrome. New York: Grune & Stratton, 1969:478:568.

37. Boshes RA, Davis JM. Medical side effects of psychoactive drugs. In: Berger PA, Brodie HK, eds. American handbook of psychiatry. Vol 8. New York: Basic Books, 1986.

38. Lieberman J, Kane JM, Johns CA. Clozapine guidelines for clinical management. J Clin Psychiatry 1989;58:329–338.

39. Davis JM, Janicak, PG, Linden R, Moloney J, Pavkovic I. Neuroleptics and psychotic disorders. In: Coyle JT, Enna SJ, eds. Neuroleptics: neurochemical, behavioral, and clinical perspectives. New York: Raven Press, 1983.

40. Kane JM, Honigfeld G, Singer J, et al. Clozapine for the treatment resistant schizophrenic. A double blind comparison versus chlorpromazine/benztropine. Arch Gen Psychiatry 1988;45:789.

CHAPTER 6

Indications for Antidepressant Therapy

Major Depression

EPIDEMIOLOGY

Klerman and Weisman (1989) reported an increasing rate of major depressive disorder (MDD) in cohorts born after World War II (1). This observation was associated with several factors, including:

- A *lowering of the age of onset*, with an increase in the late teenage and early adult years
- An *increase in the rates of depression* for all ages in the years between 1960 and 1975
- A *persistent gender effect*, with the risk of depression consistently two to three times higher among women than men across all adult ages
- A *persistent family effect*, with the risk about two to three times higher in first-degree relatives as compared with controls
- The suggestion of a *narrowing in the differential risk to men and women* because of a greater increase in the risk of depression among young men.

DIAGNOSTIC CRITERIA

A major depressive episode consists of mood changes accompanied by neuroveg- etative **symptoms on a daily basis for at least 2 weeks.** Our nosology also lists inclusion and exclusion criteria for MDD (Table 6.1; Appendices I and J), but there are problems with these.

First, this classification takes a *"Chinese menu" approach,* in that a patient needs only one criteria in category A, at least four of eight in category B, and should have none in category C. Thus, substantially different symptom clusters may still meet criteria for the same diagnosis. This approach increases diagnostic heterogeneity and impedes research by including patients in clinical trials with similar syndromic diagnoses but with different symptom constellations, and possibly with different pathophysiologies. The more immediate impact is to impair prediction about the natural outcome and to complicate the choice of appropriate treatment strategies. Improved diagnostic criteria would require the presence of the complete neurovegetative syndrome to meet the diagnosis of MDD. Otherwise, one could code conditions as a partial MDD, or use a completely different designation. Nonetheless, the Diagnostic and Statistical Manual, 3rd edition, revised (DSM-III-R) is an advance over the earlier system, which

Table 6.1.
DSM-III-R Diagnostic Criteria for a Major Depressive Episode

- Presence of at least 5 of the following symptoms during the same 2-week period (nearly every day), representing a change from previous functioning; at least one symptom is either (*a*) depressed mood, or (*b*) loss of interest or pleasure; exclude symptoms due to a physical condition, mood-incongruent delusions or hallucinations, incoherence, or marked loosening of associations.
  - Depressed mood (irritable mood in children and adolescents)
  - Markedly diminished interest or pleasure in almost all activities
  - Significant weight loss or gain (failure to attain expected weight gain in children)
  - Insomnia or hypersomnia
  - Observable psychomotor agitation or retardation
  - Fatigue or loss of energy
  - Feelings of worthlessness or excessive or inappropriate guilt (which may be delusional)
  - Diminished ability to think or concentrate, or indecisiveness
  - Recurrent thoughts of death, recurrent suicidal ideation, plans, or attempts
- Symptoms are not initiated or maintained by organic factor
- Symptoms do not result from uncomplicated bereavement
- Delusions or hallucinations are not present for as long as 2 weeks in the absence of prominent mood symptoms
- Not superimposed on schizophrenia, schizophreniform disorder, delusional disorder, or psychotic disorder not otherwise specified

                          Melancholic Type
- The presence of at least 5 of the following:
  - Loss of interest or pleasure
  - Lack of reactivity to usually pleasurable stimuli
  - Depression worse in the morning
  - Early awakening (at least 2 hours)
  - Observable psychomotor retardation or agitation
  - Significant weight loss or gain
  - No significant personality disturbance before first major depressive episode
  - One or more previous major episodes; previous good response to psychotropics or somatic therapy resulting in complete or nearly complete recovery

                          Seasonal Pattern (SAD)
- Regular temporal relationship between the onset of an episode (bipolar or major depression) and a particular 60-day period of the year
- Full remissions (or switch from depression to mania or hypomania) also occur within a particular 60-day period of the year
- Occurrence of at least 3 episodes of mood disturbance in 3 separate years (at least 2 consecutive) that demonstrated temporal seasonal relationship
- Seasonal episodes of mood disturbance outnumber nonseasonal episodes by more than 3:1

Adapted from American Psychiatric Association. Diagnostic and statistical manual of mental disorders. 3rd ed, revised. Washington, D.C.: American Psychiatric Association, 1987.

essentially based the diagnosis on the presence of a depressed mood alone.

The reliance on a syndromic diagnosis of MDD rather than a symptomatic diagnosis is important for prognostic and hence, for treatment planning purposes. The use of syndromes comes from factor analysis of characteristics that distinguished drug versus placebo responders in clinical trials conducted in the early 1960s, when depressed mood was the singular criterion for entry. From these studies, a mood change alone was highly predictive of a placebo response, while the presence of neurovegetative signs and symptoms predicted a poor response to placebo.

An additional problem with the DSM-III-R criteria is the *short duration* In earlier nosologies (e.g., Washington University criteria), a minimum of 4 weeks was required. In double-blind, placebo-controlled trials, a duration of less than 3 months is often associated with a higher placebo response rate. **Thus, the longer an episode, the greater the clinician's confidence that a patient will need and will respond to medical intervention.**

DIFFERENTIAL DIAGNOSIS

A depressive episode may result from a diverse group of psychiatric and nonpsychiatric conditions (Table 6.2), which differ in their natural course as well as in their response to treatment. Hence, a differential diagnosis is critical to the workup of an episode.

Masked Depression

The first step is the recognition that a depressed mood is not synonymous with a depressive episode. Conversely, an episode of depression may not present with a mood complaint, but rather with associated symptoms such as insomnia or somatic complaints. This is particularly true for the elderly and for those seen in primary care settings. Even when a mood complaint is prominent it may not be described as "depressed" but instead, as "irritable" or "anxious." Thus, patients with MDD may present with a variety of complaints other than depressed mood, including:

- Insomnia
- Fatigue
- Somatic complaints, such as headache or gastrointestinal distress.

If the physician does not recognize that an MDD underlies such complaints, this could lead to costly but unnecessary tests, as well as to a delay in effective treatment. Complaints may also vary by age group. Common symptomatic issues are listed in Table 6.3.

Table 6.2.
Diagnostic Indications for Antidepressants (DSM-III-R-Categories)

- Mood disorders
  - Major depression
    - Single or recurrent
    - With or without melancholia
    - Seasonal pattern
  - Bipolar disorders
    - Depressed
    - Mixed
  - Cyclothymia
  - Dysthymia (or depressive neurosis)
- Psychotic disorders not elsewhere classified—schizoaffective disorder, depressed phase
- Organic mental disorder
  - Primary degenerative dementia with depression
  - Multi-infarct dementia with depression
  - Amphetamine or similarly acting sympathomimetic intoxication withdrawal
  - Organic mood disorder (e.g., reserpine-induced depression)

Table 6.3.
Presenting Complaints of Depression beyond the Typical Symptoms

- Prepubertal children
  - Somatic complaints
  - Agitation
  - Anxiety
  - Phobias
- Adolescents
  - Substance abuse
  - Antisocial behavior
  - Restlessness
  - Truancy and other school difficulties
  - Promiscuity
  - Rejection hypersensitivity
  - Poor hygiene
- Adults
  - Somatic complaints, particularly CV, GI, GU
  - Low back pain or other orthopaedic symptoms
- Elderly
  - Cognitive deficits
  - Pseudodementia
  - Somatic complaints as described above for adults

Subsyndromal Mood Disorders

Some patients present with a condition other than MDD (e.g., alcohol abuse), but the history often suggests the possibility of an underlying affective condition. Thus, a positive family history in first-degree relatives or reports consistent with an earlier but apparently resolved depressive episode may be critical to making the proper diagnosis. These patients may also have positive results on biological markers associated with MDD (e.g., the dexamethasone suppression test (DST), the thyrotropin-releasing hormone (TRH) test, or shortened rapid eye movement (REM) latency on the electro-oculogram). In addition, a substantial percentage respond to antidepressant (AD) therapy.

Treatment-Resistant Depression

We define treatment nonresponse as the persistence of a significant depression for at least 6 weeks despite appropriate treatment. For example, a course of treatment with a serotonin reuptake inhibitor (SRI) at the minimum effective dose or a tricyclic antidepressant (TCA) at therapeutic plasma concentrations (see also Therapeutic Drug Monitoring in Chapter 7) (2).

Incorrect diagnosis is the most common cause for AD nonresponse. Two common examples include: dual depression, in which a superimposed MDD improves with AD therapy but dysthymic symptoms persist and are mistaken for unimprovement; and second, affective disturbances associated with alcohol or drug abuse, which may persist even though symptoms of the MDD improve with drug therapy.

Noncompliance with the medication regimen is the next most common factor, and when suspected, therapeutic drug monitoring can be useful.

Subtherapeutic doses are often prescribed, especially by nonpsychiatrists. Preskorn et al. (1991) have noted that about 50% of depressed patients are prescribed doses of standard ADs that produce plasma tricyclic antidepressant (TCA) levels outside of the putative therapeutic ranges for such medications (2).

Time on treatment is another issue. Even though patients can show improvement at 2–3 weeks, many require at least 6 weeks before an adequate response. If, however, there has not been at least partial benefit by 4 weeks, we recommend an alternate strategy.

Treatment approaches for nonresponders are discussed in more detail in Alternate Treatment Strategies in Chapter 7.

TYPES OF DEPRESSIVE DISORDERS

There are several ways to subtype mood disorders (Table 6.4). *One system distinguishes functional psychiatric disorders from other medical conditions.* In the DSM-III-R, the latter are referred to as *organic mood disorders,* which is misleading because it implies that other mood disorders are not "organic" and/or are not medical conditions. Neither conclusion is accurate because, like other medical "organic" disorders, these conditions have an associated morbidity and mortality. As clinical neuroscience provides a better un-

Table 6.4.
Subtypes of Depressive Disorder

- Bipolar depression vs. unipolar depression
- Psychotic vs. nonpsychotic
- Primary psychiatric vs. secondary to other medical conditions
- Uncomplicated vs. complicated by other co-morbid disorders
- Phenomenology: melancholic, "atypical," psychotic
- Family pattern: familial = spectrum, sporadic
- Biological markers: DST, TRH-TSH, REM

derstanding of their pathophysiology, the "organic" basis will become more apparent. Thus, it is likely that the forthcoming DSM-IV will drop the distinction between "functional" and "organic" forms of mood disorders, and instead distinguish depressions that are primarily psychiatric versus those that are primarily nonpsychiatric, medical conditions.

A *second model is the primary versus secondary dichotomy* (see Secondary Type, later in this chapter).

Both the primary, psychiatric versus nonpsychiatric, medical disorder dichotomy, as well as the uncomplicated versus complicated dichotomy will be considered.

Primary Type:
Major Depressive Disorder

Bipolar versus Unipolar

The crucial element of both a bipolar and a unipolar disorder is the occurrence of an affective episode. The critical distinction is that *bipolar disorder* includes both hypomanic/manic and depressive episodes, whereas a *unipolar disorder* includes only depressive episodes.

After nonpsychiatric conditions have been ruled out, the clinician should determine whether the patient has a unipolar or a bipolar disorder (presenting for the first time with a depressive episode). Although this differentiation can be difficult, there are some clues that should help, including:

- The *younger* the patient is, the greater the chance that the course will have a bipolar disorder on longitudinal follow-up
- A *positive family history* for bipolar disorder, particularly in first-degree relatives
- A *hypomanic phase prior* to the onset of the depressive episode.

Hypomania consists of a disturbance in the same neurovegetative functions found in depression; however, they are qualitatively different. Moreover, they generally are not viewed as a problem by the patient. This means that patients are unlikely to complain spontaneously about such an episode, and the clinician will have to be alert and to screen for its occurrence.

Although hypomanic and manic episodes will be discussed comprehensively in Chapter 9, it is important to note that the disturbance in mania (and hypomania), as well as in depression, includes the same core symptoms, differing only in the direction of change. Unipolar patients may also present with classic melancholia or atypical (nonclassic) symptoms, with the latter, in particular, overlapping considerably with hypomania. Similarly, bipolar patients in a depressive phase may demonstrate classic or nonclassic symptoms (see Table 6.5).

Subtypes of Major Depressive Disorder

There are three subtypes of major depressive disorder: *melancholia,* or classic depression; *atypical* or nonclassic depression; and *psychotic* depression. These three subtypes have construct validity based on differences in:

- *Phenomenology* (Table 6.5)
- *Family history* of the illness, especially in first-degree relatives
- *Age of onset* distributions
- *Response rates* to specific types of drug or somatic therapies
- Incidence of positive *biological markers.*

There are several reasons to acknowledge these different subtypes:

- Melancholia is considered the classic (or typical) depressive disorder; thus,

Table 6.5.
Signs and Symptoms of Different Types of Affective Episodes

Sign/Symptom	Melancholia	"Atypical" or Nonclassic Depression	Hypomania
Mood	Depressed Anxious Irritable	Irritable Anxious Depressed	Irritable Euphoric
Affect	↓ Reactivity	↑ Reactivity	↑ Reactivity
Energy (subjective)	↓	↓	↑
Activity (objective)	↓	↑	↑
Sleep	↓	↑	↓
Appetite	↓	↑	↓
Sex drive	↓	↓	↑
Concentration/attention	↓	↓	↓
Interest	↓	↓	↑
Leaden paralysis		↑	↓
Rejection hypersensitivity		↑	

From Preskorn SH, Burke M. Somatic therapy for Major depressive disorder: Selection of an antidepressant. J Clin Psychiatry 1992;53(9;Suppl):5–18. Copyright 1992, Physicians Postgraduate Press.

nonclassic types can be misdiagnosed (e.g., as a personality disorder), because frequent and prominent symptoms include irritability, demandingness, and hostility.

- *Psychotic episodes* may be misdiagnosed as schizophrenia in younger patients or dementia with paranoia in the elderly.
- *Failure to identify the specific subtype may delay the most effective treatment,* particularly with psychotic depression.
- Failure to consider *differing natural courses* does not allow the clinician to anticipate sequelae or to respond quickly when they occur.

Patients with these different subtypes also differ in terms of the likelihood that they will demonstrate abnormalities on various biological tests for MDD. Thus, these markers are most likely to be positive in psychotic depressions and least likely to be positive in "atypical" MDD, with melancholia having an incidence somewhere between these two groups.

The fact that these tests are most often positive in psychotic MDD is also consistent with the observation that they predict a *low* placebo response.

Melancholia (Classic Depression). The features that distinguish melancholia from the other subtypes of MDD include:

- A *profoundly depressed* mood and appearance
- *Anhedonia*
- Accompanying feelings of *helplessness, worthlessness,* and *guilt* over imagined "sins"
- Problems with initial, middle, and terminal (or early morning awakening) *insomnia*
- Significant *anorexia,* often with appreciable *weight loss* (usually 20 or more pounds)
- Obvious psychomotor *retardation* or *agitation*
- An *absence of mood reactivity*
- A *diurnal variation* in the severity of symptoms

- Age of onset in the *mid-40s*
- *Female:male ratio* of 2:1.

This disorder tends to occur most often in patients with a positive family history of depression, although it can occur in the absence of such a history.

Atypical (Nonclassic Depression). Another subtype has been termed "atypical" MDD to denote that the clinical presentation is different from that of the classic form, namely:

- *Hypersomnia* rather than insomnia
- *Hyperphagia* rather than anorexia
- *Psychomotor agitation* rather than psychomotor retardation
- *Anxious or irritable mood* rather than dysphoria
- *A younger age of onset* than for melancholia, with a mean in the mid-20s
- *Female:male ratio* of about 3–4:1.

In addition, these patients often exhibit *rejection hypersensitivity,* and a *"leaden paralysis."* They may be misdiagnosed as having a personality disorder because of the associated irritability and demandingness. The presence of longstanding irritability and hostility may reflect a chronic depressive disorder and not necessarily "character" pathology. With this type of MDD, the patient tends to have a family pattern that has been designated "depressive-spectrum." Here, first-degree female relatives experience depression, while male relatives exhibit alcohol abuse or other unstable character traits reminiscent of antisocial personality disorder.

Nonclassic patients (especially males) may be at greater risk for sedative-hypnotic abuse. If the clinician is cognizant of these probabilities, he/she can take preventive steps (e.g., education about sedative-hypnotics). **The identification of** the nonclassic forms, as well as their differences in clinical presentation, has substantial implications for their differential treatment (see Chapter 7).

Psychotic or Delusional Depression. Psychotic depression is often characterized by the presence of mood-congruent delusions or hallucinations (the symptom is consistent with the mood state). Age of onset tends to follow a bimodal distribution, occurring either in the young or the old. Younger patients often have a family history of bipolar disorder. The female:male ratio tends to approximate 1:1. This disorder usually has fewer psychotic symptoms than mania or schizophrenia, most often a single, mood-congruent hallucination or delusion. Delusions are more common than hallucinations, which is why the term "delusional depression" has also been used. There is no apparent prognostic significance whether the patient presents with delusions or hallucinations. Examples include the belief:

- That one *has cancer* as a punishment from God for some earlier perceived sin
- That one *is bankrupt* because of fiscal irresponsibility
- That others have malicious intent toward one because one is *perceived as evil*
- That one is of very little value and *should cease to exist.*

The last two examples are often referred to as nihilistic delusions, frequently seen in older patients, who may even be convinced that they are already dead and their bodies have started to decay.

While the presence of delusions is usually clear, they may lead to a false diagnosis of schizophrenia in younger patients or dementia with paranoia in the elderly. Nihilistic delusions may be more subtle,

particularly in the elderly, appearing as a profound sense of worthlessness and despair. When probed further, the delusional quality of their thinking becomes more evident, facilitating the appropriate therapeutic intervention. When a patient has failed AD monotherapy and demonstrates significant feelings of worthlessness and hopelessness, the possibility of a psychotic MDD should be entertained.

Aronson et al. (1988) reported a retrospective study of 52 delusionally depressed patients, suggesting that there may be various subgroups: bipolar, early onset; unipolar; and possibly a late onset unipolar group (3). As with previous reports, there was a remarkably high rate of psychotic relapse in those patients who manifested psychotic symptoms at the index admission (i.e., depression or mania with psychotic features). Further, they found that psychotic features were more common in bipolar than in unipolar depression.

Treatment Implications. In 1975, Glassman et al. noted that delusionally depressed patients did not do well on imipramine alone, but did respond well with electroconvulsive therapy (ECT) (4). This study also ruled out low plasma levels as a possible explanation. In performing a statistical analysis of the published data and comparing the response rates of psychotic and nonpsychotic depressed patients treated with heterocyclics (HCAs), Chan et al. (1987) found that those with psychotic features had a substantially poorer response rate in every study (5). The results of these studies (which included 1054 patients) combined with the Mantel-Haenszel test showed that 67% of the nonpsychotic patients improved on HCAs alone, whereas only 35% of those with psychosis improved (see Table 6.6) (5–16). This difference was highly significant (chi square $= 104.2$; df $= 1$; $p < 2 \times 10^{-24}$).

A related factor is the nature of the severity of an episode. Typically, psychotic depressions are more severe and may require more than monotherapy, solely because of this; however, the National Institute of Mental Health (NIMH) Collaborative Study data revealed the *severely ill nonpsychotic* depressive patients may fare as poorly as their psychotic counterparts (17).

Antidepressant-antipsychotic combinations, antipsychotics alone, or HCAs alone have been compared in psychotically depressed patients, with the improvement rate for the combination better than for antipsychotics or HCAs alone (18). Amoxapine, which is metabolized to a neuroleptic, may have a particular advantage here. So far, however, there have been only limited data on comparisons between amoxapine and either ECT or combined pharmacological treatment (19). A disadvantage regarding this agent is its ability to cause extrapyramidal symptoms and tardive dyskinesia. Due to the ability of its metabolite to block dopamine (DA) receptors, the use of amoxapine in *nonpsychotic* patients is not recommended. Since depressive disorders are often recurrent, sustained AD therapy is often necessary. The question of how long to continue the antipsychotic is less certain. With an agent like amoxapine, which is in essence a combination treatment, the clinician does not have the option of "discontinuing" the antipsychotic component. For this reason, we would prefer using an antipsychotic plus an antidepressant other than amoxapine. **Because there is evidence that psychotically depressed patients have an excellent response to ECT, Janicak et al. (1989) recommend this therapy or an antipsychotic-antidepressant combination as the treatments of choice (20).**

Table 6.6.
Literature Review of Psychotic and Nonpsychotic Depressed Patient Response to Tricyclic Antidepressants[a]

Study	Psychotic				Nonpsychotic			Difference % Recovery
	Responders N	%	Nonresponders N		Responders N	%	Nonresponders N	
Friedman, 1961	0	0	8		11	65	6	65
Hordern, 1963	4	15	23		89	81	21	66
Simpson, 1976	8	53	7		31	86	5	33
Glassman, 1977								
adequate plasma levels	3	33	6		19	95	1	62
inadequate plasma levels	3	38	5		6	27	16	−11
Avery, Winokur, 1977	2	9	20		18	25	53	16
Davidson, 1977	0	0	3		3	100	0	100
Avery, Lubrano, 1979	72	40	109		174	68	82	28
Charney, Nelson, 1981	2	22	7		32	80	8	58
Brown, 1982	3	17	15		17	74	6	57
Nelson, 1984	2	15	11		7	58	5	43
Howarth, Grace, 1985	21	62	13		9	41	13	−21
Chan, 1987	7	44	9		48	81	11	37
Summary Results	127	35%	236		464	67%	227	32

[a]Adapted from Chan CH, Janicak PG, Davis JM, et al. Response of psychotic and nonpsychotic depressed patients to tricyclic antidepressants. J Clin Psychiatry 1987;48:197–200. Copyright 1992, Physicians Postgraduate Press.

Primary Type:
Other Depressive Disorders

Dysthymia (Depressive Neurosis)

Dysthymia represents a chronic but less severe form of depression. Depressed mood and partial neurovegetative symptoms are typically present for sustained periods (e.g., years). The major differences between this condition and MDD are the duration of the mood disorder; the absence of feelings of low self-esteem, worthlessness, hopelessness; and the absence of a full neurovegetative syndrome.

There are still many questions about this condition, including:

- Is it a fundamentally *different condition* from MDD?

- Does it share a common *pathophysiology and/or etiology*?
- Is it the *residual* of an incompletely remitted MDD episode?
- Is it the *sequelae* of an MDD episode that did not receive prompt and aggressive treatment?

If the answer to the last question is positive, dysthymia could represent a phenomenon consistent with the concept of "learned helplessness" and would underscore the importance of early detection and aggressive therapy of MDD.

Dual Depression

Patients who meet criteria for both MDD and dysthymia are referred to as having a "double" or "dual" depression. This term, however, should not be used for a first episode until an adequate trial of at least three different classes of ADs, or two classes of drug and ECT have been tried. Retrospective distortion is common in these patients, who may report having always been depressed, but remit completely with adequate therapy. Assuming a valid designation of "dual" depression, most clinicians will manage the neurovegetative syndrome with medication while simultaneously using psychotherapeutic approaches specifically developed for mood disorders (e.g., cognitive or interpersonal psychotherapy for dysthymia).

Mixed Anxiety and Depression

Fogelson et al. (1988) note that the most frequent combinations of anxiety and mood disorders include:

- *Panic disorder* and major depression
- *Panic attacks* and major depression
- *Obsessive-compulsive disorder* and major depression
- *Generalized anxiety* and major depression (21).

Frequently, distinguishing between depressive and anxiety disorders is difficult because patients present with an admixture of symptoms. This issue has gained considerable attention because the DSM-IV must be compatible with the International Classification of Diseases, Clinical Modification (ICD-CM) system, which includes a category termed "mixed anxiety and depression." There are, however, many unanswered questions about this category, including its incidence, etiology, natural course, and treatment response, especially as distinguished from MDD alone or various anxiety disorders alone (21a).

Clarifying the actual incidence is complicated by two issues. The first has to do with the structure of assessments, such as the Hamilton Anxiety and Depression Rating Scales, that were developed to quantitate severity, as well as treatment-related changes, but not to determine diagnosis. Nevertheless, these scales are often used for the latter purpose in clinical trials requiring preset scores to determine enrollment. Because the scales were not designed for diagnostic purposes, they have substantial overlap, giving the impression that depressive and anxiety disorders frequently present with a mixture of symptoms.

The second issue is that many primary care physicians have difficulty distinguishing between depressive disorders and anxiety disorders. This has led to the impression that patients in a general medical setting are more likely to have an admixture of symptoms, rather than a clearly defined condition. The fact that depressed patients have anxiety symptoms and that anxiety-disordered patients have depressive symptoms as assessed by the Hamilton scales is used to support this clinical impression. This ignores the fact that these scales were developed to quantitate symptoms *only after a definitive syndromic diagnosis had been made.*

Rather than postulating a new category, there may be a better explanation for this phenomenon of mixed symptoms. Patients are frequently not forthright about psychiatric-related complaints due to the associated stigma. Further, in the primary care setting, the amount of time a physician can spend with a patient is limited. Thus, given a reluctant historian, the ability to make the proper diagnosis is severely limited.

Making an appropriate diagnosis is also complicated by the minimal psychiatric training many primary care physicians receive. This is compounded by the fact that many practicing primary care physicians received their only formal exposure to psychiatry at a time when diagnosis was not emphasized. This latter point deserves some elaboration. Psychiatry has undergone fundamental philosophical changes in the last 20 years. At the beginning of the 20th century, most specialties had adopted the medical model as their guiding principle for diagnosis. In this model, empirically based diagnoses are the cornerstone upon which the understanding and treatment of medical illnesses are based. In contrast, the psychoanalytic approach, which dominated psychiatry until the early 1970s, espoused principles of ego psychology, believed to be common to all psychiatric conditions. With this philosophy, the cause for all conditions was known and the treatment was the same, making diagnosis less important.

Given this context, it is not surprising that general physicians find psychiatric differential diagnosis difficult. Whether there is a unique condition consisting of mixed anxiety and depression is not known, but before it is added to our nomenclature, there should be evidence supporting its construct validity. The standard tests of such validity are:

- Demonstration of a *unique clustering* of signs and symptoms
- *Reproducibility* over time (i.e., temporal stability)
- *Unique course of illness*
- *Predictability of treatment response*
- Evidence of a *common pathophysiology or etiology* (e.g., does it breed true within a given family?)

Whereas such data exist for MDD and the various anxiety disorders, this is not true for the proposed mixed category.

There are also possible adverse consequences to establishing such a category. First, it may contribute to an even more casual practice of making differential diagnosis by providing an ill-defined syndrome in which patients with complaints of depression and/or anxiety can be readily placed. Thus, such a categorization could contribute to a decreased recognition of MDD; place patients at greater risk for sequelae such as suicide; and delay the implementation of effective treatment.

While there is considerable overlap in drug therapies for depressive and anxiety-related disorders, there are also important differences. For example, there is no convincing evidence that benzodiazepines are effective for MDD, and indeed such medications may increase the risk of a serious or successful suicide attempt, secondary to behavioral disinhibition. Despite this problem, benzodiazepines are often the first-line treatment in the primary care setting for patients with anxiety symptoms, regardless of their psychiatric diagnosis. Finally, such a category could impede research by blurring the distinctions between MDD and anxiety-related disorders, creating a heterogenous rather than homogeneous grouping of patients for clinical studies. In terms of treatment, monotherapy with an antidepressant (e.g., SRI) is often sufficient to control symptoms while also clarifying the diagnosis (see also Chapter 7).

Panic Associated with Major Depression. About 25% of patients with major depression have associated past or current panic attacks. The adverse consequences of severe anxiety have been relatively unrecognized, but the recent concern about the possible association between panic symptoms and suicidality dramatically underscores this problem. Panic episodes have four major components:

- *Physical complaints*, such as tachycardia, dyspnea, dizziness, flushing, tremor, and sweating

- *Cognitive complaints,* usually characterized as a sense of catastrophic fear of dying or losing control or going "crazy"
- *Affective symptoms,* including terror, heightened arousal, marked anticipatory anxiety, and secondary depression
- *Behavioral symptoms,* such as withdrawal, excessive dependency, and phobic avoidance.

Depressed patients with panic symptoms may also develop another complication, namely, *agoraphobia.*

Standard doses of heterocyclics (HCAs), especially in the earliest phases of therapy, can heighten anxiety, irritability, and restlessness because panic-disordered patients are extremely sensitive to their stimulating properties. As a result, it is best to start with low doses (e.g., 10–25 mg/day imipramine), using a gradual upward titration, as tolerated. Thus, a slower titration schedule in the earliest phases of treatment, and/or the judicious addition of an anxiolytic may be helpful.

Avoiding drugs that lower the threshold for panic symptoms, such as caffeine or over-the-counter stimulants, may also help. Some phobic symptoms are managed by in vivo exposure or cognitive therapy. In general, the best approach is a combination of pharmacotherapy and psychotherapy, in particular, cognitive behavioral techniques.

> *Case Example.* A 39-year-old female suffering from chronic dysthymia with a mixture of panic and phobic symptoms had been in psychotherapy for several years. She was resistant to a trial with antidepressants because of a history of sensitivity to various medications. She finally agreed to start imipramine at 25 mg qhs. After one dose, she experienced a prolonged period of anxiety and agitation, leading to an entire night without sleep. She called the next day to report this reaction and refused to continue medication. Subsequently, she again agreed to begin a trial of imi-

pramine, but this time the dosage was only 10 mg/day. She tolerated this dose well and was able to gradually increase the AD to a maximum of 125 mg over a 6- to 9-month period. At that point, there was a clinically significant improvement in dysthymia and a complete resolution of her phobic and panic symptoms.

This particular case illustrates the hypersensitivity to HCAs in some patients with mixed anxiety and depression. Starting at a very low dose and using a gradual incremental schedule allowed the patient to acclimate to imipramine's side effects and, ultimately, to achieve the intended benefit.

Seasonal Affective Disorder

Seasonal affective disorder (SAD) is a recurrent depressive illness that regularly coincides with particular seasons (22, 23). Such a phenomenon is consistent with the influence of seasonal and other environmental factors on mood changes, which have been described for over 2 millennia. The two predominant presentations have bimodal peaks of depression onset, either in the spring or in the fall. The spring-onset type (SOSAD) is usually more severe, albeit less frequent, and is associated with a greater risk of suicide, hospitalization, and the need for somatic therapies (i.e., ECT). The fall-onset type (FOSAD) is more common, results in less severe depressive episodes, is typically managed on an outpatient basis, and poses less danger of suicide. *Full remission in the summer months is a diagnostic criteria for FOSAD in the DSM-III-R,* with patients noting significant increases in energy and productivity during this period. As many as 25% actually meet clinical criteria for hypomania, perhaps precipitated by a sudden resolution of the depressive episode in the late winter-early spring period (see Table 6.1 for DSM-III-R criteria).

Epidemiology. SAD appears to have a prevalence rate of about 4–6%, with a female:male ratio of about 4:1. Another 20% of the population describe symptoms consistent with SAD that do not meet diagnostic criteria for severity. There appears to be a correlation with age, such that the mean age of onset is in the mid-20s, with older people less susceptible, particularly those over 55 years.

Although there appears to be a familial pattern, there are no definitive data demonstrating a hereditary component. Studies from four different centers have found a greater incidence of mood disorders in the first-degree relatives of SAD patients. For example, Rosenthal found a family history of mood disorders in 55% and of alcoholism in 36% of 294 subjects studied (24). The majority of patients (i.e., about 80%) tend to be females, young, white, and in the middle-to-upper middle class socioeconomically. Many fall in the mild-to-moderate level of severity in terms of their depression, and few have previous histories of antidepressant therapy or hospitalization for their mood disturbance. Severity of episodes may relate to their length, which varies from an average of 5 months in Maryland to 6 months in the Chicago area, perhaps reflecting differences in latitude and the relative length of winter.

Clinical Presentation. Rosenthal et al. (25) have described SAD as a major depressive disorder but noted that many who suffer from this condition present with atypical symptoms, including:

- *Increased* rather than decreased *sleep*
- *Increased* rather than decreased *appetite*, with increased food intake
- *Carbohydrate craving*
- Marked *increases in weight*.

as well as more typical symptoms, such as:

- *Decreased energy* or fatigue
- Mixed *anxiety/depression*
- Social *withdrawal*.

Reports vary as to the predominant picture, which ranges from one quite similar to unipolar recurrent disorder to that more consistent with an atypical depressive disorder or a Bipolar II disorder (Table 6.5). Complaints usually involve a diminution in energy, followed by an increased need for sleep, increased appetite and weight, and a lack of involvement or interest in one's activities. Only toward the end of the episode onset does the patient become aware of the depressed mood and such classic symptoms as poor concentration, feelings of self-worthlessness, and multiple somatic complaints. Insomnia often develops over the next 1–2 months. Whereas this atypical picture is more characteristic of the early phases of the illness, reminiscent of certain bipolar subtypes, the affective episode appears to evolve toward a more classic depressive syndrome as it progresses over multiple seasons.

In a recent review, Wehr and Rosenthal noted differences and similarities between SOSAD and FOSAD (26). Specifically, vegetative signs were often of the opposite type, with atypical symptoms predominating in FOSAD and more typical and more severe symptoms in SOSAD. Further, studies indicate that FOSAD may be precipitated by light deficiency and responds to treatment with bright light (BL). Contributing factors to SOSAD are less well established, but some preliminary data indicate that heat may be one possible triggering mechanism. At higher latitudes, FOSAD tends to be longer and more severe. In contrast, SOSAD is more severe at lower latitudes. Preliminary results of a three-center study indicate that the ratio of FOSAD to

SOSAD increases with increasing latitudes (27).

Conclusion. Blehar and Rosenthal (23) in their report and summary of a NIMH-sponsored workshop on recurrent FOSAD concluded that:

- Evidence for the *syndromal validity* of SAD is strong and perhaps even stronger than for other established diagnoses, such as dysthymia
- Preliminary evidence supports *phototherapy* as an effective treatment for SAD; however, its mechanism of action is not understood
- *Circadian hypotheses* have been most frequently used to explain the mechanism of action of BL therapy, as well as the pathophysiology of SAD; however, results are inconclusive.

Secondary Type: Complicating Disorders

A *second model of mood disorder subtypes is the primary versus secondary dichotomy, which distinguishes a primary depressive disorder from a syndrome chronologically secondary to another psychiatric or medical condition.* Here, the term "secondary" simply designates the timing of the disorder in reference to another psychiatric or medical problem. The concept of "secondary" is not meant to suggest causality, although such an inference is often assumed. This dichotomy found its major use in identifying mood disorders alone, versus those associated with another "comorbid" psychiatric condition, such as alcohol dependence. This distinction is valuable because mood disorders complicated by another illness have a poorer natural prognosis, and a poorer response to therapy.

Before making a definitive diagnosis of a primary depression or concluding the exis-

tence of treatment resistance, one must consider the possibility of another concurrent, confounding, medical or psychiatric disorder, in addition to depression.

Medical Disorders

Physical problems that may complicate or underlie a depressive condition include:

- Subclinical *hypothyroidism*
- *Malabsorption* due to various gastrointestinal conditions (e.g., Crohn's disease)
- Unrecognized *malignancies*
- Chronic *renal failure*
- Coexisting *dementia*
- *Autoimmune disorder* (e.g., systemic lupus erythematosus (SLE))
- *Influenza*.

Most of these conditions are chronic and debilitating, with their underlying mechanisms not well understood. Postulated relationships include demoralization and depression due to the anorexia and malaise caused by profound systemic effects. These disorders may also affect the amine systems that mediate the depressive syndrome.

Malignancies, particularly of neural crest origin, are known to affect brain function adversely through remote (presumably hormonal) effects on neural tissue. For example, ovarian adenocarcinoma can selectively induce a profound cerebellar syndrome due to the selective death of Purkinje cells (presumably from a neurotoxic hormonal factor). Such phenomena simply illustrate the complicated nature of central nervous system (CNS) functioning and the need to be cautious about explanations in the absence of systematic data.

Brain lesions that produce depression can be divided into structural and biochemical. Any disease that produces a mass lesion or deficit in the frontal lobes can cause a depressive syndrome, and typically, the occurrence and severity is correlated with proximity to the tip of the frontal pole rather than to the extent of motor function loss. The most extensively studied lesions are *strokes,* but *tumors* and *plaques,* related to multiple sclerosis, can produce similar results.

Lesions on the left side, closer to the tip of the frontal lobe, are the most likely to produce depression. Such lesions result in bilateral cortical depletion of CNS amines, again implicating these neurotransmitters in the pathogenesis. Further, treatments that potentiate norepinephrine transmission have been effective in reversing such syndromes.

Biochemical lesions that induce depressive syndromes include such classic examples as *Parkinson's* and *Huntington's* diseases, especially early in their courses. These disorders involve derangements of central amine systems (i.e., in Parkinson's there is a disturbance in both dopamine and norepinephrine; in Huntington's, dopamine is affected as well as other nonbiogenic amine neural circuits). Antidepressants and ECT, which potentiate central neurotransmission, have effectively relieved depression associated with Parkinson's disease.

Treatment of these disorders has received less systematic study, in part because these patients are more diverse in terms of their health status, leading to potentially complicating alterations in the pharmacokinetics and pharmacodynamics of antidepressants.

As with any decision to initiate an AD trial, it should be based upon the potential risks and benefits. The limited evidence that exists indicates that both drugs and ECT can be used safely and effectively in such patients when appropriate allowances are made for health status. Empirical trials are wanting but clearly warranted.

Concurrent Psychiatric Disorders

These include *schizoaffective or delusional unipolar disorders* that require combination therapy (e.g., antipsychotic/antidepressant and/or mood stabilizer). Certain *mixed bipolar states* require lithium and may do poorly with an AD only. Patients with *"comorbid" depression and panic disorder* often do not tolerate heterocyclic ADs during the first few weeks because of their stimulating effects. This is also true of serotonin reuptake inhibitors, such as fluoxetine.

Personality disorders can also complicate management (e.g., borderline disorder with a superimposed MDD). As noted earlier, *dual depression* occurs in patients who have chronic dysthymic disorder and then experience a superimposed MDD.

Concurrent Psychosocial Issues

Significant *psychosocial stressors* that are not addressed and ameliorated are frequently assumed to contribute to persistent depressive symptomatology, despite adequate pharmacological intervention. In such situations, supportive, interpersonal, and cognitive therapy may be necessary adjuncts to medication.

Drug-Induced Syndromes

Conditions mimicking MDD can occur secondary to a wide variety of prescribed and illicit agents. With some drugs, the syndrome occurs as a direct and immediate effect. For example, the antihypertensive agents acutely antagonize central biogenic amine neurotransmitter systems and include such drugs as:

- *Reserpine*
- α-Methyldopa

This phenomenon is one of the pillars of the biogenic amine hypothesis. An intriguing finding with reserpine is that those susceptible to a depressive syndrome while on this agent also have an increased likelihood of a personal or family history of MDD, in comparison with those who are not susceptible. This finding suggests an interaction between a constitutional predisposition and the biochemical effects of this drug. Because depression is a common disorder, we would expect some cases to occur by chance alone with every medical drug (e.g., depression has been reported in patients on clonidine, propranolol, calcium antagonists, etc.). This, however, could be coincidence, or there could be a causal relationship, but either possibility remains to be proven.

Other agents can also produce a depressive syndrome after lengthy and/or repeated use. This is generally true with certain drugs of abuse, such as psychostimulants and sedative-hypnotics. Again, antagonistic effects on biogenic amines appear critical in the pathophysiology of the resultant depression.

Acutely, *psychostimulants* (e.g., cocaine, amphetamines) act as indirect agonists of biogenic amines, causing their release and inhibiting their neuronal reuptake. Repeated exposure, however, causes a depletion of central amines, similar to the action of reserpine. The syndrome produced by cocaine is initially reversible with the addition of higher doses, but over time, profound neurotransmitter depletion occurs that cannot be ameliorated by further drug increases. This phenomenon has been termed "burnout," and creates a vicious cycle critical to the addiction potential of this agent, as well as to other psychostimulants. The first step in treatment is to discourage abuse through education. When the condition is more advanced, treatment often involves detoxifi-

cation with an antidepressant (e.g., desipramine), which potentiates the effects of any remaining central biogenic amines. ADs have also been used to reduce cocaine craving, and thus, to decrease the likelihood of relapse.

Alcohol abuse and dependence is the most common cause of drug-induced depressive syndromes. As with psychostimulants, its effect requires chronic, sustained exposure, but unlike with psychostimulants, symptoms generally occur as a result of withdrawal and are reversed by its reinstitution. Gradual depletion of central amines, particularly serotonin, appears to be an important pathogenic factor. With chronic exposure, alcohol produces a decrease in cerebrospinal fluid 5-HIAA and an increased density of 5-HT_2 receptors in the neocortex, similar to the findings observed in at least a subset of naturally occurring depressive disorders. Thus, chronic alcohol exposure may produce a phenocopy of MDD because it causes a derangement in central neurotransmitter systems similar to that underlying mood disorders.

Other *sedative-hypnotics* (e.g., benzodiazepines) are also capable of producing a phenomenologically similar syndrome during the withdrawal phase of addiction, but the mechanisms responsible are not well understood. The possibility that common mechanisms are involved is supported by the fact that a depression induced by one class of sedative-hypnotics can be reversed by another class. For example, benzodiazepines can reverse the syndrome induced by alcohol withdrawal.

Other Disorders

Both heterocyclics and SRIs may also be useful for other mood and non-mood disorders (see Tables 6.7 and 6.8).

Table 6.7.
Indications for Antidepressants: Other Mood Disorders

• Primary degenerative dementia, with depression	• Late luteal phase dysphoric disorder
• Multi-infarct dementia, with depression	• Postpartum depression
• Organic mood syndrome	• Adjustment disorder with depressed mood
	• Bereavement

Table 6.8.
Indications for Antidepressants: Other Non-Mood Psychiatric and Medical Conditions

• Sleep disorders (see Chapters 11 and 12)	• Substance abuse disorder
• Insomnia	• Cocaine craving
• Somnambulism	• Certain paraphilias
• Night terrors	• Pain syndromes
• Sleep apnea	• Headaches (e.g., intractable migraine)
• Narcolepsy (including cataplexy)	• Bone pain secondary to metastases
• Functional enuresis	• Somatoform pain disorder (see Somatoform
• Anxiety disorders (see Chapters 11, 12, and 13)	Disorder in Chapter 13)
• Phobic disorders	• Chronic pain
• Panic disorder	• Gastrointestinal
• Obsessive-compulsive disorder	• Irritable bowel syndrome
• Generalized anxiety disorder	• Peptic ulcers
• Post-traumatic stress disorder	• Genitourinary
• Eating disorders (see The Eating-Disordered Patient in Chapter 13)	• Enuresis
• Bulimia	• Cardiovascular
• Anorexia	• Arrhythmias
• Attention deficit disorder with or without hyperactivity (see The Child and the Adolescent Patient in Chapter 14)	• Miscellaneous
	• Mild immune dysfunction
	• Some dermatologic disorders

Suicide

Depressive disorders include some of the most common and serious psychiatric conditions. They are categorized together because of a similar constellation of signs and symptoms. Approximately one of ten Americans will suffer a major depressive episode in their lifetime, and one of 20 will have recurrences, with women twice as likely as men to experience an episode. There is evidence to suggest a subtype with a familial pattern in which women are three to four times more likely to develop depression whereas men tend to develop alcohol abuse and/or dependence (28). Depression's impact on patients and their families is profound, with suicide the most severe sequela. **In this respect, depressive disorders are a major health care problem, contributing to 70% of suicide-related deaths (with a 15% mortality risk due to suicide in untreated recurrent major episodes).**

EPIDEMIOLOGY

Suicide is the eighth leading cause of death in the United States for all ages. Among teenagers and young adults, it is the third most common cause of death. Approximately 40,000–50,000 Americans die every year by their own hand. **Thus, suicide claims more lives annually in the United States than leukemia or kidney disease, and also seriously affects relatives, friends, and coworkers who were close to the suicide victim.** Suicide potential is the highest among middle-aged men and women; is more prevalent among whites; and is frequently preceded by work or legal problems, which themselves could be the result (as opposed to the cause) of antecedent and often untreated psychiatric disorders.

There has been an alarming increase in the rate of suicide over the past 30 years, especially for young men, both white and black. Suicide deaths in this cohort (i.e., the ages of 18–30 years) increased nearly 150% between 1960 and 1980, paralleled by increased substance abuse and depressive disorders as well. A possible new factor is the report of social contagion, as evidenced by clusters or miniepidemics of suicide that mimic the original method.

ASSESSMENT OF SUICIDE POTENTIAL

Clinicians may be reluctant to ask about suicidal ideation because of their own discomfort with the topic or for fear of offending the patient. The latter virtually never occurs when the topic is approached in a stepwise, empathic manner. Instead, such an approach typically generates relief and appreciation that the clinician has recognized the seriousness of a patient's complaints. The first step is to elicit the depressive symptoms and acknowledge a patient's distress. Next, the examiner empathically inquires whether these symptoms have ever led to feelings that life is not worth living. At this point, patients will often spontaneously discuss suicide. If not, they may acknowledge that life seems hopeless and bleak, allowing the clinician to inquire about any death wishes or thoughts about taking one's life. The importance of a clinician's sensitivity to the potential for suicide is borne out by studies showing that many victims (more than 70%) visit a physician within 2 months preceding their death (29). Because suicide is usually the result of a treatable illness, its identification and appropriate management can avert an unnecessary tragedy.

RISK FACTORS

Although direct inquiry about suicide is the single most critical part of an evaluation, one should also ask about other risk factors associated with completed suicides. Although there is no fail-safe method for identifying all patients at serious risk, knowledge of these factors can help estimate its likelihood.

Psychiatric-Related Risk Factors

By far the most important contributor is a serious psychiatric disorder, with major depressive disorder, bipolar disorder, schizophrenia, and substance abuse most closely associated with suicide. The male:female ratio is less pronounced among psychiatric patients than in the general population, with a higher rate in unmarried psychiatric patients living alone. The lifetime probability of death by suicide in various psychiatric disorders is estimated to be between 10% and 15%.

This contrasts with less than a 1% lifetime probability in those without a psychiatric disorder.

Black et al. (1987) looked at suicide in subtypes of major mood disorders and compared them to the general population in Iowa (30). They found an increased risk in all psychiatric groups, except for female patients with bipolar mood disorder, which was associated with a lower risk in comparison to unipolar disorders. Seventy-three percent of all suicides occurred during the first few years of follow-up. This trend was particularly pronounced in primary unipolar females and bipolar males.

Beck et al. (1990) reported that *hopelessness* was the MDD symptom most often associated with suicide (31). This finding was replicated by Fawcett et al. (1987), who found that hopelessness with anhedonia, mood cycling within an episode, loss of mood reactivity, and psychotic delusions were high-risk factors for a subsequent suicide (32). *Negative life events* often precede suicide (e.g., the death of a loved one, or humiliating events, such as financial ruin).

Johnson et al. (1990) found that the lifetime rate of suicide attempts with uncomplicated *panic disorder* was about 7%, consistently higher than the general population without a psychiatric disorder (i.e., about 1%); but similar for uncomplicated major depression (i.e., a suicide attempt rate of about 7.9%) (33). They concluded that panic disorder, either uncomplicated or as a "comorbid" illness, led to a risk of suicide attempts comparable to those of major depression ("comorbid" or uncomplicated). Their data were derived from an Epidemiologic Catchment Area study, with a probability sample of more than 18,000 adults living in five United States communities.

In a second review of these data, Weissman et al. (1989) found that 20% of patients with panic disorder and 12% of those with panic attacks had made suicide attempts (34). These results could not be explained by the coexistence of major depression, nor the presence of alcohol or drug abuse. They concluded that panic disorder or attacks were associated with an increased risk of suicidal ideation and attempts.

One-quarter to one-half of all completed suicides were by psychiatric patients who had a history of *a prior attempt*. Thus, the majority of those who attempted suicide did not ultimately go on to complete the act, with estimates placing the ratio of attempters to completers at approximately 8:1. The absence of a suicide attempt history does not guarantee or substantially reduce the risk of suicide if the other risk factors are present. Suicide completions usually occur on the first or second attempt; thus, multiple attempters (i.e., greater than five) are at greater risk for *future attempts* rather than completion.

In summary, the risk factors for suicide in *psychiatric patients* include:

- *Male sex*
- *Middle age*, in contrast to the general population, where the elderly are at greatest risk
- *Race:* whites are at a much higher risk than blacks
- *Depression and schizophrenia*—the primary psychiatric diagnoses associated with successful suicide attempts
- *History of suicide attempt* (but not multiple attempts)
- *Undesirable life events*
- *Hospitalization*
- The *6- to 12-month period after discharge* (this interval risk is particularly true among women in the first 6 months following hospitalization).

Treatment-Related Risk Factors

One naturalistic study compared the incidence of suicidal behavior to the dose of HCA and found the rate was 22% for low doses (i.e., less than 75 mg/day) but decreased progressively as the AD dose was increased (i.e., 11% at 75–149 mg/day; 1% at 150–249 mg/day; and 0.5% at 250+ mg/day) (35). This finding is even more remarkable when one considers that the more severely ill patients would be receiving the higher doses.

Epidemiologic Risk Factors

Those who complete suicide tend to be middle aged or older and suffer from a depressive disorder. Younger individuals who commit suicide usually suffer from a schizophrenic or bipolar disorder. The risk factors are:

- For suicide attempts:
  - *Female*
  - Recent *stressful life event*
  - *Impulsivity*
  - *Previous attempts.*
- For suicide deaths:
  - *Male*
  - A *psychiatric disorder*
  - A *family history* of suicide.
- For suicide deaths in patients under the age of 30:
  - *White males and American Indians,* who appear to be at high risk
  - *Depression* and other mood disorders
  - Current *substance abuse*
  - *Eating disorders*
  - A history of *prior attempts* (but not more than five)
  - Social *contagion* (perhaps most critical in American Indians)
  - A *family history.*

Generally, the clinical and psychosocial factors that combine to increase the risk of suicide have a high sensitivity but a low specificity. Because only a small minority who meet these criteria successfully complete suicide, the clinician's task of accurately assessing risks is exceedingly difficult.

History-Related Risk Factors

One risk factor is counterintuitive and, therefore, deserves special mention. Most individuals who die from suicide do so on their first or second attempt. Thus, the absence of a prior attempt should not minimize concern about its risk. In fact, the absence of previous attempts in a first-time, profoundly depressed middle- or late-life patient who has other risk factors (as discussed) should increase rather than diminish concern.

There are also data that those who make multiple attempts (i.e., greater than four) are a different population than those who will die from suicide. Multiple suicide attempters tend to be younger and to have a diagnosis other than a depressive disorder (e.g., antisocial personality, histrionic or borderline personality). Although they are likely to make future attempts, they do not constitute a substantial proportion of those who die from suicide.

Medical Risk Factors

It appears that most patients with medical disorders who commit suicide, even those with terminal disorders, have concurrent treatable major depression. Patients with *respiratory diseases* are three times more likely to commit suicide than other medical patients. Those on *hemodialysis* or who suffer from *cancer* also constitute high-risk groups, in comparison with the general population.

Substance Abuse-Related Risk Factors

The relationship between alcohol abuse and suicide has been recognized for many years, with at least one in five suicide victims being intoxicated at the time of their death. Alcohol may lower inhibitions, serving as a precipitant to the act; and/or the disease of alcoholism itself could be a risk factor. Alcohol also induces biochemical changes (e.g., lowers CSF 5-HIAA and decreases 5-HT_2 receptors in the neocortex), similar to changes observed in at least a subset of depressive disorders. Thus, alcohol may aggravate or contribute to the pathophysiology that mediates the depressive syndrome and leads to suicide completions.

Roy et al. (1990) studied approximately 300 alcoholics, of whom 20% *attempted suicide* (36). In comparing the attempters with nonattempters, there were a number of predictors, including:

- *Younger females*
- *Lower socioeconomic status*
- Consumption of *greater amounts*
- Onset of alcohol-related problems at an *earlier age*
- An apparent increase in *additional lifetime psychiatric diagnoses,* including:
  - Major depression
  - Panic disorder
  - Phobic disorder
  - Generalized anxiety disorder
  - Antisocial personality disorder
  - Substance abuse
- Significantly more *first- or second-degree alcoholic relatives.*

Estimates of the lifetime risk of suicide in alcoholics were reviewed by Murphy and Wetzel (1990), who concluded that the current estimate of 11–15% was not tenable based on a more careful examination of the data, and was probably more in the range of 2–3.4% (37). This still contrasts with the 1.3% annual incidence in the United States. Much of the increase, however, could be related to another Axis I diagnosis (e.g., bipolar disorder).

The characteristics of alcoholic *patients who committed suicide* include:

- Male
- 20–40 years old
- Concurrent abusers of alcohol plus other drugs (e.g., opiates, sedatives, psychostimulants, amphetamines, cocaine).

The relationship between suicide and *other drugs of abuse* typically involves a pattern of chronic use; an earlier age of onset; and a prior history of drug overdose. Often there is a childhood history of hyperactivity, parental abuse; or family history of depression, suicide, and/or alcoholism. As with alcohol, other substances can decrease inhibition or markedly impair judgment, turning a gesture into a successfully completed suicide. **Clinicians should assume that patients with a history of substance abuse are at a higher risk for impulsive behavior that may place them or others in jeopardy.** In obtaining a history, specific questions, in addition to suicidal ideation or behavior include:

- Prior *drug overdoses*
- *Accidents*
- Serious *risk-taking behavior*
- *Legal* difficulties
- Recent *increasing pattern of abuse*
- Recent *interpersonal losses.*

Because maintaining a drug habit often involves criminal activities, one should inquire about access to guns and/or other lethal weapons, which should be removed from the home, if at all possible, especially if the clinician thinks there is a serious risk of suicide in the near future.

Biological Risk Factors

There are a number of biochemical findings associated with suicide. For example, there has been a recent focus on the 5-HT system, with findings such as:

- *Lower CSF 5-HIAA* concentrations in those who attempt violent and impulsive suicide
- *Lower brain serotonin or 5-HIAA* concentrations in suicide victims
- *Increased density of serotonin receptors* (particularly 5-HT$_2$ receptors in the neocortex), consistent with decreased activity of presynaptic serotonin.

The clinical implications of such data point to a relationship between abnormalities in the central serotonin system and self-injurious behavior. These findings have led to an interest in developing specific drugs that alter 5-HT activity, in an effort to treat suicidality, impulsivity, and aggressivity independent of any specific psychiatric disorder. Central serotonin function can be enhanced by agents such as lithium and various reuptake inhibitors, including fluoxetine, sertraline, paroxetine, and clomipramine. Prospective controlled trials are needed to test for efficacy in this regard, both in depressive as well as other psychiatric disorders.

In summary, the issue of suicide should always be considered in depressed patients and gently but thoroughly explored during the initial evaluation. Subsequent reinquiry is also critical, given the increased incidence of suicide during the early phases of treatment and recovery.

OTHER CAUSES OF DEATH

Depressive disorders can lead to death in other ways (see Table 6.9). For example, depressed individuals are more prone to accidents, due to impaired concentration and attention. They also often attempt to self-medicate, particularly with alcohol or other sedative agents, which may lead to death due to organ toxicity, as well as accidents. Psychotic depressive patients may act irrationally, putting themselves at greater physical risk. Although rare today, patients have died of severe malnutrition secondary to catatonic symptoms that precluded the ability to care for their basic needs.

Depressive disorders can also cause substantial morbidity. Thus, injury and illness occur secondary to suicide attempts, accidents, substance abuse, malnutrition, or irrational behavior due to psychosis. Failure to seek medical attention for intercurrent medical disorders may occur because of apathy, feelings of guilt, or low self-esteem. Finally, impaired concentration and attention, a lack of energy, or anhedonia can all substan-

Table 6.9.
Hidden Cost of Not Treating Major Depressive Disorder

Mortality	Patient Morbidity	Societal Cost
• 30,000–35,000 suicides per year • Accidents due to impaired concentration and attention • Death due to illnesses that can be sequelae (e.g., alcohol abuse)	• Suicide attempts • Accidents • Associated illnesses • Lost jobs • Failure to advance • Substance abuse	• Dysfunctional families • Absenteeism • Decreased productivity • Job-related injuries • Adverse effect on quality control

tially impair psychosocial functioning (e.g., failure to advance in one's career or in school; job loss; social isolation; dysfunctional home life, including divorce).

Other Costs of Major Depression

Attempts have been made to calculate the societal cost of MDD in terms of health care utilization, absenteeism from work, decreased productivity, job-related injuries, and adverse effects on quality control because of impaired concentration and attention. In a prospective study of 3000 patients, depression was related to poorer physical health and increased health care utilization (38). In the same study, employed individuals had a five times greater risk of using disability days. In another study, disability because of major depression was similar to or worse than chronic medical illnesses such as hypertension, diabetes mellitus, and arthritis (39).

Based on such data, the societal cost of depressive disorders is estimated to be $26 billion annually. Even this figure does not represent the full economic impact. A more complete estimate should include the cost of decreased work productivity, the effect of lost jobs, and failure to advance in one's career or education. Such an estimate should also consider the effect of depressive disorders on parenting skills and family functioning. A 15-year follow-up study found that 80% of depressed individuals had a poor outcome (i.e., committed suicide, remained ill, or experienced a recurrence) without effective treatment (40).

REFERENCES

1. Klerman GL, Weissman MM. Increasing rates of depression. JAMA 1989;261:2229–2235.

2. Preskorn S, Fast GA. Therapeutic drug monitoring for antidepressants: efficacy, safety and cost effectiveness. J Clin Psychiatry 1991;52:23–33.

3. Aronson TA, Shukla S, Hoff A, Cook B. Proposed delusional depression subtypes: preliminary evidence from a retrospective study of phenomenology and treatment course. J Affective Disord 1988;14:69–74.

4. Glassman AH, Kantor SJ, Schostak M. Depression, delusions and drug response. Am J Psychiatry 1975;132:716–719.

5. Chan CH, Janicak PG, Davis JM, Altman E, Andriukaitis S, Hedeker D. Response of psychotic and nonpsychotic depressed patients to tricyclic antidepressants. J Clin Psychiatry 1987;48:197–200.

6. Friedman C, De Mowbray MS, Hamilton V. Imipramine (Tofranil) in depressive states: a controlled trial with in-patients. J Ment Sci 1961;107:948–953.

7. Hordern A, Holt NF, Burt CG, Gordon WF. Amitriptyline in depressive states: phenomenology and prognostic considerations. Br J Psychiatry 1963;109:815–825.

8. Simpson GM, Lee JH, Cuculic Z, Kellner R. Two dosages of imipramine in hospitalized endogenous and neurotic depressives. Arch Gen Psychiatry 1976;33:1093–1102.

9. Glassman AH, Perel JM, Shostak M, Kantor SJ, Fleiss JL. Clinical implications of imipramine plasma levels for depressive illness. Arch Gen Psychiatry 1977;34:197–204.

10. Avery D, Winokur G. The efficacy of electroconvulsive therapy and antidepressants in depression. Biol Psychiatry 1977;12:507–523.

11. Davidson JRT, McLeod MN, Kurland AA, White HL. Antidepressant drug therapy in psychotic depression. Br J Psychiatry 1977;131:493–496.

12. Avery D, Lubrano A. Depression treated with imipramine and ECT: the De Carolis study reconsidered. Am J Psychiatry 1979;136:559–562.

13. Charney DS, Nelson JC. Delusional and nondelusional unipolar depression: further

evidence for distinct subtypes. Am J Psychiatry 1981;138:328–333.

14. Brown RP, Frances A, Kocsis JH, Mann JJ. Psychotic vs. nonpsychotic depression: comparison of treatment response. J Nerv Ment Dis 1982;170:635–637.

15. Nelson WH, Khan A, Orr WW. Delusional depression, phenomenology, neuroendocrine function and tricyclic antidepressant response. J Affective Disord 1984;6:297–306.

16. Howarth BG, Grace MGA: Depression, drugs, and delusions. Arch Gen Psychiatry 1985;42:1145–1147.

17. Kocsis JH, Croughan JL, Katz MM, Butler TP, Secunda S, Bowden CL, Davis JM. Severe major depression without psychotic features. Am J Psychiatry 1990;147:621–624.

18. Spiker DG, Weiss JC, Dealy RS, Griffin SJ, Hanin I, Neil JF, Perel JM, Rossi AJ, Soloff PH. The pharmacological treatment of delusional depression. Am J Psychiatry 1985;142:430–436.

19. Anton RF, Burch EA. Amoxapine versus amitriptyline combined with perphenazine in the treatment of psychotic depression. Am J Psychiatry 1990;147:1203–1208.

20. Janicak PG, Easton M, Comaty JE, Dowd S, Davis JM. Efficacy of ECT in psychotic and nonpsychotic depression. Convulsive Ther 1989;5:314–320.

21. Fogelson DL, Bystritsky A, Sussman N. Interrelationships between major depression and the anxiety disorders: clinical relevance. Psychiatr Ann 1988;18:158–167.

21a. Boulenger JP, Lavallée YS. Mixed anxiety and depression. Diagnostic issues. J Clin Psychiatry 1993;54(1, Suppl):3–8.

22. Lahmeyer HW. Seasonal affective disorders. Psychiatr Med 1991;9:105–114.

23. Blehar MC, Rosenthal NE. Seasonal affective disorders and phototherapy: report of a National Institute of Mental Health-Sponsored Workshop. Arch Gen Psychiatry 1989;46:469–474.

24. Rosenthal NE, Wehr TA. Seasonal affective disorders. Psychiatr Ann 1987;17:670–674.

25. Rosenthal NE, Sack DA, Gillin JC, Lewy AJ, Goodwin FK, Davenport Y, Mueller PS, Newsome DA, Wehr TA. Seasonal affective disorder: a description of the syndrome and preliminary findings with light therapy. Arch Gen Psychiatry 1984;41:72–80.

26. Wehr TA, Rosenthal NE. Seasonality and affective illness. Am J Psychiatry 1989;146:829–839.

27. Rosen LN, Moghadam LZ. Patterns of seasonal change in mood and behavior: an example from a study of military wives. Milit Med 1991;156:228–230.

28. Winokur G. The development and validity of familial subtypes in primary unipolar depression. Pharmacopsychiatry 1982;15:142–145.

29. Robins E. The final months. New York: Oxford University Press, 1981.

30. Black DW, Winokur G, Nasrallah A. Suicide in subtypes of major affective disorder: a comparison with general population suicide mortality. Arch Gen Psychiatry 1987;44:878–880.

31. Beck AT, Brown G, Berchick RJ, Stewart BL, Steer RA. Relationship between hopelessness and ultimate suicide: a replication with psychiatric outpatients. Am J Psychiatry 1990;147:190–195.

32. Fawcett J, Scheftner W, Clark D, Hedeker D, Gibbons R, Coryell W. Clinical predictors of suicide in patients with major affective disorders: a controlled prospective study. Am J Psychiatry 1987;144:35–40.

33. Johnson J, Weissman MM, Klerman GL. Panic disorder, comorbidity, and suicide attempts. Arch Gen Psychiatry 1990;47:805–808.

34. Weissman MM, Klerman GL, Markowitz JS, Ouellette R. Suicidal ideation and suicide attempts in panic disorder and attacks. N Engl J Med 1989;321:1209–1214.

35. Keller MB, Klerman GL, Lavori PW, Fawcett JA, Coryell W, Endicott J. Treatment received by depressed patients. JAMA 1982;248:1848–1855.

36. Roy A, Lamparski D, DeJong J, Moore V, Linnoila M. Characteristics of alcoholics who attempt suicide. Am J Psychiatry 1990;147:761–765.

37. Murphy GE, Wetzel RD. The lifetime risk of suicide in alcoholism. Arch Gen Psychiatry 1990;47:383–392.

38. Broadhead WE, Blazer DG, George LK, Tse CK. Depression, disability days, and days lost from work in a prospective epidemiologic survey. JAMA 1990;264:2524–2528.

39. Wells KB, Stewart A, Hays RD, Burnam A, Rogers W, Daniels M, Berry S, Greenfield S, Ware J. The functioning and well-being of depressed patients. JAMA 1989;262:914–919.

40. Kiloh LG, Andrews G, Neilson M. The long-term outcome of depressive illness. Br J Psychiatry 1988;153:752-757.

CHAPTER 7

Treatment with Antidepressants

History

Disturbances in mood are one of the most pervasive human experiences. The lifetime expectancy for the development of a more serious mood disorder ranges between 3 and 8% for the general population. Treatment of these disorders has been revolutionized by the introduction of mood stabilizing drugs, whose modern era dates back to the early 1950s. As a result, there have been two major outcomes: the availability of relatively safe and efficient therapies for more severe depressions; and, through an understanding of the mechanism of action of these drugs, the unraveling of the pathogenesis, and ultimately the etiology, of major mood disorders. Completing the circle, a better appreciation of the underlying mechanisms has led to the development of even more specific, effective, and safer drug treatments.

The antidepressant properties of both the tricyclics and the monoamine oxidase inhibitors (MAOIs) were chance discoveries. Thus, imipramine was first developed as a potential antipsychotic; but when Dr. Kuhn (1958) tested the clinical efficacy of this agent, he found that it only benefited depressed schizophrenic patients (1). This

prompted him to employ it for depression only. Iproniazid was developed as an antitubercular drug, but the observation that euphoria was a side effect led George Crane to conduct clinical trials, which found it useful in purely depressed patients (2). A year later, Nathan Kline, following up on this observation, reported positive results when he administered iproniazid to another depressed group (3).

Paralleling these clinical developments were basic pharmacological studies that noted that reserpine (4–7; Bunney WE Jr, Davis JM, et al. unpublished data) and α-methyldopa produced depression in patients treated for hypertension (8–10). The fact that the MAOIs and tricyclic antidepressants functionally increased norepinephrine activity, while reserpine lowered its activity, led Schildkraut (1965) and Bunney and Davis (1965) to independently formulate the norepinephrine hypothesis of depression (11, 12). This same line of reasoning was also applied to serotonin (13, 14).

Given two effective classes of antidepressants, pharmacologists developed animal models to screen new compounds in an attempt to predict efficacy. Thus, Everett developed the *dopa test,* while others found that antidepressants reversed reserpine- or tetrabenazine-induced sedation in rodents (15–17). The *learned helplessness* test is another paradigm in which an animal is put in an impossible situation and eventually gives up (18–20). For example, a dog repeatedly shocked and unable to escape gives up trying, even though an exit is subsequently available to him. A similar model is a test in which animals are dropped into a tank of water (21, 22). At first they actively try to escape by swimming for a given amount of time, but then give up and just float. Antidepressants cause the animals in both paradigms to struggle longer before capitulating. Norepinephrine and/or serotonin were hypothesized to be the mediating transmitters in these behavioral models.

Since many have suggested that the beneficial effect of antidepressants is based on their ability to block the reuptake of norepinephrine and/or serotonin, pharmaceutical companies screen potential antidepressants for their ability to block neurotransmitter reuptake. Partially as a result of this paradigm (i.e., reuptake blockade), the industry has developed agents that can specifically block norepinephrine reuptake, serotonin reuptake, or both.

REFERENCES

1. Kuhn R. The treatment of depressive states with G-22355 (imipramine hydrochloride). Am J Psychiatry 1958;115:459–464.
2. Crane GE. Iproniazid (Marsilid) phosphate, a therapeutic agent for mental disorders and debilitating disease. Psychiatry Res Rep 1957;8:142–152.
3. Kline NS. Clinical experience with iproniazid (Marsilid). J Clin Exp Psychopath 1958;19(suppl 1):72–78.
4. Ayd Jr FJ. Drug-induced depression—fact or fallacy. New York Journal of Medicine 1958;58:354–356.
5. Faucett RL, Litin EM, Achor RWP. Neuropharmacologic action of rauwolfia compounds and its psychodynamic implications. Arch Neurol Psychiat 1957;77:513–518.
6. Jensen K. Depression in patients treated with reserpine for arterial hypertension. Acta Psychiat Neurol Scand 1959;34:195–204.
7. Lemieux G, Davignon A, Genest J. Depressive states during rauwolfia therapy for arterial hypertension. Can Med Assoc J 1956;74:522–526.
8. Dollerey CT, Harington M. Methyldopa in hypertension: clinical and pharmacological studies. Lancet 1962;i:759–763.
9. Smirk H. Hypotensive action of methyldopa. Br Med J 1963;7:146–155.
10. Sourkes TW. The action of α-methyldopa in the brain. Br Med Bull 1965;21:66–69.
11. Schildkraut JJ. The catecholamine hypothesis of affective disorders: a review of supporting evidence. Am J Psychiatry 1965;122:509–522.
12. Bunney Jr WE, Davis JM. Norepinephrine in depressive reactions. Arch Gen Psychiatry 1965;13(6):483–494.
13. Coppen A, Prange AJ, Hill C, Whybrow PC, Noguera R. Abnormalities of indolamines in affective disorders. Arch Gen Psychiatry 1972;26:474–478.
14. Lapin IP, Oxenkrug GF. Intensification of the central serotonergic processes as a possible determinant of the thymoleptic effect. Lancet 1969;i:132–136.
15. Everett GM. The dopa response potentiation test and its use in screening for antidepressant drugs. In: Garattini S, Dukes MNG, eds. Antidepressant drugs. Amsterdam: Excerpta Medica, 1967.
16. Sulser F, Bickel MH, Brodie BB. The action of desmethylimipramine in counteracting sedation and cholinergic effects of reserpine-like drugs. J Pharmacol Exp Ther 1964;144:321–330.
17. Sulser F, Owens ML, Dingell JV. In vivo modification of biochemical effects of reserpine by desipramine in the hypothalamus of the rat [Abstract]. Pharmacologist 1967;9:213.
18. Seligman ME, Maier SF. Failure to escape traumatic shock. J Exp Psychol 1967;74:1–9.
19. Overmier JB, Seligman MEP. Effects of inescapable shock upon subsequent escape and avoidance learning. Journal of Comparative and Physiological Psychology 1967;63:23–33.

20. Seligman ME. Learned helplessness. Ann Rev Med 1972;23:407–412.
21. Porsolt RD, Anton G, Blavet N, et al. Behavioral despair in rats. A new model sensitive to antidepressant treatments. Eur J Pharmacol 1979;47:379–391.
22. Porsolt RD. Behavioral despair. In: Enna SJ, Malik JB, Richelson E, eds. Antidepressants: neurochemical, behavioral, and clinical perspectives. New York: Raven Press, 1981.

Mechanism of Action

Antidepressants are not euphoriants or stimulants. Thus, while they can markedly benefit depressed patients, they have little or no effect on nondepressed individuals. For example, when an MAOI is used to treat hypertension, most patients deny any cognitive or mood effect, although a few experience sedation, mild euphoria, and/or insomnia. In contrast, amphetamines are potent stimulants and euphoriants, but are usually ineffective for severe depressions.

The fact that antidepressants (ADs) counteract depression without altering normal mood states impels us to consider theories about their mechanism of action, as well as the biological basis for depression.

Indeed, hypotheses regarding the biological mechanisms subserving mood disorders have developed from observations on the clinical effects of drug and somatic therapies in humans, as well as drug-induced behavioral changes in animals (1). For the purpose of discussion, current theories can be divided into several categories:

• Neurotransmitter-receptor
• Membrane/cation
• Neurophysiological
• Biological rhythms
• Neuroendocrine
• Immunological
• Genetic.

We emphasize that these theories are not mutually exclusive. Thus, a *genetically* determined *membrane* defect could produce a dysregulation in the *neurotransmitter-receptor* interaction. This in turn may impact *second messenger systems* within target neural circuits, resulting in a disturbance of *biological rhythms,* such as *neuroendocrine* function.

NEUROTRANSMITTER AND RELATED HYPOTHESES
Monoamine Theories of Depression
Catecholamine Hypothesis

This theory, first promulgated in the mid 1960s, postulated a diminished activity of catecholamines in the central nervous system (CNS) (e.g., norepinephrine (NE)) (see references 11 and 12 at end of previous section). Conversely, mania was explained as a relative increase in their activity.

The ascending NE pathway in the CNS begins with projections from the locus coeruleus, an anatomical site encompassing about 5000 neurons (containing 85–90% of central norepinephrine stores) that project to the:

• Hippocampus
• Cerebral cortex
• Amygdala
• Lower brain stem center (which controls sympathetic output).

It is the effect of antidepressants on this system that is believed to subserve their efficacy. While various agents may enhance, inhibit, or modulate NE activity, the heterocyclics (HCAs) and MAOIs increase this transmitter's activity, by two different mechanisms. HCAs generally block the reuptake pump mechanism that recovers NE from the synaptic cleft shortly after the drug reaches the transporter. Thus, reuptake inhibition is occurring during both the acute and the chronic phases of therapy. Interestingly, clinical effects usually occur during the chronic phase. MAOIs, by contrast, interfere with enzymatic deamination. In either case, the outcome is increased NE concentrations.

The earliest investigations of this hypothesis considered the major metabolite(s) of NE (e.g., 3-methoxy-4-hydroxyphenylacetic acid (MHPG)) in cerebrospinal fluid (CSF), plasma, and urine. The purpose was to elucidate the biological mechanism(s) subserving mood disorders; to develop potential markers to facilitate diagnosis; and to aid in the prediction of treatment response. While promising, this line of inquiry has been impeded by various methodological obstacles (e.g., the relative contribution of peripheral versus central sources, etc.) and conflicting results. For example, most studies find that CSF MHPG in depressed patients is identical to that in normal controls. Since it is in equilibrium with plasma MHPG, however, the failure to find low CSF or plasma MHPG does not negate the NE hypothesis, because CSF MHPG may not be an accurate reflection of NE activity in the CNS.

The Depression-type (D-type) score, developed as a predictive tool by Schildkraut, Schatzberg, Mooney et al., exemplifies the most comprehensive attempt to pursue this line of investigation (2). Janicak et al. summarized this issue while reporting negative results on the predic-

tive value of urinary MHPG in unipolar depressed patients treated with standard ADs (3). Thus, since the value of MHPG as a marker has not been clearly established (e.g., it has not been studied as a predictor of response for many of the newer ADs), we believe that currently its routine commercial use is not warranted (4).

In animals, *chronic treatment* (i.e., for several days or weeks) with heterocyclics, monoamine oxidase inhibitors, and electroconvulsive therapy coincides more closely with the time course to maximum response (5–8). This time frame coincides with the most consistent adaptive change (i.e., a reduced sensitivity of postsynaptic receptors, leading to diminished adenylate-cyclase activity). In the original hypothesis, depression was postulated to be secondary to decreased NE levels or release, or subsensitive receptors. A *downregulation (or reverse catecholamine) hypothesis* has subsequently been proposed to explain the decreased numbers of postsynaptic β_2-adrenergic receptors in peripheral tissues (e.g. leukocytes) after chronic antidepressant treatment. Thus, depression, rather than the result of a *hypoadrenergic state*, may be due to a *hyperadrenergic state* (i.e., increased levels or release, or supersensitive receptors are the critical event(s)). This hypothesis was further supported by the neuropharmacological effects of chronic antidepressant treatment, which decreased:

- Brain *tyrosine hydroxylase* and norepinephrine
- Postsynaptic β-adrenergic receptor sensitivity and density
- The basal firing rate of NE neurons in the *locus coeruleus*.

Within this context, the original theory may still be valid, since a defect in presynaptic neurotransmission should result in a compensatory *upregulation* of postsynaptic receptors. Thus, normalization of presynaptic activity should down-regulate (or "normalize") postsynaptic receptor function.

In addition, β-adrenergic receptors are increased in the brains of suicide victims, as are the number of α_2-adrenergic receptor binding sites in the brain of suicide completers and in the platelets of depressed patients (9). The implication of the latter is that the pathological increased activity of these autoreceptors may reduce NE output secondary to a short loop, negative feedback mechanism. Furthermore, Crews and Smith (1978) found the α_2-adrenergic receptors adapted (i.e., down-regulated) to 3 weeks of treatment with desipramine, ultimately enhancing NE transmission (10).

On balance, these actions could support a decrease rather than an increase in the functional state of CNS NE transmission, since depression can be conceptualized as a state of supersensitive catecholamine receptors secondary to decreased NE availability. This reasoning is consistent with the original hypothesis of diminished NE functioning, with antidepressants returning receptors to a more normal state of sensitivity. Siever and Davis (1985) have further elaborated on this concept by suggesting the possibility of dysregulation in the homeostatic mechanisms of one or more neurotransmitter systems, culminating in an unstable or erratic output (11).

Indolamine Hypothesis

The second neurotransmitter implicated in the monoamine theory was *serotonin (5-HT)*. Indeed, Bunney and Davis (1965) noted that 5-HT may also be a candidate:

> There are other neurohumors which may play a role in depressive.... Serotonin, like NEP, is effected by antidepressants and is

decreased by the two drugs producing depression. It is premature to argue that one and not the other is important in human depression, since both are implicated by indirect evidence and both may be important. The evidence on NEP is summarized here. The evidence on serotonin is an equally likely candidate (11a).

This neurotransmitter is contained in a few pathways, of which the midbrain raphe nuclei to the limbic-septal area (e.g., hippocampus and amygdala) is probably the most important. Serotonin abnormalities are widely reported in patients with depression, especially those with suicidal behavior.

Several lines of evidence support 5-HT involvement in depression and include:

- Decreased levels of *5-HT or its metabolite (5-HIAA)*, as well as decreased imipramine binding and increased 5-HT_2 binding sites in postmortem suicide brains (12)
- Increased 5-HT_2 receptor binding sites in the platelets of depressed and suicidal patients (12)
- *Decreased 5-HIAA CSF levels in living*, depressed patients who attempt suicide by violent means (13)
- *Decreased 5-HT reuptake in the platelets* (V_{max}) of depressed patients linked to a decrease in the number of platelet imipramine binding sites (14)
- Blunting of the maximal *prolactin response to i.v. tryptophan* (the precursor of 5-HT) in depressed patients. Similar results have also been observed with fenfluramine and m-chlorophenyl-piperazine (mCPP) (15)
- p-*chlorophenylalanine* (PCPA), which decreases 5-HT synthesis, reverses the clinical efficacy of antidepressants (16, 17)
- Depletion of plasma tryptophan precursors may reverse antidepressant-induced remissions (18)

- *Tryptophan and 5-hydroxytryptophan (5-HTP)*, the precursors of 5-HT, may have antidepressant effects, alone or in combination with other drugs (19)
- Analogous to β-adrenergic receptor down-regulation, *antidepressants* reduce 5-HT receptor number but not their affinity (20)
- Electroconvulsive therapy (ECT) potentiates *prolactin response to TRH*, which is mediated by serotonin (21)
- Electroconvulsive shock (ECS) enhances functional activity and binding characteristics of $5\text{-}HT_2$ *receptors* in postmortem studies on animals (22).

Partial Agonists

In the context of the receptor-ligand model, the role of partial agonists has been clarified more recently. In essence, these ligands are partially stimulatory to a receptor in the absence of the natural, fully stimulating ligand. Paradoxically, in the presence of the natural ligand, partial agonists reduce the degree of stimulation, in that they compete with full agonists (e.g., 5-HT) for binding sites, and in essence function as an antagonist.

In this context, Eison (1990) argues for a common underlying pathology for anxiety and depression. In support of this position, he cites the *azaspirones* (e.g., buspirone, gepirone, tandospirone, ipsapirone), which appear to exert their beneficial effects by modulating the activity of 5-HT through partial agonism of $5\text{-}HT_{1A}$ receptors (23). In support of their antidepressant effects, he notes that members of this class can down-regulate $5\text{-}HT_2$ receptors, as well as desensitize presynaptic, $5\text{-}HT_{1A}$ autoreceptors. He notes that $5\text{-}HT_{1A}$ receptors are also found postsynaptically, and azaspirones may affect postsynaptic receptors differently than their presynaptic counterparts (i.e., buspirone is only a partial agonist of postsynaptic receptors). He concludes that in a given context of 5-HT activity (i.e., up or down), these drugs may be able to normalize neurotransmission, which is excessive in anxiety disorders and deficient in depressive disorders.

Other Neurotransmitters

Other neurotransmitter systems have also been implicated in depression, including: γ-aminobutyric acid (GABA), the opiods, and in particular, dopamine (DA).

Dopamine. Randrup first postulated a role for dopamine in depressive disorders (24). More recently, a reanalysis of the data from several groups has found evidence for a bimodal distribution of CSF homovanillic acid (HVA) levels in depressed patients, with one group comparable to normal controls and the other with decreased levels (5). Roy and colleagues (1992) also reported on the potential predictive value of lower urinary HVA output in depressed patients who attempted suicide versus those who did not (25). Both reports indicate a decreased turnover in DA.

Consistent with earlier studies, Muscat et al. (1992) reported on chronic exposure to mild unpredictable stress in rats as a model to study the AD-reversible decreases in the consumption of palatable sweets (26, 27). Using this model they found that DA agonists (i.e., quinpirole, bromocriptine) administered intermittently had the same positive effects as tricyclic antidepressants (TCAs). They further postulate that the infrequent, intermittent administration of dopamine agonists (e.g., psychostimulants) may avoid problems with tolerance and abuse while providing a clinically relevant antidepressant strategy.

A recent report by Kapur and Mann (1992) comprehensively reviews the role of DA in depressive disorders (27). They discuss several lines of evidence including:

- The lower CSF HVA levels in some depressed patients
- An increased incidence of depression in Parkinson's disease as well as in patients receiving DA-depleting or antagonistic agents
- The antidepressant effect of agents that enhance DA transmission
- The ablility of various classes of ADs and ECS to enhance DA effects in animal models.

Interaction Theories of Depression
Permissive Hypothesis

It is now evident that a single neurotransmitter theory does not suffice to explain all known evidence. As a result, models that include two or more systems have been developed to encompass their modulatory interactions. One of the most cogent is the "permissive" hypothesis, which proposes that a decreased function in central serotonin transmission sets the stage for either a depressive or manic phase (28). This circumstance itself is not sufficient to produce the mood disturbance, however, with superimposed aberrations in norepinephrine function required to determine the phase of an affective episode (i.e., decreased 5-HT and decreased NE subserves depression; decreased 5-HT and increased NE subserves mania). Data from animal studies to support this theory include:

- *5,6-dihydroxytryptamine (5,6,DHT) lesions* of the serotonin nuclei are known

to attenuate the reduction in β-noradrenergic receptor binding induced by chronic tricyclic treatment (29, 30)
- *6-hydroxydopamine (6-OHDA) lesions,* which destroy 5-HT neurons in the dorsal and ventral bundles as well as the locus coeruleus, block the enhanced locomotor responses to quipazine after repeated ECS.

Adrenergic-Cholinergic Balance Hypothesis

A second interaction theory postulates an imbalance between the cholinergic and the noradrenergic systems (31). The central cholinergic system consists of projections primarily from the nucleus basalis. A relative increase in this system's activity in comparison to central norepinephrine activity, is thought to play a role in producing depression. Conversely, a decrease relative to central NE activity is thought to play a role in producing mania. Clinically, agents with cholinomimetic effects (e.g., precursors, cholinergic agonists, cholinesterase inhibitors) have shown some benefit in mania (see Alternate Treatment Strategies in Chapter 10). Cholinergic abnormalities are also thought to underlie some of the abnormal sleep patterns (e.g., decreased rapid eye movement (REM) latency, increased REM density) found in depression. Also consistent with this theory is evidence that ECT:

- Decreases brain acetylcholine (Ach) levels
- Increases choline acetyltransferase activity, the enzyme most prominently involved in Ach breakdown
- Causes release of CSF acetylcholine
- Produces cholinergically mediated electroencephalogram (EEG) slowing following a series of treatments.

Bidimensional Model

Proponents of this hypothesis identify three types of abnormal neurochemistry:

- Causative
- Phenomenological ("expressive")
- Epiphenomenological (possible useful state markers).

As others before them, Emrich and colleagues propose that a single neurochemical imbalance is not sufficient to explain many of the inconsistencies and contradictions in studies with various mood stabilizers (32). Instead, they speculate that several neurotransmitter imbalances relating to different brain areas should be anticipated.

The possible differing mechanisms of action of three mood stabilizers (i.e., lithium, valproic acid (VPA), carbamazepine (CBZ)) are incorporated into a bidimensional model of mood regulation which postulates two "gating zones" (one for depression and one for mania). These zones are thought to be subserved by different neurochemical abnormalities, leading to a situation where both could be impacted by certain agents (i.e., mood stabilizers), or alternatively, could individually be affected by unidirectional compounds (e.g., HCAs).

Second Messenger Dysbalance Hypothesis

Receptors are glycoproteins imbedded in the lipid bilayer of neuronal membranes, and can detect minute amounts of specific ligands (e.g., neurotransmitters; hormones). The ligand-receptor interaction sets in motion a transduction system (e.g., an enzyme; ion channel) that orchestrates various intracellular biochemical events.

More recently, investigators have looked beyond the receptor-ligand binding relationship to study intraneuronal events stimulated by this interaction. Two primary areas are the adenylate-cyclase (AC) and the phosphoinositol (PI) second messenger systems. **Such investigations have led to the postulation that functional disturbances in intraneuronal signal transmission distal to the receptors of classic neurotransmitters (i.e., the first messengers) are pathogenetically important in mood disorders** (33). Further, it suggests that these disorders are caused by a dysfunction in the "crosstalk" between major intraneuronal signal amplification systems (e.g., adenylate-cyclase and the phospolipase C systems). Thus, depression may result from a diminished functioning in cyclic monophosphate (c-AMP)-mediated effector cell responses, together with an absolute or relative dominance of the inositol triphosphate/diacylglycerol-mediated responses. Mania is conceptualized as resulting from the reverse circumstances.

Membrane/Cation Hypothesis

The resting membrane potential; monoamine transport and reuptake; and other functions of the cellular membrane are partially related to cation transport mechanisms. This hypothesis proposes that there is a deficiency in one or more of these transport functions; that such a deficit is genetically determined; and that the resulting membrane dysfunction predisposes to a mood disorder.

The steady state distribution of lithium has provided some evidence to support this hypothesis. Thus, it has been shown that patients with bipolar illness have a higher mean intra/extracellular red blood cell (RBC) to lithium ratio, as do their first-degree relatives (34, 35). These findings have led to speculation about genetic control of the lithium ratio and its role in the pathogenesis, as well as pharmacotherapy, of mood disorders.

BIOLOGICAL RHYTHM HYPOTHESIS

Halberg (1968) has postulated a desynchronization of circadian rhythms in depression; while Goodwin (1982) has found a phase advance in the rhythms of depressed patients, and Schulz and Lund (1985) a diminished amplitude (36–38). Perhaps most interesting is the ability of antidepressants to alter these rhythms, possibly by binding to receptor sites in the suprachiasmatic nucleus (39).

A clear example is the disturbance in the sleep-wake cycle that constitutes one of the hallmarks of depression. Thus, several non-REM components are disrupted, including:

- A decrease in *total sleep time*
- An increase in *sleep onset* latency
- A decrease in the *arousal* threshold
- An increase in *wakefulness*
- *Terminal insomnia* (early morning awakening).

as well as REM-related phenomena such as:

- A decrease in *REM onset* latency
- An increase in *REM density*
- A *redistribution of REM sleep* to earlier in the sleep phase.

These last three culminate in a state of "REM pressure," which can be viewed as a state of hyperarousal (29).

Theories explaining the mechanism of action of phototherapy and the biological basis of seasonal affective disorder (SAD) are also related to this area of investigation (i.e., infraradian rhythm disturbances) (see also Bright Light Phototherapy in Chapter 8). For example, Skewerer and colleagues reported that *plasma norepinephrine levels* in SAD were inversely related to the

level of depression, and these levels increased proportionally to the degree of therapeutic improvement (40). Depue et al., in reporting their work on the possible role of *dopamine* in SAD, noted that basal serum prolactin values did not change as a function of season or after successful phototherapy (41). Further, these values remained significantly lower in comparison to control subjects, suggesting they could serve as a trait marker for this disorder.

These findings do not exclude the possibility that the central *serotonin system* is also involved, given its influence on prolactin levels. In this regard, there is some data indicating an antidepressant response to dietary L-tryptophan and *d*-fenfluramine, an indirect serotonin agonist (42). In an open trial, Jacobsen reported a euphoric, energized reaction in 10 SAD patients given infusions of the serotonin agonist mCPP (43). Finally, Lacoste and Wirz-Justice found evidence for seasonal rhythms in serotonin levels in their healthy controls, with the winter values significantly lower than their summer counterparts (44).

NEUROENDOCRINE HYPOTHESES

Cortisol hypersecretion, blunted growth hormone and prolactin responses, blunted thyrotropin-stimulating hormone (TSH) response to thyrotropin-releasing hormone (TRH), reduced luteinizing hormone secretion, and disturbances in β-endorphin, vasopressin, and calcitonin have all been associated with depression.

As summarized by Gold and colleagues (1988), acute behavioral and physiological changes that occur in the *general adaptational syndrome* are almost identical to those seen in the depressive syndrome (45). They suggest that melancholia may be conceptualized as an acute generalized stress response that has escaped the normal regulatory restraints. Further, they implicate a dysregulation in glucocorticoid activity, which typically antagonizes corticotropin-releasing hormone (CRH) neurons, as well as the locus ceoruleus-NE system, in addition to mediating immunosuppression. This activity would normally restrain or counter-regulate the effectors of the stress response, precluding excessive or extended activation.

Dysregulation of the hypothalamic-pituitary-adrenal axis is thought to cause a disturbance of the circadian rhythm of cortisol. Depression is associated with failure of feedback mechanisms to regulate cortisol secretion, resulting in high cortisol levels. The relationship between cortisol secretion and depression can be investigated through the use of the dexamethasone suppression test (DST), since approximately 50% of patients with symptoms of major depressive disorder show nonsuppression of cortisol. Further, we as well as other investigators have noted that patients who are improved but continue to have an abnormal DST result may be at a higher risk for relapse or suicidal behavior (46, 47).

Dysregulation of the hypothalamic-pituitary-thyroid axis causes a reduction in thyroid function. There may be a relationship between an abnormal thyroid-stimulating hormone response to thyrotropin-releasing hormone and depressive symptoms. Thus, unipolar patients undergoing the TRH-TSH test (which measures the difference between baseline TSH and peak postinfusion TSH after they are given synthetic TRH) reportedly have a blunted response while bipolar, depressed patients have an elevated response (see also Role of the Laboratory in Chapter 1).

IMMUNOLOGICAL HYPOTHESIS

Two hypotheses about the relationship between mood and the immune system have been the suggestions that depression may alter immunologic function; or that an unidentified infectious process (e.g., viral) may induce affective disturbances. In support of the former postulate, Bartrop et al. (1977) and Schleifer et al. (1983) both reported suppression of the immune system following a period of bereavement (48, 49).

More recently, Schleifer et al. (1989) found significant age-related immunological differences between their group of 91 unipolar depressed patients and a group of matched controls. Specifically, mitogen responses and the number of T4 lymphocytes did not increase in the depressed group with advancing age, as was the case with the normal controls (50). The impact of elevated cortisol levels on this phenomenon also needs further clarification.

While the results of several lines of investigation have generally been inconclusive, there may be subtypes of depressive disorders that affect immune function. Further, the question of a possible causative infectious process has yet to be adequately addressed.

GENETIC HYPOTHESIS

The evidence available from family, twin, and adoption studies supports the existence of a genetic factor(s) in the development of a primary mood disorder.

There is clearly a higher incidence of both bipolar and apparent unipolar disorders in first-degree relatives of bipolar patients. We say "apparent" because "unipolar" patients from bipolar families may simply have not yet experienced a manic phase. Families of unipolar patients, however, show a higher incidence of unipolar, but not bipolar disease. Given that unipolar and bipolar disorders are inherited separately suggests that there are at least two variations of mood disorders. We do not know where the gene (or genes) for the disorders are located, however, or how such aberrant genes translate into a mood disorder. Linkage studies using recombinant deoxyribonucleic acid (DNA) techniques have examined possible loci for association with mood disorders (e.g., the X or 11th chromosome) (51). Further confirmation is required, however, and it is possible that other loci may also be implicated (52). A more precise statement about the mode of genetic transmission, its contribution to pathogenesis, and environmental interactions is currently not possible.

In an effort to find a biological process that may identify a specific genotype, differences in various enzymes, (e.g., monoamine oxidase, dopamine β-hydroxylase (DBH), and catechol-O-methyltransferase (COMT)), have also been investigated.

Both unipolar and bipolar disorders tend to be recurrent and progressive. Post (1992) postulates that early episode stress-related alterations in gene expression may subserve long-lasting changes in stress responsivity, episode sensitization, and differences in pharmacosensitivity as a function of the longitudinal course of an illness. He further proposes that adequate drug prophylaxis may interrupt the phenomenon of "episodes begetting episodes," since subsequent exacerbations may overwhelm or circumvent a previously effective treatment(s) (53).

CONCLUSION

Since the original catecholamine hypothesis, which attempted to elucidate the biological mechanisms subserving mood disorders, there has been a gradual evolution from consideration of a single neurotransmitter system to the modulating interactions of various neurotransmitters. Most recently, the effects these "first messenger" systems have upon receptor subtypes and the intraneuronal "second messenger" or signal amplification system in post-synaptic cells have been explored.

Further, many of these neurotransmitters subserve or intimately interact with a number of neuroendocrine, circadian rhythm, and neurophysiological activities, which may be dysregulated in mood disorders. Genetic defects may well be the basis for such pathology.

REFERENCES

1. Richelson E. Biological basis of depression and therapeutic relevance. J Clin Psychiatry 1991;52(suppl 6):4–10.
2. Mooney JJ, Schatzberg AF, Cole JO, Samson JA, Waternaux C, Gerson B, et al. Urinary 3-methoxy-4-hydroxy phenylglycol and the Depression-Type Score as predictors of differential responses to antidepressants. J Clin Psychopharmacol 1991;11(6):339–343.
3. Janicak PG, Davis JM, Chan C, Altman E, Hedeker D. Failure of urinary MHPG levels to predict treatment response in patients with unipolar depression. Am J Psychiatry 1986;143:1398–1402.
4. Davis JM, Bresnahan DB. Psychopharmacology in clinical psychiatry. In: Hales RE, Frances AJ, eds. Psychiatry update. American Psychiatric Association Annual Review. Vol 6. Washington DC: American Psychiatric Press, 1987.
5. Vetulani J, Stawarz RJ, Dingell JV, Sulser F. A possible common mechanism of action of antidepressant treatments: reduction in the sensitivity of the nonadrenergic cyclic AMP-generating system in the rat limbic forebrain. Naunyn-Schmiedebergs Archives of Pharmacol 1976;293(2):109–114.
6. Banerjee SP, Kung LS, Riggi SJ, Chanda, SK. Development of beta-adrenergic receptor subsensitivity by antidepressants. Nature 1977;268(5619):455–456.
7. Pandey GN, Heinze WJ, Brown BD, Davis, JM. Electroconvulsive shock treatment decreases beta-adrenergic receptor sensitivity in rat brain. Nature 1979;280;234–235.
8. Pandey GN, Janicak PG, Javaid, JI, Davis JM. Increased ^{3}H-clonidine binding in the platelets of patients with depressive and schizophrenic disorders. Psychiatry Res 1987;28:73–88.
9. Pandey, GN, Pandey SC, Janicak PG, Marks RC, Davis JM. Platelet serotonin-2 receptor binding sites in depression and suicide. Biol Psychiatry 1990;28:215–222.

10. Crews FJ, Smith CB. Presynaptic alpha receptor subsensitivity after longterm antidepressant treatment. Science 1978;202:322–324.

11. Siever LJ, Davis KL. Overview: toward a dysregulation hypothesis of depression. Am J Psychiatry 1985;142:1017–1031.

11a. Bunney WE, Davis JM. Norepinephrine in depressive reactions. Arch Gen Psychiatry 1965;13:483–494.

12. Stanley M, Mann JJ. Increased serotonin-2 binding sites in frontal cortex of suicide victims. Lancet 1983;i:214–216.

13. Asberg M, Schalling D, Traskman-Bendy L, Wagner A. Psychobiology of suicide, impulsivity and related phenomena. In: Meltzer HY, ed. Psychopharmacology: the third generation of progress. New York: Raven Press, 1987:655–668.

14. Tuomisto J, Tukiainen E. Decreased uptake of 5-hydroxytryptamine in blood platelets from depressed patients. Nature 1976;262:596–598.

15. Price LH, Charney DS, Delgado PL, Heninger GR. Serotonin function and depression: neuroendocrine and mood responses to intravenous L-tryptophan in depressed patients and healthy comparison subjects. Am J Psychiatry 1991;148:1518–1525.

16. Shopsin B, Freedman E, Gershon S. PCPA reversal of tranylcypromine effects in depressed patients. Arch Gen Psychiatry 1976;33:811–819.

17. Shopsin B, Gershon S, Goldstein M, Freedman E, Wilk S. Use of synthesis inhibitors in defining a role for biogenic amines during imipramine treatment in depressed patients. Psychopharmacol Commun 1975;1:239–249.

18. Delgado PL, Charney DS, Price LH, Landis H, Heninger GR. Serotonin function and the mechanism of antidepressant action: reversal of antidepressant induced remission by rapid depletion of plasma tryptophan. Arch Gen Psychiatry 1990;47:411–418.

19. Van Praag HM. Management of depression with serotonin precursors. Biol Psych 1981;16:291–310.

20. Peroutka SJ, Snyder SH. Longterm antidepressant treatment decreases spiroperidol-labelled serotonin receptor binding. Science 1980:210;88–90.

21. Aperia B, Thoren M, Wetterberg L. Prolactin and thyrotropin in serum during ECT in patients with major depressive illness. Acta Psychiatr Scand 1985;72:302–308.

22. Stockmeier CA, Kellar KJ. In vivo regulation of the serotonin-2 receptor in rat brain. Life Sci 1986;38:117–127.

23. Eison MS. Azapirones: mechanism of action in anxiety and depression. Drug Therapy 1990;Aug(suppl):3–8.

24. Randrup A, Munkvad I, Fog R, et al. Mania, depression and brain dopamine. In: Essman WB, Valzelli L, eds. Current developments in psychopharmacology. New York: Spectrum Publications 1975:207–209.

25. Roy A, Karoum F, Pollack S. Marked reduction in indices of dopamine metabolism among patients with depression who attempt suicide. Arch Gen Psychiatry 1992;49:447–450.

26. Muscat R, Papp M, Willner P. Antidepressant-like effects of dopamine agonists in an animal model of depression. Biol Psychiatry 1992;31:937–946.

27. Kapur S, Mann JJ. Role of the dopaminergic system in depression. Biol Psychiatry 1992;32:1–17.

28. Prange Jr AJ, Wilson IC, Lynn CW, Alltop LB, Stikeleather RA. L-Tryptophan in mania. Arch Gen Psychiatry 1974;30:56–62.

29. Stockmeier CA, Martino AM, Kellar KJ. A strong influence of serotonin axons on β-adrenergic receptors in rat brain. Science 1985;230:323–325.

30. Janowski A, Okada F, Manier DH, Applegate CD, Sulser F, Streranka LR. Role of serotonergic input in the regulation of the β-adrenergic receptor–coupled adenylate cyclase system. Science 1982;218:900–901.

31. Janowsky DS, El-Yousef MK, Davis JM, Serkerke HJ. A cholinergic-adrenergic hypothesis of mania and depression. Lancet 1972;2:632–635.

32. Emrich HM, Wolf R. Recent neurochemical and pharmacological aspects of the pathogenesis and therapy of affective psychoses. Pharmacol Toxicol 1990;66(suppl 3):5–12.

33. Wachtel H. The second messenger dysbalance hypothesis of affective disorders. Pharmacopsychiat 1990;23:27–32.

34. Dorus E, Pandey GN, Shaughnessy R, Gaviria M, Val E, Ericksen S, Davis JM. Lithium transport across red blood cell membrane: a cell membrane abnormality in manic-depressive illness. Science 1979;205:932–934.

35. Pandey GN, Dorus E, Davis JM, Tosteson DC. Lithium transport in human red blood

cells: genetic and clinical aspects. Arch Gen Psychiatry 1979;36:902–908.

36. Halberg F. Physiological considerations underlying rhythmicity with special reference to emotional illness. In: de Ajuriaguerra JG, ed. Cycles biologique et psychiatrie. Paris: Geneve & Masson, 1968.

37. Goodwin, FK, Wirz-Justice A, Wehr T. Evidence that the pathophysiology of depression and the mechanism of action of antidepressant drugs involve alterations in circadian rhythms. Adv Biochem Psychopharmacol 1982;31:1–11.

38. Schulz H, Lund R. On the origins of early REM episodes in the sleep of depressed patients; a comparison of 3 hypotheses. Psychiatry Res 1985;16:65–77.

39. Wirz-Justice A, Krauchi K, Morimasa T, Willener R, Feer H. Circadian rhythm of ^{3}H-imipramine binding in the rat suprachiasmatic nuclei. Eur J Pharacol 1983;87:331–333.

40. Skewerer RB, Duncan C, Jacobsen FM, Sack DA, Tamarkin L, Wehr TA, Rosenthal NE. The neurobiology of seasonal affective disorder and phototherapy. J Biol Rhythms 1988;3:135–153.

41. Depue RA, Arbisi P, Spoont MR, Ainsworth RT. Dopamine functioning in the behavioral facilitation system and seasonal variation in behavior: normal population and clinical studies. In: Rosenthal NE, Blehar MC, eds. Seasonal affective disorders and phototherapy. New York: Guilford Press, (in press).

42. O'Rourke D, Wurtmann JJ, Brzeskinski A, Abou-Nader T, Marchant P, Wurtman RJ. Treatment of seasonal affective disorder with d-fenfluramine. Ann N Y Acad Sci 1987;499:329–330.

43. Jacobsen FM, Sack DA, Wehr TA, Rogers S, Rosenthal NE. Neuroendocrine response to 5-hydroxytryptophan in seasonal affective disorder. Arch Gen Psychiatry 1987;44:1086–1091.

44. LaCoste V, Wirtz-Justice A. Seasonal variation in normal subjects: an update of variables current in depression research. In: Rosenthal NE, Blehar MC, eds. Seasonal affective disorders and phototherapy. New York: Guilford Press, 1989.

45. Gold PW, Goodwin FK, Chrousos GP. Clinical and biochemical manifestations of depression: relation to the neurobiology of stress. Parts 1 and 2. N Engl J Med 1988; 319(6):348–353 and 1988;319(7):413–420.

46. Dysken MW, Pandey GN, Chang SS, Hicks R, Davis JM. Serial postdexamethasone cortisol levels in a patient undergoing ECT. Am J Psychiatry 1979;136(10):1328–1329.

47. The APA Task Force on Laboratory Tests in Psychiatry. The DST: an overview of its current status in psychiatry. Am J Psychiatry 1987;144:1253–1262.

48. Bartrop RW, Lazarus L, Luckhurst E, Kiloh LG, Penny R. Depressed lymphocyte function after bereavement. Lancet 1977;i:834–836.

49. Schleifer SJ, Keller SE, Camerino M, Thornton JC, Stein M. Suppression of lymphocyte stimulation following bereavement. JAMA 1983;250(3):374–377.

50. Schleifer SJ, Keller SE, Bond RN, Cohen J, Stein M. Major depressive disorder and immunity: role of age, sex, severity and hospitalization. Arch Gen Psychiatry 1989;46:81–87.

51. Gershon ES, Berrettini W, Nurnberger Jr J, Goldin LR. Genetics of affective illness. In: Meltzer HY, ed. Psychopharmacology: the third generation of progress. New York: Raven Press, 1987:481–491.

52. Berretini WH, Goldin LR, Gelernter S, Gejman PV, Gershon ES, Detera-Wadleigh S. X-chromosome markers and manic-depressive illness: rejection of linkage to x$_q$28 in nine bipolar pedigrees. Arch Gen Psychiatry 1990;47:366–373.

53. Post RM. Transduction of psychosocial stress into the neurobiology of recurrent affective disorder. Am J Psychiatry 1992;149:999–1010.

Treatment Planning

Most psychiatric disorders are chronic, often involve more than one episode, and rarely are curable in the sense that pneumonia is "cured." Nonetheless, symptoms may go into prolonged remission with effective treatment. Some disorders may take an episodic course, encompassing discrete episodes interspersed with asymptomatic or clearly less symptomatic intervals. A more chronic course involves continuous symptoms that wax and wane, or alternatively, steady deterioration.

A traditional distinction between mood disorders and schizophrenia was that the former were most often episodic whereas the latter was a chronic condition, often characterized by progressive worsening. Emil Kraepelin based the distinction between these two illnesses on the fact that remissions early in the course of mood disorders were common; by contrast, this was rare in schizophrenia. Recent data, however, has shown that some major depressive disorders can also be chronic and may even show a deteriorating pattern (1).

Treatment planning should take the issue of chronicity into account, and will necessarily differ for a first occurrence versus a recurrent disorder with no or only brief well intervals. Even the treatment of a chronic persistent course will differ, based on whether there is an acute exacerbation or a period of relative quiescence.

TREATMENT SETTING

The first step is to decide on the appropriate treatment environment (e.g., a hospital unit or an outpatient setting), keeping in mind several variables while making this decision. Proper assessment must also consider the *living situation and social support system,* which may or may not be able or willing to accommodate the patient.

All patients must be assessed for *active suicidal ideation or behavior,* as described in the section on Suicide in Chapter 6. Next, the presence of *psychosis* should be determined (e.g., hallucinations; delusions), as well as cognitive slowing, which may present as a thought disorder. With a

psychotic depression, patients may inadvertently endanger themselves and/or others by reason of an overt act or impaired judgment. Severity of an episode should also be assessed in terms of the *ability to care for oneself.* For example, with *catatonia,* it is obvious that patients are unable to function independently. Even if the presentation is less dramatic, the depressed patient may still be sufficiently impaired, requiring a care provider (or being in a structured setting) during the lag phase preceding the onset of antidepressant action to assure their safety and well-being.

Hospitalization may also be appropriate if the treatment plan involves observation, testing, or treatment that cannot be accomplished on an outpatient basis. For example, although ECT can be done without hospitalization, patients are usually admitted (at least initially), due to the level of care and sophistication required to properly administer this therapy, while ascertaining whether any unexpected complications arise.

If a patient needs hospitalization, the next decision involves the type of unit. For example, an intensive care setting is required for the actively suicidal, the overtly psychotic, or the profoundly impaired patients to insure their safety. Typically, treatment begins on an intensive care or short-term evaluation unit in larger, highly specialized psychiatric facilities. When the patient's condition improves, the person is transferred to a less structured unit in anticipation of discharge to an outpatient setting.

DEVELOPING RAPPORT

Once a treatment setting is established, the clinician can then begin active treatment, which for MDD invariably requires drug intervention. The proper use of pharmacotherapy, however, does not begin and end with the prescription, which, while necessary, is in some ways less consequential.

Most importantly, developing rapport with the patient is critical to all phases of diagnosis and treatment. Patients must feel comfortable with and confident in their physician. Otherwise, they will be less candid during the diagnostic and treatment phases, with undetected noncompliance a possible consequence.

THE PLACEBO RESPONDER

The issue of placebo response must always be considered, since several controlled studies have shown that 15 to 50% of depressed patients on placebo demonstrate improvement (2). Those figures encompass:

- Improvement for various *internal or external reasons*
- *Spontaneous recovery* with the passage of time
- Improvement caused by the *nondrug aspects of treatment*
- The *suggestive effect* of a dummy tablet
- *Clinician bias* in an uncontrolled trial.

Premorbid neurotic personality is also associated with a *higher placebo response,* as well as fluctuating symptoms with day-to-day variation, and high mood reactivity (3). While these findings have been replicated in several studies, they do not preclude an empirical trial of an antidepressant in a patient with some of these characteristics. Instead, such findings are one aspect to consider in a comprehensive treatment plan.

Conversely, certain factors repeatedly surface as predictors of a *low placebo response:*

- The presence of a *full vegetative syndrome* of major depressive disorder

- The *severity* of symptoms (sleep, appetite, psychomotor retardation)
- The *presence of positive biological markers* (e.g., dexamethasone nonsuppression, REM latency on sleep polysomnography, TSH blunting upon challenge with TRH infusion)
- The *duration of the current depressive episode* (greater than 3 months' duration)
- The *chronicity of the illness since first diagnosed* (i.e., either recurrent or chronic depressive illness).

Educational level, insight into illness, and likability (as reported by the physician) have also been correlated with poor placebo response (4). Any of these factors would support the use of drug therapy in the overall treatment strategy.

ADEQUACY OF TREATMENT

An adequate AD trial involves an adequate dose for an adequate period of time. For the tricyclics, therapeutic drug monitoring (TDM) can confirm a safe and effective dose. For other antidepressants, such information is not available or does not materially help beyond titrating the dose based on response and how well the drug is tolerated. Adequate duration is at least 4–6 weeks, due to these agents' delayed onset of action; however, early positive effects often predict later response. By contrast, no effect after 2–3 weeks usually indicates an unsatisfactory outcome.

The possible responses to an adequate trial include:

- Full *remission*
- *Partial* response
- *Nonresponse*
- Development of *adverse effects* that preclude an adequate trial

• Treatment *discontinuation* for other reasons.

If the depressive episode does not remit after an adequate trial, sequential trials with alternate antidepressants (usually from a different class) or use of an augmenting agent are the most common strategies. The choice of AD is usually based on the alternative having a different spectrum of activity (i.e., ideally, based upon data that patients who failed on one class of ADs still may respond to an alternate agent). If the patient was benefitting, but developed intolerable adverse effects, the clinician may either choose another member of the same class, with a different side-effect profile, or add another medication to ameliorate the adverse effect. If the patient has a partial response, the clinician may switch to another agent or attempt to potentiate the response by adding an augmenting drug (e.g., lithium).

COPHARMACY FOR DEPRESSION

Most antidepressants have a delayed onset of action and patients may not experience substantial symptom relief for 2 or more weeks. Hence, additional medications may be appropriate during the early phase of treatment to provide more rapid symptomatic relief. One common example is the concurrent use of benzodiazepines (BZDs) to relieve associated insomnia or severe anxiety. While several controlled trials find that the addition of a BZD enhances improvement during the early phases (i.e., first week) of treatment, by 4 weeks those on ADs only have also achieved comparable results.

There are drawbacks as well as benefits in utilizing copharmacy. Anxiolytics expose patients to a potentially addictive medication, as well as possibly lowering behavioral inhibition in the suicidal pa-

tient or aggravating the depressive syndrome itself (see Chapter 6). When these agents are cautiously used in carefully selected patients, primarily on an as-needed basis, these risks are minimal. Patients should always be informed of the potential risks of copharmacy, and some may elect not to take such medications, even if the possibility of an adverse event is small. These drugs can also impair mental alertness and coordination, endangering the patient and/or others (e.g., on a job that involves operating dangerous equipment). BZDs, in particular, potentiate the effects of alcohol, so patients should be warned about this interaction, as well as assessed for their propensity to drink while taking them.

MAINTENANCE THERAPY

Major depressive disorder is frequently a recurrent illness, thus treatment is divided into three phases:

• *Acute,* to quell an exacerbation
• *Maintenance,* to prevent a relapse into the current episode
• *Prophylaxis,* to prevent recurrence after at least 6 months of full remission from a prior episode.

Maintenance drug therapy is mandatory following successful induction of a remission, while prophylaxis is reserved for those patients who have experienced one or more serious episodes. Thus, treatment planning must not only consider the demonstrated efficacy, tolerability, and safety of a treatment for the induction of remission but for the maintenance of remission as well. The same considerations apply for prophylactic therapy.

Following remission of an acute episode, maintenance treatment should continue for at least 6–12 months to prevent relapse in the patient without a prior history. During this interval, the acute dose should be maintained rather than reduced. After 4 months, the dose may be gradually tapered and discontinued by the sixth month. After a single episode there is a 50-50 chance of a recurrence within the first few months; but with each recurrence, the likelihood of future episodes increases (e.g., after three episodes, the likelihood of recurrence is over 90%) (5). In the patient with a single episode, the best predictor of increased risk of recurrence is a positive family history. Thus, if there are one or more first-degree relatives with a history of MDD, the chance of recurrence increases, and extending maintenance treatment to 1 year or more is appropriate (2).

Longitudinal studies find that most patients will experience a recurrence. If a patient has subsequent but infrequent, mild depressive episodes, the adverse effects of drug therapy may outweigh its prophylactic value. Conversely, patients with more frequent, severe, or suicidal recurrences will clearly benefit from indefinite drug maintenance. Where to draw the line is often a matter of clinical judgment.

PROPHYLACTIC THERAPY

Prophylaxis refers to the prevention of recurrent episodes, rather than preventing relapse of a recently remitted depression. Prophylaxis involves the indefinite continuation of medication, usually over many years. Ultimately, the decision is the patient's, since the patient is the one who must contend with adverse effects, expense, the nuisance of taking medication, and the psychological issues inherent in any drug therapy for a mental disorder. The clinician should provide the best information and guidance available to help make the decision, based on:

- The *history*, including the number of prior episodes
- The *severity* of prior episodes, including suicidality
- The *duration of the well interval(s)* between episodes
- The presence of any persistent albeit *minor symptoms* between full episodes
- How an episode *evolves*.

In terms of this last issue, if the patient is able to recognize certain symptoms that serve as a harbinger of a developing recurrence, aggressive intervention may be requested and instituted before an episode fully develops. Conversely, if the episodes have short prodromes or develop insidiously, continuous prophylactic therapy would be more appropriate. **In the end, only the fully informed patient can decide whether to take medication indefinitely or risk a recurrence by discontinuing the antidepressant.**

REFERENCES

1. Janicak PG, O'Connor E. Major affective disorders: issues involving recovery and recurrence. Current Opinion in Psychiatry 1990;3:48–53.
2. Brown W, Dornseif B, Wernicke J. Placebo response in depression: a search for predictors. Psychiatry Res 1988;26:259–264.
3. Kiloh L, Ball J, Garside R. Prognostic factors in treatment of depressive states with imipramine. Br Med J 1962;1:1225–1227.
4. Downing R, Rickels K. Physicians' prognosis in relationship to drug and placebo response in anxious and depressed psychiatric outpatients. J Nerv Ment Dis 1973;156(2):109–129.
5. Keller MB, Shapiro RW, Lavori PW, Wolfe N. Relapse in major depressive disorder: analysis with the life table. Arch Gen Psychiatry 1982;39:911–915.

Management of an Acute Depressive Episode

EFFICACY FOR ACUTE TREATMENT

The treatment of major depression in psychiatry is analogous to the treatment of many conditions in general medicine, in that patients with these various disorders can benefit from several classes of medications with different mechanisms of action and/or adverse effects. The development of newer agents with unique spectra of activity requires the parallel development of specific strategies for their optimal use. After a review of the efficacy literature, we will suggest such a model to manage the depressed patient.

The efficacy of standard antidepressants for major depression is supported by about 400 well-controlled studies, as well as many more partially controlled or open trials. Overall, response to the heterocyclics in treating nonpsychotic depression is approximately 65%, with recent evidence suggesting that monoamine oxidase inhibitors may be comparably effective (see Table 7.1). By contrast, the placebo response rate was about 35% across all these studies (1).

In severely depressed patients, these agents produce a striking improvement in behavior and a marked lessening of depression, generally beginning 3 to 10 days after their initiation. The rate of response is linear over time, with a "half-life to improvement" of about 10–20 days. Consequently, patients who do not demonstrate satisfactory response after an adequate trial for a 4- to 6-week period, probably will not. The degree of response in the first 2 weeks of treatment may predict the ultimate outcome, with 65 to 80% of depressed patients substantially benefited by HCAs during this period, in contrast to only 20 to 40% of those on placebo (2).

We have provided a summary of the results from double-blind, random-assignment studies (usually class I or II designs) comparing heterocyclic, serotonin reuptake inhibitor (SRI), and MAOI antidepressants to placebo or to each other for the acute treatment of depression. Each study was reviewed, and a global judgment made, based on all the evidence presented, as to whether a given drug was more effective than placebo or another control therapy.

First Generation Antidepressants

Imipramine

Studies comparing imipramine to placebo (including 2649 depressed patients)

Table 7.1.
Combined Antidepressants versus *Placebo:* Acute Treatment

Number of Studies	Number of Subjects	Responders (%)		Difference (%)	Chi Square	p Value
		Drug (%)	Placebo (%)			
		Combined Cyclic Antidepressants				
79	5159	62.8	35.9	26.9	365	$< 10^{-40}$
		Combined MAO Inhibitors				
16	1697	66	32	35	49.9	2×10^{-12}

found that 68% on active drug were substantially improved, compared to only 40% on placebo (i.e., an average drug-placebo difference of 28%) (see Table 7.2). Imipramine was more effective than, or at least equal to placebo, in all studies; but placebo was never found to be better than imipramine. Generally, those studies that failed to show a definite active drug effect suffered from methodological inadequacies such as insufficient dose, inappropriate rating scales, and small, nonhomogenous patient populations (e.g., significant numbers of psychotic, schizoaffective, or neurotic patients). The probability of these results occurring by chance alone was nonexistent when calculated by the Mantel-Haenszel test.

We noted that despite a clear advantage for drug over placebo, about 30% of patients on imipramine remained unimproved, indicating the need for alternate treatment methods in many of these patients.

Amitriptyline

Most studies comparing amitriptyline to placebo found the drug to be superior (see Table 7.2). Those comparing it to imipramine found these two agents to be equally effective (Table 7.3) No studies found amitriptyline to be less effective than imipramine; and two double-blind studies showed amitriptyline (200 mg) to be superior to imipramine (200 mg) (3, 4). This finding, however, may be an artifact, in that the imipramine group included more delusional patients, who generally respond poorly to monotherapy with any

Table 7.2.
Heterocyclic Antidepressants Versus *Placebo:* Acute Treatment

Drug	Number of Studies	Number of Subjects	Responders (%) Drug (%)	Placebo (%)	Difference (%)	Chi Square	p Value
First Generation							
Imipramine	50	2649	67.5	39.8	27.7	184.0	$< 10^{-40}$
Amitriptyline	8	292	60	26	34	30.9	3×10^{-8}
Second Generation							
Amoxapine	10	386	67	49	18	12.4	4×10^{-4}
Trazodone	13	824	59	28	32	93.3	1×10^{-22}
Bupropion	4	425	55	29	26	26.6	2×10^{-7}
Mianserin	5	336	60	28	31	31.0	2×10^{-8}
Lofepramine	3	135	79	48	31	4.6	0.02

Table 7.3.
Summary of Controlled Double-Blind Studies of Heterocyclic Antidepressants

Drug	Number of Studies in Which the Effect Was More than Placebo	Equal to Placebo	More than Imipramine	Equal to Imipramine	Less than Imipramine
Imipramine	30	14	—	—	—
Amitriptyline	9	2	2	5	0
Desipramine	3	2	0	6	1
Nortriptyline	4	0	0	0	0
Doxepin	2	0	0	3	0
Protriptyline	2	0	0	2	0
Trimipramine	1	0	2	0	0
Maprotiline	2	2	0	10	0

Adapted from Klein DF, Davis JM. Diagnosis and drug treatment of psychiatric disorders. Baltimore: Williams & Wilkins, 1969:193–194.

antidepressant. When imipramine and amitriptyline were administered in different dose ratios—maximum dose of imipramine 240 mg/day and amitriptyline 150 mg/day—they were again found to be equally effective, raising the possibility that amitriptyline is slightly more potent than imipramine on a milligram per milligram basis.

Desipramine and Nortriptyline

Based on comparisons with imipramine and amitriptyline, desipramine and nortriptyline (secondary amines) are comparable in efficacy to their tertiary-amine parent compounds and clearly superior to placebo (Table 7.3). Clinically, they are often preferred to the tertiary amine compounds because of their less bothersome side-effect profiles. The introduction of newer compounds (e.g., SRIs) with even fewer adverse effects, however, has made this distinction less clinically relevant.

Doxepin

Doxepin was found to be superior to placebo and equal to other tricyclics (Table 7.3). Virtually all subjects were outpatients with mixed anxiety and depression, rather than inpatients with MDD. In spite of this methodological limitation, a reasonable conclusion is that doxepin has significant antidepressant properties. Three studies comparing doxepin with imipramine, amitriptyline, and clomipramine found it to be equal to the other drugs, but there was a trend favoring imipramine (5–7). While typical doses were 200 to 300 mg/day, it is possible that doxepin is less potent than imipramine, and slightly higher doses may be necessary to achieve optimal benefit. Alternatively, since doxepin has the highest first-pass effect of all the tricyclic antidepressants, higher doses (about one-third higher) may be needed to achieve comparable plasma drug levels.

It is difficult to interpret the specificity of this drug for mixed anxiety-depression because the beneficial effect could be a result of an anxiolytic without antidepressant properties or an antidepressant without anxiolytic properties. Thus, studies can show a drug to be more effective than placebo but fail to answer by which mechanism (i.e., antidepressant or anxiolytic).

Protriptyline

This tricyclic drug is superior to placebo and equivalent to standard HCAs in outpatient populations, although it is a more potent agent on a per milligram basis (i.e., average daily dose is 20–60 mg/day) (Table 7.3). This may be due in part to its low first-pass effect and long half-life, so that patients develop substantially higher plasma levels per milligram dose taken.

Trimipramine

Several small, double-blind studies show trimipramine to be superior to placebo and comparable to other standard tricyclics (Table 7.3). There was a trend in one large, carefully controlled study favoring amitriptyline, but it did not supply data on percent improvement, so it was not included in our analysis (8). Considering all the data, we would conclude that trimipramine is equal in effect to other TCAs.

Second Generation Antidepressants

Since the advent of the prototypic tricyclic antidepressants in the 1950s, there has been a persistent quest for agents that would be equally effective with fewer sedative, anticholinergic, and cardiovascular effects; as well as less likely to be fatal when taken in overdose. This search has produced a number of:

- Monocyclic, bicyclic, tricyclic, and tetracyclic antidepressants
- Other compounds structurally unrelated to existing antidepressants
- More specific reuptake inhibitors of serotonin
- Less toxic MAOIs.

In general, efficacy has been comparable to that of their predecessors (see Table 7.4).

Amoxapine

Amoxapine has been found effective in several double-blind studies (Tables 7.2 and 7.4). It is a dibenzoxazepine derivative that has both norepinephrine and serotonin reuptake inhibiting properties.

A few reports also indicate that the antipsychotic properties of its active metabolite, 8-hydroxyamoxapine, may benefit psychotically depressed patients as well (9). This metabolite has considerable dopamine receptor binding properties (i.e., radioreceptor bioassays on patients given amoxapine have found activity levels similar to patients on standard antipsychotics); a chemical structure similar to loxapine; and effects similar to antipsychotics, including:

- Dopamine blockade
- Extrapyramidal side effects; tardive dyskinesia
- Elevated prolactin
- Transitory suppression of avoidance reaction
- Inhibition of stereotyped behavior induced by amphetamines.

Long-term use of amoxapine has produced tardive dyskinesia, as substantiated by several case reports (10).

- Advantages:
  - Low sedating and anticholinergic activity
  - May be used as monotherapy for psychotic depression
  - Possibly a more rapid onset of action.
- Potential disadvantages:
  - D_2 blockade—leading to extrapyramidal symptoms
  - Inability to titrate antidepressant from antipsychotic effect
  - May be lethal with overdose.

Maprotiline

This agent has been extensively studied in double-blind trials. Two found it clearly superior to placebo and two found trends in the same direction ($p < 0.001$, combined data) (see Table 7.3) (11–14).

Table 7.4.
New versus *Standard Antidepressants:* Acute Treatment

Drug	Number of Studies	Number of Subjects	Responders (%)		Difference (%)
			New AD (%)	Standard AD (%)	
Amoxapine	19	784	79	73	6
Maprotiline	20	1638	73	72	1
Trazodone	18	913	62	58	4
Bupropion	4	293	71	72	−1
Mianserin	15	1155	58	64	−6
Lofepramine	4	160	55	60	−5
Clomipramine	6	350	61	62	−1

Over 1,600 patients have been randomly assigned to either maprotiline or a standard HCA: 660 on maprotiline did well and 247 showed minimal improvement, no change, or worsened. For the HCAs (usually imipramine or amitriptyline) 640 patients did well and 255 showed minimal improvement, no change, or worsened. In summary, 73% did well with maprotiline and 72% with a standard AD. Combining these data with the Mantel-Haenszel test indicated no difference in efficacy (see Table 7.4).

- Advantages:
  - Low anticholinergic effect
  - Sedative properties may be useful for agitation
  - Does not antagonize antihypertensive effects of clonidine.
- Potential disadvantages:
  - Increased incidence of seizures
  - Overdoses are lethal
  - Long half-life
  - Increased incidence of rash.

Trazodone

This agent has been widely studied. A review of several random-assignment, well-controlled trials found it to be 32% more effective than placebo and a nonsignificant 4% more effective than standard HCAs (Tables 7.2 and 7.4). The therapeutic dose is 200–600 mg/day, and it has fewer anticholinergic adverse effects, but excessive sedation may limit the total dose. The absolute milligram dosage is higher than for other HCAs, with some patients needing 400–600 mg to achieve adequate response.

This agent represents a new class of antidepressants that block 5-HT$_2$ receptors, inhibit 5-HT reuptake, and down-regulate NE receptor sites. Trazodone, however, is not as potent an inhibitor of 5-HT reuptake as fluoxetine, sertraline, or paroxetine.

- Advantages:
  - No anticholinergic effects
  - Sedating; useful for agitation and hostility in geriatric patients
  - May be used as a hypnotic agent
  - Relative safety with overdose.
  - No quinidine-like effect
- Potential disadvantages:
  - Not antiarrhythmic
  - May induce/exacerbate ventricular arrhythmia (not proven)
  - Priapism
  - Postural hypotension.

Bupropion

Bupropion has been found to be an effective antidepressant in several double-blind studies (see Tables 7.2 and 7.4) (15). It is neither an uptake inhibitor nor an MAOI, but in rodents, high doses will produce a down-regulation of postsynaptic β-noradrenergic receptors (16). Bupropion is not self-administered in animals when using the paradigm for amphetamine-like drugs. This agent, as well as nomifensine and psychostimulants, are of interest because they probably work through a dopamine mechanism and often help patients who do not respond to standard TCAs.

- Advantages:
  - Nonsedating
  - Low incidence of anticholinergic adverse effects
  - No weight gain
  - No electrocardiographic changes or hypotension
  - Low toxicity with overdose.
- Potential disadvantages:
  - Overstimulation, insomnia, tremor
  - May induce perceptual abnormalities, psychosis

- Increased incidence of seizures, particularly in patients with eating disorders.

Mianserin

Three double-blind studies revealed mianserin to be clearly superior (about 42%) to placebo, but 15 studies found it slightly less effective (about 6%) than standard HCAs (Tables 7.2 and 7.4).

Mianserin is a tetracyclic compound that has some interesting properties. It does not inhibit the reuptake of NE, 5-HT, or dopamine, and is not an MAOI. Mianserin appears to act through a presynaptic α_2-adrenergic mechanism to increase NE turnover. Thus, the effects of mianserin are consistent with the NE theory, which is of particular interest because its mechanism of action is quite different from that of other standard antidepressants.

Lofepramine

Well-controlled studies have found this agent to be superior to placebo and comparable to amitriptyline, imipramine, and maprotiline (17). It may be better tolerated than earlier HCAs, especially by the elderly. Desipramine is its major metabolite (see Tables 7.2 and 7.4).

Serotonin Reuptake Inhibitors

During the last two decades there has been increasing evidence that serotonin neurotransmission is diminished during an episode of depression. Drugs that modify 5-HT activity by inhibiting the reuptake carrier have been the most productive line of inquiry thus far.

Zimelidine was the first serotonin reuptake inhibitor available for clinical use, but in 1982 was withdrawn worldwide due to toxicity (18). Among HCAs, *clomipramine* is one of the more selective reuptake inhibitors of serotonin. Since plasma levels of its demethylated metabolite (which primarily works through the NE system) exceed those of the parent compound, however, therapeutic action cannot be solely attributed to serotonin reuptake inhibition. More selective SRIs that have undergone extensive investigation include: citalopram, fluoxetine, fluvoxamine, paroxetine, and sertraline. *Fluoxetine* (Prozac, Dista Products) was introduced in 1988; *sertraline* (Zoloft, Pfizer) in early 1992; and *paroxetine* (Paxil, SmithKline Beecham) in early 1993.

Clomipramine

Clomipramine has been approved by the FDA for the treatment of obsessive-compulsive disorder (OCD) but is also used in the United State, Europe, Canada, England, and, indeed, most of the world as an antidepressant as well. In six random-assignment, double-blind studies, this agent was equal in efficacy to standard tricyclics, with a side-effect profile comparable to other TCAs (Table 7.4).

Fluoxetine

There is a substantial body of evidence indicating that fluoxetine is clearly better than placebo and equal in effect to standard antidepressants (Tables 7.5 and 7.6). It may also be an effective anti-obsessive and anti-panic agent as well (see also Obsessive-Compulsive Disorder in Chapter 13) (19).

Sertraline

Several studies have found this agent superior to placebo and comparable to the HCAs (Tables 7.5 and 7.6) (20). It appears to be effective in patients with moderate or severe depression, with or without melancholia, with low or high anxiety, with or without insomnia, with psychomotor agitation or psychomotor retardation. Studies of continuation therapy demonstrated efficacy up to 8 weeks in patients who responded to an initial 8 weeks of acute therapy (21). It also appears to be effective and well tolerated in the elderly.

This agent is a highly selective and potent inhibitor of 5-HT reuptake (e.g., four to five times more potent than fluoxetine). Further, it appears to have little binding affinity for other receptors when studied in vitro. Unlike fluoxetine, its principal metabolite is considerably less active than the parent compound.

Paroxetine

Paroxetine has been compared in double-blind studies with placebo, imipramine, amitriptyline, doxepin, clomipramine, dothiepin, mianserin, and fluoxetine. With few exceptions, its overall antidepressant efficacy was superior to placebo and equal to the comparison antidepressant (see Tables 7.5 and 7.6 (22). In addition, it was equally effective in the presence or absence of anxiety, agitation,

retardation, and reactive and endogenous features (23). Several studies have found that paroxetine is highly effective in reducing anxiety, a common symptom in depressive illness (24).

This agent is a phenylpiperidine derivative that potently and selectively inhibits synaptosomal reuptake of serotonin, but has virtually no affinity for the reuptake inhibition of noradrenaline and other neurotransmitter amines.

Fluvoxamine

Currently available in Europe, fluvoxamine has been reported to be superior to placebo and equal to imipramine (see Tables 7.5 and 7.6) (25). It has been studied for both its antidepressant and anti-obsessive properties (see also Chapter 13).

Citalopram

This agent is available in Europe, with controlled studies finding it comparable to maprotiline and amitriptyline (see Table

Table 7.5.
SRIs versus *Placebo:* Acute Treatment

Drug	Number of Studies	Number of Subjects	Responders (%)		Difference (%)	p Value
			SRI (%)	Placebo (%)		
Fluoxetine	7	897	60	33	27	10^{-13}
Sertraline	2	545	79	48	31	10^{-11}
Paroxetine	9	649	65	36	29	10^{-14}
Fluvoxamine	3	125	67	42	25	0.008

Table 7.6.
SRIs versus *Standard Antidepressants:* Acute Treatment

Drug	Number of Studies	Number of Subjects	Responders (%)		Difference (%)
			SRI (%)	Standard AD (%)	
Fluoxetine	16	1549	63	64	−1
Sertraline	2	320	73	74	−1
Paroxetine	11	393	81	83	−2
Fluvoxamine	4	137	70	66	+4
Citalopram	6	347	73	74	−1

7.6) (26–28). Approval by the Food and Drug Administration is expected in the near future.

Monoamine Oxidase Inhibitors

There are two types of monoamine oxidase (i.e., A and B), which represent different proteins. MAO-A selectively deaminates serotonin and norepinephrine, while MAO-B selectively deaminates benzylamine and phenylethylamine. Certain substrates (e.g., tyramine, tryptamine, and dopamine) are deaminated by both types.

Important intraspecies differences are found in the relative proportions of MAO-A or MAO-B in tissues (e.g,, human brain has more MAO-B (about 70%) activity, and rat brain more MAO-A). After administration of an MAOI, intracellular levels of endogenous amines (e.g., NE) increase, but levels of amines not usually found in humans (tryptamine and phenylethylamine) also increase, followed by a compensatory decrease in amine synthesis because of feedback mechanisms. Levels of other amines or their metabolites (i.e., false transmitters) rise in storage vesicles and may displace true transmitters, while presynaptic neuronal firing rates decrease. After 3 to 6 weeks, brain serotonin may return to normal levels and norepinephrine levels may decrease. There is a compensatory decrease in the number of α_2 and β receptors, including β-adrenergic receptor–related functions (e.g., norepinephrine-stimulated adenyl cyclase).

Interest in drugs that inhibit monoamine oxidase, and an increase in their use, has been spurred, not only by controlled studies that document their antidepressant efficacy but also by the recent demonstration of their benefit in the treatment of:

- *Atypical* depression
- *Mixed anxiety and depressive disorders*
- *Panic disorder,* with or without agoraphobia
- *Eating disorders,* particularly bulimia (due to required dietary restrictions, this may not be a feasible therapy in many of these patients).

Iproniazid was the first widely prescribed MAOI. The discovery that the drug can produce rare but dangerous liver toxicity led to the synthesis of the other *hydrazine* MAOIs, such as isocarboxazid, nialamide, and phenelzine; and the *nonhydrazine* MAOIs, tranylcypromine and pargyline.

Most presently available MAOIs are irreversible inhibitors of the enzyme, forming a chemical bond with part of the enzyme or the flavin adenine dinucleotide (FAD) cofactor. When treatment is stopped, inhibition continues for a time until MAO levels return to normal as new enzyme is synthesized. Thus, phenelzine, isocarboxazid, and tranylcypromine are all irreversible, nonselective MAOIs. *Clorgyline,* however, is an irreversible, selective MAO-A inhibitor; *moclobemide* is a reversible, selective MAO-A inhibitor; *L-deprenyl* is an irreversible, selective MAO-B inhibitor; and *pargyline* is a relatively selective, irreversible MAO-B inhibitor.

While the half-life of an MAOI is short (hours), the half-life of MAO inhibition is about 2 weeks because it takes that long for new enzyme to be synthesized. Some have speculated that phenelzine may be metabolized by acetylation and that there are two hereditary types (i.e., slow and fast acetylators), with slow acetylators presumably having a greater degree of MAO inhibition. There is only limited support for the theory that slow acetylators have a better response; while other investigators find no difference (29). More importantly, there is no evidence that phenelzine is indeed acetylated.

Selective and Reversible Monoamine Oxidase Inhibitors

More recently, both selective and reversible MAOIs have been developed to minimize the complications of earlier generation agents (30). Specifically, these selective, reversible MAO inhibitors have *minimal interactions with tyramine,* markedly diminishing the need for the dietary restrictions that plague the use of mixed A, B inhibitors. Collaborative clinical trials of the reversible inhibitors of monoamine oxidase A (RIMAs) in Europe have included over 2000 patients, many hospitalized for more severe, endogenous depressive episodes (31). The best studied of this group is *moclobemide,* which has been equal in efficacy to standard HCAs and superior to placebo (Tables 7.7 and 7.8). In comparison trials to the tricyclics, the onset of effect with RIMAs was also more rapid in some cases.

If Type A inhibitors prove to be as efficacious as other MAOIs and non-MAOIs, there is no doubt that some clinicians will prescribe them with increasing frequency, especially for the elderly. In addition, if there is minimal risk of adverse interactions with tyramine and other substances (e.g., sympathomimetics), medical-legal concerns about their use will be practically nonexistent.

Other RIMAs under investigation include:

- Brofaromine
- Cimoxatone
- Toloxatone.

Table 7.7 summarizes the characteristics of several of these agents, which are either clinically available or under study.

Table 7.7.
Classes of MAO Inhibitors

MAOI	Selectivity	Substrate	Reversibility
Clorgyline	MAO-A	Serotonin	no
Moclobemide		and norepinephrine	yes
Brofaromine			yes
Cimoxatone			yes
Toloxatone			yes
Selegiline	MAO-B	Phenylethlyamine	no
Pargyline		and benzylamine	no
Phenelzine	MAO A,B	Tyramine and	no
Tranylcypromine		dopamine and	no
Isocarboxazid		tryptamine	no

Table 7.8.
MAO Inhibitors versus *Placebo:* Acute Treatment

Drug	Number of Studies	Number of Subjects	Responders (%) MAOI (%)	Placebo (%)	Difference (%)	Chi Square	*p* Value
Phenelzine	8	429	56	43	14	7.9	0.005
Moclobemide	6	535	65	24	41	87.2	10^{-20}

- Advantages:
  - *No nonspecific biochemical or pharmacological actions*
  - Antidepressant effect attributed to effect on *isoenzyme MAO-A only;* therefore, lesser propensity to cause *tyramine potentiation*
  - Effective in *endogenous and atypical depression*
  - No correlation between *plasma concentrations* and response; therefore, monitoring is not necessary.
- Potential Disadvantages:
  - *Adverse effects:* loss of appetite, nausea, and other GI disturbances; insomnia
  - Effective *dosage* is quite variable
  - Shorter *duration* of action
  - *Idiosyncratic responses* occur from time to time
  - Substantially *different pharmacodynamic profiles* from earlier MAOIs.

Efficacy: Monoamine Oxidase Inhibitors

At one time, the tricyclics were thought to be more effective than the MAOIs, but recent investigation has found these two classes equally effective (32). The poorer showing in some of the earlier studies was the result of subtherapeutic doses of MAOIs administered to treatment-resistant populations (e.g., psychotic depressions, which are not usually responsive to any form of monotherapy).

The efficacy of phenelzine and tranylcypromine has now been well established by several large, double-blind studies, which found them equal to the comparative standard tricyclics and clearly superior to placebo (see Tables 7.8 and 7.9) (33). Other studies indicate that atypical depressions may respond better to MAOIs, and typical depressions to tricyclics; however, most find that their similarities are more obvious than their differences (34). One research group has suggested that anergic, bipolar patients respond particularly well to tranylcypromine and other MAOIs (35). Extensive clinical experience indicates the MAOIs are often effective when HCAs have failed.

Other Drug Therapies
Psychomotor Stimulants

Cocaine, amphetamine, dextroamphetamine, methylphenidate, and pemoline are classified as psychomotor stimulants, producing an acute euphoria in controls as well as a wide variety of responses in psychiatric patients. The stimulants are also effective in postponing the deterioration in psychomotor performance that often accompanies extreme fatigue, a property that may be useful in some carefully selected cases.

Table 7.9.
Summary of Controlled Double-Blind Studies of MAO Inhibitors

Drug	Number of Studies in Which the Effect Was				
	More than Placebo	Equal to Placebo	More than Imipramine	Equal to Imipramine	Less than Imipramine
Phenelzine	11	4	0	4	3
Tranylcypromine	2	1	0	3	0
Isocarboxazid	2	4	0	2	2
Pargyline	2	0	0	0	0

Adapted from Klein DF, Davis JM. Diagnosis and drug treatment of psychiatric disorders. Baltimore: Williams & Wilkins, 1969:207–208.

While there is no doubt that amphetamine or other psychomotor stimulants induce an initial euphoria, there is considerable doubt that they can serve as long-lasting antidepressants. For example, cocaine produces a euphoria almost immediately after i.v. injection and within a few minutes after intranasal administration, but the euphoria, as well as the tachycardia, decrease at a slightly faster rate than the level of plasma cocaine. A second dose given 1 hour later fails to produce a similar level of euphoria or tachycardia, suggesting a rapid-acting tachyphylaxis.

Amphetamines. One British study found amphetamine to be no different than placebo in the treatment of depressed outpatients (36); a second found amphetamine *less effective* than phenelzine and no better than placebo (37); and a Veteran's Administration (VA) study found dextroamphetamine no more effective than placebo in hospitalized depressed patients (38). Uncontrolled clinical evidence indicates that amphetamine may occasionally be of value; but, except for a mild, early, transient benefit, there is no evidence that it can ameliorate moderate to severe conditions.

Methylphenidate. The authors have encountered some patients refractory to all other therapies who had a dramatic, full, rapid, and sustained response to methylphenidate. One study found methylphenidate effective in treating mildly depressed outpatients, particularly those who drank three or more cups of coffee a day (39). A replication study did not find a drug-placebo difference on the physician's ratings, but did demonstrate one for the patients' subjective assessment of improvement (40). Another blind study of methylphenidate found improvement in an outpatient group (41). Finally, two out of three trials of methylphenidate in apa-

thetic, senile geriatric patients showed that this drug produced more improvement than placebo (42). To date, no evidence indicates that it is beneficial in cases of moderate to severe depression.

Complications. All psychostimulants can cause jitteriness, palpitations, and psychic dependence. Depression may arise after their discontinuance, and high doses can produce a florid psychosis. On occasion, even small doses of amphetamine can precipitate psychotic episodes in those with an underlying predisposition (e.g., schizophrenic disorder).

Summary. Five studies of amphetamine for depression were clearly negative, with none finding it more effective than placebo. Although there were occasional hints of efficacy, in one study amphetamine was even less effective than placebo.

The results with methylphenidate, however, are more impressive. Two out of three studies found a significant effect and the third found improvement on the patients' subjective evaluation. Although amphetamine and methylphenidate are similar in their pharmacology, they differ in some respects. Amphetamine releases dopamine from newly synthesized pools (α-methyl-p-tyrosine-sensitive pool); whereas methylphenidate releases dopamine from storage sites (reserpine-sensitive sites). It is possible that this pharmacological difference could be related to methylphenidate's apparent greater efficacy. We would note that there are also isolated reports of depressed patients who fail to respond to standard antidepressants but do well on low doses of stimulants.

Lithium

This agent has been found superior to placebo, particularly as an acute treatment for the depressed phase of a bipolar disorder (see Table 7.10). Mendels et al. (1979) reviewed and, more recently, Souza et al. (1991) statistically combined the data from many of the same trials. Their results also indicate that the marginal evidence for lithium's acute antidepressant effect was in the bipolar depressed patient group (43,44).

The use of lithium as an augmentation to standard ADs has been the most effective strategy in partially responsive depressive episodes (see Alternate Treatment Strategies later in this chapter).

Antipsychotics

There are several studies addressing the possible antidepressant effects of antipsychotics (e.g., chlorpromazine, thioridazine, chlorprothixene); however, interpretation of their results is complicated by the inclusion of patients with anergic schizophrenia, psychotic depression, or compensation neurosis (see Table 7.11) (45). In general, antipsychotics seemed better for anxious or hostile, rather than retarded depressions. By contrast, a VA random-assignment, double-blind study found that imipramine was superior to placebo for retarded depression (46). It is not clear how to translate this finding into a clinically meaningful strategy for treating depression.

Benzodiazepines

BZDs have been used for the treatment of depression because their sedative effects can reduce insomnia, agitation, and anxiety, symptoms that frequently accompany depressed states. Considerable evidence also indicates that major depression may accompany panic and agoraphobic disorders (47–49). *When depression pre-*

Table 7.10.
Lithium versus *Placebo:* Acute Treatment

Disorder	Number of Studies	Number of Subjects	Responders (%)		Difference (%)	Chi Square	*p* Value
			Lithium (%)	Placebo (%)			
Unipolar Depression	4 (Uncontrolled)	79	39	27	12	0.5	NS
Unipolar Depression	1 (Controlled)	27	57	38	19	0.9	NS
Bipolar Depression	2 (Controlled)	38	76	35	41	5.5	0.02

Table 7.11.
Summary of Controlled Double-Blind Studies of Antipsychotics for Depression

Drug	Number of Studies in Which the Effect Was:				
	More than Placebo	Equal to Placebo	More than Imipramine	Equal to Imipramine	Less than Imipramine
Chlorpromazine	3	0	0	3	0
Thioridazine	0	0	0	1	0
Chlorprothixene	0	0	0	1	0

Adapted from Klein DF, Davis JM. Diagnosis and drug treatment of psychiatric disorders. Baltimore: Williams & Wilkins, 1969:272–276.

cedes the onset of panic disorder, clinical experience suggests a better response to antidepressants than to BZDs, although no studies have directly addressed this issue (50). Conversely, available evidence indicates that when depression occurs after the onset of panic disorder, effective treatment with either a BZD or a tricyclic may result in concomitant improvement of both the panic and depressive symptoms (48, 51). It is important to note that some have reported depression as a adverse effect of BZD treatment.

Compared to HCAs, BZDs have a rapid onset of action; they have fewer unpleasant adverse effects; and are considerably less toxic than the HCAs or MAOIs. Despite these advantages, however, BZDs (with the possible exception of alprazolam, discussed below) generally appear devoid of true antidepressant effects. When the results of several well-controlled studies, totalling 1275 patients, were summarized, the overall response to BZDs was 51%, versus 73% for standard ADs. This generated a highly significant difference ($p < 10^{-16}$) on the Mantel-Haenzsel test in favor of the antidepressants (see Table 7.12).

Schatzberg and Cole reviewed 20 controlled studies of BZDs used in the treatment of a mixed profile of depressions and also concluded that while anxiety and insomnia may be significantly relieved, core depressive symptoms (e.g., psychomotor retardation and diurnal variation) remain essentially unchanged (52). Some positive resolutions were seen in depressions associated with a high level of anxiety, but there was little evidence for efficacy in more severe depressions without prominent anxiety.

Cassano et al. reviewed a series of studies comparing a tricyclic antidepressant to a BZD for "neurotic" and "endogenous" depressions, as well as anxiety states (53). Again, they concluded that BZDs were effective in reducing insomnia, agitation, and anxiety, and had some effect in elevating mood and improving social adjustment, but were not effective in improving core depressive symptoms. Further, "endogenous" patients treated with BZDs often appeared to experience residual symptomatology.

Noting that these findings suggest that BZDs could be useful adjuncts to HCAs, Klerman nevertheless cautioned about this approach, since these agents have been reported to aggravate depression; possibly increase the risk of suicide; and may lead to a more chronic syndrome (54–58). By contrast, Fawcett et al. suggest that treatment with anxiolytics may decrease suicidal behavior in anxious, depressed patients (59). It is possible that a depressed patient can become worse (and perhaps more suicidal) because of inadequate therapy with a BZD, which generally have no antidepressant effects. Such a scenario could lead to an association between suicide and BZD treatment on a statistical basis.

In addition, when BZDs are used with tricyclics to control insomnia, patients may experience some withdrawal symptoms (dysphoric mood, agitation, increased insomnia) when they have trough blood lev-

Table 7.12.
Benzodiazepines versus _Standard Antidepressants:_ Acute Treatment

Number of Studies	Number of Subjects	Responders (%) BZD (%)	Responders (%) Standard AD (%)	Difference (%)	Chi Square	p Value
19	1275	51	72	21	65.3	6×10^{-16}

els the next day. They may then take a higher dose on following nights, leading to increased physiological and psychological dependence, prolongation of depressive states, and social disability.

Alprazolam. During early clinical trials, alprazolam was noted to have an unexpected antidepressant effect. Since then, a number of controlled studies have compared alprazolam with standard HCAs (imipramine, amitriptyline, doxepin, desipramine) (60–73). Study patients were carefully diagnosed as suffering from a major depressive episode, and most were treated as outpatients. In most of these studies (up to 6 weeks' duration), alprazolam was reported to exert an antidepressant effect equal to that of the comparison AD and superior to that of placebo, when the latter was used. One study involving 504 outpatients found alprazolam effective regardless of patients' initial anxiety, depressive subtype, or level of psychomotor retardation (64).

10.0   An important criticism of most of these studies is that the average daily tricyclic dosages were less than 150 mg and were compared to relatively high average daily alprazolam doses (e.g., 2.5 mg to over 4 mg). In one study that employed therapeutic tricyclic dosages (i.e., desipramine, 229.8 ± 60.5 mg/day), however, no significant differences in antidepressant efficacy were reported (70).

Three other studies, in which average daily tricyclic doses ranged from 190 mg to 243 mg, reported that comparison tricyclics (imipramine and amitriptyline) were more effective than alprazolam (63, 65, 71). Although alprazolam-treated patients showed initial improvement, by the end of the study periods (24 days to 6 weeks), tricyclic-treated patients showed greater improvement. In another 6-week trial comparing alprazolam to placebo in patients with a major depressive disorder, there were no statistical differences between groups at any time during the study (74).

A meaningful comparison of the various studies is difficult because of the many variables from one study to another. Although most studies have reported efficacy equal to tricyclics and even those finding a greater efficacy for the tricyclic have also found some improvement with alprazolam, it remains unclear whether alprazolam is a useful alternative to established drug treatments for major depression.

Most depressive episodes are likely to last for several months. Assuming alprazolam does exert a true antidepressant effect that is sustained for 6 weeks, its long-term effectiveness is unknown since no study to date has exceeded 6 weeks' duration. Available data do suggest, however, that if a patient has an apparent antidepressant response to alprazolam, it occurs early in treatment (even if it is not sustained). **Thus, although early response may not be predictive of continuing benefit, lack of a prompt response does suggest that alprazolam will not be effective and should be discontinued.**

Some researchers have stated that alprazolam's antidepressant effects do not appear to be explained by its sedative or hypnotic effects, while others have suggested that since depression rating scales include so many items related to anxiety, much of the improvement attributed to alprazolam may result from its anxiolytic effects (61, 75). Potter et al., noting that generalized anxiety disorder may be difficult to differentiate from a major mood disorder, state that uncertain diagnosis, however, does not constitute an indication for the use of alprazolam (76). In addition, since the reported antidepressant effect with alprazolam was obtained with relatively high dosages, there is no justification for treating a depressed patient with anxiolytic dosages in the hope that the lower dose will also exert an antidepressant effect.

Interestingly, the authors found that this agent down-regulated β-adrenergic receptors when given in high doses to rats (77). What is needed to confirm its antidepressant action is a patient population with unequivocal depressive illness assessed with a depression-specific scale.

Adinazolam. This triazolobenzodiazepine is used in Europe and is under investigation here. Several well-controlled studies have found it comparable to standard HCAs (i.e., imipramine, amitriptyline) and superior to placebo (78).

Complications. BZDs may exacerbate depression and possibly increase suicide risk. Case reports and clinical trials also indicate that BZD treatment of generalized anxiety and panic may result in emergence of depression (79–90). In some of these reports depression is ill defined, but in others it met DSM-III criteria for a major depressive disorder, requiring treatment with an antidepressant (89, 90). Depression has been reported with a variety of BZDs (alprazolam, bromazepam, clonazepam, diazepam, lorazepam), but there is no evidence that one is more likely than another to cause this syndrome.

Risk may be increased in patients with low trait anxiety or when higher than usual BZD doses are used (83, 86, 87, 89, 90). Depression may abate if dosage is decreased, although discontinuation and treatment with an antidepressant may be required (86, 89, 90).

Alprazolam has no significant anticholinergic or cardiovascular effects, but in almost all studies reporting adverse effects, alprazolam-induced sedation was comparable to or greater than that of the tricyclic. In one comparison with desipramine, drowsiness led to motor vehicle accidents in two of 16 outpatients taking alprazolam and re-

quired discontinuation in another three (67). Definitive data are lacking on the potential for tolerance and dependence when used in the treatment of depression. The risk of dependency could increase with continued use and/or higher dosages. Goldberg et al. reported one alprazolam patient who, against instructions to taper the medication, abruptly discontinued it and suffered a seizure (69). **It should be noted that the triazolobenzodiazepines probably have the highest withdrawal seizure rate of all BZDs, and possibly of all psychotropics.**

Novel Compounds

Buspirone. This 5-HT_{1A} partial agonist belongs to a class called the azaspirodecadiones and is FDA-labelled as an anxiolytic. Early open trials that indicated that buspirone, as well as others in its class (e.g., gepirone), may be effective antidepressants have been supported by subsequent double-blind studies (91, 92).

Nefazodone. This compound has a chemical structure related to trazodone and is the first of a new group that incorporates both 5-HT reuptake properties plus 5-HT_2 receptor blockade (93–97). There is some evidence from controlled trials that this agent is an effective AD with a favorable side-effect profile.

Nefazodone has some unusual pharmacological properties, not only inhibiting serotonin reuptake, but also blocking 5-HT_2 receptors. It may be that the antidepressant effect of serotonin agents is due to mediation 5-HT_{1A} transmission in the absence (or even the blockade) of 5-HT_2 transmission. In this scenario, nefazodone may be even more specific in affecting a subtype of serotonin receptor than the standard SRIs.

This agent has been examined in several double-blind studies and has been found equally effective to other comparative ADs. It has not demonstrated sedating or stimulatory properties.

S-Adenosyl-L-Methionine. S-Adenosyl-L-Methionine (SAM) is a naturally occurring substance whose primary role appears to be that of a methyl donor in the CNS (98). Since it participates in the metabobolism of various biogenic amines implicated in the pathogenesis of depressive disorders, there have been several investigations that indicate that it may be an effective antidepressant with minimal adverse effects.

We performed a Mantel-Haenszel test on three studies comparing SAM to placebo, and found this agent was significantly better (i.e., chi square $= 26.0$; $p < 3 \times 10^{-7}$) (99). A second Mantel-Haenszel test on nine studies comparing SAM to standard ADs revealed a chi square of 6.7 ($p < 0.01$). Thus, 109 of 142 SAM-treated patients and 80 of 124 HCA-treated patients were classified as responders (i.e., a 12% difference favoring SAM).

Thus, results of a literature review and meta-analyses were consistent with our preliminary findings, all of which show a greater efficacy for SAM over placebo and comparable efficacy to HCAs. Furthermore, adverse effects with this agent were generally negligible in comparison to those associated with HCAs. While there was a trend in most studies favoring SAM over the HCAs, the number of subjects was small. Further, the significant difference with the meta-analysis was based principally on the results of two studies, suggesting caution in its interpretation.

Unfortunately, difficulties in developing a stable oral preparation of this drug have impeded its development for routine clinical use.

CHOICE OF ANTIDEPRESSANT

When selecting an antidepressant, the following should always be considered:

- *Monodrug therapy* is preferable whenever possible
- *Safety and tolerability*, keeping in mind that these are different concepts (i.e., a treatment may be safe but poorly tolerated, while another is well tolerated but with a low margin of safety)
- *Class and spectrum of activity* of a given AD
- *Likelihood of pharmacokinetic or pharmacodynamic interactions*, with the goal of minimizing adverse interactions with other drugs or medical conditions
- *Ease of administration* (to maximize patient compliance)
- *Confidence in its use*, generally based upon:
  - Years of patient exposure
  - Number and quality of controlled trials, including data on effectiveness for severe, as well as milder, episodes
  - Number and variety of patients treated in terms of age, health status, and concurrent medications
- *Cost and cost-effectiveness*
- When *psychotic symptoms* are present, a combination of AD plus AP or a trial with ECT should be instituted.

Certain clinical variables are also helpful in choosing a drug for an initial trial, including:

- If the patient (or perhaps a family member) has had a *previous positive response* to a particular drug, it should be considered as a first choice.
- If patients have predominant symptoms of *insomnia and/or psychomotor agitation,* a more sedating drug (e.g., amitriptyline, doxepin, or trazodone) may benefit initially, but could be problematic later in therapy (i.e., cause excessive sedation once sleep normalizes).
- In psychomotorically *retarded* patients, some recommend a less sedating drug (e.g., protriptyline, desipramine,

bupropion, fluoxetine, sertraline), but definitive evidence is lacking.

- Patients with *cardiovascular disorders* or those predisposed to *anticholinergic adverse effects* (e.g., elderly or diabetic patients) do best on drugs low in these effects (e.g., desipramine, trazodone, bupropion, buspirone, fluoxetine, sertraline, or paroxetine).
- Depressed patients with an *eating disorder* (i.e., anorexia, bulimia) or a history of *seizures* should not take bupropion or maprotiline because of an increased risk of seizures.
- *Highly suicidal* patients should be given agents posing less risk of lethality with overdose (e.g., sertraline, trazodone).

Antidepressant Classes

With the above issues in mind, the clinician can begin to formulate a logical and systematic approach to antidepressant therapy. At present there are six major classes available, which can be categorized on the basis of their structure and/or presumed mechanism of action:

- *HCAs,* which block the neuronal reuptake of norepinephrine and/or serotonin
- *Serotonin reuptake inhibitors*
- *Monoamine oxidase inhibitors,* which increase the concentration of several biogenic amines
- *Aminoketones* (e.g., bupropion), whose most potent known effect is neuronal dopamine reuptake blockade, but whose mechanism of action is unknown
- *Triazolopyridines* (e.g., trazodone), which have mixed effects on the serotonin system, with the predominant effect being 5-HT_2 receptor blockade
- *5-HT_{1A} receptor partial agonists* (e.g., buspirone), marketed as anxiolytics, but which also have proven AD properties, especially with higher doses

The benefit of having several different classes to choose from includes their presumed differing mechanisms of action (i.e., their range of antidepressant activity is not completely overlapping), as well as differing tolerability and safety. Knowledge about these differences can then be used to tailor drug treatment, thus optimizing outcome.

HCAs adjusted by clinically determined dose titration alone will produce at least a partial response in 60–70% of depressed patients, and a full remission in 20–40%. When the dose is adjusted using therapeutic drug monitoring (TDM), the full remission rate may be higher (100).

Serotonin reuptake inhibitors have response and remission rates equal to the HCAs. The dose-response curve (i.e., a plot of the percentage of patients who will respond or remit) is generally flat, such that higher initial doses do not increase the overall response or remission rates. Currently, there is no evidence for a clinically useful plasma concentration/response relationship with the SRIs.

Those who fail to respond to one SRI may respond to another or to an HCA, and vice versa. Thus, these two broad spectrum classes can be used in a sequential strategy to adequately treat the majority of patients.

Unfortunately, designs that maintain some patients on their original medication as a control for time on treatment, have not been conducted. The side-effect profiles of these two classes also differ substantially, hence, patients who do not tolerate one class frequently do well on the other.

The other classes of antidepressants are generally used to treat a smaller percentage of patients, due in part to the rate of response and relatively low dropout rates associated with the two primary classes. One exception is atypical depression, which may preferentially benefit from an initial MAOI trial.

Heterocyclics

Starting with a standard HCA such as *imipramine*, a typical dose is 25 mg 3 times daily. Dose may be increased by 25 mg every 2 or 3 days, as tolerated, and can usually be increased to 150 mg/day by the end of the first week in healthy adults. *The elderly, medically compromised, those hypersensitive to side effects, or those with associated panic disorder may require lower doses and more gradual increases* (see discussion in Chapter 6).

The dose of most HCAs may be increased to a maximum of 300 mg/day or until there is adequate response (4–6 weeks). The ultimate total daily dose can vary dramatically, with some patients requiring as little as 50 mg/day and others 300 mg/day or more. One approach to determine the optimal amount of required drug is to obtain a plasma level after at least 1 week on 100–150 mg/day and then adjust the dose accordingly. Doses exceeding the recommended upper limit should also be followed with TDM to avoid significant toxicity, with the final dose striking a balance between benefit and adverse effects. Once established, most or all of the medication can be given once daily, usually 1 hour before bedtime; however, it is better not to exceed 150 to 200 mg of a TCA at one time. In such cases, 50 to 150 mg may be given in the morning, with the remainder taken at bedtime.

Serotonin Reuptake Inhibitors

An alternative approach is to start with an SRI (see Table 7.13). *Fluoxetine* can be started at 10–20 mg every morning, monitoring for response over the next several weeks, and then, if necessary, adjusting the amount up or down.

This agent has a favorable adverse-effect profile, with minimal sedating, hypotensive, and anticholinergic effects, and may cause weight loss rather than weight gain. It is modestly stimulating and appears safe for patients with cardiovascular disease (e.g., no prolongation of cardiac conduction), but this question has yet to be thoroughly tested.

Sertraline is the second SRI approved by the FDA. Starting dose is 50 mg/day, which can be raised after the first 1–2 weeks, if necessary, by 50 mg/week, to a maximum of 200 mg/day (50–100 mg in the elderly), with once daily dosing well tolerated. Other clinically relevant issues include:

- Taking the dose after the evening meal, since its rapid absorption is further enhanced by food and it does not interfere with sleep
- Bioavailability is higher after multiple doses
- Steady state is achieved within 7 days, and then no further accumulation
- Most common adverse effects are:
  - Nausea; diarrhea or loose stools
  - Tremor
  - Dysomnia (e.g., insomnia, somnolence)
  - Dry mouth.

This agent has significantly fewer anticholinergic, antihistaminic, and cardiovascular adverse effects than the TCAs; as well as a low risk of toxicity in overdose.

Table 7.13.
SRIs: Dose Regimens

Drug	Usual Starting Dose (mg)	Usual Daily Dose (mg)
Clomipramine	25	100–250
Fluoxetine	10–20	20–60
Sertraline	50	100–200
Paroxetine	20	20–50
Fluvoxamine	50	150–300

Paroxetine is well absorbed from the gastrointestinal tract; undergoes first-pass metabolism; is extensively distributed into tissues; and is excreted as pharmacologically inactive polar metabolites. At therapeutic concentrations, plasma protein binding is approximately 95%. Steady-state plasma concentrations generally occur within 7 to 14 days, with no further accumulation. Terminal phase half-life is about 1 day, but wide intersubject variability has been observed. Bioavailability is higher after multiple than single doses, but is unaffected by the presence or absence of food, fat content of food, or coadministration with milk. There are no controlled studies of the relationship between plasma concentrations and clinical efficacy or adverse effects. Paroxetine has not been associated with clinically significant changes in electrolyte balance or hematologic, renal, hepatic, and metabolic parameters.

From dose-ranging studies, it has been determined that 10 mg/day is not significantly more effective than placebo and that 20 mg/day is the optimal starting dose. In addition, the upper limit of the clinically effective range, with no significant increase in toxicity is about 50 mg/day (40 mg/day in the elderly). Since the dose-response curve is flat across the range of 20 mg to 40 mg, most patients will respond well to 20 mg/day; some, however, may require higher doses, which should be increased by increments of 10 mg at no less than weekly intervals. Since the average elimination half-life of paroxetine is approximately 24 hours, once-daily dosing is adequate. Although antidepressant efficacy does not appear to be affected by the timing of its ingestion, evening administration has been associated with sleep interference and daytime somnolence. The manufacturer thus recommends morning administration (data on file, SmithKline Beecham).

Summary.

For the two most recently released SRIs, sertraline and paroxetine, comparable characteristics include:

- Inactive metabolites
- Half-lives of about 24 hours
- More selective than fluoxetine for 5-HT reuptake blockade.

All the SRIs have a *flat* dose-response curve; therefore, it is best to keep a patient on the starting dose for 2–4 weeks prior to increasing it. The rationale is that while the response versus dose curve is flat, side effects do increase with dose, and these drugs are expensive (see also Pharmacokinetics later in this chapter).

Monoamine Oxidase Inhibitors

MAOIs may be the treatment of choice for atypical (or nonclassic) depressive disorders. As noted in Chapter 6, features of this subgroup usually include:

- *Reversed diurnal variation* in mood (i.e., worse in the afternoon or evening)
- *Mood reactivity*
- *Variability in the same depressive episode,* from irritability to mild dysphoria to severe depression
- *Hypersomnia; hyperphagia*
- *Somatization*
- *Rejection hypersensitivity*
- *Anxiety,* including panic episodes

Starting doses of various MAOIs include:

- *Phenelzine.* Give 15 mg twice daily; daily dose range = 45–90 mg
- *Tranylcypromine.* Give 10 mg twice daily; daily dose range = 20–40 mg
- *Isocarboxazid.* Give 10 mg twice daily; daily dose range = 20–60 mg

- *Moclobemide.* Give 100–200 mg daily tid (450 mg upper dose for outpatients).

Major depression (unipolar or bipolar). MAOIs may also be a second choice for MDD, improving response in nonpsychotic depressed patients whose symptoms fail to respond to HCAs or SRIs and for whom ECT is not yet warranted.

These agents may also be used in *geriatric patients*, with average dose ranges similar to that for younger adults; however, lower initial amounts are indicated (see The Elderly Patient in Chapter 14). In general, geriatric patients should initially receive one-half the adult dose. For example, phenelzine may be started at 15 mg 2 or 3 times daily in the healthy younger adult but should be started at 15 mg once daily in the elderly. Dose adjustments in the geriatric patient should be made less frequently than in the younger adult, and weekly changes should be sufficient to minimize untoward effects. MAOIs should not be used above 60 mg/day in this age group. The new RIMAs may be the preferred agents if early benefit and safety profiles hold up.

Dysthymia. MAOIs may improve mood state and resolve vegetative symptoms, although the relative merits of MAOIs and HCAs in the treatment of dysthymia have not been defined. In general, dysthymic states do not respond as well as major depressive episodes to pharmacological intervention.

Cyclothymia is a cyclical mood state characterized by alternating episodes of dysthymia and hypomania. As with bipolar disorders, lithium may be the drug of choice. If depressive episodes recur, however, a trial of a heterocyclic or MAOI, in addition to lithium, may be indicated. There are no systematic data to suggest that MAOIs are of benefit in the treatment of cyclothymic states.

Contraindications for MAOIs

Physical conditions that may preclude the use of MAOIs include:

- Advanced *renal disease*
- *Pheochromocytoma*
- Significant *hypertension*

Cautious use is required with disorders in the following organ systems:

- *Hepatic*
- *Cardiovascular*
- *Respiratory* (e.g., asthma; chronic bronchitis)
- *Ocular* (e.g., narrow-angle glaucoma).

If a patient does not respond to one MAOI or there appears to be a loss of efficacy over time, it may be reasonable to try a second. When switching from a hydrazine-based MAOI (e.g., phenelzine or isocarboxazid) to a nonhydrazine MAOI (e.g., tranylcypromine), one should wait at least 2 weeks. For example, the nonhydrazine MAOI **tranylcypromine has NE reuptake inhibitory and sympathomimetic effects similar to dextroamphetamine and may cause a toxic reaction if initiated within 2 weeks following MAO inhibition by another agent** (101).

If a patient is to be switched to an HCA (e.g., amitriptyline), an MAOI should be discontinued for 2 weeks before beginning the new treatment. Since recovery of the MAO enzyme following irreversible inhibition takes up to 2 weeks, sympathomimetic agents given during that time may increase the risk of toxicity.

Special caution should be taken when switching from fluoxetine, as well as other SRIs, to an MAOI. Three fatalities are known to have followed initiation of tranylcypromine shortly after fluoxetine had been stopped (102). Fluoxetine and its metabolite desmethylfluoxetine (norfluoxetine) potentiate the accumulation of serotonin at nerve terminals and may produce a *"central serotonin syndrome"* (see Adverse Effects later in this chapter).

Because of the long elimination half-life of fluoxetine (2–3 days) and its active metabolite, norfluoxetine (7–9 days), at least 5 weeks should elapse after fluoxetine discontinuation before an MAOI is initiated. To avoid such drug-drug interactions, the newer subclass of RIMAs may become the MAOIs of choice.

CONCLUSION

Regardless of the specific agent, it is important to watch for improvement in target symptoms. Psychomotor agitation or retardation often improve first, followed by concentration and increased capacity for interpersonal contact. The patient's family (or nursing staff) may recognize an improvement before the patient does. Interestingly, the patient's subjective sense of depression, anhedonia, and hopelessness may not improve until the 4–6th week of treatment.

Figure 7.1 summarizes the strategy we would follow for patients who fail to adequately respond initially (see also Alternate Treatment Strategies later in this chapter).

Table 7.14 summarizes the various factors to consider when choosing a specific class of antidepressant.

Maintenance/Prophylaxis

EFFICACY LITERATURE REVIEW

The amount of data on maintenance antidepressant therapy is substantial and growing. Thus far, the HCAs, fluoxetine, sertraline, and paroxetine have data from double-blind, placebo-controlled studies to support their value as maintenance therapies for MDD (see Table 7.15) (21, 103–106). Only TCAs have such data for prophylactic therapy, a fact that is in part logistical, since such studies require years to complete, and recently released agents have not been available long enough for adequate study.

The fact that there is any data on maintenance and prophylactic therapy is remarkable. Such studies are expensive, fraught with problems, and are not required for registration purposes in the United States; hence, there is little incentive to conduct them. The existing data, however, supports the HCAs and the SRIs as first-line maintenance therapies.

The decision to employ prophylactic therapy should be based on the:

• *Severity* of the depressive episode
• *Frequency* of past depressions
• Risk of *suicide*
• Risk of potential *adverse effects.*

Antidepressants do not prevent relapses into mania, perhaps even precipitating a manic phase. For these reasons, lithium (with or without concomitant ADs) is the prophylaxis of choice for bipolar-related depressions. Carbamazepine and valproic acid may also be useful in the prevention of recurrent mood disorders. If there is a reasonable hint of bipolarity (e.g., a family history of bipolar illness, a prior hypomanic episode, or drug-induced hypomania), lithium, CBZ, or VPA should

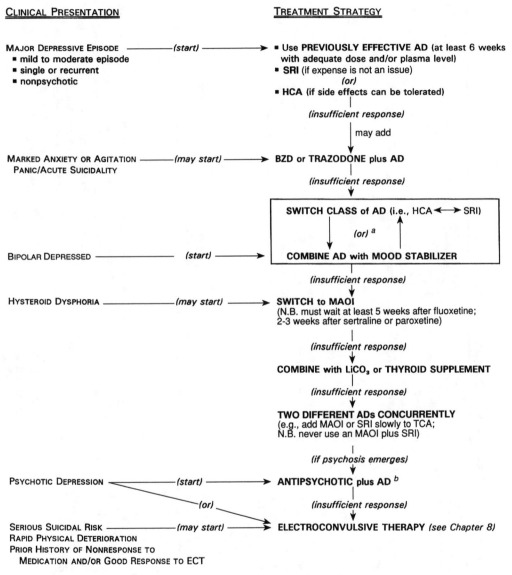

CLINICAL PRESENTATION

TREATMENT STRATEGY

MAJOR DEPRESSIVE EPISODE ———— *(start)* ————→
- mild to moderate episode
- single or recurrent
- nonpsychotic

- Use **PREVIOUSLY EFFECTIVE AD** (at least 6 weeks with adequate dose and/or plasma level)
- **SRI** (if expense is not an issue)
  (or)
- **HCA** (if side effects can be tolerated)

(insufficient response)

may add

MARKED ANXIETY OR AGITATION ———— *(may start)* ————→ **BZD or TRAZODONE plus AD**
PANIC/ACUTE SUICIDALITY

(insufficient response)

SWITCH CLASS of AD (i.e., HCA ←——→ SRI)

(or) [a]

BIPOLAR DEPRESSED ———————————— *(start)* ————→ **COMBINE AD with MOOD STABILIZER**

(insufficient response)

HYSTEROID DYSPHORIA ———————— *(may start)* ————→ **SWITCH to MAOI**
(N.B. must wait at least 5 weeks after fluoxetine; 2-3 weeks after sertraline or paroxetine)

(insufficient response)

COMBINE with LiCO$_3$ or THYROID SUPPLEMENT

(insufficient response)

TWO DIFFERENT ADs CONCURRENTLY
(e.g., add MAOI or SRI slowly to TCA; N.B. never use an MAOI plus SRI)

(if psychosis emerges)

PSYCHOTIC DEPRESSION ———————— *(start)* ————→ **ANTIPSYCHOTIC plus AD** [b]

(or)

(insufficient response)

SERIOUS SUICIDAL RISK ———————— *(may start)* ————→ **ELECTROCONVULSIVE THERAPY** *(see Chapter 8)*
RAPID PHYSICAL DETERIORATION
PRIOR HISTORY OF NONRESPONSE TO
  MEDICATION AND/OR GOOD RESPONSE TO ECT

[a] Initially switching class of AD or combining with mood stabilizer is based on clinician's judgement

[b] Amoxapine alone may be an alternative

Figure 7.1. Strategy for the management of an acute major depressive episode.

Table 7.14.
Considerations When Selecting an Antidepressant: Comparison of Classes

Consideration	TCAs (e.g., nortriptyline)	SRIs (e.g., sertraline)	Triazolopyridines (e.g., trazodone)	Aminoketones (e.g., bupropion)	MAOIs (e.g., tranylcypromine)
Likelihood of response	High	Equivalent to TCA in outpatients	Less than TCAs	Less than TCAs	Less than TCAs
Unique spectrum of activity	Can work in SRI failures	Can work in TCA failures	None demonstrated	Can work in TCA failures	Can work in TCA failures
Maintenance of response	Evidence from controlled studies	Evidence from controlled studies	None demonstrated	None demonstrated	None demonstrated
Safety	Serious systemic toxicity can result from overdose, either acute ingestion or from gradual accumulation due to slow clearance	No serious systemic toxicity demonstrated	Minimal serious systemic toxicity due to acute overdose	Seizures as primary acute systemic toxicity due to acute overdose, easily managed in medical setting	Serious systemic toxicity can result from acute ingestion
Tolerability	Generally good with secondary amine TCAs; much superior to tertiary amine TCAs	Generally good, especially if dose is kept to effective minimum dose	Sedation and cognitive slowing are frequently problems even at effective minimum dose	Generally good, especially if dose is kept to effective minimum dose	Generally good, except for the occurrence of hypotension and the dietary restrictions
Pharmacokinetic interactions	Can be affected by other drugs (e.g., SRIs) to a clinically significant extent but do not affect other drugs	Can inhibit oxidative metabolism of a variety of drugs, but considerable differences among class in terms of magnitude and duration of affect. No known effect of other drugs on SRIs that is clinically significant	Neither is affected by other drugs nor affects other drugs in a clinically significant way	Can be affected by SRIs (e.g., fluoxetine) and probably others in a potentially clinically significant way. No known effect on the metabolism of other drugs	Neither is affected by other drugs nor affects other drugs in a clinically significant way

Pharmacodynamic interactions	Multiple due to the large number of effects of TCAs. Can be agonistic (additive or potentiating) or antagonistic. Such interactions are more likely and more significant with tertiary as opposed to secondary amines	See MAOI interaction. May occur with other serotonin agonists. Fluoxetine can have agonistic interaction with dopamine agonists in terms of extrapyramidal effects. Minimal experience with sertraline in this regard	Can have interaction with other agents with decreased arousal or impaired cognitive performance. Can interact with adrenergic agents affecting blood pressure regulation. Complex interactions with other serotonin-active agents	Can have interactions with dopamine agonists and antagonists	Clinically significant interactions with: Tyramine and sympathomimetic agents on blood pressure Serotonin-active agents, inducing the central serotonin syndrome
Physician confidence	Excellent due to extensive database in terms of human exposure (e.g., patient-years of exposure, total number of patients exposed, variety of patients exposed)	Excellent due primarily to efficacy and safety profile. Less extensive database in terms of human exposure compared to TCAs but rapidly expanding	Satisfactory due to substantial database in terms of human exposure. Concerns are with spectrum of activity and tolerability	Reserved due to less extensive database concerning human exposure coupled with concerns about safety due to seizure risk	Caution due to safety concerns, primarily about patient compliance with dietary restrictions
Ease of administration	Excellent, generally can be administered once a day	Excellent for sertraline and paroxetine due to once-a-day administration. Good for fluoxetine, typically administered once a day, but long half-life of parent compound and active metabolite can make dose titration difficult	Satisfactory but requires multiple dosing for antidepressant effect	Satisfactory but requires multiple dosing for antidepressant effect	Satisfactory, but clinical practice is to generally give in divided doses

From Preskorn SH, Burke M. Somatic therapy for major depressive disorder: selection of an antidepressant. J Clin Psychiatry 1992; 53(9,suppl):5–18. Copyright 1992, Physicians Postgraduate Press.

Table 7.15.
Antidepressants versus *Placebo:* Maintenance Therapy

Number of Studies	Number of Subjects	Relapsed (%)		Difference (%)	Chi Square	p Value
		AD (%)	Placebo (%)			
18	2225	23	50	27	150	10^{-34}

always be considered (see Chapter 10 for more detailed discussion).

CHOICE OF TREATMENT

Maintenance Phase: Heterocyclics

Preventing relapse is of critical importance in the life course of major depressive disorder, and every effort should be made to assure patient compliance. Maintenance therapy should be continued for 6–12 months after an acute episode, with recent data indicating that acute doses equivalent to 200 mg of imipramine may be optimal (105, 106).

After 6–12 months, medications can usually be tapered over a period of several weeks to avoid autonomic rebound. If symptoms reemerge, medication should be reinstated and maintained for 3–6 additional months before an attempt is made to taper them again. In patients with recurrent unipolar depressions, indefinite maintenance antidepressants may be required.

Maintenance Phase: SRIs

Fluoxetine, sertraline, and paroxetine have also been shown to significantly prevent relapse when compared to placebo, in several controlled trials (21,103,104).

Maintenance Phase: Monoamine Oxidase Inhibitors

Patients should be maintained on MAOIs for a period of at least 6 months. If there is a history of recurrent depressive episodes following discontinuation, MAOI therapy may be extended for two years or more, as long as the patient is closely supervised and shows no significant adverse effects or toxicity. There is evidence that a few patients maintained on MAOIs for periods of 6 months or more may experience loss of therapeutic effect, correlating with a decrease in adverse effects such as anorexia and insomnia (107). Tolerance to the hypotensive effects does not seem to develop, however. Waning of therapeutic efficacy can be compensated for by increasing the dose, but the extent of increase may be limited by adverse effects, particularly hypotension.

Prophylactic Phase: HCAs and MAOIs

Depression is often a recurrent disorder, with the rate of relapse linear over time. Therefore, the question arises as to whether continued treatment will prevent relapse.

There are excellent data from several collaborative trials that tricyclics prevent relapse, as well as one small study showing that MAOIs also do so (108, 109). When the data for TCAs was statistically combined, it confirmed that active drug therapy can successfully prevent relapse. Several independent controlled studies have also shown that maintenance TCAs prevent the recurrence of depression in patients with multiple relapses (110–119). For example, a British collaborative group divided amitriptyline or imipramine responders into two groups: one continued on tricyclics at 75 mg to 100 mg/day, and the other was placed on placebo. After 15 months, 22% of the tricyclic maintenance group had relapsed, compared to 50% of those on placebo. In two of these studies, patients were initially treated with ECT, and in the others with tricyclics. Maintenance tricyclics or placebo were then administered in a double-blind, random-assignment design. As noted above, since antidepressants may precipitate manic attacks and/or induce rapid cycling, their use should be carefully evaluated, and if employed, they should be used only on a short-term basis in bipolar patients and/or combined with a mood stabilizer.

In 1974, investigators studied the role of psychotherapy in maintenance treatment, finding it ineffective for preventing relapse, but helpful in improving social adjustment (120). This study defined a qualitatively different role for drugs in the treatment of depression (i.e., both psychological and drug treatments are important, since they act through different mechanisms).

Maintenance/Prophylaxis: Lithium

In bipolar depressed patients, lithium (with or without concurrent antidepressants) is the maintenance treatment of choice, with carbamazepine or valproic acid as potential alternatives (see also Maintenance/Prophylaxis in Chapter 10). Maintenance lithium has also been shown to prevent some relapses in recurrent unipolar depression (Table 7.16).

Souza and Goodwin (1991) studied the prophylactic value of lithium by combining data from both controlled and uncontrolled studies assessing this agent's benefit over 3 months to 5 years (44). Lithium was significantly more effective than placebo in 263 unipolar depressed patients studied in eight controlled trials ($p < 0.0001$). In the uncontrolled studies there was a similar effect size, corresponding to an improvement rate of 70% for the lithium-treated versus only 35% for the placebo-treated group. When lithium was compared to other ADs as a potential prophylactic therapy, there was a nonsignificant trend favoring lithium. Only two studies compared lithium alone to lithium plus imipramine, with their pooled results favoring the combination ($p < 0.02$).

An earlier study of 40 unipolar depressed patients by this same group found a cumulative probability of recurrence over 2 years to be 0.08 with lithium and 0.58 without lithium (121). They concluded that the outcome strongly supported the value of lithium prophylaxis in unipolar depression in contrast to this agent's lack of acute efficacy in this group.

CONCLUSION

Two issues have emerged from the literature on maintenance treatment for depressive disorders. First, the condition is often recurrent and debilitating. Second, ADs (in doses comparable to acute treatment levels) with or without various psychotherapeutic approaches, can favorably alter the longitudinal course. See Figure 7.2 for the strategy we would recommend.

Our approach to both acute and mainte-

Table 7.16.
Lithium versus *Placebo*: Maintenance Therapy (Recurrent Unipolar Depression)

Number of Studies	Number of Subjects	Relapsed (%)		Difference (%)	Chi Square	p value
		Lithium (%)	Placebo (%)			
8	287	41	75	34	34.7	3×10^{-9}

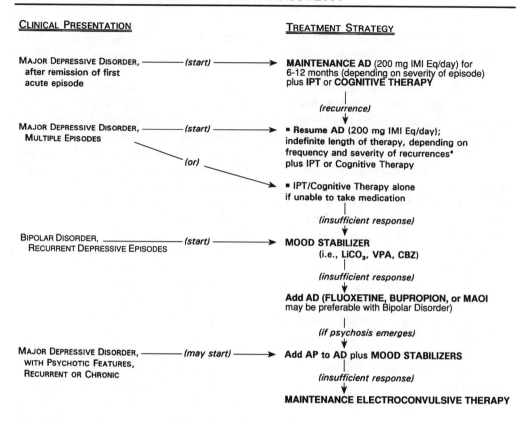

Figure 7.2.   Maintenance strategy for the management of recurrent and/or chronic depression.

nance therapy is consistent with the recently published American Psychiatric Association guidelines for the treatment of MDD in adults (122).

REFERENCES

1. Davis JM, Janicak PG, Wang Z, Gibbons R, Sharma R. The efficacy of psychotropic drugs. Psychopharmacol Bull 1992;28:151–155.
2. Appleton WS, Davis JM. Practical clinical psychopharmacology. New York: Medcomb Publishing, 1973.
3. Burt CG, Gordon WF, Holt NF, Hordern A. Amitriptyline in depressive states: a controlled trial. J Ment Sci 1962;108:711–730.
4. Hordern A, Holt NF, Burt CG, Gordon WF. Amitriptyline in depressive states: phenomenology and prognostic considerations. Br J Psychiatry 1963;109:815–825.
5. Hasan KZ, Akhtar MI. Double blind clinical study comparing doxepin and imipramine in depression. Curr Ther Res 1971;13:327–336.
6. Grof P, Saxena B, Cantor R, Daigle L, Hetherington D, Haines T. Doxepin versus amitriptyline in depression: a sequential double-blind study. Curr Ther Res 1974;16:470–476.
7. Linnoila M, Seppala T, Mattila M, Vihko R, Pakarinen A, Skinner T. Clomipramine and doxepin in depressive neurosis: plasma levels and therapeutic response. Arch Gen Psychiatry 1980;37:1295–1299.
8. Rickels K, Gordon PE, Weiss CC, Bazilian SE, Feldman HS, Wilson DA. Amitriptyline and trimipramine in neurotic depressed patients: a collaborative study. Am J Psychiatry 1970;127:208–218.
9. Wilson C et al. A double-blind clinical comparison of amoxapine, imipramine and placebo in the treatment of depression. Curr Ther Res 1977;22:620–627.
10. Fann WE, Davis JM, Domino E, Smith

RC. Tardive dyskinesia: research and treatment. New York: Spectrum Medical, 1980.

11. VanDer Velde C. Maprotiline versus imipramine and placebo in neurotic depression. J Clin Psychiatry 1981;42:138–141.

12. Rouillon F, Phillips R, Serrurier D, et al. Rechutes de depression unipolaire et efficacite de la maprotiline. L'Encephale 1989;15:527–534.

13. Jukes AM. A comparison of maprotiline (Ludiomil) and placebo in the treatment of depression. J Int Med Res 1975;3(suppl 2):84–88.

14. McCallum P, Meares R. A controlled trial of maprotiline (Ludiomil) in depressed outpatients. Med J Aust 1975;2:392–394.

15. Soroko FE et al. Bupropion hydrochloride, a novel antidepressant agent. J Pharmacol (in press).

16. Pandey GN, Davis JM. Treatment with antidepressants, sensitivity of beta receptors and affective illness. New York: John Wiley & Sons, 1980.

17. d'Elia et al. Comparative clinical evaluation of lofepramine and imipramine. Psychiatric aspects. Acta Psychiatr Scand 1977;55(1):10–20.

18. Björk K. The efficacy of zimeldine in preventing depressive episodes in recurrent major depressive disorders—a double-blind placebo-controlled study. Acta Psychiatr Scand 1983;68(suppl):182–189.

19. Beasley CM, Sayler ME, Bosomworth JC, Wernicke JF. High-dose fluoxetine: efficacy and activating-sedating effects in agitated and retarded depression. J Clin Psychopharmacol 1991;11:166–174.

20. Reimherr FW, Chouinard G, Cohn CK, Cole JO, Itil TM, LaPierre YD, Masco HL, Mendels J. Antidepressant efficacy of sertraline: a double-blind, placebo- and amitriptyline-controlled, multicenter comparison study in outpatients with major depression. J Clin Psychiatry 1990;51(12, suppl B):18–27.

21. Doogan DP, Caillard V. Sertraline in the prevention of depression. Br J Psychiatry 1992;160:217–222.

22. Feighner JP, Boyer WF. Paroxetine in the treatment of depression: a comparison with imipramine and placebo. J Clin Psychiatry 1992;53(2, suppl):44–47.

23. Rasmussen J. Overview of efficacy, tolerability, and safety of paroxetine: a potent, selective inhibitor of serotonin reuptake. Presented at "Biological markers of depression: state of the art," Liege, June 1990.

24. Kiev A. A double-blind, placebo-controlled study of paroxetine in depressed outpatients. J Clin Psychiatry 1992; 53(suppl):27–29.

25. Guy W, Wilson WH, Ban TA, King DL, Manov G, Fjetland OK. A double-blind clinical trial of fluvoxamine and imipramine in patients with primary depression. Drug Dev Res 1984;4:143–153.

26. Milne RJ, Goa KL. Citalopram: a review of its pharmacodynamic and pharmacokinetic properties, and therapeutic potential in depressive illness. Drugs 1991;41(3):450–477.

27. Bouchard JM, Delaunay J, Delisle JP, et al. Citalopram vs maprotiline. A controlled, clinical multicentered trial in depressed patients. Acta Psychiatr Scand 1987;76:583–592.

28. Gravem A, Amthor F, Astrup C, et al. A double blind comparison of citalopram and amitriptyline in depressed patients. Acta Psychiatr Scand 1987;75:478–486.

29. Johnstone EC. The relationship between acetylator status and inhibition of monoamine oxidase, excretion of free drug and antidepressant response in depressed patients on phenelzine. Psychopharmacologia 1976;46:289–294.

30. Lecrubies Y, Guelfi JD. Efficacy of reversible inhibitors of monoamine oxidase-A in various forms of depression. Acta Psychiatr Scand 1990;360(suppl):18–23.

31. Berwish NJ, Amsterdam JD. An overview of investigational antidepressants. Psychosomatics 1989;30:1–17.

32. Greenblatt M, Grosser GH, Wechsler H. Differential response of hospitalized depressed patients to somatic therapy. Am J Psychiatry 1964;120:935–943.

33. Quitkin F, Rifkin A, Klein DF. Monoamine oxidase inhibitors: a review of antidepressant effectiveness. Arch Gen Psychiatry 1979;36:749–760.

34. Rowan PR, Paykel ES, Parker RR. Phenelzine and amitriptyline: effects on symptoms of neurotic depression. Br J Psychiatry 1982;140:475–483.

35. Thase ME, Mallinger AG, McKnight D, Himmelhoch JM. Treatment of imipramine-resistant recurrent depression, IV: a double-blind crossover study of tranylcypromine for anergic bipolar depression. Am J Psychiatry 1992;149:195–198.

36. Wheatley D. Amphetamines in general practice: their use in depression and anxiety. Semin Psychiatry 1969;1:163–173.

37. Hare RH, Dominian J, Sharpe L. Phenelzine and dexamphetamine in depressive illness. Br Med J 1962;1:9–12.

38. Overall JE, Hollister LE, Pokorny AD, Casey JF, Katz G. Drug therapy in depressions. Clin Pharmacol Ther 1961;3:16–22.

39. Hesbacher PT. Pemoline and methylphenidate in mildly depressed outpatients. Clin Pharmacol Ther 1970;11:698–710.

40. Rickels K, Ginrich Jr RL, McLaughlin W, Morris RJ, Sablasky L, Silverman H, Wentz HS. Methylphenidate in mildly depressed outpatients. Clin Pharmacol Ther 1972;13:595–601.

41. Robin AA, Wiseberg S. A controlled trial of methylphenidate (Ritalin) in the treatment of depressive states. J Neurol Neurosurg Psychiatry 1958;21:55–57.

42. Kaplitz SE. Withdrawn apathetic geriatric patients responsive to methylphenidate. J Am Geriatr Soc 1975;23:271–276.

43. Mendels J, Ramsey TA, Dyson WL, Frazer A. Lithium as an antidepressant. Arch Gen Psychiatry 1979;36:845–846.

44. Souza FGM, Goodwin GM. Lithium treatment and prophylaxis in unipolar depression: a meta-analysis. Br J Psychiatry 1991;158:666–675.

45. Hollister LE, Overall JE, Shelton J, Pennington V, Kimbell I, Johnson M. Drug therapy of depression. Amitriptyline, perphenazine, and their combination in different syndromes. Arch Gen Psychiatry 1967;17:486–493.

46. Overall JE, Hollister LE, Meyer F, Kimball Jr I, Shelton J. Imipramine and thioridazine in depressed and schizophrenic patients. Are there specific antidepressant drugs? JAMA 1964;189:605–608.

47. Lesser IM. The relationship between panic disorder and depression. J Anxiety Dis 1988;2:2–16.

48. Lesser IM, Rubin RT, Pecknold JC, et al: Secondary depression in panic disorder and agoraphobia. I. Frequency, severity, and response to treatment. Arch Gen Psychiatry 1988;45:437–443.

49. Grunhaus L, Harel Y, Krugler T, Pande AC, Haskett RF: Major depressive disorder and panic disorder. Clin Neuropharmacol 1988;11:454–461.

50. Lesser IM. The treatment of panic disorders: pharmacologic aspects. Psychiatric Annals 1991;21:341–346.

51. Klerman GL, Argyle N, Deltito JA, Roth M. The effects of alprazolam, imipramine, and placebo on the depressive symptoms associated with panic disorder. J Clin Psychopharmacol (in press).

52. Schatzberg AF, Cole JO. Benzodiazepines in depressive disorders. Arch Gen Psychiatry 1978;24:509–514.

53. Cassano GB, Castrogiovanni P, Conti I. Drug responses in different anxiety states under benzodiazepine treatment: some multivariate analyses for evaluation of Rating Scale for Depression scores. In: Garratini E, Mussini S, Randall LO, eds. The benzodiazapines. New York: Raven Press, 1973.

54. Klerman GL. The use of benzodiazepines in the treatment of depression. International Drug Therapy Newsletter 1986;21: 37–38.

55. Baldessarini RJ. Drugs and the treatment of psychiatric disorders. In: Gilman AG, Goodman LS, Gilman A, eds. The pharmacological basis of therapeutics. New York: Macmillan, 1980.

56. Ryan HW, Merrill FB, Scott GE, et al. Increase in suicidal thoughts and tendencies. JAMA 1968;203:135–137.

57. Weissman MM, Klerman GL. The chronic depressive in the community: unrecognized and poorly treated. Compr Psychiatry 1977;18:523–531.

58. Weissman MM, Myers JK, Thompson WD. Depression and its treatment in a US urban community. Arch Gen Psychiatry 1981;38: 417–421.

59. Fawcett J. Targeting treatment in patients with mixed symptoms of anxiety and depression. J Clin Psychiatry 1990;51(11 suppl):40–43.

60. Fabre LF, McLendon DM. A double-blind study comparing the efficacy and safety of alprazolam with imipramine and placebo in primary depression. Curr Ther Res 1980;27:474–482.

61. Feighner JP, Aden GC, Fabre LF, et al. Comparison of alprazolam, imipramine and placebo in the treatment of depression. JAMA 1983;249:3057–3064.

62. Ansseau M, Ansoms C, Beckers G, et al. Double-blind clinical study comparing alprazolam and doxepin in primary unipolar depression. J Affective Disord 1984;7:287–296.

63. Lenox RH, Shipley JE, Peyser JM, et al. Double-blind comparison of alprazolam versus imipramine in the inpatient treatment of major depressive illness. Psychopharmacol Bull 1984;20:79–82.

64. Rickels K, Feighner JP, Smith WT. Alpra-

zolam, amitriptyline, doxepin and placebo in the treatment of depression. Arch Gen Psychiatry 1985;42:134–141.

65. Rush AJ, Erman MK, Schlesser MA, et al. Alprazolam vs amitriptyline in depressions with reduced REM latencies. Arch Gen Psychiatry 1985;42:1154–1159.

66. Imlah NW. An evaluation of alprazolam in the treatment of reactive or neurotic (secondary) depression. Br J Psychiatry 1985; 146:515–519.

67. Remick RA, Fleming JAE, Buchanan RA, et al. A comparison of the safety and efficacy of alprazolam and desipramine in moderately severe depression. Can J Psychiatry 1985;30:597–601.

68. Weissman MM, Prusoff BA, Kleber HD, et al. Alprazolam (Xanax) in the treatment of major depression. In: Burrows GD, ed. Clinical and pharmacological studies in psychiatric disorders. London: John Libbey, 1985.

69. Goldberg SC, Ettigi P, Schulz PM, et al. Alprazolam versus imipramine in depressed out-patients with neurovegetative signs. J Affective Disord 1986;11:139–145.

70. Rickels K, Chung HR, Csanalosi IB, et al. Alprazolam, diazepam, imipramine, and placebo in outpatients with major depression. Arch Gen Psychiatry 1987;44:862–866.

71. Fawcett J, Edwards JH, Kravitz HM, Jeffries H. Alprazolam: an antidepressant? Alprazolam, desipramine, and an alprazolam-desipramine combination in the treatment of adult depressed outpatients. J Clin Psychopharmacol 1987;7:295–310.

72. Overall JE, Biggs J, Jacobs M, Holden K. Comparison of alprazolam and imipramine for treatment of outpatient depression. J Clin Psychiatry 1987;48:15–19.

73. Eriksson B, Nagy A, Starmark JE, Thelander U. Alprazolam compared to amitriptyline in the treatment of major depression. Acta Psychiatr Scand 1987;75:656–663.

74. Borison RL, Sinha D, Geber S, et al. Double-blind evaluation of alprazolam versus placebo in outpatients with major depression. Biol Psychiatry 1989;25:54a.

75. O'Shea B. Alprazolam: just another benzodiazepine? Ir J Psychol Med 1989;6:89–94.

76. Potter WZ, Rudorfer MV, Manji H. The pharmacologic treatment of depression. N Engl J Med 1991;325:633–642.

77. Hu H-Y, Davis JM, Heinze WJ, Pandey GN. Effect of chronic treatment with antidepressants on beta-adrenergic receptor binding in guinea pig brain. Biochem Pharmacol 1980;29:2895–2896.

78. Feighner JP. A review of controlled studies of adinazolam mesylate in patients with major depressive disorder. Psychopharmacol Bull 1986;22(1):186–191.

79. Hicks F, Robins E, Murphy G. Comparison of adinazolam, amitriptyline, and placebo in the treatment of melancholic depression. Psychiatry Res 1987;23:221–227.

80. Gundlach R, Engelhardt DM, Hankoff L, et al. A double-blind outpatient study of diazepam (Valium) and placebo. Psychopharmacologia 1966;9:81–92.

81. McDowall A, Owen S, Robin AA. A controlled comparison of diazepam and amylobarbitone in anxiety states. Br J Psychiatry 1966;112:629–631.

82. Rao AV. A controlled trial with "Valium" in obsessive compulsive state. J Indian Med Assoc 1967;42:564–567.

83. Hall RCW, Joffe JR. Aberrant response to diazepam: a new syndrome. Am J Psychiatry 1972;129:738–742.

84. Lader MH, Petursson H. Benzodiazepine derivatives—side effects and dangers. Biol Psychiatry 1981;12:1195–1201.

85. Fontaine R, Annable L, Chouinard G, et al. Bromazepam and diazepam in generalized anxiety: a placebo-controlled study with measurement of drug plasma concentrations. J Clin Psychopharmacol 1983;3:80–87.

86. Wilkinson CJ. Effects of diazepam (Valium) and trait anxiety on human physical aggression and emotional state. J Behav Med 1985;8:101–114.

87. Fontaine R, Mercier P, Beaudry P, et al. Bromazepam and lorazepam in generalized anxiety: a placebo-controlled study with measurement of drug plasma concentrations. Acta Psychiatr Scand 1986;74:451–458.

88. Pollack MH, Tesar GE, Rosenbaum JF, et al. Clonazepam in the treatment of panic disorder and agoraphobia: a one-year follow-up. J Clin Psychopharmacol 1986;47:475–476.

89. Lydiard RB, Laraia MT, Ballenger JC, Howell EF. Emergence of depressive symptoms in patients receiving alprazolam for panic disorder. Am J Psychiatry 1987;144:664–665.

90. Lydiard RB, Howell EF, Laraia MT, et al. Depression in patients receiving lorazepam for panic. Am J Psychiatry 1989;146; 629–631.

91. Robinson DS, Rickels K, Feighner J, Fabre Jr LF, Gammans RE, Shrotriya RC, Alms DR, Andary JJ, Messina ME. Clinical effects of the 5-HT$_{1A}$ partial agonists in depression: a composite analysis of buspirone in the treatment of depression. J Clin Psychopharmacol 1990;10(3 suppl):67S–76S.

92. Jenkins SW, Robinson DS, Fabre Jr LF, Andary JJ, Messina ME, Reich LA. Gepirone in the treatment of major depression. J Clin Psychopharmacol 1990; 10(suppl):77S–85S.

93. Fontaine R, Ontiveros A, Faludi G, Elie R, Roberts D, Ecker J. A study of nefazodone, imipramine, and placebo in depressed outpatients. Biol Psychiatry 1991;29:3–38.

94. Feighner JP, Pambakian R, Fowler RC, Boyler WF, D'Amico MF. A comparison of nefazodone, imipramine and placebo in patients with moderate to severe depression. Psychopharmacol Bull 1989;25:219–221.

95. Fontaine R, Ontiveros A, Faludi G, Elie R, Roberts D, Ecker J. A study of nefazodone, imipramine, and placebo in depressed outpatients. Biol Psychiatry 1991;29:3–38.

96. Weise C, Fox I, Clary C, Schweizer E, Rickels K. Nefazodone in the treatment of outpatient major depression. Biol Psychiatry 1991;29:03–33.

97. Yocca FD, Hyslop DK, Taylor DP. Nefazodone: a potential broad spectrum antidepressant. Trans Am Soc Neurochem 1985; 16:115.

98. Stramentinoli G, Catto E, Algeri S. The increase in Sadenosyl-L-methionine (SAMe) concentration in rat brain after its systemic administration. Commun Psychopharmacol 1977;1:89–97.

99. Janicak P, Lipinski J, Davis JM, Altman E, Sharma RP. Parenteral SAMe in depression: literature review and preliminary data. Psychopharmacol Bull 1989; 25(2):238–242.

100. Perry PJ, Pfohl BM, Holstad SG. The relationship between antidepressant response and TCA plasma concentrations. Clin Pharmacokinet 1987;13:381–392.

101. Nies A. Monoamine oxidase inhibitors. In: Paykel ES, ed. Handbook of affective disorders. New York: Guilford Press, 1982.

102. Feighner JP, Boyer WF, Tyler DL, Nebrosky RJ. Adverse consequences of fluoxetine-MAOI combination therapy. J Clin Psychiatry 1990;51(6):222–225.

103. Montgomery SA, Dufour H, Brion S, Gailledreau J, Laqueille X, Ferrey G, Moron P, Parant-Lucena N, Singer L, Danion JM, Beuzen JN, Pierredon MA. The prophylactic efficacy of fluoxetine in unipolar depression. Br J Psychiatry 1988;153(suppl 3):69–76.

104. Eric L. A prospective, double-blind, comparative, multicentre study of paroxetine and placebo in preventing recurrent major depressive episodes [Abstract]. Biol Psychiatry 1991;29(11S): 254S–255S.

105. Frank E, Kupfer DJ, Perel JM, et al. Three-year outcomes for maintenance therapies in recurrent depression. Arch Gen Psychiatry 1990;47:1093–1099.

106. Kupfer DJ, Frank E, Perel JM et al. Five year outcome for maintenance therapies in recurrent depression. Arch Gen Psychiatry 1992;49:769–773.

107. Georgotis A, McCue RE. Relapse of depressed patients after effective continuation therapy. J Affective Disord 1989; 17:159–164.

108. Robinson D, Lerfald SC, Binnett B, et al. Continuation and maintenance treatment of major depression with the monoamine oxidase inhibitor phenelzine: a double-blind placebo-controlled study. Psychopharmacol Bull 1991;27:31–40.

109. Georgotas A, McCue RE, Cooper TB. A placebo controlled comparison of nortriptyline and phenelzine in maintenance therapy of elderly depressed patients. Arch Gen Psychiatry 1989;46:783–786.

110. Kane JM, Quitkin FM, Rifkin A, et al. Lithium carbonate and imipramine in the prophylaxis of unipolar and bipolar II illness. Arch Gen Psychiatry 1982;39:1065–1069.

111. Prien RF, Kupfer DJ, Mansky PA, et al. Drug therapy in the prevention of recurrences in unipolar and bipolar affective disorders. Arch Gen Psychiatry 1984;41:1096–1104.

112. Coppen A, Montgomery SA, Gupta RK, Bailey JE. A double-blind comparison of lithium carbonate and maprotiline in the prophylaxis of the affective disorders. Br J Psychiatry 1976;128:479–485.

113. Coppen A, Ghose K, Rama Rao VA, Bailey J, Peet M. Mianserin and lithium in the prophylaxis of depression. Br J Psychiatry 1978;133:206–210.

114. Bialos D, Giller E, Jatlow P, Docherty J,

Harkness L. Recurrence of depression after discontinuation of long-term amitriptyline treatment. Am J Psychiatry 1982;139:325–329.

115. Coppen A, Gupta R, Montgomery S, Bailey J. A double blind comparison of lithium carbonate and Ludiomil in the prophylaxis of unipolar affective illness. Pharmacopsychiatry 1976;9:94–99.

116. Quitkin FM, Kane J, Rifkin A, et al. Lithium and imipramine in the prophylaxis of unipolar and bipolar II depression: a prospective, placebo-controlled comparison. Psychopharmacol Bull 1981;17:142–144.

117. Stein MK, Rickels K, Weise CC. Maintenance therapy with amitrptyline: a controlled trial. Am J Psychiatry 1980;137:370–371.

118. Kay DWK, Fahy Y, Garside RF. A seven-month double-blind trial of amitriptyline and diazepam in ECT-treated depressed patients. Br J Psychiatry 1970;117: 667–671.

119. Mindham RHS, Howland C, Shepherd M. An evaluation of continuation therapy with tricyclic antidepressants in depressive illness. Psychol Med 1973;3:5–17.

120. Prien RF, Kupfer DJ. Continuation drug therapy for major depressive episodes: how long should it be maintained? Am J Psychiatry 1986;143:18–23.

121. Souza FGM, Mander AJ, Goodwin GM. The efficacy of lithium in prophylaxis of unipolar depression: evidence from its discontinuation. Br J Psychiatry 1990;157:718–722.

122. American Psychiatric Association. Practice guidelines for MDD in adults. Am J Psychiatry 1993;150(4, Suppl):1–26.

Pharmacokinetics

THERAPEUTIC DRUG MONITORING

Therapeutic drug monitoring enhances the clinician's ability to rationally adjust the dose of antidepressants, increasing their therapeutic efficacy and reducing adverse events. This is in part because patients have substantial interindividual differences in their drug metabolism and elimination rates (up to 40-fold), and may obtain widely different plasma concentrations on standard doses of the same medication. TDM not only allows the clinician to identify subtherapeutic levels but also potentially toxic plasma concentrations, which may occur at levels two to three times above the therapeutic range. Such toxicity can be serious, and at times even fatal, due primarily to the effects on brain and heart.

As elaborated in Chapters 1 and 3, the basic principle underlying TDM is that a threshold plasma concentration is needed at an effector site to initiate a pharmacodynamic response. While the effector site is the CNS for psychotropics, in vivo measurement of brain tissue is obviously not feasible. Plasma concentrations of drugs such as the TCAs, however, have been shown to correlate well with CNS concentrations (1).

TDM must always be used in conjunction with sound clinical judgment, since drug concentration is not the sole determinant of clinical response. Thus, interindividual differences exist in tissue sensitivity that contribute to a wide variance in response (e.g., nuisance side effects, therapeutic response, or toxicity).

TDM can be seen as a refinement in the titration dose/response approach, in which medication adjustment is based on a balance between efficacy and adverse effects. Since it may take several weeks for certain psychotropics to achieve the steady state plasma levels required to assess response, TDM provides guidelines for more quickly optimizing the dose.

The antidepressants most extensively

studied with regard to TDM are the TCAs, which have been the first-line pharmacotherapy for depression over the last 30 years.

Pharmacokinetics of TCAs

TCAs are pharmacologically complex. They are slowly but generally completely absorbed from the small bowel; enter the portal blood; pass through the liver, where there is significant first-pass metabolism (40 to 70%); and then enter the systemic circulation for distribution. These agents are generally highly protein-bound (75 to 95%), as well as highly lipophilic, with a large volume of distribution. Their half-lives range from 16 to 126 hours.

TCAs are metabolized in the liver by three pathways:

- N-demethylation
- N-oxidation
- Aromatic hydroxylation.

The ratio of parent drug to desmethylated metabolite at steady state has been reported to range from 0.47 to 0.70 for imipramine:desipramine and from 0.83 to 1.16 for amitriptyline:nortriptyline. These typical ratios can be used to distinguish between an acute overdose (increased ratios) versus a steady state situation (normal ratios).

TCA Plasma Concentration and Response Relationship

Studies have attempted to demonstrate a relationship between concentration and antidepressant response for:

- Nortriptyline
- Desipramine
- Amitriptyline
- Imipramine.

While a comprehensive review of all studies of the plasma concentration/ antidepressant response relationship of TCAs is beyond the scope of this chapter, Perry et al. (1987) have recently summarized this literature using logistic regression analysis (2). Their results are discussed in the following paragraphs. One of the limitations of such a study is that cut-off points are chosen based on a data set and not independently verified. This may bias the results in favor of a relationship between plasma level and clinical response.

Nortriptyline. Studies demonstrate a curvilinear plasma concentration/antidepressant response relationship, with an optimum range of 50 to 150 or 170 ng/ml depending on the study. Perry finds that within this range, 70% of patients with primary major depressive disorder experience complete remission (e.g., a final Hamilton Depression Rating Scale score equal to or less than 6) versus only 29% of patients who have plasma concentrations outside this range (i.e., below or above 50–170 ng/ml). Of note, the response rate is generally higher in the lower end of this range than at the upper limit. This observation may be relevant to the often asked question: "If my patient has gotten somewhat better but is in the middle of nortriptyline's range (e.g., 75–125 ng/ml), should I push the dose up?" Under these circumstances, we would recommend augmenting the drug with lithium or thyroid supplement rather than further adjusting the dose. Alternatively, if the clinician wants to adjust the dose, a modest reduction might be attempted.

Desipramine. Desipramine studies demonstrate a threshold concentration/ antidepressant response relationship. The "therapeutic window" for desipramine according to their analysis was about 110–160 ng/ml. Thus, there was a remission rate of 59% within, versus 20% outside this range.

Amitriptyline. The results for this tertiary amine tricyclic are less convincing.

Its optimal range may be based on both efficacy and data demonstrating that CNS and cardiac toxicity, as well as dropout rates for adverse effects, are a function of its plasma levels. With this in mind, the optimum range for this medication may be about 80–150 ng/ml. Thus, Perry found a nonsignificant trend, with a remission rate of 48% within, versus 29% outside this range was found by Perry et al.

Imipramine. Imipramine did not show a curvilinear relationship between concentration and antidepressant response in adult patients, with a threshhold relationship best fitting the data. A curvilinear relationship has been described for imipramine, however, when used in children. Based on their analysis, the upper end for optimum antidepressant response to imipramine was close to the threshold for CNS and cardiac toxicity. Thus, the upper limit to the therapeutic range is a function of toxicity rather than reduced efficacy, as with other TCAs. The threshold proposed from the Perry meta-analysis is 265 ng/ml, with a remission rate of 42% above this threshold versus 15% below it.

Some of this text's authors partially disagree with the analysis of Perry, feeling that the data better supports a plasma threshold level/clinical response relationship for desipramine and amitriptyline. But it is instructive how little difference this makes in the clinical interpretation. If a patient has a plasma level below the threshold (or therapeutic window), the patient may be noncompliant or a fast metabolizer, and compliance should be assured or the dose should be increased, respectively. For a nonresponder without significant adverse effects in the low normal range (i.e., only slightly above the threshold level or lower end of a therapeutic window) we suggest raising the dose. If a patient has a very high plasma level and has not responded, we would switch to another drug, attempt lithium or thyroid potentiation, or lower the dose. In patients above the range in which most tend to respond, we would be concerned about toxicity and lower the dose.

Perry would suggest that patients are nonresponders because of too high a plasma level. If the threshold model is more appropriate, we would also be concerned about a moderately high level causing adverse effects and would probably switch to another agent, while others lower the dose for a week or so to see if a better response could be achieved.

A summary of the plasma concentration/efficacy data with these four TCAs supports the use of TDM, at least once, as a routine aspect of therapy for major depressive disorder. The data are consistent across three of these agents that optimal plasma levels are associated with a greater likelihood of full remission after 4 weeks. **Translated into clinical terms, Perry finds a 1.7- to 3-fold increase in clinical response to tricyclic antidepressants if the depressed patient obtains an optimal TCA plasma level** (2).

Use of TDM to Increase Safety of TCAs

Studies have also focused on issues of TDM and enhanced safety to avoid CNS or cardiac toxicity, as well as catastrophic outcomes.

Plasma Concentration and CNS Toxicity

The relationship between TCA plasma concentration and central nervous system toxicity has been well established. The incidence varies from 1.5–13.3% (mean of 6%) when hospitalized patients take doses of 400–450 mg/day without the benefit of TDM-based dose adjustment (3). Furthermore, these symptoms often evolve insidiously, such that they mimic the depressive episodes that the medications are being used to treat (4). An *increase in affective symptoms* (e.g., deterioration in mood, poor concentration, social withdrawal, and lethargy) may be the earliest warning signs of impending CNS toxicity. *Motor symptoms* (e.g., tremor and ataxia) frequently develop next, followed by *psychosis* (e.g., thought disorder, delusions, and hallucinations). All of these may lead the clinician to erroneously conclude that the depressive episode is worsening, prompting an increase in the TCA dose or the addition of an antipsychotic. The latter in turn can increase the TCA plasma levels by inhibiting metabolism, further exacerbating toxicity. The last stage in the evolution of TCA-induced CNS toxicity is *delirium* (e.g., memory impairment, agitation, disorientation, and confusion) and/or *seizures*. The use of TDM can detect the slow metabolizer, who is at greater risk for developing this scenario.

Preskorn and Jerkovich (1990), using meta-analysis, demonstrated that TCA-induced CNS toxicity is concentration-dependent (3). The risk was 13 times higher when the plasma levels exceeded 300 ng/ml and 37 times higher when they exceeded 450 ng/ml. **Interestingly, peripheral anticholinergic effects, (e.g., blurry vision, dry mouth, and constipation) were reported as more significant than expected in only 8% of the toxic patients.**

In patients who are not neurologically compromised, plasma concentrations of less than 250 ng/ml rarely present with CNS manifestations. As this threshold concentration is exceeded, however, patients develop asymptomatic, nonspecific EEG abnormalities (5). With concentrations beyond 450 ng/ml, however, the risk of seizures, in addition to delirium, clearly increases (6).

TCA-induced seizures typically have no prodrome and are a single generalized motor seizure that lasts several minutes. The incidence of seizures during treatment with standard doses is estimated at 0.5% in nonepileptic patients (7). In a review of 8 cases of TCA-induced seizures during routine chemotherapy, none had significant risk factors other than elevated plasma levels: the mean was 734 ± 249 ng/ml, with a range of 438–1200 ng/ml (6). Consistent with this finding, Tamayo et al. reported two cases of TCA-induced seizures in patients who had mean plasma concentrations of 1209 ± 485 ng/ml (a range of 805–1776 ng/ml) (8).

Unlike TCA-induced delirium and seizures, *coma* rarely develops, due to the gradual development of toxic concentrations, and because clinicians stop the drug when a patient becomes excessively somnolent. Nevertheless, the minimum threshold for developing coma is estimated to be about 1000 ng/ml, based on data from acute overdose cases (9). It should be kept in mind that the TCA plasma levels in these cases were not at steady state. Still, this demonstrates that the CNS toxicity is concentration-dependent and underscores the importance of early detection and prevention.

Plasma Concentration and Cardiovascular Toxicity

The cardiovascular effects of TCAs have been well documented, and the mechanisms underlying these effects elucidated by in vitro and in vivo animal studies (10). Since the cardiac effects of TCAs are concentration-dependent, with the possible exception of orthostatic hypotension and tachycardia, TDM may help avoid iatrogenic cardiotoxicity.

While conduction disturbances are more likely to occur in those predisposed to cardiac disease, data demonstrate that these effects also occur in healthy individuals if the appropriate threshold is exceeded. In healthy middle-aged subjects, TCA plasma concentrations of less than 200 ng/ml rarely induce intracardiac conduction defects. At 200 ng/ml, however, slowing of the His bundle-ventricular system routinely occurs (11). At concentrations above 350 ng/ml, first degree atrioventricular (AV) block was found to occur in 70% of physically healthy patients on desipramine or imipramine (12–14). Although there have been no published studies on the incidence of cardiac arrhythmia or sudden death in physically healthy subjects during standard TCA therapy, studies of overdoses find that arrhythmias occur at a mean concentration of 1275 ± 290 ng/ml and arrest at a mean concentration of 1700 ± 150 ng/ml (9). These cardiac effects probably occur at lower plasma concentrations under steady state conditions, since equilibrium between the plasma and the tissue compartment has not been reached in an acute overdose.

Composite analysis of treatment studies permits a better understanding of the various CNS and cardiac effects in patients during TCA therapy as a function of the plasma level achieved. Thus:

- Both are *unlikely* to occur at therapeutic concentrations.
- Their *incidence and severity* increases as a function of the degree to which the plasma levels exceed the therapeutic concentration.
- They can cause serious *morbidity and mortality* at high concentrations.
- They can develop *insidiously,* and simple inquiry about adverse effects may miss their presence.
- Both toxicity curves are shifted to the left in the *elderly* (see Chapter 3).

Sudden Death. The usefulness of TDM has been underscored by the recent spate of sudden deaths for which autopsy revealed no cause except sudden cardiac arrest and markedly elevated postmortem TCA plasma and tissue levels. The authors are now aware of 20 such cases in which acute overdose was ruled out at autopsy. In some instances, malpractice suits have been filed alleging failure to diagnose TCA toxicity, specifically citing failure to use TDM to adjust the dose. Court awards in favor of the plaintiffs have totaled $1.5 million. Clinicians should be aware that significant postmortem changes in TCA plasma levels may occur, and interpretation must be done cautiously. Sudden death is common and may only be coincidentally associated with a drug the patient was taking. But, if a patient has a toxic TCA level, the clinician has a legal problem, given the adverse effects of TCAs on cardiac conduction.

Techniques for Therapeutic Drug Monitoring of TCAs

Generally, the physician starts with a standard TCA dose (e.g., 50–75 mg/day of nortriptyline) in a physically healthy adult. After 1 week, the vast majority of patients will be at steady state. A blood sample is then drawn 10–12 hours after the last dose to ensure that absorption and distribution of the drug are complete and because virtually all the data on optimal concentration ranges are based on this post-dose time interval. If the sample cannot be drawn at 10–12 hours, obtaining it later is better than earlier, since these drugs have half-lives around 24 hours. If the level is drawn at 16 hours rather than 10–12 hours, the drug is only 4 hours into its second half-life, and while this sample will underestimate the 10–12 hour level, the magnitude of the error is small. In contrast, too early a sample can overestimate the 10–12 hour level in a less predictable way.

Single-dose prediction strategies have also been established for TCAs, such as nortriptyline, allowing for a more rapid prediction of the dose required to achieve therapeutic plasma concentrations (15). Nomograms have been developed in which a 25 mg test dose of nortriptyline is given and then blood is drawn 24, 36, or 48 hours later to obtain plasma concentrations. This data is then plotted on the nomogram to estimate the dose that would achieve a therapeutic plasma concentration. The utility of this approach is limited, however, since errors in technique (e.g., imprecise timing of blood draw) can be magnified, leading to miscalculations of the required dose.

Therapeutic Drug Monitoring of Other Antidepressants
Fluoxetine

Fluoxetine is well absorbed from the GI tract and undergoes hepatic biotransformation to its active metabolite, norfluoxetine. Plasma concentration/clinical response studies have not demonstrated a positive correlation (16, 17).

Given fluoxetine's long half-life, it takes many weeks to reach steady state concentration (C_{SS}) (16–21). The same issue may explain the occurrence of late adverse effects with this agent.

Since these factors make it difficult to rapidly titrate to the optimal dose, the clinician is in the difficult situation of waiting at least a month to determine efficacy or adjusting the dose well before C_{SS} has been reached.

Since fluoxetine inhibits the hepatic P-450 oxidase system, a 4- to 6-fold increase in TCA or bupropion plasma levels can occur when fluoxetine is used concurrently or if these other ADs are initiated immediately after fluoxetine discontinuation. As outlined above, the toxicity of elevated TCA or bupropion plasma levels can be quite serious. **Therefore, TDM may be especially important if other psychotropics are used in conjunction with fluoxetine, as well as sertraline and paroxetine.**

Monoamine Oxidase Inhibitors

Phenelzine has been studied for the treatment of anxiety, phobic and obsessive-compulsive disorders, as well as typical and atypical depressions. Its antidepressant efficacy has been correlated with an 80–85% inhibition of the MAO enzyme. Studies by Ravaris replicated by the authors indicate that 60 mg/day are usually needed to inhibit MAO by at least 80% (22, 23). While monitoring of platelet MAO inhibition during treatment may permit more optimal dosing, the assay is not readily available commercially. This fact, coupled with the infrequent use of MAOIs, has hampered their widespread application.

Bupropion

Bupropion shows considerable interindividual variability in plasma levels, even among physically healthy patients. Still, studies indicate a relationship between trough steady-state plasma concentrations of 50–100 ng/ml and optimal response, while higher levels of the parent compound and its metabolites are associated with a poorer outcome (24, 25).

The risk of seizure with bupropion has been estimated at 4 per 1000, and several observations suggest that it may be concentration-dependent (26). These observations include:

- The incidence of seizures is *dose-related* (and hence must be concentration-related)
- Seizures typically *occur within days of a dose change* and a *few hours after the*

last dose, suggesting that peak plasma concentrations play a role

- Individuals with *lean body mass* such as anorexic-bulimic patients have an increased risk.

Unfortunately, early studies correlating bupropion dose with seizure activity did not measure its three active metabolites, which accumulate at plasma concentrations of 2–10 times that of the parent compound and may correlate more closely with the risk of seizure (27). At this time, TDM for bupropion might be valuable in assessing compliance and to avoid (or at least mitigate) seizure risk. Routine TDM with bupropion, however, cannot be recommended given the lack of data; the inability to measure all three metabolites, as well as the parent compound; and uncertainty about the proper timing to obtain samples.

Trazodone

There is only limited information on trazodone. A recent study suggested, however, that a threshold concentration in the elderly may be 650 ng/ml, with a range between 300 and 1600 ng/ml (28). Additional research is warranted.

CONCLUSION

There are three possible relationships between plasma concentration and efficacy:

- *None or a poor* relationship between plasma level and therapeutic response
- A *threshold* for therapeutic response, such that below this level there is less likelihood of response and above it there is a good chance for response
- An inverted U-shaped or *therapeutic window*

All three relationships occur with cyclic antidepressants. The various courses of action utilizing the results of TDM may include:

- *Plasma levels seem adequate* but there is insufficient clinical response: *try another agent*
- *Plasma levels are low* and there is insufficient response: *increase the dose*
- *Plasma levels are high,* and there is insufficient clinical response or severe adverse effects: *reduce the dose or try another agent*
- *One or more trials* with standard TCAs at adequate blood levels are not effective: consider an MAOI; lithium or thyroid augmentation; an SRI; or electroconvulsive therapy (see also Alternate Treatment Strategies later in this chapter)
- Nonresponse on adequate blood levels with *obsessive-compulsive* symptoms (or disorder): consider *clomipramine* or other 5-HT reuptake inhibitors (e.g., fluoxetine, sertraline, paroxetine).

REFERENCES

1. Glotzbach RK, Preskorn SH. Brain concentrations of tricyclic antidepressants: single-dose kinetics and relationship to plasma concentration in chronically dosed rats. Psychopharmacology 1982;78:25–27.
2. Perry PJ, Pfohl BM, Holstad SG. The relationship between antidepressant response and tricyclic antidepressant plasma concentrations. Clin Pharmacokinet 1987;13:381–392.
3. Preskorn SH, Jerkovich GS. Central nervous system toxicity of tricyclic antidepressants: phenomenology, course, risk factors, and role of therapeutic drug monitoring. J Clin Psychopharmacol 1990;10:88–94.
4. Preskorn SH. Therapeutic drug monitoring of tricyclic antidepressants: a means of avoiding toxicity. Psychopharmacol Bull 1989;7:237–243.
5. Preskorn SH, Othmer S, Lai C, et al. Tricyclic antidepressants and delirium. J Clin Psychiatry 1982;139:822–823.
6. Preskorn SH, Fast GA. Tricyclic antidepressant-induced seizures and plasma drug concentration. J Clin Psychiatry 1992;53:160–162.
7. Lowry MR, Dunner FJ. Seizures during tricyclic therapy. Am J Psychiatry 1980;127:1461–1462.

8. Tamayo M, deGatta F, Gutierrez JR, et. al. High levels of tricyclic antidepressants in conventional therapy: determinant factors. Int J Clin Pharmacol Ther Toxicol 1988;26(10):495–499.

9. Petit JM, Spiker DG, Ruwitch JF, et. al. Tricyclic antidepressant plasma levels and adverse effects after overdose. Clin Pharmacol Ther 1977;21:47–51.

10. Preskorn SH, Irwin H. Toxicity of tricyclic antidepressants: kinetics, mechanisms, intervention: a review. Clin Psychiatry 1982;143:151–156.

11. Vohra J, Burrows G, Hunt D, et al. The effects of toxic and therapeutic doses of tricyclic antidepressant drugs on intracardiac conduction. Eur J Cardiol 1975;3:219–227.

12. Rudorfer MB, Young RC. Desipramine: cardiovascular effects and plasma levels. Am J Psychiatry 1980;137:984–986.

13. Veith RC, Friedel RO, Bloom B, et. al. Electrocardiogram changes and plasma desipramine levels during treatment. Clin Pharmacol Ther 1980;27:796–802.

14. Preskorn SH, Weller E, Weller R, et al. Plasma levels of imipramine and adverse effects in children. Am J Psychiatry 1983;140:1332–1335.

15. Katz IR, Simpson GM, Jetanandoni V, et al. Steady-state pharmacokinetics of nortriptyline in the frail elderly. Neuropsychopharmacology. 1989;2(3):229–236.

16. Preskorn SH, Silkey B, Beber J, Darey C. Antidepressant response and plasma concentrations of fluoxetine. Ann Clin Psychiatry 1991;3(1):61–65.

17. Kelly MW, Perry PJ, Holstead SG, et al. Serum fluoxetine and norfluoxetine concentration and antidepressant response. Ther Drug Monit 1989;11(2):165–170.

18. Stark R, Hardison CD. A review of multicenter controlled studies of fluoxetine vs. imipramine and placebo in outpatients with major depressive disorder. J Clin Psychiatry 1985;45(3)Sec 2:53–58.

19. Brenner JD. Fluoxetine in depressed patients: a comparison with imipramine. J Clin Psychiatry 1984;45:414–419.

20. Feighner JP. A comparative trial of fluoxetine and amitriptyline in patients with major depressive disorder. J Clin Psychiatry 1985;46:369–372.

21. Chouinard G. A double-blind controlled clinical trial of fluoxetine and amitriptyline in the treatment of outpatients with major depressive disorder. J Clin Psychiatry 1985;46(3)Sec 2:32–37.

22. Ravaris CL, Nies A, Robinson DS, et al. A multiple-dose, controlled study of phenelzine in depression-anxiety states. Arch Gen Psychiatry 1976;33:347–350.

23. Bresnahan DB, Pandey GN, Janicak PG, Sharma R, Boshes RA. MAO inhibition and clinical response in depressed patients treated with phenelzine. J Clin Psychiatry 1990;51:47–50.

24. Preskorn SH. Antidepressant response and plasma concentrations of bupropion. J Clin Psychiatry 1983;44(5)Sec 2:137–139.

25. Golden RN, DeVane CL, Laizure SC, et al. Bupropion in depression, II: The roles of metabolites in clinical outcome. Arch Gen Psychiatry 1988;45:145–149.

26. Davidson J. Seizures and bupropion: a review. J Clin Psychiatry 1989;50:256–261.

27. Preskorn SH, Fleck RJ, Schroeder, DH. Therapeutic drug monitoring of bupropion. Am J Psychiatry 1990;147:12,1690–1691.

28. Monteleone P, Gnocchi G. Evidence for a linear relationship between trazodone levels and clinical response in depression in the elderly. Clin Neuropharmacol 1990;13(suppl 1):584–589.

Alternate Treatment Strategies

TREATMENT-RESISTANT DEPRESSION

Two major problems complicating the question of treatment-resistant depression are inappropriate diagnosis and inadequate treatment. A recent study found that only 3.5% of over 6000 newly diagnosed depressed patients had received appropriate antidepressant treatment (i.e., absolute resistance) based upon dose and duration criteria (1). Hence, a substantial number of "treatment-resistant" cases may actually be the result of inadequate therapy (i.e., relative resistance). For example, in the MacEwan and Remick (1988) study, 70% of those defined as treatment-unresponsive achieved complete remission with an adequate trial of a heterocyclic, MAO inhibitor, or ECT (2). Patients who truly fail to respond to an adequate trial of one antidepressant now have the option of newer agents whose activity does not necessarily overlap with earlier generation compounds (e.g. SRIs; RIMAs).

Guscott and Grof (1991) list a series of variables critical to the understanding and management of refractory depression (3), presented here with minor modifications:

- Is the *diagnosis correct?* (e.g., both incorrect diagnosis or subtype, such as atypical depression)
- Does the patient have a *psychotic* depression?
- Has the patient received *adequate treatment?* (dose and duration)
- Do *adverse effects* preclude adequate dosing?
- Is the patient *compliant?*
- Was a rational, *stepwise approach* used?
- How was *outcome measured?*
- Is there a *coexisting medical or psychiatric disorder* (e.g., substance abuse) that interferes with response to treatment?
- Are there *other factors in the clinical setting* that interfere with treatment?

Also of concern are the effects that nonresponse may have on the *clinician,* including:

- *Avoidance* of the patient (e.g., countertransference)
- *Affective disturbances*, resulting in feelings of dysphoria, anger, and decreased tolerance for patients' complaints

- An increased tendency to add or to *switch diagnosis to an Axis II disorder.*

Guscott and Grof consider the vast majority of these patients only *relatively refractory* and analogize this situation to other medical disorders, such as asthma, which is often underdiagnosed and undertreated. Thus, like asthma, morbidity and mortality associated with depression are increasing worldwide. Ironically, these complications occur at a time when the understanding of their pathophysiology has greatly advanced over the last 2 decades, and when appropriate diagnosis and aggressive drug therapy can improve outcome. Guscott and Grof recommend giving careful attention to an adequate treatment trial, using a rational, stepwise model, like those often used in other medical specialties to treat asthma, essential hypertension, and rheumatoid arthritis.

White and Simpson (1987) caution that patients intolerant to heterocyclics should not be considered resistant, since another AD with a different profile (e.g., an SRI), can often bring about remission (4). Other strategies include a second trial using an HCA with a different biochemical profile; evidence for this approach, however, is very weak. Finally, Paykel et al. (1987) emphasize that, in addition to pharmacotherapy, other therapeutic modalities—including social support; environmental manipulation; and family, cognitive, or dynamic psychotherapy—are often helpful in managing these patients (5).

It is also important to note that patients tend to improve with time, and the level of depression fluctuates from day to day. Sometimes when a second drug is added, improvement may have occurred simply because of the passage of time but be falsely attributed to the additional drug. It is virtually impossible to do controlled studies in treatment nonresponders, since so many improve with the first treatment. Also, there are many drugs and combinations used, so that to get an adequate homogeneous sample of nonresponders to any given treatment would require a very large collaborative study mechanism.

Specific Strategies to Manage Treatment Resistance

There are three major options available with true treatment nonresponse (6):

- When there has been no benefit, stop the current antidepressant and *initiate a trial with an unrelated agent* (e.g., switch from an HCA to an SRI or MAOI)
- When there has been partial response
  - *Potentiate* the effects of the current agent with *lithium, thyroid hormone* (e.g., T_3), or an *anticonvulsant* (e.g., carbamazepine or valproic acid)

     or

  - Concurrently use *two different classes of ADs* (e.g., HCA plus MAOI).

Again, we emphasize that the combination of an MAOI plus an SRI should never be attempted.

In support of the first option, an analysis of data from studies in which hospitalized, severely depressed patients were included indicates that *paroxetine* was significantly better than placebo and as effective as comparison antidepressants in producing clinical response (7, 8). In two studies involving a total of 50 patients unresponsive to conventional antidepressants, a majority responded well to 6 weeks' treatment with paroxetine (9, 10). When adequate trials of an HCA and an SRI have failed, many advocate switching to an *MAO inhibitor,* particularly in *atypical depression,* where this class may be the treatment of choice.

Potentiation strategies, such as *lithium augmentation* of standard antidepressants, have been reported to significantly benefit previously treatment-resistant and psychotic depressions, particularly in bipolar patients (11, 12). There is a substantial case report literature reporting that many patients have benefited when lithium was added to an ongoing TCA. Often these results occurred rapidly, sometimes with very low doses of lithium. While the results of controlled trials have not been as dramatic, they still support this approach, which should be seriously considered for the treatment-resistant patient. More recently, Pope and colleagues reported on five refractory depressions who improved when lithium was added to fluoxetine (13). There is also data from a limited number of controlled studies, particularly in women, that adding T_3 may bring a nonresponder into remission.

Finally, the combination of a *tricyclic plus MAO inhibitor* should be done by a physician skilled in the use of these combinations and familiar with their potential adverse effects and interactions. For example, while desipramine is not recommended in combination with an MAOI, other heterocyclics plus MAOIs can be effective and safe in certain selected refractory, or partially responsive patients. Once the dose of the heterocyclic is established, the MAOI should be slowly added. **Never attempt the reverse order without a 2-week delay.** It may also be prudent to lower the heterocyclic dose slightly before starting the MAOI. An example might be the addition of phenelzine to amitriptyline, starting with an initial dose of 15 mg with subsequent dose increments weekly if needed. The total dose of an MAOI, used in combination with heterocyclics, is usually lower than when used alone (e.g., 30–60 mg/day). When the combination is discontinued, the MAOI should be stopped first.

If patients still show an insufficient response, there is some support for the following *combined treatment* strategies:

- TCA plus *SRI* (13a, 13b)
- AD plus *BZD*
- AD plus *antipsychotic*
- AD plus *psychostimulants* (e.g., amphetamine, methylphenidate)
- HCA, MAOI, or SRI plus *precursors* (e.g., L-tryptophan; currently removed from the market because of problems with eosinophilia myalgia syndrome)
- *Lithium* plus *CBZ or VPA*

Patients suffering from a *psychotic depression* do not benefit from a single heterocyclic or an MAO inhibitor and usually require the combination of an antidepressant/antipsychotic or ECT. There is limited evidence that amoxapine, whose primary active metabolite (8-hydroxy amoxapine) has antipsychotic-like properties, can also be used (14).

Depression associated with panic attacks may benefit from the combination of an antidepressant/anxiolytic or the use of a serotonin reuptake inhibitor (e.g., fluoxetine, sertraline, or paroxetine), which may have antipanic properties separate from their antidepressant effects.

Post and Kramlinger (1989) have also suggested that *lithium added to carbamazepine* may be useful in treatment-resistant mood disordered patients (15). One possible basis for this approach is that carbamazepine, which has a tricyclic ring structure similar to imipramine, may sensitize postsynaptic serotonin receptors in a similar way to standard drugs such as imipramine. A mood stabilizer (e.g., lithium, CBZ, VPA) plus AD may benefit some rapid cycling or mixed bipolar patients, attenuating the propensity to switch from mania to depression.

Alternate primary monotherapies include:

- ECT
- Lithium, carbamazepine, or VPA
- Buspirone
- Psychostimulants
- Stereotactic surgery

ECT should be considered for more severe forms of depression (e.g., those associated with melancholic and psychotic features, particularly when they pose an increased risk for self-injurious behavior) or when there is a past, well-documented history of nonresponse or intolerance to pharmacological intervention. There is limited data that bipolar depressed patients may be at risk for a switch to mania when given a standard heterocyclic. A mood stabilizer alone (i.e., lithium, CBZ, VPA), or in combination with an antidepressant, may be the drugs of choice in these patients. Some elderly patients and those with acquired immunodeficiency syndrome (AIDS) may also benefit from low doses of a *psychostimulant* only (e.g., amphetamine or methylphenidate) (see also The HIV-infected Patient in Chapter 14). Selected, truly treatment-resistant patients (particularly bipolar) with severe disorders unresponsive to any pharmacological or somatic intervention (e.g., ECT, bright light therapy, and sleep deprivation) may benefit from a *stereotactic tractotomy* of the subcaudate nucleus (16). Figure 7.1 summarizes the strategy for a patient insufficiently responsive to standard therapies.

Drug-Induced Depressive Syndromes

Treatment of these disorders is first directed at the causative agent (e.g., reserpine, α-methyldopa). Withdrawing the offending compound and providing supportive care may be all that is required, with the symptoms dissipating in days to weeks. When such conservative measures are unsuccessful, most clinicians initiate an antidepressant.

With drugs that produce a depression after chronic exposure (e.g., alcohol), detoxification is instituted, in addition to supportive care and therapy for substance dependency. While most alcoholics will experience depression immediately after the cessation of heavy and prolonged consumption, the majority will remit within 2 weeks following detoxification and supportive care (see The Alcoholic Patient in Chapter 14). For those who do not, it is likely there had been a pre-existing depressive disorder, which itself can lead to substance dependency, since patients frequently self-medicate prior to seeking professional intervention. This possibility should be evaluated through a review of the patient's personal medical/psychiatric history, as well as family history. The recovering patient who remains depressed after appropriate treatment of the abstinence syndrome should be given an antidepressant trial. Treatment planning should take into account the patient's physical status, especially as it may affect the pharmacokinetics and pharmacodynamics of the agent selected.

Role of Psychosocial Therapies

Since this book focuses on psychopharmacotherapy, it is not intended to review exhaustively the role of psychotherapy. Nonetheless, some form of counseling is usually necessary during the treatment of MDD. Broadly defined, psychotherapy covers a wide range of modalities, from simple education and supportive counseling to insight-oriented dynamically based therapy.

Since no illness occurs in a vacuum, medications should never be prescribed as the sole treatment. There is a fluid interaction between an individual and that individual's illness (e.g., life situations may aggravate the illness and vice versa). In addition, these disorders affect the way people think about themselves, as well as how other people view them. While the good practitioner is always cognizant of these issues, they are especially important in psychiatric disorders because of the difficulty patients have in separating themselves from the illness and its associated social stigma. Thus, patients may be able to view an illness such as cancer, as something that has happened to them and therefore as something distinct from themselves. This distancing is much more difficult with a psychiatric disorder, since it affects the fundamental processes (e.g., mood and cognition) that define oneself. This statement is particularly germane to MDD since it often involves feelings of guilt, worthlessness, low self-esteem, helplessness, and hopelessness. These symptoms, coupled with the delayed onset of drug action, make education and supportive counseling imperative.

A series of controlled outpatient studies has compared psychotherapy, tricyclics with psychotherapy, and a control group. The last consisted of patients who called for emergency appointments only (demand-only psychotherapy), a "low-contact" or a placebo group (17–20). The combined therapies had a greater efficacy on certain outcome measures than either treatment by itself, thus appearing to augment each other. Other studies found a clear therapeutic effect from ADs, but failed to find group therapy very helpful (21).

The first step in any psychotherapeutic process is education. Information should be given in a supportive manner, while also exploring whether life situations are aggravating the condition or vice versa. If medication is indicated, the patient should know why and what can be reasonably expected from this course of action. This should include an explanation of:

- *How medications* are believed to *work* for their condition
- *How to take* them
- What *life activities*, if any, need to be altered while on the medication
- The potential *adverse effects*, as well as what to do when they occur.

Education does not stop at this point, but is an ongoing process throughout treatment. Since MDD impairs concentration and attention, it is useful to repeat this information several times during the initial period (e.g., at follow-up visits). It is often helpful to query the patient about what has been explained and then clarify or expound on issues as indicated. **It is critically important to avoid patient discouragement by balancing optimism with the acknowledgement that antidepressants generally have a delayed onset of action.** It is also prudent to explain other options, especially if the first medication trial is unsuccessful. Thus, it is crucial to reassure the patient prior to the first AD trial that if unsuccessful, there is a good chance

of responding to an alternate therapy. Patients understand and accept the concept of empirical trials. Educating and involving them in the decision-making process is not only "politically correct," but also therapeutic because this:

- Addresses feelings of *loss of control* and *inadequacy*
- Makes a patient an *active participant* of the treatment
- Enhances *compliance*.

Education should continue even after the depressive episode has remitted. Thus, an explanation of the value of maintenance and prophylactic therapy, as well as when it is appropriate to discontinue treatment, is important. The early signs of relapse should be explained to both the patient and close family members or friends, if appropriate. The goal is to reduce the likelihood of relapse or recurrence, which when detected early will dictate a prompt reinstitution of therapy. This is based on the hope that early intervention will shorten the duration of an episode and lessen its consequences (22).

If there are more complicated problems or persistent personal issues, then formal psychotherapy may be indicated. That decision needs to be made within the context of an individual's specific situation. When possible, a recommendation for more intense psychotherapy should be reserved until there has been a reasonable opportunity to assess response to drug therapy plus education/supportive counseling. Many life situations that seem insurmountable become quite manageable when a depressive episode has remitted. This caveat is particularly important during the first episode in a patient with a good premorbid history and an illness duration of less than 1 year. It is also applicable to recurrent MDD when there has been a good return to psychosocial functioning between episodes.

REFERENCES

1. McCombs JS, Nichol MB, Stimmel GL, Sclar DA, Beasley CM Jr, Gross LS. The cost of antidepressant drug therapy failure: a study of antidepressant use patterns in a Medicaid population. J Clin Psychiatry 1990;51(6)suppl:60–69.
2. MacEwan WG, Remick RA. Treatment-resistant depression: a clinical perspective. Can J Psychiatry 1988;33:788–792.
3. Guscott R, Grof P. The clinical meaning of refractory depression: a review for the clinician. Am J Psychiatry 1991;148:695–704.
4. White K, Simpson G. Treatment resistant depression. Psychiatr Ann 1987;17:274–278.
5. Paykel ES, Van Waerkom AE. Parmacologic treatment of resistant depression. Psychiatr Ann 1987;17:327–331.
6. Nemeroff CB. Augmentation regimens for depression. J Clin Psychiatry 1991; 52(5)suppl:21–27.
7. Byrne MM. Meta-analysis of early phase II studies with paroxetine in hospitalized depressed patients. Acta Psychiatr Scand 1989;80(suppl 350):138–139.
8. Dunbar GC, Stoker MJ. Paroxetine in the treatment of severe (melancholic) depression. Presented at the 5th World Congress of Biological Psychiatry, Florence, June 1991.
9. Tyrer P, Marsden CA, Casey P, et al. Clinical efficacy of paroxetine in resistant depression. J Psychopharmacol 1987;1:251–257.
10. Gagiano CA, Mueller PGM, Fourie J, et al. The therapeutic efficacy of paroxetine: (a) an open study in patients with major depression not responding to antidepressants; (b) a double-blind comparison with amitriptyline in depressed outpatients. Acta Psychatr Scand 1989;80(suppl 350):130–131.
11. Heninger GR, Charney DS, Sternberg DE. Lithium carbonate augmentation of anti-depressant treatment. Arch Gen Psychiatry 1983;40:1335–1342.
12. Nelson JC, Mazure CM. Lithium augmentation in psychotic depression refractory to combined drug treatment. Am J Psychiatry 1986;143:363–366.
13. Pope HG, McElroy SL, Nixon RA. Possible synergism between fluoxetine and lithium in refractory depression. Am J Psychiatry 1988;145:1292–1294.
13a. Nelson JC, Mazure CM, Bowers MB, Jatlow PI. A preliminary open study of the combination of fluoxetine and desimipramine for rapid treatment of major depression. Arch Gen Psychiatry 1991;48:303–307.
13b. Weiberg JB, Rosenbaum JF, Biederman J, Sachs GS, Pollack MH, Kelly K. Fluoxetine added to non-MAOI antidepressants converts nonresponders to responders: a preliminary report. J Clin Psychiatry 1989;50:447–449.
14. Anton RF, Burch EA. Amoxapine versus amitriptyline combined with perphenazine in the treatment of psychotic depression. Am J Psychiatry 1990;147:1203–1208.
15. Post RM, Kramlinger KG. The addition of lithium to carbamazepine. Antidepressant efficacy in treatment-resistant depression. Arch Gen Psychiatry 1989;46:794–800.
16. Poynton A, Bridges PK, Bartlett JR. Resistant bipolar affective disorder treated by stereotactic subcaudate tractotomy. Br J Psychiatry 1988;152:354–358.
17. Klerman GL, Dimascio A, Weissman M, Prusoff B, Paykel ES. Treatment of depression by drugs and psychotherapy. Am J Psychiatry 1974;131:186–191.
18. Weissman MM, Klerman GL, Paykel ES, Prusoff B, Hanson B. Treatment effects on the social adjustment of depressed patients. Arch Gen Psychiatry 1974;30:771–778.
19. Klerman GL, Weissman MM, Rounsaville BJ, Chevron ES. Interpersonal psychotherapy of depression. New York: Basic Books, 1984.
20. Weissman MM, Jarrett RB, Rush JA. Psychotherapy and its relevance to the pharmacotherapy of major depression: a decade later (1976–1985). In: Meltzer HV, ed. Psychopharmacology: the third generation of progress. New York: Raven Press, 1987:1059–1069.
21. Coui L, Lipman RS, Derogatis LR, Smith JE III, Pattison JH. Drugs and group psychotherapy in neurotic depression. Am J Psychiatry 1974;131:191–198.
22. Kupfer DJ, Frank E, Perel JM. The advantage of early treatment intervention in recurrent depression. Arch Gen Psychiatry 1989;46:771–775.

Adverse Effects

Patient years of exposure to the TCAs is orders of magnitude greater than for any other class of antidepressant. Thus, their safety and tolerability in different types of patients with different illnesses and on different combinations of medications have been observed and documented for many years. The next substantial database is for trazodone, which has been marketed since 1982 and at one time was the most widely prescribed brand-name antidepressant in the United States. Although the SRIs have been available for a shorter period of time than the MAOIs or bupropion, their clinical database is substantially larger due to their greater acceptance.

An important aspect of proper pharmacotherapy is management of adverse effects, since most ADs are comparable in efficacy. Thus, use of psychological support and/or a change to a less problematic medication often makes adequate dosing possible. Conversely, insufficient flexibility or problem solving in the face of adverse effects may preclude adequate treatment. Table 7.17 lists the common potential adverse effects of these agents, as well as their relative severity.

Accurate identification of antidepressant-induced adverse effects is problematic, since many of these adverse reactions (e.g., fatigue, dry mouth, dizziness, constipation, sweating, tremor, nausea and vomiting, drowsiness, insomnia, and sexual impotence) are also associated with depression. Further, while some symptoms may have been present before the initiation of medication, others could emerge spontaneously, unrelated to ongoing drug therapy. Therefore, studies employing placebo control groups are important to determine if the frequency of a given adverse effect, occurring in conjunction with the administration of an AD, is greater than its base rate in a comparable, nonmedicated population.

HETEROCYCLIC ANTIDEPRESSANTS

Secondary amine TCAs (e.g., nortriptyline, desipramine) are better tolerated and somewhat safer than their tertiary amine parent compounds (e.g., amitriptyline, imipramine) (1, 2). This is due to differences in the relative potencies of several pharmacological actions, which include their binding affinity for:

- *Muscarinic acetylcholine receptors,* which mediates their atropine-like effects
- *Histamine receptors,* which may mediate their sedative and possibly the weight gain effects
- α-Adrenergic receptors, which mediate their orthostatic hypotensive effects (3).

In addition, their ability to stabilize electrically excitable membranes (i.e., quinidine-like properties) through inhibition of $Na^+:K^+$ ATPase, is the action most likely responsible for their most important adverse effect, cardiotoxicity (4).

Since tertiary amine TCAs are more potent than secondary amine TCAs in all these actions, the latter are generally safer and better tolerated. In addition, data from plasma level studies show that the secondary amines are more potent antidepressants than their parent compounds, so that lower concentrations can be used, increasing tolerance and safety (5). These facts explain why the secondary amines are

Table 7.17.
Adverse Effects of Antidepressants[a]

Drugs	Sedation	Anticholinergic	Orthostatic Hypotension	Cardiac Conduction Effects
HETEROCYCLICS				
Amitriptyline	High	High	Moderate	High
Imipramine	Moderate	Moderate	High	High
Doxepin	High	Moderate	Moderate	Moderate
Desipramine	Low	Low	Low	Moderate
Nortriptyline	Moderate	Moderate	Low	Moderate
Trimipramine	High	High	Moderate	High
Protriptyline	Low	Moderate	Low	Moderate
Clomipramine	High	High	Low	Moderate
Maprotiline	Moderate	Moderate	Low	Moderate
SEROTONIN REUPTAKE INHIBITORS				
Fluoxetine	Very low	None	Very low	Very low
Sertraline	Low	None	None	Very low
Paroxetine	Low	None	None	Very low
DIBENZOXAZEPINES				
Amoxapine	Low	Low	Low	Low
TRIAZOLOPYRIDINES				
Trazodone	High	Very low	Moderate	Low
AMINOKETONES				
Bupropion	Low	Very low	Very low	0
TRIAZOLOBENZODIAZEPINES				
Alprazolam	High	Very low	Very low	0
MONOAMINE OXIDASE INHIBITORS				
Phenelzine Tranylcypromine Isocarboxazid	As a class, orthostatic hypotension, dizziness, headache, drowsiness, overstimulation (hypomania, insomnia, anxiety), constipation, nausea, diarrhea, abdominal pain			

[a]Adapted from Ward M. Appendix B. In: Flaherty J, Davis JM, Janicak PG, eds. Psychiatry: diagnosis and therapy. Norwalk, CT: Appleton & Lang, 1993:493–494.

increasingly used by clinicians, paralleled by a decline in the use of the tertiary amine compounds.

We would emphasize that secondary amine TCAs can also be toxic when taken in overdoses, and this issue must always be considered when treating a patient who poses a substantial suicide risk. Further, despite their lower potential for adverse effects, they can cause sufficient anticholinergic, antihistaminic, and orthostatic problems to require discontinuation. In such patients, the clinician can monitor plasma drug levels to achieve the optimum range for response while minimizing the emergence of intolerable adverse effects.

The most troublesome problems with HCAs involve:

- The cardiovascular system
- The cholinergic system
- The noradrenergic system
- The central nervous system
- Overdose-related issues.

Cardiovascular Effects

Soon after the TCAs were introduced, it was noted that fatal overdoses were usually secondary to heart block or ventricular arrhythmias (6). This observation led to the concern that, in vulnerable patients, these drugs might produce similar complications at therapeutic plasma concentrations. Over the past 25 years, however, prospective trials have led to a more accurate understanding of their cardiac effects. The best way to review the present state of knowledge is to categorize these effects as follows:

- Orthostatic hypotension (significant)
- Conduction delays; arrhythmias (significant)
- Contractility impairment (not significant at usual clinical doses).

Orthostatic Hypotension

One of the most frequent and potentially serious adverse effects of HCAs (as well as MAOIs) is orthostatic hypotension. This effect leads to discontinuation of AD therapy in about 10% of healthy depressed patients. Further, fractures, lacerations, possible myocardial infarction, and sudden death have all been reported, especially in the elderly.

By far, the most studied drug is *imipramine*. There is less complete data for other HCAs. Existing studies, however, strongly imply that hypotension also occurs with *amitriptyline* and *desmethylimipramine*. It is interesting that little is known about *doxepin's* potential to lower blood pressure, although it is widely used. *Nortriptyline* is the only TCA currently on the market for which a reduced risk of orthostasis has clearly been documented. Thus, one study reported that this effect was negligible in 40 healthy, middle-aged depressed patients, and another clearly documented a reduced risk (7).

Both the rate and the magnitude of drug-induced hypotension increase dramatically with depressed patients suffering from cardiac disease. In 25 depressed patients with preexisting congestive heart failure, imipramine-induced orthostasis was approximately 50% (8). In contrast, of 21 patients without preexisting congestive failure treated with therapeutic plasma concentrations of nortriptyline, only one developed this problem. Furthermore, 19 of these 21 patients had previous trials of imipramine, with 8 experiencing falls on this agent.

Mechanism. The mechanism(s) underlying this effect is not clear, but various investigators have implicated:

- *Peripheral* α-adrenergic blockade
- Enhanced stimulation of *central* α-adrenergic receptors
- *Direct* adrenergic vasodilation.

Trazodone, which is equally potent in this regard, also causes postural hypotension, but nortriptyline, which is apparently more benign, also blocks α_1 receptors to the same degree.

The fact that a drug possesses a given property in vitro or in vivo, while presumptive evidence, does not necessarily mean that its therapeutic or adverse effects are mediated by that property. What is needed is direct evidence in humans that postural hypotension is caused by the α-adrenergic blocking properties of these drugs.

Interestingly, a significant risk factor for the development of orthostasis with imipramine may be depression itself. For example, one study found that of 22 nondepressed cardiac patients with some degree of congestive heart failure (i.e., mean ejection fraction 33% by radionuclide angiography) who were treated with imipramine for control of their arrhythmia, only one (4%) discontinued the medication because of orthostasis (9, 10). This rate contrasts with a 50% incidence of hypotension among melancholic patients with a similar degree of left-ventricular impairment treated with comparable plasma concentrations of imipramine. Muller et al. (1961) also found that 24 of 37 depressed cardiac patients experienced significant hypotension in contrast to none of the heart patients without depression (11).

Treatment. Patients should always be warned of this possible adverse effect and instructed to arise carefully from a lying or sitting position by dangling their feet before standing or sitting; or quickly lying down when feeling faint. Since falls resulting in broken bones or concussions can occur, such common sense precautions are important.

When hypotension remains problematic, support hose, salt, and fluids can also be used. Some recommend the use of the mineralocorticoid fluorohydrocortisone (Florinef, 0.025 to 0.05 mg twice a day).

Conduction Delays; Arrhythmias

Sudden death has occurred in patients with preexisting heart disease on antidepressant therapy. It may be difficult, however, to separate a causally related drug effect from a cardiovascular incident precipitated by other factors and only by

chance coincident with drug therapy. Further, Roose (1992), who has summarized the literature, noted that major depressive disorder occurs frequently after a myocardial infarct and may adversely affect the recovery process (12).

Early reports on imipramine noted that some patients developed first-degree heart block, as well as other bundle branch patterns; but it took almost 15 years to clarify that these conduction delays were the only adverse effects at therapeutic plasma concentrations. It is now well documented that increased PR, QRS, or QT intervals occur with all standard HCAs, at or slightly above their therapeutic plasma levels.

Electrophysiological studies have confirmed that the HCAs exert their major effect on the His-ventricular (HV) interval. Although they frequently prolong PR and QRS intervals in depressed patients with a normal pretreatment ECG, it is important to realize that such moderate increases are not, by themselves, clinically significant. This propensity to reduce conduction velocity, however, raises the question of whether those with preexisting disorders would be at increased risk to develop symptomatic AV block. This concern was supported by the frequency of AV block after overdose, and by case reports of patients with preexisting bundle branch block who developed two-to-one block when treated with imipramine.

Roose et al. (1987) recently completed a prospective study of 41 depressed patients with first-degree AV or bundle branch block (or both) who were compared to 151 patients with normal pretreatment ECGs (13). Both groups were treated with therapeutic plasma concentrations of imipramine or nortriptyline. The rate of two-to-one AV block was significantly higher (9%) in patients with preexisting bundle branch block, as compared with the rate (0.7%) in those with normal pretreatment ECGs ($p <$ 0.05 by Fisher's Exact Test). In fact, the one patient with a normal pretreatment ECG who developed two-to-one AV block had an abnormal His conduction, apparent only by catheterization.

It has been established that therapeutic plasma concentrations of TCAs have powerful and clinically significant antiarrhythmic activity (14). Imipramine and nortriptyline (and probably other HCAs) share electrophysiological properties characteristic of type I (A, B) compounds (e.g., quinidine, procainamide, and disopyramide) and are even used occasionally in cardiac patients free from depression, exclusively for the control of arrhythmia.

Because overdoses can cause severe arrhythmias, it had been previously thought that these drugs were contraindicated in patients with preexisting problems. A drug, however, may not produce the same cardiovascular effect at a therapeutic versus a toxic plasma concentration. In one study, 17 of 22 nondepressed cardiac patients with ventricular arrhythmias had more than 75% premature ventricular contraction (PVC) suppression after imipramine treatment (15). Particularly important from the cardiologist's perspective, imipramine also suppressed PVCs with complex features, a more serious type of rhythm disturbance. Significant reductions also occurred in the frequency of bigeminy (85% ± 45%), pairs (89% ± 30%), and ventricular tachycardia (99% ± 2%). It should be noted that combining similar agents (e.g., imipramine plus quinidine) may produce a *proarrhythmic* effect.

Contractility Problems. Until recently, it had been widely assumed that HCAs adversely affected left-ventricular function (LVF). The method used to assess LVF was the systolic time interval, a measurement partly dependent on the QRS duration. Since HCAs prolong QRS, their effect is probably due to their impact on conduction, and not on LVF.

The introduction of radionuclide angiography has provided a more reliable means of assessing drug effects on LVF. Using this methodology, relatively low doses of imipramine and doxepin did not impair LVF in 17 depressed patients; however, only a few had ejection fractions below 40%. Subsequently, Glassman et al. (1983) reported radionuclide data on 15 depressed patients with moderate to severe LVF impairment (mean ejection fraction 33%) treated with therapeutic plasma concentrations of imipramine (16). Although imipramine had no deleterious effect on any measure of LVF, as previously discussed, it produced intolerable orthostatic hypotension in about 50%. This finding was replicated in a second series of 10 depressed patients with heart failure (mean pretreatment ejection fraction 31%), who also had no change in any measure of LVF when treated with therapeutic plasma concentrations of imipramine. Thus, while many patients with CHF appear to tolerate TCAs, the number of reports is limited, and decisions to use these agents should be on a case-by-case basis.

In summarizing the relationship between TCA therapy and cardiovascular effects, Roose and Glassman (1984) concluded that TCAs:

- Are *antiarrhythmic* agents and are effective in patients with ventricular ectopic activity
- Do not have an adverse effect on *cardiac output,* even in those with CHF
- *Slow conduction,* which places patients with bundle branch block (BBB) at risk to develop conduction complications (17).

Anticholinergic Effects

Typical autonomic effects resulting from the anticholinergic properties of these agents include:

- Dry mouth
- Loss of visual accommodation; aggravation of narrow-angle glaucoma (rarely)
- Palpitations; tachycardia; dizziness
- Urinary hesitancy or retention; constipation; rarely paralytic ileus (may be severe or even fatal)
- Edema
- Memory impairment

Dry mouth is the most common autonomic adverse effect, and patients should be alerted to its possible occurrence. *Profuse sweating,* especially at night, can also occur; but the precise mechanism is unknown. *Dental caries* have been reported when patients attempt to relieve dry mouth by ingesting hard candy or soft drinks; therefore, sugar-free substances should be recommended. Finally, there is a loss of the bacteriostatic effects of saliva, predisposing the patient to increased risk for oral infections.

These autonomic adverse effects are usually mild and typically become less bothersome after the first few weeks of treatment. In any event, they can be controlled by adjusting the drug dosage. Bethanechol (Urecholine) (25–50 mg) given 3–4 times a day can reverse the urinary retention.

Using in vitro assay techniques to measure the binding of agents to muscarinic receptors in the brain, intestine, or other tissue, it was found that amitriptyline has the strongest anticholinergic properties, doxepin is intermediate, and desipramine the weakest (18). In vitro and animal studies have shown that trazodone, fluoxetine, sertraline, and paroxetine have essentially no anticholinergic adverse effects. Consis-

tent with their pharmacology, clinical studies find that they produce no more anticholinergic problems than placebo. While it is not known to what degree in vitro preparations correlate with in vivo activity, one can assume a positive correlation.

Central Anticholinergic Syndrome

This toxic reaction is manifested by:

- Florid visual hallucinations
- Loss of immediate memory
- Confusion
- Disorientation.

Diagnosis is based on the typical symptom picture and reversibility by physostigmine, an agent that increases brain acetylcholine, thus overcoming the atropine blockade. Discontinuance of anticholinergics usually ends the problem within a day or so. Rarely, in selected cases, physostigmine can produce a dramatic reversal, but it should not be used hastily, as error in diagnosis or too much of this drug may produce a cholinergic toxic syndrome.

Withdrawal Syndrome

There is no withdrawal problem with the TCAs of the type seen with narcotics, alcohol, or sedatives. Instead, abrupt discontinuation of 150–300 mg/day or more of a tricyclic, especially after 3 or more months of treatment, can induce an autonomic rebound (i.e., gastrointestinal disturbances, autonomic symptoms, anxiety, agitation, and disrupted sleep). The incidence varies, depending on dosage and duration of consumption. The higher the daily dosage and the longer it has been ingested, the more likely the occurrence. Onset usually begins by 48 hours after abrupt discontinuation in some, but not all, patients. These symptoms may be related to the anticholinergic potency of the

TCA. Withdrawal of the drug produces a state of muscarinic receptor supersensitivity, resulting in "cholinergic overdrive." If abrupt withdrawal is necessitated by a switch to hypomania or mania, temporary benztropine therapy can minimize the risk of autonomic symptoms. Generally, antidepressants should be discontinued by gradual taper.

Noradrenergic Effects

Jitteriness, tachycardia, and tremor can occur early in the course of treatment, particularly in patients with comorbid panic attacks. TCAs may cause a persistent, fine, rapid *tremor,* particularly in the upper extremities. Desipramine and protriptyline may be the most common offenders. Propranolol (60 mg/day) may help and is unlikely to worsen depression. Alternatively, switching to a drug with less NE activity may also help.

Central Nervous System Effects

Insomnia has been reported, especially in the elderly, but it is usually transitory and responds to morning dosing or switching to a more sedating antidepressant. While all these drugs produce sedation, there are quantitative differences. For example, amitriptyline, doxepin, and trazodone are more sedating than desipramine, nortriptyline, and protriptyline. Patients should be cautioned that the sedation produced by alcohol may add to or potentiate the drug's sedative effects. The pharmacological mechanism for sedation is not well understood, with 5-HT_1, H_1, or H_2 receptor blockade all implicated.

While more "stimulating" antidepressants (e.g., protriptyline, fluoxetine, or certain MAOIs) do not potentiate alcohol, they can produce insomnia. To minimize this problem, the dose may be given ear-

lier in the day. TCAs may cause episodes of schizophrenic *excitement* (very rare), confusion, or mania, usually in patients so predisposed, suggesting that a preexisting disorder must be present for these drugs to exert any psychotomimetic effects.

In addition to large overdoses of these drugs, amounts used clinically may occasionally produce *seizures.* Since convulsions may be unrelated to drug treatment, however, their origin should always be carefully evaluated. Preskorn and Fast (1992) found that the only risk factor associated with seizures in eight patients on routine TCA therapy was an elevated plasma level (mean = 734 ± 249 ng/ml; range = 438–1200 ng/ml) (19). This may be less of a problem with agents such as trazodone.

Maprotiline and bupropion cause more seizures than agents such as imipramine, amitriptyline, and nortriptyline. Thus, the relative rate of seizure occurrence (reported seizures divided by market share) is 6 to 30 times higher with maprotiline, which can cause seizures in doses only slightly above the recommended range. This has prompted some clinicians to start with a low dose (75 mg/day, or in elderly patients, even less), gradually increasing it by 25 mg increments over 2 or more weeks (remembering that the drug has a half-life of about 48 hours). Average doses in outpatients are 150 mg, with a maximum of 225 mg.

In a review of 37 reported cases, Davidson (1989) found that the risk of seizures with bupropion appeared to be higher with doses above the recommended maximum (i.e., 450 mg/day) (20). An increased risk of seizures was also noted in eating-disordered patients (i.e., bulimics) on bupropion, leading to its temporary withdrawal from the market.

Twitching, dysarthria, paresthesia, peroneal palsies, and *ataxia* may also occur in rare instances. Disturbances of *motor function* are uncommon, and most likely to occur in the elderly.

Overdose

HCAs are now the third most common cause of drug-related deaths, exceeded only by alcohol-drug combinations and heroin (21). Although it is well known that these agents can be fatal, the mechanism and the most appropriate therapeutic interventions are less clear.

An overdose of an imipramine-type antidepressant produces a clinical picture characterized by:

- Temporary agitation; confusion; convulsions
- Hypotension, tachycardia, conduction delays
- Manifestations of anticholinergic blockade
  - Bowel and bladder paralysis
  - Disturbance of temperature regulation
  - Mydriasis
  - Delirium.

Patients may progress to *coma* (generally lasting less than 24 hours) often complicated by shock and respiratory depression. Although a tricyclic-induced coma is usually short in duration, it can result in death secondary to cardiac arrhythmias.

The most characteristic and serious sequelae of overdose involve disturbances in cardiac *conduction and repolarization*. These disturbances are manifested clinically by:

- AV block
- Intraventricular conduction defects
- Prolongation of the QT interval.

As conduction times are prolonged, the chance of developing reentry arrhythmias grows. Malignant ventricular arrhythmias are uncommon in mild or moderate overdoses, but are more likely in severe cases.

All of these signs and symptoms may be present to some degree or may be absent, depending on the quantity of drug(s) ingested. The lethal dose has been estimated to be about 10 to 30 times the daily dose level. It is clear that all of the standard tricyclics can be fatal in overdose, and the same is true for some of the newer HCAs, such as maprotiline (by a different mechanism) and amoxapine. In a recent series of 32 fatal ingestions, 14 victims died on the way to the hospital, 9 were alive on arrival but already had major symptoms, and the remaining 9 arrived without major symptoms, but developed them within 2 hours of arriving (22). All deaths from the direct toxicity of the drug occurred within the first 24 hours.

Disturbances of cardiac rhythm (e.g., tachycardia, atrial fibrillation, ventricular flutter, and AV or intraventricular block) are the most frequent causes of death. Thus, management of cardiac function is critical. If the patient survives the early phase, recovery without sequelae is probable, and vigorous resuscitative measures are important. A major clinical problem is determining when a patient is no longer in danger. Many with mild overdose have been hospitalized unnecessarily or for inordinately prolonged periods because of this concern. Late deaths (2 to 5 days after overdose) have been seen; however, most of these involved complications that had presented earlier and were expected (23, 24). It appears that if a patient has not developed any major symptoms after 6 hours (depressed level of consciousness, hypotension, depressed respiration, seizures, conduction block, or arrhythmia), it is unlikely he or she will do so. While clinicians need to know about the rare possibility of late death, some degree of common sense is required when a decision is necessary regarding the discontinuation of more intensive medical care.

While the literature indicates that seizures and arrhythmias are associated with TCA plasma levels above 1000 ng/ml, the QRS duration might be a better early predictor than plasma levels. For example, in a series of 49 TCA overdoses, seizures occurred only in cases with a QRS duration above 0.10 second, and ventricular arrhythmia was seen with a QRS greater than 0.16 second (25). Thus, for acute overdose the ECG may provide a reliable and quick measure of risk with TCA drugs; however, how well a QRS of less than 0.10 predicts ultimate safety or how long after ingestion the ECG must be followed, is uncertain.

The most frequent cardiovascular effects of an acute overdose are tachycardia and hypotension. The hypotension is partially related to a relative volume depletion, but correction does not bring complete resolution. While radionuclide and catheterization studies have shown that HCAs do not impair LVF, either at therapeutic plasma levels or with overdose, data are not available for victims who died. One study describes two cases of fatal overdose in which ventricular pacing produced regular ventricular depolarization but minimal cardiac output, suggesting that at very high concentrations, HCAs might directly impair the myocardium (as demonstrated in animal studies) (26).

CNS toxicity is a serious problem with *maprotiline*, and the probable mechanism of death rather than cardiac complications. *Trazodone* is probably benign, as documented by a substantial number of overdoses occurring without death. *Fluoxetine, sertraline, paroxetine,* and *bupropion* appear safe (e.g., no seizures have been reported with fluoxetine overdose), but have not yet had extensive use, so this conclusion must be regarded as tentative.

Treatment

The one principle about which there is no dispute is aggressive interventions to rapidly remove the drug. The contents of the stomach should be emptied in any suspected HCA overdose, since once absorbed, dialysis has not been successful in removing these drugs. Treatment should include:

• Induced vomiting or gastric aspiration
• Lavage with activated charcoal
• Anticonvulsants (such as intravenous diazepam)
• Coma care
• Support of respiration
• Attention to cardiac effects.

A slurry of activated charcoal given repeatedly through a nasogastric tube, following the initial emptying of the stomach, greatly accelerates tricyclic elimination, probably due to the large enterohepatic circulation that is interrupted by the repeated charcoal (27). While encouraging, this technique has been subjected to only limited study in actual cases of overdose.

Treatment with quinidine or similar drugs might be considered for ventricular arrhythmias, but if the physician realizes that the HCAs themselves are type I antiarrhythmic agents, *the dangers of this procedure* become apparent. Although systematic studies are not yet available, it would seem reasonable to treat these victims as one would treat quinidine overdoses (i.e., with hypertonic sodium bicarbonate and pacing). This therapeutic regimen should significantly increase the percentage of surviving patients, or at least, ensure that the treatment will not unintentionally exacerbate the problem. Tachycardia is generally not a problem, and the use of physostigmine to counteract it is controversial.

Miscellaneous Adverse Effects
Weight Gain

Many antidepressants cause weight gain, possibly by decreasing the basal metabolic rate; but the exact mechanism is unknown. For those with this problem, fluoxetine, sertraline, paroxetine, trazodone, and bupropion may be better options. Indeed, some have lost weight on fluoxetine, leading to the potential marketing of this agent as an anorectic.

Sexual Dysfunction

Priapism is an abnormal, painful, and persistent erection, not related to sexual arousal that can be caused by a variety of conditions (e.g., neurological, hematological, local trauma, and scorpion or black widow spider bites). Its occurrence also has been associated with various drugs, including:

- Antipsychotics, such as chlorpromazine and thioridazine
- Drugs of abuse, such as marijuana or cocaine
- Antihypertensives, such as guanethidine and hydralazine
- Antidepressants, such as trazodone.

Its occurrence should be considered an acute medical emergency, and in the first few hours after an episode, the patient should be closely monitored. Increased penile tumescence should lead to immediate discontinuation of the drug and consultation with a urologist. If the condition persists, retained blood can lead to edema and eventual fibrosis of the corpora, at times culminating in impotence. Such an emergency requires direct injection into the cavernous bulbosa or surgical detumescence (28). As this adverse effect is rare, many specialists have not had extensive experience, and it may be useful to contact the medical staff of the drug's manufacturer to help find an experienced urologist.

Hypersensitivity Effects

Skin reactions occur early in therapy, but often subside with reduced dosage. Jaundice, which can also occur early, is of the cholestatic type, similar to that attributed to chlorpromazine. Agranulocytosis is a very rare complication, as are cases of leukocytosis, leukopenia, and eosinophilia. There are no data on the incidence of tricyclic-induced agranulocytosis, except to note that it is very rare.

SEROTONIN REUPTAKE INHIBITORS

Fluoxetine was the first SRI marketed in the United States, in 1988. Since then, sertraline and paroxetine have also been approved, while others are likely to be marketed in the next few years. There is less data in terms of patient-years experience with these medications in comparison to the HCAs, but such information is rapidly growing due to their widespread acceptance. While clinical trials comparing SRIs to tertiary amine TCAs found the newer agents to have better-tolerated side-effect profiles, these differences were less evident when they were compared to secondary amine TCAs (29–34). The most important advantage of the SRIs is the absence of severe adverse effects (e.g., cardiac conduction delays, seizures, postural hypotension) and death from overdose.

The side-effect profiles of SRIs and TCAs are generally different, with those related to the former most consistent with serotonin agonism (30–32, 35). The most frequent complications include:

- Headache; dizziness
- Nausea; loose stools; constipation

- Somnolence; or insomnia
- Sweating; tremor; dry mouth.
- Anxiety; restlessness.

Whereas infrequent adverse effects include:

- Weight gain
- Inhibition of ejaculation and/or orgasm
- Bruxism; myoclonus; parasthesia

The management of the most common adverse effects includes:

- *Nausea.* Usually transient and dose-related. May improve with:
  - Dose reduction
  - Symptomatic measures (e.g., food, antacids)
- *Anorexia.* More pronounced in overweight patients and those with carbohydrate craving. May lead to abuse in patients with bulimia or anorexia nervosa. Possibly more common with fluoxetine.
- *Increased anxiety and nervousness.* Occurs early in treatment, especially in patients with prominent anxiety symptoms. May improve with support, dose reduction, or concomitant treatment with a benzodiazepine. May be less marked with paroxetine.
- *Tremor.* May improve with:
  - Dose reduction
  - A β-blocker
  - A benzodiazepine.

These adverse effects rarely require discontinuation, and several are dose-related (e.g., anxiety, tremor, and nausea) (35, 36). As with all other classes of antidepressants, the SRIs often have a delayed onset of action, but unlike TCAs, the effective dose can be given from the beginning, rather than by gradual titration. Realizing these facts can help to minimize adverse effects by resisting the temptation to increase the dose within the first 2 to 3 weeks of treatment.

In addition to a different side-effect profile, SRIs differ from TCAs by virtue of their wider safety margin, since they have not been found to cause life-threatening toxic effects (e.g., patients having survived acute ingestion of amounts equal to ten times the daily dose) (30). For this reason, some clinicians prefer these drugs in patients who may be a significant suicide risk.

This rationale, however, has been recently brought into question by concerns that fluoxetine (and by inference other SRIs) might increase the likelihood of suicide in some patients (37, 38). An analysis of clinical trial experience with several SRIs does not reveal an increased incidence of suicide attempts or completions in comparison to patients who were randomly assigned to placebo or a TCA (35, 39, 40). An excellent review by Mann and Kapur (1991) concludes that depressed patients are at greater risk by virtue of their disorder; the overall incidence of suicide does not differ significantly among the various types of ADs; but there may be a subgroup of patients more susceptible to certain adverse effects of SRIs such as agitation and akathisia, perhaps predisposing them to a paradoxical increase in suicidal ideation or behavior (39). They further postulate that the biochemical mechanism may be a temporary decrease in firing rates of presynaptic 5-HT neurons. Careful monitoring of such symptoms and requesting the patient to inform the clinician immediately upon their emergence may be the best way to prevent such potential sequelae.

MONOAMINE OXIDASE INHIBITORS

Despite contrary impressions, MAOIs are generally well tolerated if patients observe the restricted diet and avoid medications that contain sympathomimetic amines. Thus, adverse effects are rarely a treatment-limiting problem. MAOIs also fall between TCAs and SRIs in terms of overdose risk. Major toxic reactions to MAOIs are uncommon but require immediate discontinuation and symptomatic treatment.

Hypotension

In the absence of a dietary indiscretion, the primary problem is a decrease in blood pressure, which can be appreciable and must be carefully managed to avoid precipitating a hypertensive rebound (41–44). While most often orthostatic in nature, a general reduction in blood pressure can be seen in some patients. This adverse effect may present as fatigue or decreased motivation. Hence, the unsuspecting clinician may erroneously interpret it as a worsening of the depressive episode. Monitoring the blood pressure (both lying and standing) at every visit and making arrangements for blood pressure checks between seeing the physician is advisable until the optimal dose has been established with regard to efficacy, safety, and tolerability.

One pharmacological theory of the mechanism underlying postural hypotension is the false transmitter theory. Tyramine may be metabolized to an inactive metabolite (i.e., octopamine) that partially fills the NE storage vesicles with a false (inactive) transmitter, but definitive proof is lacking.

The dose of MAOI can sometimes be reduced, but this adverse effect often occurs at the minimal therapeutic dose. A good *fluid* intake plus increased *salt* intake, support *stockings,* and a *mineralocorticoid* (e.g., fluorohydrocortisone at doses of 0.3 to 0.8 mg) can alleviate the problem.

Hypertensive Crisis

Hypertensive crisis is fortunately rare but nonetheless a severe and potentially fatal complication. It results from the interaction of MAOIs and tyramine-containing foods or sympathomimetic drugs. Prodromal symptoms include:

- Sharply *elevated blood pressure*
- Severe occipital *headaches*
- *Stiff neck*
- *Sweating*
- Nausea and *vomiting.*

Because of this risk, a patient's ability to comply with the dietary restrictions should be carefully evaluated before starting treatment. Hospitalized patients should be placed on a tyramine-free diet and outpatients should be questioned about their history of compliance, suicidal potential, and ability to comprehend the dietary restrictions, which should be given in writing. Patients who cannot follow directions accurately or who may be manipulative or suicidal should not be considered for treatment with MAOIs.

Table 7.18 lists foods and drugs to be avoided while the patient is taking MAOIs. For a complete description of the tyramine content of foods and beverages, see Shulman et al (1989) (45). Recent case reports indicate that alcohol-free beer may pose a significant risk as well (45a). It may be helpful to recommend that the patient keep a diary and record any untoward events that follow ingestion of certain foods or drinks. In this way, a personalized diet can be constructed while making the patient more aware of those foods that pose a risk.

Written instructions in case of an adverse reaction usually require that the patient be directed to an emergency room for evaluation, monitoring, and treatment.

Table 7.18.
Dietary and Drug Restrictions for Monoamine Oxidase Inhibitors[a]

Foods	Drugs
HIGH tyramine content per serving—MUST BE AVOIDED	Stimulants
Aged cheese, (e.g., English stilton, cheddar, camembert, blue)	Decongestants
Yeast products	Antihypertensives
Pickled or salted herring, snails	
Aged meats, processed meats, any nonfresh meats	Antidepressants
Chicken liver or beef liver (more than 2 days old)	Imipramine
Broad bean pods (fava beans)	Desipramine
Sauerkraut	Fluoxetine
Banana peel	Bupropion
Licorice	Narcotics
	Meperidine
MODERATE tyramine content per serving—LIMITED AMOUNTS	Dextromethorphan
ALLOWABLE	Pressor agents
Soy sauce	General anesthetics
Sour cream	Sedatives
Cyclamates, monosodium glutamate	Hypoglycemics
LOW tyramine content per serving—PERMISSIBLE	Over-the-counter
Pasteurized cheeses, cream cheese	preparations
Distilled spirits (in moderation)	containing
Caffeine-containing beverages (e.g., coffee, tea, cola drinks)	caffeine or other
Fresh liver (less than one serving per day)	stimulants,
Smoked fish (salmon, carp, whitefish)	(e.g., ephedrine)

[a]Adapted from Janicak PG et al. Pharmacological treatment of depression. In: Flaherty J, Davis JM, Janicak PG, eds. Psychiatry: diagnosis and therapy. Norwalk, CT: Appleton & Lang, 1993:54–61.

Nonspecific treatment of a hypertensive crisis includes:

- Discontinuance of the MAOI
- Acidification of the urine to hasten elimination
- Maintenance of glucose and temperature balance.

To control hypertension, *phentolamine,* 5 mg intravenously, is recommended, with repeated doses of 0.25–0.5 mg intramuscularly every 4–6 hours. Alternatively, *chlorpromazine,* 50 mg intramuscularly followed by 25 mg intramuscularly every 1–2 hours, or *nifedipine,* 10 mg, bitten and placed under the tongue, may be used to control the crisis. Blood pressure should be monitored closely to avoid overcompensation and hypotensive episodes.

We studied platelet MAO levels after phenelzine was discontinued and found that the half-life of MAO regeneration was about 5 days (46). Nevertheless, one reliable patient required hospitalization for a hypertensive crisis precipitated by cheese ingested 12 days after phenelzine discontinuation. Patients should be asked to follow dietary restrictions for at least 2 weeks after discontinuation to allow regeneration of enzymes.

Recently, the FDA approved the MAO-B inhibitor L-deprenyl for use in Parkinson's disease. At the lower dose range it does not interact with tyramine, but there is serious doubt about its antidepressant properties at these levels. Other selective and/or reversible MAOIs will be available in the near future, holding out the promise of a much safer generation of drugs. As noted earlier, *moclobemide*, a reversible and selective MAO-A type inhibitor (RIMA), may become the MAOI of choice, if approved in the United States.

Central Serotonin Syndrome

This is a toxic hyperserotonergic event that is thought to result from hyperstimulation of brainstem and spinal cord 5-HT_{1A} receptors (47). It is characterized by the following symptoms:

- Gastrointestinal
  - Abdominal cramping
  - Bloating
  - Diarrhea
- Neurological
  - Tremulousness
  - Myoclonus
  - Dysarthria
  - Incoordination
  - Headache
- Cardiovascular
  - Tachycardia
  - Hypotension
  - Hypertension
  - Cardiovascular collapse—death
- Psychiatric
  - Hypomanic symptoms
  - Racing thoughts
  - Pressure of speech
  - Elevated or dysphoric mood
  - Confusion
  - Disorientation
- Other
  - Diaphoresis
  - Elevated temperature
  - Hyperthermia
  - Hyperreflexia.

Hyperpyrexia and death may be the outcome of this rare drug-drug interaction, which occurs primarily between MAOIs and SRIs (but also with certain HCAs and demerol). Therefore, it is mandatory to wait at least 1 week before switching from an SRI to an HCA, and at least 5 weeks when switching from fluoxetine to an MAOI, particularly tranylcypromine. It is probably safe to use a drug-free period of only a few days when switching from a tricyclic to an MAOI. If the syndrome develops, management consists of discontinuation of the offending agents and waiting for resolution. While not adequately documented in humans, methysergide (5-HT antagonist) or propranolol (a 5-HT_{1A} antagonist) may be helpful.

Hepatotoxicity

This is an uncommon reaction, most frequently associated with iproniazid, a hydrazine-based MAOI that has been removed from general use. The reaction seemed to be related to the liberation of free hydrazine and does not occur with nonhydrazine MAOIs. The risk of hepatotoxicity with currently available hydrazine MAOIs (phenelzine, isocarboxazid) is extremely low.

Miscellaneous Adverse Effects

Other reactions include a *lupus-like syndrome* (again, primarily associated with iproniazid); *rash;* and total *suppression of REM sleep.*

Like most antidepressants and lithium, the MAOIs can also cause *weight gain.* As they do not affect cholinergic receptors, they produce less constipation, dry mouth, and blurred vision, typically associated with the tricyclics. MAOIs do produce some similar adverse effects, particularly urinary hesitancy, possibly because of their adrenergic effects.

The most common MAOI *behavioral toxicity* is the precipitation of a hypomanic or manic episode; but restlessness, hyperactivity, agitation, irritability, and confusion can also occur. Rare cases of paranoid psychosis have been reported.

OTHER ANTIDEPRESSANT CLASSES

Triazolopyridines

Trazodone, the only marketed triazolopyridine, also has a side-effect profile that differs substantially from other antidepressants. It has minimal anticholinergic or serotonin agonistic effects but can cause orthostatic hypotension. *Sedation and cognitive slowing are the most frequent dose-limiting adverse effects* (35, 48, 49). Although trazodone has little direct action on the heart, *aggravation of arrhythmias has been reported* in patients with preexisting ventricular conduction disorders, but there are no controlled studies (50–52). Again, the association may have been coincidental. Like the SRIs, trazodone is nonlethal in overdoses and has a *wide safety margin.*

Concerns about *priapism* invariably arise when trazodone is discussed. This adverse effect is *rare, occurring in only 1 out of 6000 treated males* (53, 54). If the patient is informed of this possibility and discontinues the drug promptly, priapism usually resolves without further intervention. While earlier persistent cases were treated surgically, this approach carries a 50% chance of permanent impotence, and pharmacological intervention via *direct injections into the cavernous bulbosa* is preferable (55, 56). Using this approach, the chance of permanent impotence is quite low and depends on the duration of symptoms prior to treatment (57). This latter fact is another reason to fully inform the male patient on trazodone, so that early detection and intervention can be implemented.

Aminoketones

Bupropion, the only marketed aminoketone antidepressant, also has a side-effect profile different from the other classes of antidepressants. It is essentially devoid of anticholinergic, antihistaminic, and orthostatic hypotensive effects. Its principal adverse effects include:

- Restlessness
- Activation
- Tremors
- Insomnia
- Nausea (58).

These adverse effects bear some similarity to those of the SRIs. While these adverse effects rarely require discontinuation, aggravation of psychosis and seizures by this agent do (59–62).

Seizures occur at a rate of 4 per 1000 patients when the dose is kept below 450 mg/day in those without known risk factors (59, 63). The pathogenesis of bupropion-induced seizures may be in part pharmacokinetically mediated (64). This conclusion is based upon several observations:

- Incidence of seizures is *dose-dependent*
- Seizures generally *occur within days of a dose increase*
- Seizures generally *occur within the first few hours after the dose*
- Bulimic patients with increased *lean body mass* may be at higher risk for seizures.

Bupropion undergoes extensive biotransformation in man to three metabolites that have pharmacological activity (65). During treatment, these metabolites accumulate in concentrations several times higher than the parent compound (66). There is some case material suggesting that high plasma levels of these metabolites, particularly hydroxybupropion, may be associated with an increased incidence of serious adverse effects, as well as poorer antidepressant response (64). Based upon these observations, the safe and effective use of bupropion might be enhanced by TDM to rationally adjust the dose, but further research is needed to test the clinical utility of this approach.

Bupropion falls between TCAs and SRIs in terms of safety in overdose. Death is a rare possibility with an overdose of bupropion alone due to the absence of adverse effects on the cardiovascular or the respiratory systems (58). Seizures may occur but are readily treatable in a hospital setting.

ADVERSE EFFECTS RELATED TO PHARMACOKINETIC INTERACTIONS

Tricyclic Antidepressants

TCAs do not generally interfere with the metabolism of other drugs, with the possible exception of *valproic acid,* whose metabolism is induced by amitriptyline and perhaps other TCAs (Vanvalkenburg C, personal communication). In contrast, *TCA metabolism can be induced by cigarette smoking and regular alcohol ingestion as well as by a number of drugs,* including:

- Barbiturates
- Carbamazepine
- Phenytoin
- Valproic acid (4, 67, 68).

While the effect of cigarette smoking is usually trivial (i.e., about a 15% induction), the effect of other agents can be clinically significant (i.e., 50 to 100% change) (69, 70). *TCA metabolism can also be inhibited* by several types of agents, including:

- Cimetidine
- Antipsychotics
- At least some SRIs, such as fluoxetine (71–73).

Both enzyme induction and inhibition are clinically important because the antidepressant and the toxic effects of TCAs are concentration-dependent (5, 74). The clinician must be alert to this effect *on initiation and discontinuation of any agent* capable of inducing or inhibiting the metabolism of concomitantly prescribed medications.

Serotonin Reuptake Inhibitors

SRIs differ substantially in terms of their ablility to alter the metabolism of other drugs. Based on in vitro testing using isolated *hepatocytes and debrisoquine as a model drug,* the rank order of SRIs for producing such effects is: *paroxetine > fluoxetine = norfluoxetine > sertraline;* however, there are limitations to such tests (74a). First, the absolute potency may vary depending upon factors such as the in vitro hepatocyte preparation and the model drug chosen. Second, the effect may be concentration-dependent, so that it is important to know what concentrations are expected in the clinical setting and how they relate to the in vitro findings. Relative to this point, patients on fluoxetine (20 mg/day) achieve plasma concentrations of the parent compound and its active metabolite, norfluoxetine, an order of magnitude higher than the plasma concentrations of sertraline (50 mg/day) or paroxetine (20 mg/day) (19, 73, 75, 76). Thus, the in vitro findings cannot be directly extrapolated to the clinical setting; rather, they are useful screening procedures to determine whether there is the potential for a pharmacokinetic interaction.

Based upon case reports and formal studies, the in vitro effect of fluoxetine on CYPIID6 does have clinical relevance in terms of *raising the plasma concentrations* of a variety of coprescribed medications or their metabolites, including:

- *TCAs*
- *Bupropion*
- 2-Ketobenzodiazepines (e.g., *diazepam*)
- Some triazolobenzodiazepines (e.g., *alprazolam*)
- Some *antipsychotics*
- *Carbamazepine and valproic acid* (64, 71, 77).

From the case reports with TCAs, this interaction can vary substantially among patients (*ranging from a 2- to 10-fold increase in TCA plasma levels*) and possibly resulting in serious toxicity.

In a double-blind, parallel design in normal volunteers, the effect of 21 days of treatment with fluoxetine (20 mg/day) or sertraline (50 mg/day) in combination with desipramine (50 mg/day) was studied (19). Fluoxetine caused an average 350% increase in plasma desipramine levels by day 21, whereas sertraline caused less than a 30% increase. This effect persisted for more than 21 days after fluoxetine's discontinuation but had resolved after 7 days off sertraline, consistent with the difference in their half-lives. In a separate study, paroxetine (20 mg/day) caused a 3-fold increase in the half-life and a 5-fold decrease in the total clearance of desipramine in normal volunteers (78). Further study is needed to determine whether similar effects occur with other medications whose metabolism is dependent in part upon the CYPIID6 hepatic isoenzyme.

Aminoketones

Bupropion does not appear to have clinically significant pharmacokinetic effects on other drugs. Its metabolism, however, can be slowed by fluoxetine, leading to an increased accumulation of hydroxybupropion (64). This interaction has been associated with increased motor (e.g., catatonia-like reactions), as well as behavioral toxicity (e.g., mental confusion and excitement). Consistent with this pharmacokinetic interaction, patients on the combination of fluoxetine and bupropion *experience seizures at about 50% lower doses* than those on bupropion alone (79).

Triazolopyridines

Trazodone does not have clinically significant pharmacokinetic interactions with other drugs, undergoes rapid biotransformation, has a half-life of 3–9 hours, and its metabolic pathway is not appreciably affected by other drugs (49). The case reports of modest elevations of trazodone plasma levels in the presence of fluoxetine are probably the result of sampling error rather than a true interaction (80).

MAOIs also do not have clinically significant pharmacokinetic interactions and are also rather promptly biotransformed and eliminated. The reason for their persistent effects is not due to a sustained presence of the drug but rather to their irreversible deactivation of the MAO enzyme (81). Thus, to reestablish normal monoamine oxidase activity, following discontinuation of currently marketed agents, requires resynthesis of the enzyme. As noted earlier, reversible MAOIs (e.g., moclobemide) have been marketed in some European countries and are under development in the United States. If approved in this country, they would eliminate this protracted recovery time.

ADVERSE EFFECTS RELATED TO PHARMACODYNAMIC INTERACTIONS

Tricyclic Antidepressants

Due to the multiple actions of TCAs (especially the tertiary amines), they additively interact with a number of other medications, producing:

- *Anticholinergic* effects (e.g., benztropine, thioridazine)
- *Antihistaminic* effects (e.g., diphenhydramine)
- *Anti-α₁adrenergic* effects (e.g., prazosin)
- *Anti-arrhythmic* effects (e.g., quinidine).

Tertiary amines, more than secondary amines, also potentiate the central nervous system effects of alcohol. Patients need to be aware of this so that they avoid drinking while taking these medications, especially when engaged in activities that require attention and coordination.

Serotonin Reuptake Inhibitors

SRIs have fewer pharmacodynamic interactions than the TCAs, and do not potentiate alcohol, perhaps even slightly antagonizing its acute CNS effects (82). Nevertheless, there are some important adverse interactions. For example, SRIs influence dopamine cell firing in the substantia nigra through their effects on serotonin input to this nucleus. The net result is that they can cause extrapyramidal side effects (EPS) (71). The most common are *akathisia* and *tremors*. The same mechanism is probably responsible for their interaction with other agents that affect central motor systems. Thus, the SRIs can potentiate the *tremor* seen with lithium carbonate and *EPS* caused by antipsychot-

ics, bupropion, and psychostimulants (71, 83).

Given their profound effects on *central serotonin mechanisms in the brain stem*, the SRIs can interact with other central serotonin agonists to produce a neurotoxic syndrome, as noted earlier (47). Although this reaction typically is mild and self-limiting once the offending agents are discontinued, it can be serious, with fatalities having been reported. Since the most profound reactions have been reported when MAOIs have been added to SRIs (84, 85), such combination therapy is to be avoided. Other agents that have been reported to produce this reaction in combination with SRIs include:

- Tryptophan
- 5-Hydroxytryptophan
- Meperidine.

The clinician needs to be aware of the long half-life (i.e., several days) of fluoxetine since the potential for this reaction remains present until its active metabolite, norfluoxetine, has been cleared, which can take 6 weeks or more.

Monoamine Oxidase Inhibitors

MAOIs have the most serious pharmacodynamic interactions of any antidepressant class. They potentiate the *hypertensive effects of most sympathomimetic amines, as well as tyramine*, which is the reason for the avoidance of over-the-counter preparations containing such agents, in addition to the tyramine-free diet (86, 87). As discussed above, MAOIs in combination with *SRIs, tryptophan, 5-hydroxytryptophan, and some narcotic analgesics*, can also cause the *central serotonin syndrome* (47). MAOIs can also significantly potentiate the sedative and respiratory depressant effects of narcotic analgesics.

Aminoketones

Consistent with its most potent known mechanism of action, bupropion is an indirect dopamine agonist via its inhibition of the dopamine neuronal reuptake pump (88, 89). Hence, bupropion can *potentiate the effects of other dopamine agonists.* This interaction does not typically cause serious problems and may even be advantageous in specific instances such as patients with Parkinson's disease plus a depressive disorder.

Triazolopyridines

Trazodone does have some pharmacodynamic interactions with other drugs, but these are usually minor. Due to its *sedative properties,* trazodone can potentiate the effects of other CNS depressants, much like tertiary amine TCAs do. The sedative effects of trazodone have also been used to treat the insomnia that can occur early during MAOI or SRI treatment, with few, if any, reports of adverse interactions (90).

CONCLUSION

In choosing an antidepressant, the clinician must consider that some adverse effects are potentially quite serious. For example, the TCAs are frequently lethal when taken in overdose. Patients with preexisting heart block may have their cardiac status significantly worsen with TCAs. Falls from postural hypotension are associated with a significant morbidity (e.g., hip or skull fractures). Sedation can interfere with work activities, and anticholinergic properties can interfere with mental function, especially in the elderly. Seizures can be alarming and dangerous. Toxicity occurs with an acute overdose or, occasionally, in a patient who is a slow metabolizer with plasma levels creeping silently upward over time. Many adverse effects also occur with normal doses and plasma levels. This means that the clinician must start with a relatively low dose and gradually increase it as appropriate. Advantages of the newer SRIs are simplicity of use and more importantly, freedom from some of the more disasterous adverse effects of the TCAs.

REFERENCES

1. Baldessarini R. Current status of antidepressants: clinical pharmacology and therapy. J Clin Psychiatry 1989;50:117–126.
2. Richelson E. Pharmacology of antidepressants in use in the United States. J Clin Psychiatry 1982;43(11)sec 2:4–11.
3. Preskorn S. Tricyclic antidepressants: the whys and hows of therapeutic drug monitoring. J Clin Psychiatry 1989;50(7, suppl):34–42.
4. Preskorn S, Irwin H. Toxicity of tricyclic antidepressants—kinetics, mechanism, intervention: a review. J Clin Psychiatry 1982;43:151–156.
5. Preskorn S, Fast G. Therapeutic drug monitoring for antidepressants: efficacy, safety and cost effectiveness. J Clin Psychiatry 1991;52(6):23–33.
6. Williams RB, Shertu C. Cardiac complications of tricyclic antidepressant therapy. Ann Intern Med 1971;74:395–398.
7. Glassman AH, Roose SP. Cardiovascular effects of tricyclic antidepressants. Psychiatr Ann 1987;17:340–347.
8. Roose SP, Glassman AH, Giardina EGV, Johnson LL, Walsh BT, Woodring S, Bigger JT Jr. Nortriptyline in depressed patients with left ventricular impairment. JAMA 1986;256:3253–3257.
9. Giardina EGV, Bigger JT Jr, Glassman AH. Comparison between imipramine and desmethylimipramine on the electrocardiogram and left ventricular function. Clin Pharmacol Ther 1982;31:230.
10. Giardina EGV, Johnson LL, Vita J, Bigger JT Jr, Brem RF. Effect of imipramine and nortriptyline on left ventricular function and blood pressure in patients treated for arrhythmias. Am Heart J 1985;109:992–998.

11. Muller OF, Goodman N, Bellet S. The hypotensive effect of imipramine hydrochloride in patients with cardiovascular disease. Clin Pharmacol Ther 1961;2:300–307.
12. Roose SP. Modern cardiovascular standards for psychotropic drugs. Psychopharmacol Bull 1992;28:35–43.
13. Roose SP, Glassman AH, Giardina EGV, Walsh BT, Woodring S, Bigger JT Jr. Tricyclic antidepressants in depressed patients with cardiac conduction disease. Arch Gen Psychiatry 1987;44:273–275.
14. Bigger JT, Giardina EGV, Perel JM, Kantor SJ, Glassman AH. Cardiac antiarrhythmic effect of imipramine hydrochloride. N Engl J Med 1977;296:206–208.
15. Giardina EGV, Bigger JT Jr, Glassman AH, Perel JM, Kantor SJ. The electrocardiographic and antiarrhythmic effects of imipramine hydrochloride at therapeutic plasma concentrations. Circulation 1979;60:1045–1052.
16. Glassman AH, Johnson LL, Giardina EGV, Walsh BT, Roose SP, Cooper TB, Bigger JT Jr. The use of imipramine in depressed patients with congestive heart failure. JAMA 1983;250:1997–2001.
17. Roose SP, Glassman AH. Cardiovascular effects of TCAs in depressed patients with and without heart disease. J Clin Psychiatry Monograph Series 1989;7(2):1–18.
18. Richelson E. Review of antidepressants in the treatment of mood disorders. In: Dunner OL, ed. Current psychiatry therapy. Philadelphia: WB Saunders, 1993;232–239.
19. Preskorn SH, Fast GA. Tricyclic antidepressant induced seizures and plasma drug concentration. J Clin Psychiatry 1992;53:160–162.
20. Davidson J. Seizures and buproprion: a review. J Clin Psychiatry 1989;50:256–261.
21. Glassman AH, Davis JM. Overdose with tricyclic drugs. Psychiatr Ann 1987;17:410–411.
22. Callaham M, Kassel D. Epidemiology of fatal tricyclic antidepressant ingestion: implications for management. Ann Emerg Med 1985;14:1–9.
23. Sedal L, Korman MG, Williams PO, et al. Overdose of tricyclic antidepressants; a report of two deaths and a prospective study of 24 patients. Med J Aust 1972;2:74–79.
24. Sunshine P, Yaffe SJ. Amitriptyline poisoning; clinical and pathological findings in a fatal case. Am J Dis Child 1963;106:501–506.
25. Boehnert MT, Lovejoy Jr FH. Value of the QRS duration versus the serum drug level in predicting seizures and ventricular arrhythmias after an acute overdose of tricyclic antidepressants. New Engl J Med 1985;313:474–479.
26. Sedal L, Korman MG, Williams PO, et al. Overdose of TCAs: a report of two deaths and a prospective study of 24 patients. Med J Aust 1972;2:74–79.
27. Swartz CM, Sherman A. The treatment of tricyclic antidepressant overdose with repeated charcoal. J Clin Psychopharmacol 1984;4:336–340.
28. Preskorn S, Burke M. Somatic therapy for major depressive disorder: selection of an antidepressant. J Clin Psychiatry 1992;53(9, suppl):5–18.
29. Bech P. Clinical effects of selective serotonin reuptake inhibitors. In: Dahl S, Graham L, eds. Clinical pharmacology in psychiatry. From molecular studies to clinical reality. Berlin/Heidelberg: Springer-Verlag, 1989:81–93.
30. Benfield P, Heel R, Lewis S. Fluoxetine: a review of its pharmacodynamic and pharmacokinetic properties and therapeutic efficacy in depressive illness. Drugs 1986;32:481–508.
31. Boyer W, Feighner J. An overview of fluoxetine, a new serotonin-specific antidepressant. Mt Sinai J Med 1989;56(2):136–140.
32. Rickels K, Schweizer E. Clinical overview of serotonin reuptake inhibitors. J Clin Psychiatry 1990;51(12)suppl B:9–12.
33. Stark P, Fuller R, Wong D. The pharmacologic profile of fluoxetine. J Clin Psychiatry 1985;46(3)Sec 2:7–13.
34. Fabre L, Scharf M, Turan M. Comparative efficacy and safety of nortriptyline and fluoxetine in the treatment of major depression: a clinical study. J Clin Psychiatry 1991;52:(6)suppl:62–67.
35. Beasley CM, Dornseif BE, Pultz JA, Bosomworth JC, Sayler ME. Fluoxetine versus trazodone: efficacy and activating-sedating effects. J Clin Psychiatry 1991;52(7):294–299.
36. Altamura A, Montgomery S, Wernicke J. The evidence for 20 mg a day of fluoxetine as the optimal in the treatment of depression. Br J Psychiatry 1988;153(suppl 3):109–112.
37. Teicher M, Glod C, Cole J. Emergence of intense suicidal preoccupation during fluoxetine treatment. Am J Psychiatry 1990;147(2):207–210.

38. Wirshing W, Van Putten T, Rosenberg J, et al. Fluoxetine, akathisia and suicidality: is there a causal connection? [Letter]. Arch Gen Psychiatry 1992;49:580–581.
39. Mann J, Kapur S. The emergence of suicidal ideation and behavior during antidepressant pharmacotherapy. Arch Gen Psychiatry 1991;48:1027–1033.
40. Fava M, Rosenbaum J. Suicidality and fluoxetine: is there a relationship? J Clin Psychiatry 1991;52(3):108–111.
41. Robinson D, Kurtz W. Monoamine oxidase inhibiting drugs: pharmacologic and therapeutic issues. In: Meltzer H, ed. Psychopharmacology: the third generation of progress. New York: Raven Press, 1987.
42. Rabkin J, Quitkin F, Harrison W, Tricamo E, McGrath P. Adverse reactions to monoamine oxidase inhibitors. Part I. A comparative study. J Clin Psychopharmacol 1984;4(5):270–278.
43. Ravaris CL, Robinson DS, Ives JO, Nies A, Bartlett D. Phenelzine and amitriptyline in the treatment of depression. A comparison of present and past studies. Arch Gen Psychiatry 1980;37(9):1075–1080.
44. Robinson D, Kayser A, Bennett B, et. al. Maintenance phenelzine treatment of major depression: an interim report. Psychopharmacol Bull 1986;22(3):553–557.
45. Shulman KI, Walker SE, MacKenzie S, Knowles S. Dietary restrictions, tyramine, and the use of monoamine oxidase inhibitors. J Clin Psychopharmacol 1989;9:397–402.
45a. Thakore J, Dinan TG, Kelleher M. Alcohol-free beer and the irreversible monoamine oxidase inhibitors. Int Clin Psychopharmacol 1992;7:59–60.
46. Bresnahan DB, Pandey GN, Janicak PG, Sharma R, Boshes RA, Chang SS, Gierl BL, Davis JM. MAO inhibition and clinical response in depressed patients treated with phenelzine. J Clin Psychiatry 1990;51(2):47–50.
47. Sternbach H. The serotonin syndrome. Am J Psychiatry 1991;148:705–713.
48. Bayer A, Pathy M, Ankier S. Pharmacokinetic and pharmacodynamic characteristics of trazodone in the elderly. Br J Clin Pharmacol 1983;16(4):371–376.
49. Brogden R, Heel R, Speight T, Avery G. Trazodone: a review of its pharmacological properties and therapeutic use in depression and anxiety. Drugs 1981;21(6):401–429.
50. Janowsky D, Curtis G, Zisook S, Kuhn K, Resovsky K, Le Winter M. Ventricular arrhythmias possibly aggravated by trazodone. Am J Psychiatry 1983;140(6):796–797.
51. Vitullo RN, Wharton JM, Allen NB, Pritchett EL. Trazodone-related exercise induced non-sustained ventricular tachycardia. Chest 1990;98:247–248.
52. Jefferson J. Treatment of depressed patients who have become nontolerant to antidepressant medication because of cardiovascular side effects. J Clin Psychiatry Monograph Series 1992;10(1):66–71.
53. Rudorfer M, Potter W. The new generation of antidepressants. In: Extein I, ed. Treatment of tricyclic resistant depression. Washington, DC: APA Press, 1989.
54. Warner M, Peabody C, Whiteford H, Hollister L. Trazodone and priapism. J Clin Psychiatry 1987;48(6):244–245.
55. Brindley G. Pilot experiments on the actions of drugs injected into the human corpus cavernosum penis. Br J Pharmacol 1986;87:495–500.
56. Goldstein I et al. Pharmacologic detumescence: the alternative to surgical shunting. J Urol 1986;135(4):308A.
57. Pantaleo-Gandais M, Chalbaud R, Charcon O, Plaza N. Priapism evaluation and treatment. Urology 1984;24:345–346.
58. Preskorn S, Othmer S. Evaluation of bupropion hydrochloride: the first of a new class of atypical antidepressants. Pharmacotherapy 1984;4:20–34.
59. Davidson J. Seizures and bupropion: a review. J Clin Psychiatry 1989;50:256–261.
60. Dager S, Heritch A. A case of bupropion-associated delirium. J Clin Psychiatry 1990;51:307–308.
61. Golden R, James S, Sherer M. Psychosis associated with bupropion treatment. Am J Psychiatry 1985;142:1459–1462.
62. Liberzon I, Dequardo J, Silk K. Bupropion and delirium. Am J Psychiatry 1990;147:1689–1690.
63. Johnston JA, Lineberry CG, Ascher JA, Davidson J, Khayrallah MA, Feighner JP, Stark P. A 102-center prospective study of seizure in association with bupropion. J Clin Psychiatry 1991;52(11):450–456.
64. Preskorn S. Should bupropion dosage be adjusted based upon therapeutic drug monitoring? Psychopharmacology Bull 1991;27(4):637–643.
65. Perumal A, Smith T, Suckow R, Cooper T. Effect of plasma from patients containing

bupropion and its metabolites on the up-take of norepinephrine. Neuropharmacology 1986;25:199–202.

66. Golden RN, De Vane CL, Laizure SC, et al. Bupropion in depression. II. The role of metabolites in clinical outcome. Arch Gen Psychiatry 1988;45:145–149.

67. Van Brunt W. The clinical utility of tricyclic antidepressant blood levels: a review of the literature. Ther Drug Monit 1983;5(1):1–10.

68. Vandel S, Bertschy G, Jounet J, Allers G. Valpromide increases the plasma concentrations of amitriptyline and its metabolite nortriptyline in depressive patients. Ther Drug Monit 1988;10:386–389.

69. Alexanderson B, Evans DA, Sjoqvist F. Steady-state plasma levels of nortriptyline in twins: influence of genetic factors and drug therapy. Br Med J 1969;4:764–768.

70. Moody J, Whyte S, Mac Donald A, Naylor G. Pharmacokinetic aspects of protriptyline plasma levels. Eur J Clin Pharmacol 1977;11(1):51–56.

71. Ciraulo D, Shader R. Fluoxetine drug-drug interactions I: antidepressants and antipsychotics. J Clin Psychopharmacol 1990;10(1):48–50; II. J Clin Psychopharmacol 1990;10(3):213–217.

72. Miller D, Macklin M. Cimetidine-imipramine interaction: a case report. Am J Psychiatry 1983;140(3):351–352.

73. Preskorn S. The future of psychopharmacology: needs and potentials. Psychiatr Ann 1990;20(11):625–633.

74. Preskorn S, Fast G. Tricyclic antidepressant-induced seizures and plasma drug concentration. J Clin Psychiatry 1992;53(5):160–162.

74a. Crewe HK, Lennard MS, Tucker GT, Woods FR, Haddock RE. The effect of select re-uptake inhibitors on cytochrome P450IID6 (CYP2D6) activity in human liver microsomes. Br J Clin Pharmacol 1992;34:262–265.

75. Kelly MW, Perry PJ, Holstad SG, Garvey MJ. Serum fluoxetine and norfluoxetine concentrations and antidepressant response. Ther Drug Monit 1989;11(2):165–170.

76. Tasker T, Kaye C, Zussman D, Link C. Paroxetine plasma levels: lack of correlation with efficacy or adverse events. Acta Psychiatr Scand 1990;80(suppl 350):152–155.

77. Greenblatt DJ, Preskorn SH, Cotreau MM, Horst WD, Harmatz JS. Fluoxetine impairs clearance of alprazolam but not of clonazepam. Clin Pharmacol Ther 1992;52(2):479–486.

78. Brosen K, Gram L, Sindrup S, Skjelbo E, Nielsen K. Pharmacogenetics of tricyclic antidepressants and novel antidepressants: recent developments. Clin Neuropharmacol 1992;15(suppl 1):80A–81A.

79. Rosenblatt J, Rosenblatt N. More about spontaneous post marketing reports of bupropion related seizures. Curr Affective Illness 1992;11(4):18–20.

80. Aranow RB, Hudson JI, Pope Jr HG, Grady TA, Laage TA, Bell IR, Cole JO. Elevated antidepressant plasma levels after addition of fluoxetine. Am J Psychiatry 1989;146(7):911–913.

81. Potter W, Rudorfer M, Manji H. The pharmacologic treatment of depression. N Engl J Med 1991;325(9):633–642.

82. Lemberger L, Bergstrom R, Wolen R, Farid N, Enas G, Aronoff G. Fluoxetine: clinical pharmacology and physiologic disposition. J Clin Psychiatry 1985;46(3)sec 2:14–19.

83. Salama A, Shafey M. A case of severe lithium toxicity induced by combined fluoxetine and lithium carbonate [Letter]. Am J Psychiatry 1989;146(2):278.

84. Feighner J, Boyer W, Tyler D, Neborsky R. Adverse consequences of fluoxetine-MAOI combination therapy. J Clin Psychiatry 1990;51(6):222–225.

85. Sternbach H. Danger of MAOI therapy after fluoxetine withdrawal [Letter]. Lancet 1988;ii:850–851.

86. McCabe B. Dietary tyramine and other pressor amines in MAOI regimens: a review. J Am Diet Assoc 1986;76:1059–1064.

87. Folks D. Monoamine oxidase inhibitors: reappraisal of dietary considerations. J Clin Psychopharmacol 1979;40:33–37.

88. Cooper B, Hester T, Maxwell R. Behavioral and biochemical effects of the antidepressant bupropion (Wellbutrin): evidence of selective blockade of dopamine uptake in vivo. J Pharmacol Exp Ther 1980;215:127–134.

89. Ferris R, Maxwell R, Cooper B, Soroho F. Neurochemical and neuropharmacological investigations into the mechanisms of action and bupropion hydrochloride—a new atypical antidepressant agent. In: Costa E, Racagoni B, eds. Typical and atypical antidepressants: molecular mechanisms. New York: Raven Press, 1982.

90. Jacobsen FM. Low-dose trazodone as a hypnotic in patients treated with MAOIs and other psychotropics: a pilot study. J Clin Psychiatry 1990;51:298–302.

CHAPTER 8

Treatment with ECT
and other Somatic Therapies

Electroconvulsive Therapy

Electroconvulsive therapy (ECT) is the most effective treatment for severe depressions, which are often characterized by melancholic and/or psychotic features. While primarily employed for an acute episode, it may also be a useful maintenance strategy for those with frequent relapses despite adequate pharmacotherapy. The use of electrical stimulation to induce therapeutic seizures is the safest and most efficient form of convulsive therapy (i.e., versus pharmacoconvulsive therapy). It was first attempted by Cerletti and Bini in May 1938, and until the introduction of effective pharmacotherapy, remained the primary treatment for more severe episodes of mood and psychotic disorders (1). Since then, however, this somatic therapy has been relegated to a secondary role, with patients usually undergoing trials with standard psychotropics (e.g., antidepressants, antipsychotics, lithium and other mood stabilizers, oftentimes in multiple combinations) before receiving ECT.

Uneasiness concerning the passage of electricity through the human brain to induce seizures (a phenomenon otherwise considered pathological) has contributed to the controversy surrounding this treatment. Thus, despite the lack of supporting documentation, some groups have continued to raise concerns about irreversible memory loss and associated brain damage (2). Further, during its zenith, ECT was used in a wide range of cases now deemed inappropriate. More recently, United States and United Kingdom reports find that training is often inadequate and a large proportion of facilities administer ECT improperly (3, 4). Partly as a result of these factors, strident antipsychiatry forces have attempted to eliminate or severely curtail its use. A recent example was seen in Berkeley, California, in the early 1980s, where local legislative restrictions led to a temporary ban until it was overturned by a court. By way of contrast, the attitudes of professionals regarding the use of ECT are more favorable with their increasing levels of knowledge and experience (5, 6).

Figure 8.1 outlines the role for ECT in the overall treatment strategy we have proposed throughout this book. Such circumstances include a previous good response to ECT and/or in those nonresponsive to standard pharmacotherapy or intolerant to drug adverse effects. Further, for

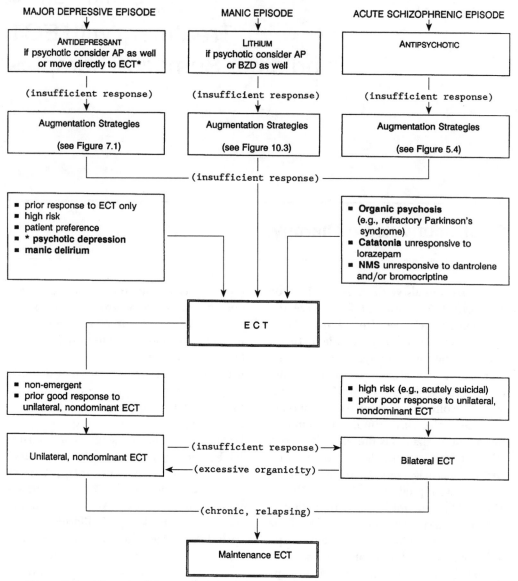

Figure 8.1.   The role of electroconvulsive therapy in the treatment of psychiatric disorders.

patients who present as high risks, either because of acute suicidality or rapid physical deterioration, this treatment may be lifesaving. Finally, in patients who express a preference for this efficient, rapidly acting, relatively short-term treatment, ECT may be an appropriate first-line therapy. For example, recent reports find significantly shortened hospital lengths of stay, as well as

overall cost, in patients with major depression who received ECT (7).

MECHANISM OF ACTION

ECT produces improvement in:

• Mood
• Sleep
• Appetite, with associated weight gain

- Sexual drive
- General interest in the environment.

The biological basis for the effects of ECT is unknown; however, most theories parallel the proposed mechanism of action of antidepressants (see also Mechanism of Action in Chapter 7).

Neurotransmitter Theories

The *amine hypothesis* of depressive mood disorders postulates a critical disruption in one or more neurotransmitters (e.g., norepinephrine (NE) or serotonin (5-HT)) culminating in a dysregulation of their activity, leading to the behavioral and vegetative symptoms. Electroshock (ECS) in animals increases NE, 5-HT, and dopamine (DA) central nervous system (CNS) synthesis. It induces a down-regulation in postsynaptic NE β_1-receptors, but interestingly and differently from tricyclic antidepressants (TCAs) and monoamine oxidase inhibitors (MAOIs), appears to up-regulate 5-HT$_2$ postsynaptic receptors (8–10). Results from both animal and human studies have been inconsistent, with potential confounds including:

- The use of brain or peripheral tissues, as well as the differential effects of ECS in animal versus ECT in human subjects, respectively
- A predominance of NE β_1-receptors in CNS and NE β_2-receptors in peripheral tissues
- Findings of receptor activity differences in normal young animals, with their own species-specific biochemistry and physiology, cannot be easily generalized to baseline and posttreatment differences in normal humans or depressed patients.

A further elaboration on these theories considers the modulating interactions among several neurotransmitter systems (e.g., the *permissive hypothesis;* the *cholinergic-adrenergic balance hypothesis*). Other neurotransmitters implicated include dopamine, γ-aminobutyric acid (GABA), and endogenous opiates, which subserve many of the vegetative functions disrupted in depressive states. One intriguing example is the connection postulated between DA, GABA, and major depression, in part based on ECT's efficacy in Parkinson's disease (see Mechanism of Action in Chapter 7) (11, 12).

Neuroendocrine Theory

Another approach considers the effects of various ligands on their receptors located in the diencephalic and mesiotemporal areas. Cell clusters in the hypothalamus coordinate the normal regulation of the vegetative functions of sleep, appetite, and sexual drive, which are typically disrupted in severe depression. In addition, the limbic area modulates many aspects of behavior and mood that are characteristically disturbed in mood disorders.

Fink and Nemeroff postulated the existence of a neuropeptide, *"antidepressin,"* that is released by diencephalic stimulation and enhances hypothalamic and perhaps limbic area function (13). Repeated ECT-induced seizures and the resultant increased levels of acetylcholine (Ach) are thought to promote the production of this putative peptide. In support of their theory, they discuss several lines of evidence. Using the analogy of the insulin/diabetes model, they note that:

- ECT enhances the production and *release of several neuropeptides* (including insulin), some of which have demonstrated transient antidepressant effects (e.g., thyrotropin-releasing hormone (TRH))
- *Vegetative* (e.g., appetite, sleep, sexual drive) *and neuroendocrine* (e.g., hyper-

cortisolism) *dysregulation*, characteristic of severe depression and mediated by centrencephalic structures, are improved by ECT

- ECT-induced increases in the *permeability of the blood-brain barrier* facilitate the distribution of neuropeptides throughout the CNS.

Neurophysiological Theories

Alterations in neurophysiological activity are subserved by many of the neurotransmitters discussed earlier in this section, as well as in Mechanism of Action in Chapter 7. After repeated seizures spaced over a given period of time (usually 2–3 times per week over a 3–5 week period), there is an increase in cerebral circulation (primarily due to increased systemic circulation) and an acute and sustained increase in cerebral metabolism. One of the most characteristic changes is a slowing in the electroencephalogram (EEG) pattern over a series of ECT, associated with increased acetylcholine activity. Increases in amplitude and decreases in frequency appear to affect thalamocortical and diencephalic structures, which may modulate recently acquired behavior, such as psychosis or melancholic features.

EEG interictal changes are characterized by a desynchronized resting configuration, leading to high-amplitude synchronized patterns, and symmetrical bursts of activity characteristic of *centrencephalic seizures*. With successive treatments there is progressive slowing in the mean frequency and increases in the mean amplitude of activity, both of which seem to be necessary but not sufficient for an antidepressant effect. Within 2–8 weeks after a course of ECT, the EEG returns to regular rhythmic alpha wave activity, comparable to baseline recordings.

Changes in *sleep architecture* include decreased rapid eye movement (REM) sleep, increased stage 4 sleep, and increased total sleep time. The authors have looked at the effects of ECT on sleep architecture in a preliminary trial of five depressed patients who underwent serial sleep studies during their course of treatments. We found that all subjects improved clinically, accompanied by a normalization of all sleep parameters (e.g., total sleep time (TST), sleep efficiency, etc.), except for REM latency, which at first became even shorter but then normalized by the end of the course of ECT (14). Although quite preliminary, we speculate that the unexpected initial decrease in REM latency might serve as a predictor of final outcome.

The *"anticonvulsant"* hypothesis has been developed to explain the efficacy of ECT as well as certain antiepileptic drugs for mood disorders. Anticonvulsants (e.g., carbamazepine (CBZ), valproic acid (VPA)) have several effects on seizure activity that include:

- Increasing the seizure *threshold*
- Decreasing the overall *duration* of a seizure episode
- Diminishing *neurometabolic response* to an episode
- Decreasing the phenomenon of *amygdaloid kindling*.

Interestingly, ECT induces the same effects (see Mechanism of Action in Chapter 10). Thus, while a given ECT treatment elicits seizure activity, the net outcome is an antiseizure effect over a course of therapy. ECS is also known to diminish the phenomenon of amygdaloid kindling in animal models (15). Similarities between such neuroelectrical, stress-induced phenomena and the longitudinal course of some bipolar disorders have been noted and have served as a heuristic, nonhomologous model for understanding the development of certain affective dysregulations (16).

Recently, Small and colleagues have promulgated the concept of *hemispheric equilibration,* which attributes efficacy to the apparent ability of ECT to restore the relative balance between right and left brain functions (17).

INDICATIONS/CONTRAINDICATIONS

As noted earlier, while it is often used as a "treatment of last resort," there are situations when ECT may be used as the primary treatment. The most recent revision of the APA Task Force Report on ECT discusses four specific situations:

- Patients who are at *high risk for suicidal behavior*
- Those who are *rapidly deteriorating,* either physically, psychologically, or both
- Those who have a *prior history of good response* to ECT and/or a poor history of response to pharmacotherapy
- Those who *prefer* to receive this treatment rather than undergo lengthy and possibly unsuccessful trials of medications with their associated adverse effects (18).

To this list we would add the issue of *delusional* (or psychotic) *depression* (see Chapters 6 and 7 also). While some have suggested that pre-ECT nonresponse to adequate pharmacotherapy is a powerful factor for predicting nonresponse to ECT (19), the authors, as well as others, have argued for its superiority over antidepressants, alone or in combination with antipsychotics for prior drug-nonresponsive, psychotic depressions (20–22). Recent support for this position comes from the discussion by Schatzberg and Rothschild (1992), who argue for separating this condition from other depressive disorders, in part due to its differential responsivity to various treatments (23).

In addition to depression, other indications for ECT include:

- *Mania* (especially manic delirium)
- *Schizophrenic* disorders (especially with "positive" symptoms)
- *Catatonia* associated with major mood disorders, schizophrenia, or organic mood disorders (e.g., systemic lupus erythematosus)
- Mood disturbances secondary to an underlying *organic process.*

Paradoxically, ECT is equally useful in both the acute manic and depressive phases of a bipolar disorder, constituting the only truly bimodal therapy available. This is not the case for lithium or the anticonvulsants, which, at best, have only relatively weak acute antidepressant effects. Drug therapies may also induce a switch from a depressed to a manic phase, while ECT can control both phases of the illness.

In *schizophrenia,* ECT, as with antipsychotic agents, is most effective in the acutely ill patient with a more recent onset of illness. Catatonia, withdrawn type, characterized by immobility and an inability to interact or maintain one's basic needs (at times posing a life-threatening situation) can dramatically resolve with ECT.

Case Example. A 31-year-old male who presented with unremitting psychotic symptoms and depressive periods marked by agitation and attempts at self-mutilation and physical assaults. He had essentially been hospitalized for the past 5 years, being treated as an outpatient for only a few months. The patient had been unsuccessfully treated with chlorpromazine, thioridazine, loxapine, lithium, amitriptyline, and diazepam. Prior to ECT he was treated with 120 mg/day of fluphenazine and continued to experience command auditory hallucinations to injure himself; persecutory and religious delusions; and increased depression and agitation. During this period the patient bit through his lip, lacerated his scrotum, and inflicted bite wounds on his hands. The oral antipsychotic was then stopped, and the patient received 15 unilateral, nondominant ECT treatments, with a resolution of his agitation and self-destructive behavior. Oral fluphenazine was then resumed and switched to the decanoate form (4.0 ml every 2 weeks). The patient was placed in a work-related day program and approximately 1 year later was doing well without rehospitalization.

Other disorders where ECT may be helpful include:

- *Organic* mental disorders
- Certain *medical* problems
  - Intractable *seizures*
  - *Parkinson's* disease
  - *Hypopituitarism*
  - *Neuroleptic malignant syndrome* (NMS).

In particular, the use of ECT during or shortly after an episode of NMS has come under scrutiny in the case report literature. A major concern has been reported fatalities associated with its use for this problem. Davis et al. recently reviewed the world's literature, identifying approximately 1000 NMS episodes in 755 patients (24). Using mortality rate as the major outcome variable, they compared patients who received nonspecific supportive treatment, specific drug treatment (i.e., dopamine agonists or dantrolene) plus supportive measures, or ECT. There was a 21% mortality rate in the nonspecific-treated group, as compared to a 9.7% rate in the specific drug-treated group, and a 10.7% mortality rate in the ECT-treated group. Further, the ECT patients who died or experienced severe adverse effects were continuing to receive concomitant high-

potency antipsychotics. An analysis of the case-controlled data indicated that ECT was clinically effective while resulting in a similar mortality rate to that with specific drug therapies and approximately half that seen with supportive treatments. While the specific drug/supportive therapy difference was statistically significant, the sample size in the ECT group was too small (i.e., 28) to reach statistical significance.

The most recent APA Task Force Report on ECT supports the concept of differing levels of relative contraindications and no longer lists "absolute" restrictions for the use of ECT (18). In particular, they caution that the following conditions may be associated with increased risk of morbidity and warrant special attention:

- *Space-occupying supratentorial cerebral lesions*
- A recent history of *myocardial infarction* and associated instability (less than 3 months)
- Recent *intracerebral bleeds*
- Bleeding or unstable *aneurysm or arteriovenous (AV) malformations*
- *Retinal detachment*
- *Pheochromocytoma*
- ASA (American Society of Anesthesiologists) classification *risk level* of 4 or 5.

When considering ECT in patients with any of these systemic conditions, a careful review of the risk-to-benefit ratio must always be conducted in conjunction with consultation from the appropriate specialists.

LITERATURE REVIEW: EFFICACY

Acute Treatment

ECT is superior in efficacy when compared to placebo, sham ECT, and active drug therapy. With the introduction of effective pharmacotherapy for severe depression, the relative efficacy of drug versus ECT was frequently studied. The authors' review of the relevant literature allowed an extrapolation of the data from selected studies for a quantitative analysis of ECT's efficacy versus other treatments for an acute depressive episode (25). The comparisons with ECT included: simulated (or sham) ECT, placebo, the standard tricyclic antidepressants, and the monoamine oxidase inhibitors (Tables 8.1 (26–31), 8.2 (32–35), 8.3 (29, 33–38), and 8.4 (28, 32–35)). We also compared the relative efficacy of the bilateral (BILAT) versus the unilateral nondominant (UND) forms of administration (Table 8.5 (21, 39–50)). A meta-analysis was computed on the data across all studies that met our a priori inclusion criteria (Tables 8.6–8.11)).

The overall efficacy of ECT was 78%, which is significantly superior to that of tricyclic antidepressants, whose overall efficacy was 64%, as well as to placebo, simulated ECT, and the monoamine oxidase inhibitors, whose overall response rates ranged from 28% to 38%. This difference was particularly striking, since many patients in the ECT-treated groups had failed previous drug trials, but the adequacy of some of these was questionable. Further, our analysis did not find a significant difference favoring BILAT over UND-ECT (i.e., only a 7% overall difference).

Maintenance Treatment

Just as drug-treated patients require maintenance management after an adequate response for an acute episode, so do acute ECT responders. Unlike with drug-responsive patients, however, maintenance management with ECT is a more complex matter, given that most received ECT because of a poor response or an intolerance to pharmacotherapy. Alternative maintenance strategies in this group include:

- *Antidepressants* that demonstrated at least partial benefit in the past
- *Lithium* or lithium-antidepressant combinations in bipolar disorders
- Combined *TCA plus antipsychotic*
- *Antipsychotic* alone (in schizophrenia)
- *Anticonvulsants,* such as CBZ or VPA, with or without other mood stabilizers
- *Maintenance ECT.*

While there is little systematic controlled data, open investigations support the potential value of maintenance ECT after an acute episode has remitted. This usually consists of a tapering schedule of single outpatient treatments, starting with a session every 1–2 weeks, and then reducing the frequency based on the patient's response. Although compliance may also be an issue with this strategy (i.e., patients are often reluctant to return as an outpatient for treatments), recent reports document its efficacy and safety in an otherwise chronic, relapsing depressed group (51, 52). Adding a sense of urgency to this issue is a recent report that patients who responded poorly to adequate *pre-ECT* pharmacotherapy may also respond poorly to *post-ECT* drug maintenance (53).

ADVANCES IN ADMINISTRATION

A number of advances in the administration of ECT have enhanced its efficacy and minimized some of the more troublesome adverse effects. They include:

- Enhanced *anesthetic* techniques
- Selected stimulus *electrode placement* (e.g., UND versus BILAT)
- Change from sinusoidal to *brief pulse* inducing currents
- Understanding of the role played by the *electrical stimulus* itself
- Improved assessment for the *adequacy of seizure activity.*

Table 8.1.
Studies Examining the Efficacy of Real ECT in Comparison to *Simulated ECT*

Study	Subjects and Diagnosis	Experimental Design	Results

Ulett G et al. (1956)	84 Inpatients
	Bipolar, depressed
	Involutional depression
	Neurotic depression
	Schizoaffective
	Other subtypes
	Schizophrenics
		Random assignment (stratified matching)
		Four groups
		  Active treatment
		    ECT (21)
		    Photo. convulsion (21)
		  Control
		    Subconvulsion (21)
		    I.v. anesthetic (21)
		Global ratings at weeks 4–5
			ECT > simulated-ECT
			"+" = improved; marked improvement; or recovered
			"–" = slightly improved; no change; worse

Brill N et al. (1959)	27 Inpatients
	Depressive diagnoses
	  Bipolar, depressed
	  Involutional
	  Psychotic
	  Reactive
	  Schizoaffective
	18–68 Years old
		Double-blind, random assignment
		Real ECT groups
		  ECT alone (7)
		  ECT plus muscle relaxant (8)
		  ECT with anesthesia (3)
		  Simulated ECT
		  Anesthesia alone (5)
		  Nitrous oxide alone (4)
		Doctors' Lorr scale
		Data combined for groups 1–3 and 4 + 5
			ECT > simulated-ECT
			"+" = improved or recovered
			"–" = no change

Harris J and Robin A (1960)	12 Inpatients
	Depressive reactions
		Double-blind, random assignment
		Three groups:
		  ECT plus placebo (4)
		  Hexobarbitone plus phenelzine (4)
		  Hexobarbitone plus placebo (4)
		Global assessment
		  1 = No change
		  2 = Slight improvement
		  3 = Moderate improvement
		  4 = Great improvement
			ECT > hexobarbitone plus placebo (after 2 weeks)
			"+" = moderate or great improvement
			"–" = slightly improved or no change

Study	Patients	Methods	Results
Fahy P et al. (1963)	50 Inpatients Endogenous or involutional depression 20–60 Years old 35 females; 25 males	Blind observations and ratings by two independent raters; random assignment Three groups: ECT (17) Imipramine 100 mg (16) Thiopentone (17) Ratings done at 3 weeks	ECT > simulated-ECT "+" = improved or recovered "−" = no change
Lambourn J and Gill D (1978)	32 Patients Depressive psychosis	Double-blind, random assignment Two groups: UND-ECT[a] (16) UND simulated-ECT (16) (Six treatments each; three times per week) Hamilton and GAS ratings	ECT = simulated-ECT "+" = 5 or more pluses on combined HAM-D and GAS scales "−" = less than 5 pluses
West E (1981)	22 Patients Primary depressive illness	Double-blind; random assignment BL ECT[a] 40 Joules Two times per week Double waveform At least six treatments per patient All patients on 50 mg of amitriptyline Crossover if no improvement after six treatments	10/11 simulated-ECT patients crossed over to real ECT No real ECT patients crossed over to simulated-ECT "+" = no switch "−" = switched

[a]BL, bilateral ECT; UND, unilateral nondominant ECT.

Table 8.2.
Studies Examining the Efficacy of ECT in Comparison to *Placebo*

Study	Subjects and Diagnosis	Experimental Design	Results
Kiloh L et al. (1960)	81 Inpatients Endogenous or involutional depression 52 Females; 29 males	Blind ratings for patients on drugs or placebo; non-blind for ECT One of three groups, in strict rotation ECT (27) Iproniazid (26) Placebo (28) Global ratings at 3–6 weeks for placebo; or 7–10 days after last ECT	ECT > placebo "+" = greatly improved; or symptom-free "−" = worse; unchanged or slightly improved
Greenblatt M et al. (1962, 1964, personal communication)	351 Inpatients at three centers Bipolar, depressed Psychotic depression Involutional depression Schizoaffective Neurotic depression	Double-blind, except for some ECT patients; random assignment Six groups: ECT (70) Imipramine (78) Desipramine (21) Phenelzine (48) Isocarboxazid (68) Placebo (67) Global ratings on a 3-point scale: Marked improvement Moderate improvement No improvement	ECT > placebo "+" = marked or moderate improvement "−" = no improvement
Shepherd M (1965)	217 Inpatients Primary depressions 40–69 Years old Females and males Patients switched to alternate treatment-nonresponders	Double-blind for medication groups; non-blind for ECT; random assignment (deteriorated patients dropped from study) Four groups: ECT (58) (4–8 treatments) Imipramine (58) Phenelzine (50) Placebo (51) Ratings for 15 symptoms; global assessment at 4 weeks	ECT > placebo "+" = good or excellent response "−" = poor or deteriorated

Table 8.3.
Studies Examining the Efficacy of ECT in Comparison to *Tricyclic Antidepressants*

Study	Subjects and Diagnosis	Experimental Design	Results
Bruce E et al. (1960)	48 Consecutive inpatients Depression	Non-blind ratings Random assignment to two groups: ECT (22) Imipramine, 225 mg (26) (three of seven IMI failures withdrawn before 4 weeks and given ECT to which they responded) Global scale at 4 weeks	ECT > imipramine "+" = good response "−" = poor response
Robin A and Harris J (1962)	31 Patients Depressed and chosen by clinician to receive ECT	Double-blind; random assignment Two groups: ECT (15) (Two times/week) plus placebo tabs Anesthetic (two times/week plus imipramine (16) Blind ratings with Hamilton Depression Rating Scale	ECT > imipramine "+" = marked or moderate improvement "−" = slight improvement; no improvement or withdrawn because of deterioration
Greenblatt M et al. (1962, 1964, personal communication)	351 Inpatients at three centers Bipolar, depressed Psychotic depression Involutional depression Schizoaffective Neurotic depression	Double-blind, (except for some ECT patients); random assignment Six groups: ECT (70) Imipramine (78) Desipramine (21) Phenelzine (48) Isocarboxazid (68) Placebo (67) Global ratings on a 3-point scale: Marked improvement Moderate improvement No improvement	ECT comparable to imipramine (perhaps more rapid in action) ECT > desipramine "+" = marked or moderate improvement "−" = unimproved

(continued)

**Table 8.3.—continued
Studies Examining the Efficacy of ECT in Comparison to *Tricyclic Antidepressants***

Study	Subjects and Diagnosis	Experimental Design	Results

Fahy P et al. (1963)	50 patients
	Endogenous or involutional depression
	20–60 Years old
	35 Females; 25 males
		Blind observations and ratings by two independent raters; random assignment
		Three groups:
		  ECT (17)
		  Imipramine 100 mg (16)
		  Thiopentone (17)
		Ratings done at 3 weeks
			ECT comparable to imipramine
			"+" = improved or recovered
			"–" = no change

Wilson I et al. (1963)	36 Inpatients
	Bipolar, depressed
	Involutional depression
	Reactive depression
	40–59 Years old; females
		Random assignment; patients blind, 2 raters blind (1 non-blind); high interrater reliability
		Four groups:
		  ECT + placebo
		  Six treatments
		    Phase I = (6)
		    Phase II = (4)
		
		  ECT + imipramine (4)
		    Six treatments
		
		  Imipramine
		    Phase I
		      Average daily dose = approx. 175 mg, plus anesthesia (6)
		    Phase II
		      Average daily dose = approx. 240 mg, without anesthesia (10)
		
		  Anesthesia plus placebo (6)
		Two scales:
		  MMPI Depression Scale (self-rated)
		  Hamilton Depression Rating Scale
			Phase I
			  ECT slightly better than imipramine
			Phase II
			  ECT equal to imipramine
			"+" = decrease in scores on HDRS and MMPI Depression Scales
			"–" = increase in scores or no change

| Shepherd M (1965) | 217 Inpatients Primary depression 40–69 Years old Females and males | Random assignment; double-blind for medication groups; non-blind for ECT Four groups: ECT (58) (4–8 treatments) Imipramine (58) Phenelzine (50) Placebo (51) (Deteriorated patients dropped from study) Ratings for 15 symptoms and global assessment at 4 weeks | ECT and imipramine were comparable Imipramine especially effective in men; but slower onset of action ECT especially effective in females "+" = good or excellent response "–" = poor or deteriorated |

Table 8.4.
Studies Examining the Efficacy of ECT in Comparison to *MAO Inhibitors*

Study	Subjects and Diagnosis	Experimental Design	Results
Harris J and Robin A (1960)	12 Inpatients Depressive reactions	Double-blind, random assignment Three groups: ECT plus placebo (4) Hexobarbitone plus phenelzine (4) Hexobarbitone plus placebo (4) Global assessment 1 = no change 2 = slight improvement 3 = moderate improvement 4 = great improvement	ECT > hexobarbitone plus phenelzine "+" = moderate or great improvement "−" = slightly improved or no change
Kiloh L et al. (1960)	81 Inpatients Endogenous or involutional depression 52 Females; 29 males	Blind ratings for patients on drugs or placebo; non-blind for ECT One of three groups, in strict rotation: ECT (27) Iproniazid (26) Placebo (28) Global ratings at 3–6 weeks for drugs; or 7–10 days after last ECT	ECT > iproniazid "+" = greatly improved; or symptom-free "−" = worse; unchanged or slightly improved

Greenblatt M et al. (1962, 1964, personal communication)	351 Inpatients at three centers Bipolar, depressed Psychotic depression Involutional depression Schizoaffective Neurotic depression	Double-blind, except for some ECT patients; random assignment Six groups: ECT (70) Imipramine (78) Desipramine (21) Phenelzine (48) Isocarboxazid (68) Placebo (67) Global ratings on a 3-point scale: Marked improvement Moderate improvement No improvement	ECT > MAOI "+" = marked or moderate improvement "−" = no improvement
Shepherd M (1965)	217 inpatients Primary depressions 40–69 Years old 169 Females; 81 males	Double-blind for medication groups; non-blind for ECT; random assignment Four groups: ECT (58) (4–8 treatments) Imipramine (58) Phenelzine (50) Placebo (51) Ratings for 15 symptoms; global assessment at 4 weeks	ECT > MAOI "+" = good or excellent response "−" = poor or deteriorated

Table 8.5.
Studies Examining the Effect of Electrode Placement on Efficacy

Study	Subjects and Diagnosis	Experimental Design	Results
Cannicott S (1962)	50 Patients Depression severe enough to warrant ECT All females	Double-blind; random assignment Two groups: BL[a] (20), mean 6.7 treatments UND[a] (30), mean 7.0 treatments Clinical global assessment Recovered Relieved Unchanged	No difference, based on clinical assessment "+" = recovered or relieved "_" = unchanged
Strain J et al. (1968)	96 Patients Bipolar, depressed Involutional psychosis Psychotic depression Depressive reaction Neurotic reaction 22–82 Years old (mean age 55 years) Males and females	Double-blind; random assignment Two groups: BL (46), mean 7.5 treatments UND (50), mean 8.4 treatments Ratings: Depression Evaluation Form Clyde Mood Scale (self-administered)	No difference, based on depression rating forms "+" = no relapse after 1 year "_" = required additional treatment or hospitalization within one year
Zinkin S and Birtchnell J (1968)	44 Patients Depressive illness	Double-blind; random assignment Two groups: BL (20), mean 8.29 treatments UND (24), mean 8.02 treatments Self-administered Depression Rating Scale	UND showed slightly greater improvement "+" = decrease in score after course of ECT "_" = increase in score after course of ECT
Halliday A et al. (1968)	52 Patients Endogenous depressives; less than 1 year's duration <65 years old Males and females	Double-blind; random assignment Three groups: BL (18), mean 5.5 treatments UND (18), mean 5.9 treatments UD[a] (16), mean 6.2 treatments	UND = BL-ECT "+" = recovered or improved "_" = no change or worse

Study	Patients	Method/Ratings	Results
Abrams R and DeVito R (1969)	21 Patients Bipolar, depressed Neurotic depression 22–55 years old Males and females	Ratings: Hamilton Depression Rating Scale Hildreth Self-Rating Scale Double-blind; random assignment Two groups: BL (11), six treatments UND (10), six treatments Hamilton Depression Rating Scale	No difference (i.e., 80% clinical recovery in both groups) "+" = recovered "–" = not recovered
d'Elia G (1970)	59 Newly admitted patients Endogenous depression	Double-blind; random assignment Two groups: BL (29), mean 6.2 treatments UND (30), mean 7.0 treatments Cronholm-Ottosson Depression Scale	No difference between UND and BL-ECT 1 month later "+" = recovered or much improved "–" = slightly improved or unchanged
Fleminger JJ et al. (1970)	36 Patients Referred for ECT because of depression Schizophrenia and organicity ruled out	Double-blind; random assignment Three groups: BL (12) UND (12) UD (12) Self-Rating Depression Inventory (D.I.) Differences in scores after 6th treatment	All three groups comparable "+" = + 5 or > "–" = < + 5
Sand-Stromgren L (1973)	100 Patients Endogenous depression 61 females; 39 males	Double-blind; random assignment Two groups: BL (48), mean 8.7 treatments UND (52), mean 8.9 treatments Scale for Severity of Depression Ten weighted factors scored on a 4-point scale (0–3)	No difference in total depression score "+" = satisfactory response based on decrease in depression "–" = unsatisfactory response

(continued)

Table 8.5.—continued
Studies Examining the Effect of Electrode Placement on Efficacy

Study	Subjects and Diagnosis	Experimental Design	Results
Heshe J et al. (1978)	51 Patients Endogenous depression	Double-blind; random assignment Two groups: BL (24) UND (27) Clinical global evaluation of depression into: Mild Moderate Severe	BL slightly better than UND 1 week after treatments were over; no difference after 3 months "+" = definite effect, or remission "–" = no effect, or doubtful
Fraser R and Glass I (1980)	27 Elderly patients Depressive illness Mean age 73 (± 6) years	Random assignment; blind independent observers Two groups: BL (15) UND (12) 4–11 treatments, based on clinical response Hamilton Depression Rating Scale	Based on scores 3 weeks after last ECT "+" = HDRS score ≤12 "–" = HDRS score >12
Sackeim H et al. (1987)	52 Patients SADS-derived, RDC diagnosis of primary major depressive disorder 18 Males; 34 females	Double-blind; random assignment Two groups: BL (27) Right Unilat (25) (Low-dose titration procedure; at least 10 treatments before classified as nonresponder) Hamilton Depression Rating Scale	BL > UND for short-term symptom reduction "+" = at least 60% reduction in HDRS; ≤16 total score; maintain 60% reduction for at least 1 week "–" = did not meet above criteria
Janicak P et al. (1989)	33 patients DSM-III diagnoses: Major depression (29) BP, depressed (3) SA, depressed (1) 16 Males; 17 females	Initial assignment: all to UND (10); then double-blind, random assignment to UND or BL; 2 patients switched from UND to BL Two groups BL (13), mean 9.5 treatments UND (20), mean 9.1 treatments Hamilton Depression Rating Scale	UND = BL "+" = ≥50% reduction in HDRS "–" = <50% reduction in HDRS

[a]BL, bilateral ECT; UD, unilateral dominant ECT; UND, unilateral nondominant ECT.

Table 8.6.
Efficacy of Real ECT in Comparison to *Simulated ECT*

Study	Real ECT[a]		Simulated ECT		Chi Square	p Value
	"+"	"−"	"+"	"−"		
Ulett G et al. (1956)	28	14	15	27	6.86	0.01
Brill N et al. (1959)	12	6	2	7	3.13	0.08
Harris J and Robin A (1960)	2	2	0	4	0.67	0.41
Fahy P et al. (1963)	12	5	8	9	1.09	0.30
Lambourn J and Gill D (1978)	8	8	8	8	0.13	0.72
West E (1981)	11	0	1	10	14.85	0.0001

Chi square for statistical method of combination	=	22
Composite p value	=	3.5×10^{-6}
Estimated difference between real ECT and simulated ECT	=	33%

[a] "+" represents a responder; "−" represents a nonresponder

Table 8.7.
Efficacy of ECT in Comparison to *Placebo*

Study	ECT		Placebo		Chi Square	p Value
	"+"	"−"	"+"	"−"		
Kiloh L et al. (1960)	24	3	3	25	30.56	<0.001
Greenblatt M et al. (1962, 1964)	65	5	43	24	15.19	<0.001
Shepherd M (1965)	49	14	23	37	18.10	<0.001

Chi square for statistical method of combination	=	62
Composite p value	=	4×10^{-15}
Estimated difference between ECT and placebo	=	42%

Table 8.8.
Efficacy of ECT in Comparison to *Tricyclic Antidepressants*

Study	ECT		TCAs		Chi Square	p Value
	"+"	"−"	"+"	"−"		
Bruce E et al. (1960)	21	1	16	10	5.96	0.01
Robin A and Harris J (1962)	12	3	3	12	8.53	0.004
Greenblatt M et al. (1962, 1964)	65	5	71	28	10.36	0.001
Fahy P et al. (1963)	12	5	10	6	0.015	0.90
Wilson I et al. (1963)	10	0	10	0	0.0002	0.99
Shepherd M (1965)	49	14	42	19	0.84	0.36

Chi square for statistical method of combination	=	22
Composite p value	=	3×10^{-6}
Estimated difference between ECT and tricyclics	=	19%

Table 8.9.
Efficacy of ECT in Comparison to *MAO Inhibitors*

Study	ECT		MAOIs		Chi Square	p Value
	"+"	"−"	"+"	"−"		
Harris J and Robin A (1960)	2	2	0	4	0.67	0.41
Kiloh L et al. (1960)	24	3	14	12	6.38	0.01
Greenblatt M et al. (1962, 1964)	65	5	30	42	39.7	<0.001
Shepherd M (1965)	49	14	19	41	24.6	<0.001

Chi square for statistical method of combination	=	75
Composite p value	=	5×10^{-18}
Estimated difference between ECT and MAOIs	=	46%

Table 8.10.
Efficacy of Bilateral ECT in Comparison to *Unilateral Nondominant ECT*

Study	Bilateral		Unilateral Nondominant		Individual Chi Square with Yate's Correction	Individual p Value
	"+"	"−"	"+"	"−"		
Cannicott S (1962)	18	2	27	3	0.231	0.75
Strain J et al. (1968)	29	17	33	17	0.008	0.90
Halliday A et al. (1968)	17	1	13	5	1.800	0.25
Zinkin S and Birtchnell J (1968)	13	7	18	6	0.154	0.75
Abrams R and DeVito R (1969)	9	2	8	2	0.203	0.75
d'Elia G (1970)	21	8	23	7	0.006	0.90
Fleminger J et al. (1970)	10	2	7	5	1.810	0.35
Sand-Stromgren L (1973)	37	11	39	13	0.000	0.95
Fraser R and Glass I (1980)	14	1	10	2	0.042	0.90
Janicak P et al. (1989)	11	2	15	5	0.050	0.82
Heshe J et al. (1978)	24	0	20	7	5.189	0.025
Sackeim H et al. (1987)	19	8	7	18	7.704	0.006
TOTAL N	222	61	220	90		

Chi square for statistical method of combination		
Mantel-Haenszel	=	4.87
Woolf-Haldens	=	2.88
Composite p value		
Mantel-Haenszel	=	0.03
Woolf-Haldens	=	NS
Estimated difference between Bilateral ECT and Unilateral Nondominant ECT	=	7%

Table 8.11.
Statistical Overview of Studies Comparing Unilateral Nondominant ECT to Bilateral ECT

	Number of Studies	Number of Subjects	Mantel-Haenszel		Woolf-Haldens		Estimated Difference: BILAT > UND
			Chi Square	p Value	Chi Square	p Value	
Studies finding no difference	10	490	0.31	NS	0.25	NS	2%
Studies finding BILAT > UND-ECT	2	103	14.2	0.0002	11.7	0.0006	32%
TOTAL RESULTS	12	593	4.87	0.03	0.29	NS	7%

ADMINISTRATION OF ELECTROCONVULSIVE THERAPY

The standard pre-ECT workup should include:

- A complete *physical and neurological* exam
- Routine *hematological* indices (e.g., complete blood count (CBC)) and serum *electrolytes*
- Review of cardiac status and *electrocardiogram (ECG)*
- Simple *tests of cognitive function.*

If deemed necessary, *spinal x-rays* (anteroposterior and lateral) to rule out severe skeletal problems may be appropriate. If such x-rays are done pre-ECT, they should be repeated post-ECT.

Informed consent must be obtained before the administration of ECT. Often, the same severity of illness that necessitates the use of ECT also impairs a patient's capacity to consent. When the patient is unable to give adequate informed consent, the clinician and the patient's family can usually obtain partial conservatorship from the court, allowing a family member to give substituted permission (see also Informed Consent in Chapter 2).

Anesthesia

Anesthetic techniques that have minimized adverse effects include the use of *muscle relaxants* and, more recently, nerve stimulators to assess adequacy of relaxation; the introduction of very *rapid acting, short-duration barbiturates;* and the use of *atropinic agents* to minimize the cardiovascular response to a combination of a seizure and anesthesia. In addition, 100% oxygenation (adequacy monitored by a pulse oximeter) with *positive-pressure ventilation* can minimize related cardiac events and memory disruption.

Electrode Placement

In comparing the relative benefit of UND versus BILAT administration, the authors found no significant difference in their overall efficacy or rate of response (as measured by the number of treatments required) with either method (21, 50). This finding supports the recent recommendations of the APA Task Force Report, which suggests clinician discretion as to the choice of administration (18). With a very severe and/or rapidly deteriorating situation or a prior history of inadequate response to UND-ECT, the authors recommend beginning with BILAT-ECT. In less urgent circumstances, however, UND-ECT is as effective, can be accomplished in approximately the same time period as BILAT-ECT, and induces less-severe short-term cognitive disruption. Further, switching to BILAT administration is always an option in a given patient if the rate or degree of response to UND-ECT is unsatisfactory.

Given the high probability of response to ECT and the potential for adverse interactions with concomitant psychotropics, we prefer to stop all medications during a course of ECT and resume drugs, as indicated, after completion of treatments. One exception may be the use of low doses of high-potency antipsychotics (e.g., haloperidol 2–5 mg/day) to control a treatment-induced acute organic syndrome or to enhance the overall benefit in certain psychotic conditions (54).

Acute Mania

A second issue is the relative benefit of BILAT versus UND-ECT for the treatment of acute mania. Milstein et al. (1987) reported on the early results of an ongoing controlled trial comparing ECT to lithium for acute mania, noting that the initial group of UND-ECT patients did not respond (55). At that point the design was changed and all subsequent patients assigned to the ECT group were then given the BILAT administration. Final results of this study indicate that the BILAT-ECT group tended to demonstrate greater improvement in comparison to lithium over an 8-week period (see Electroconvulsive Therapy in Alternate Treatment Strategies in Chapter 10) (56). While these data support the preferential use of BILAT- over UND-ECT in the treatment of acute mania, this finding has not been replicated, with Mukherjee et al. (1988) reporting no difference in efficacy with either method (57). Since these patients often constitute acute emergencies, starting with BILAT-ECT maximizes the chances for a rapid resolution of the manic episode.

Electrical Stimulus

Studies into various components of the electrical stimulus have also led to further advances. The most recent ECT devices deliver a *constant current, brief-pulse, low-energy stimulus,* in contrast to earlier devices, which used a constant-voltage, sine-wave, high energy stimulation. These newer devices require only about one-third of the energy to elicit a grand mal seizure, thus contributing to a decrease in *current density,* a critical factor underlying cognitive disturbances. There also appears to be a difference in efficacy between a stimulus that minimally surpasses the seizure threshold and those that moderately or maximally surpass it, especially in patients treated with unilateral electrode placement.

The best outcome may be achieved using a constant-current device with a brief-pulse stimulus sufficient to moderately surpass the seizure threshold, especially when using the UND placement. This will typically result in 5–40 joules of energy being delivered. For comparison, the amount of electricity used for cardiac defibrillation or cardioversion is typically in the range of 200–400 joules. With the use of the brief-pulse device and UND electrode placement, however, there may be an increased risk for suboptimal seizure activity, including missed, abortive, or inadequate seizures. Conversely, there is the possibility of prolonged seizure activity when the threshold is maximally surpassed. Such events, defined as a continuous seizure longer than 180 seconds, are aborted with 2.5–5.0 mg i.v. diazepam.

Seizure Activity

The optimal seizure duration appears to be in the range of 25–80 sec for a given treatment. A number of techniques may be employed to achieve this, in addition to an adequate delivery of energy to moderately surpass the seizure threshold. They include:

- Avoidance of concomitant drugs with *anticonvulsant activity*
- *Reduction in the anesthetic dose* of the most commonly used barbiturate, methohexital; or the use of *alternate agents* such as ketamine or etomidate
- *Preinduction hyperventilation*
- Adequate *hydration*
- Enhancement with intravenous *caffeine sodium benzoate* (500–2000 mg) given 5–10 minutes before the seizure induction (58).

Adequate monitoring of seizure activity includes the use of single- or multiple-lead recordings on the *EEG,* and/or the *unmodified limb* technique. The latter is achieved by applying a blood pressure cuff to an arm or a leg and inflating it above systolic levels after the anesthetic agent is administered but before the muscle relaxant is given. One then observes unmodified seizure activity and counts the seconds to determine the length of a seizure episode. To assure a generalized seizure, the ipsilateral limb should be used when employing the UND electrode placement.

COMPLICATIONS

Complications of ECT can be grouped under three major categories:

- *Cognitive*
- *Cardiovascular*
- *Other* effects.

Cognitive Disturbances

Short-term adverse cognitive effects, which may be more severe with BILAT administration, could delay or preclude an adequate trial with ECT. Strategies to circumvent this problem include:

- *Increasing time between treatments*
- *Switching from BILAT to UND* electrode placement
- *Adding* low-dose high-potency *antipsychotics* to manage organic delirium (e.g., haloperidol, 1–2 mg/day).

While short-term memory disruptions are less pronounced with UND administration, studies that have tested patients' memory performance several weeks to months after either BILAT or UND administration find little difference in residual deficits with either method (50). Limited data addressing the issues of efficacy and cognitive disruption with unilateral dominant (UD) versus UND or BILAT-ECT, and bifrontal versus bitemporal BILAT-ECT do not allow for definitive recommendations at this time. The authors prefer to begin with UND-ECT (using the temporal-occipital or d'Elia technique) if there are no mitigating factors, as noted earlier. If after 3–5 treatments the rate of response is not adequate, we then switch to bitemporal, BILAT administration.

Memory disturbances typically include *anterograde amnesia* (i.e., the inability to recall newly learned material) and *retrograde amnesia* (i.e., the inability to recall previously learned material). Both types can present as deficits in either the dominant or nondominant cerebral hemispheres (i.e., verbal and nonverbal anterograde and retrograde amnesia). Some patients also complain of loss of *autobiographical memories*. What is often difficult to sort out are the relative contributions from the induced seizures, the anesthesia, or the depressive illness.

The retrograde amnesia is temporally graded, in that as one goes back in time from the initiation of a course of treatments, the memory disturbance diminishes, and beyond 2 years, little or no deficits are evident. As an individual's memory recovers, the ability to recall events occurs in the reverse fashion, with those memories closest to the initiation of ECT returning last. Some recall for isolated incidents shortly before or during the course of ECT may be lost permanently, since they were probably never stored. This can also be a complication of anesthesia.

Another important aspect to this question is the cognitive dysfunction associated with severe depression. It should be noted that much of the memory effects are focused on events occurring during the illness and the period of treatment (see Abrams (1992) for a detailed analysis (59)). Thus, many depressed patients appear to suffer from severe memory disturbances prior to their course of ECT, and paradoxically appear to improve over a course of treatment. This is because improvement in the attention and concentration disruption often associated with severe depression is so significant, it overrides the organic amnesia induced by the course of seizures.

Those who receive BILAT-ECT tend to have more complaints about their memory subsequent to their course of treatment, perhaps representing an increased sensitivity to any type of memory lapse due to the greater initial disruption associated with this method. It may also represent a type of amnesia for which existing assessment scales are insufficiently sensitive. Overall, memory deficits are uncommon, rarely disabling, and are clearly outweighed by the benefits of treatment.

Cardiovascular Disturbances

In the cardiovascular system, arrhythmias and, in extreme situations, arrest may occur, usually secondary to the combination of seizure activity and anesthetic agent. The mortality rate per course of ECT treatments is in the range of 1 per 10,000 or 0.01%. This risk is less than the overall morbidity and mortality (i.e., 3–9 per 10,000) seen in severely depressed patients who go untreated or receive inadequate medication trials, and is less than the anesthetic risk for labor and delivery during childbirth. Thus, those who receive an adequate trial of ECT may actually be at a reduced risk of dying from a variety of causes.

Transient rises in blood pressure and heart rate occur with seizures, probably secondary to increased sympathetic stimulation that leads to increases in norpinephrine levels. Hypertension or increased pre-treatment heart rate are strongly predictive of peak postictal change in both heart rate and blood pressure (60). Increased parasympathetic stimulation decreases the heart rate secondary to inhibition of the sinoatrial node. Stimulation of the adrenal cortex leads to increased plasma corticosteroids and stimulation of the adrenal medulla, which may also con-

tribute to increases in blood pressure and heart rate.

Other Effects

Some experience *prolonged seizures*, defined as a duration greater than 120–180 sec. This requires continued oxygenation, control of ventilation, and an i.v. bolus of the anesthetic agent (20–40 mg methohexital) or diazepam (2.5–10 mg) to abort the seizure.

Patients may complain of *headaches, muscle aches, and nausea* associated with an individual treatment. Many also report *anticipatory anxiety* or fearfulness prior to receiving a treatment. This may require management with anxiolytics, but type and dose must be chosen carefully to avoid increasing the seizure threshold, thus undermining the adequacy of therapy.

Rarely, *prolonged apnea* may occur in those susceptible because of an inability to adequately metabolize succinylcholine (i.e., increased pseudocholinesterase levels). This requires continued positive pressure ventilation until the patient begins spontaneous respiration.

CONCLUSION

When properly administered, ECT is an effective treatment for the most severe mood and psychotic disorders encountered in clinical practice, especially those warranting hospital care. Its efficacy is even more striking given the fact that most successfully treated patients have previously been nonresponsive to one or more courses of medication. While primarily utilized for severe depression, it is also an effective antimanic therapy, and may be lifesaving in catatonic states. Further, it has been used successfully to treat other psychotic disorders and various organic conditions, such as NMS and Parkinson's disease.

REFERENCES

1. Bini L. Experimental researches on epileptic attacks induced by electric current. Am J Psychiatry 1938;94(May suppl):172–174.
2. Weiner R. Does electroconvulsive therapy cause brain damage? Behavioral and Brain Sciences 1984;7(1):1–48.
3. Fink M. New technology in convulsive therapy: a challenge in training. Am J Psychiatry 1987;144:1195–1198.
4. Pippard J, Ellam L. ECT in Great Britain, 1980: a report to the Royal College of Psychiatrists. London: Gaskell, 1981.
5. Janicak PG, Mask J, Trimakas KA, Gibbons R. ECT: an assessment of mental health professionals' knowledge and attitudes. J Clin Psychiatry 1985;46:262–266.
6. Benbow SM. Medical students and ECT: their knowledge and attitudes. Convulsive Therapy 1990;6(1):32–37.
7. Markowitz J, Brown R, Sweeney J, Mann JJ. Reduced length and cost of hospital stay for major depression in patients treated with ECT. Am J Psychiatry 1987;144:1025–1029.
8. Pandey GN, Heinz WJ, Brown BD, Davis JM. Electroconvulsive shock treatment decreases beta-adrenergic receptor sensitivity in rat brain. Nature 1979;280:234.
9. Vetulani J, Lebrecht V, Pile A. Enhancement of responsiveness of the central serotonergic system and serotonin-2 receptor density in rat frontal cortex by electroconvulsive treatment. Eur J Pharmacol 1981; 76:81.
10. Pandey GN, Pandey SC, Isaac L, Davis JM. Effect of electroconvulsive shock on $5HT_2$ and α_1-adrenoceptors and phosphoinositide signalling system in rat brain. Eur J Pharmacol (Molecular Pharmacol section) 1992;226:303–310.
11. Dysken M, Evans HM, Chan CH, Davis JM. Improvements of depression and parkinsonism during ECT: a case study. Neuropsychobiology 1976;2:81–86.
12. Faber R, Trumble MR. Electroconvulsive therapy in Parkinson's disease and other movement disorders. Movement Disorders 1991;6(4):293–303.
13. Fink M, Nemeroff C. A neuroendocrine view of ECT. Convulsive Therapy 1989; 5(3):296–304.
14. Lahmeyer HW, Janicak PG, Easton M, Davis JM. ECT's effect on sleep in major depression [Abstract]. APA New Research and Abstracts 1988;NR:69.
15. Post RM, Ballenger JC, Uhde TW, Bunney Jr WE. Efficacy of carbamazepine in manic-depressive illness: implications for underlying mechanisms. In: Post RM, Ballenger JC, eds. Neurobiology of mood disorders. Baltimore: Williams & Wilkins, 1984:777–816.
16. Post RM, Weiss SRB. Endogenous biochemical abnormalities in affective illness: therapeutic versus pathogenic. Biol Psychiatry 1992;32:469–484.
17. Small JG, Milstein V, Miller MS, Sharpley PH, Small IF, Malloy FW, Klapper MH. Clinical, neuropsychological and EEG evidence for mechanisms of action of ECT. Convulsive Therapy 1988;4:280–291.
18. APA Task Force on ECT (Richard Weiner, chair). The practice of ECT: recommendations for treatment, training and privileging. Washington D.C.: APA Press, 1990.
19. Prudic J, Sackeim H, Devanand DP. Medication resistance and clinical response to ECT. Psychiatry Res 1990;31:287–296.
20. Kantor S, Glassman A. Delusional depressions: natural history and response to treatment. Br J Psychiatry 1977;131:351–360.
21. Janicak PG, Easton, MS, Comaty JE, Dowd S, Davis JM. Efficacy of ECT in psychotic and nonpsychotic depression. Convulsive Therapy 1989;5(4):314–320.
22. Pande AC, Grunhaus LJ, Hachett RF, Gredin JF. ECT in delusional and non-delusional depressive disorder. J Affective Disord 1990;19:215–219.
23. Schatzberg AF, Rothschild AJ. Psychotic (delusional) major depression: should it be included as a distinct syndrome in DSM-IV? Am J Psychiatry 1992;149:733–745.
24. Davis JM, Janicak PG, Sakkas P, Gilmore C, Wang Z. ECT in the treatment of NMS. Convulsive Therapy 1991;7(2):111–120.
25. Janicak PG, Davis JM, Gibbons RD, Ericksen S, Chang S, Gallagher P. Efficacy of ECT: a meta-analysis. Am J Psychiatry 1985;142:297–302.
26. Ulett GA, Smith K, Gleser GC. Evaluation of convulsive and subconvulsive shock therapies utilizing a control group. Am J Psychiatry 1956;112:795–802.
27. Brill NQ, Crumpton E, Eiduson S, Grayson HM, Hellman LI, Richards RA. Relative effectiveness of various components of ECT. Archives Neurol Psychiatry 1959;81:627–635.
28. Harris JA, Robin AA. A controlled trial of phenelzine in depressive reactions. J Mental Science 1960;106:1432–1437.

29. Fahy P, Imlah N, Harrington J. A controlled comparison of ECT, imipramine and thiopentone sleep in depression. Journal Neuropsychiatry 1963;4:310–314.

30. Lambourn J, Gill D. A controlled comparison of simulated and real ECT. Br J Psychiatry 1978;133:514–519.

31. West ED. Electric convulsion therapy in depression: a double blind controlled trial. Br Med J 1981;1:155–357.

32. Kiloh LG, Child JP, Latner GA. A controlled trial of iproniazid in the treatment of endogenous depression. J Mental Science 1960;106:1139–1144.

33. Greenblatt M, Grosser GH, Wechsler H. A comparative study of selected antidepressant medications and EST? Am J Psychiatry 1962;119:144–153.

34. Greenblatt M, Grosser GH, Wechsler H. Differential response of hospitalized depressed patients to somatic therapy. Am J Psychiatry 1964;120:935–943.

35. Shepherd M. Clinical trial of the treatment of depressive illness. Br Med J 1965;1:881–886.

36. Bruce EM, Crone N, Fitzpatrick G, Frewin SJ, Gillis A, Laselles CF, et al. A comparative trial of ECT and Tofranil. Am J Psychiatry 1960;117:76.

37. Robin AA, Harris JA. A controlled comparison of imipramine and electroplexy. J Mental Science 1962;108:217–219.

38. Wilson IC, Vernon JT, Guin T, Sandifer MG. A controlled study of treatments of depression. J Neuropsychiatry 1963;4:331–337.

39. Cannicott SM. Unilateral electroconvulsive therapy. Postgrad Med 1962;38:451–459.

40. Strain JJ, Brunschwig L, Duffy JP, Agle P, Rosenbaum AL, Bidder TG. Comparison of therapeutic effects and memory changes with bilateral and unilateral ECT. Am J Psychiatry 1968;125:294–304.

41. Zinkin S, Birtchnell J. Unilateral ECT: its effects on memory and its therapeutic efficacy. Br J Psychiatry 1968;114:973–88.

42. Halliday AM, Davison K, Browne MW, Kruger LC. A comparison of the effects on depression and memory of bilateral ECT and unilateral ECT to the dominant and non-dominant hemispheres. Br J Psychiatry 1968;114:997–1012.

43. Abrams R, DeVito R. Clinical efficacy of unilateral ECT. Diseases of the nervous system 1969;30:262–263.

44. d'Elia G. Comparison of electroconvulsive therapy with unilateral and bilateral stimulation. II. Therapeutic efficiency in endogenous depression. Acta Psychiatr Scand 1970;(suppl 215):30–43.

45. Fleminger JJ, Horne DJ, Nair NPV, Nott, PN. Differential effects of unilateral and bilateral ECT. Am J Psychiatry 1970;127:430–436.

46. Sand-Stromgren L. Unilateral vs. bilateral ECT. Acta Psychiatr Scand 1973;(suppl 240):1–65.

47. Heshe J, Roder E, Theilgaard A. Unilateral and bilateral ECT: a psychiatric and psychological study of therapeutic effect and side effects. Acta Psychiatr Scand 1978;(suppl 275):4–181.

48. Fraser RM, Glass IB. Unilateral and bilateral ECT in elderly patients. Acta Psychiatr Scand 1980;62:13–31.

49. Sackeim HA, Decina P, Kanzler M, Kerr B, Maletz S. Effects of electrode placement on the efficacy of titrated, low-dose ECT. Am J Psychiatry 1987;144:1449–1455.

50. Janicak PG, Sharma RP, Israni TH, Dowd, SM, Altman E, Davis JM. Effects of UND versus BL-ECT on memory and depression: a preliminary report. Psychopharmacol Bull 1991;27(3):353–357.

51. Clarke TB, Coffey EC, Hoffman GW, Weiner RD. Continuation therapy for depression using outpatient ECT. Convulsive Therapy 1989;5(4):330–337.

52. Thienhaus OS, Margletta S, Bennett JA. A study of the clinical efficacy of maintenance ECT. J Clin Psychiatry 1990;51(4):141–144.

53. Sackeim H, Prudic J, Devanand DP, Decina P, Kerr B, Malitz S. The impact of medication resistance and continuation pharmacotherapy on relapse following response to ECT in major depression. J Clin Psychopharmacol 1990;10:96–104.

54. Abraham KR, Kulhara P. The efficacy of ECT in the treatment of schizophrenia: a comparative study. Br J Psychiatry 1987; 151:152–155.

55. Milstein V, Small JG, Klapper MH, Small IF, Miller MJ, Kellanis J. Uni- versus bilateral ECT in the treatment of mania. Convulsive Therapy 1987;3(1):1–9.

56. Small JG, Klapper MH, Kellams JJ, Miller MJ, Milstein V, Sharpley PH, Small IF. ECT compared with lithium in the management of manic states. Arch Gen Psychiatry 1988;45:727–732.

57. Mukherjee S, Sackeim HA, Lee C. Unilateral ECT in the treatment of manic episodes. Convulsive Therapy 1988;4(1):74–80.

58. Coffey CE, Figiel GS, Weiner RD, Saunders WB. Caffeine augmentation of ECT. Am J Psychiatry 1990;147:579–585.

59. Abrams R. Electroconvulsive therapy. 2nd ed. Oxford: Oxford University Press, 1992.

60. Prudic J, Sackeim HA, Decina P, Hopkins N, Ross FR, Malitz S. Acute effects of ECT on cardiovascular functioning: relations to patient and treatment variables. Acta Psychiatr Scand 1987;75:344–351.

Experimental Somatic Therapies

Psychiatry, as well as medicine in general, has had many potential "therapies" promoted with much enthusiasm, only to eventually see them fall by the wayside. While ECT has withstood both the test of time and rigorous methodological scrutiny, the same cannot be said for other somatic approaches. Nonetheless, two promising strategies (i.e., bright light phototherapy and sleep deprivation) have gained in recognition over the last several years. The authors feel that while these therapies remain in the experimental realm, there is sufficient evidence to warrant a discussion of their potential clinical utility.

BRIGHT LIGHT PHOTOTHERAPY

Animals exhibit a number of seasonal rhythms (e.g., body weight, hibernation, reproduction, and migration), with most species using the change in day length (i.e., photoperiod) to time seasonal events. Light has a dual role, both entraining a circadian photosensitivity rhythm and producing a photoperiodic response (e.g., gonadal growth). There is evidence that such seasonal changes are mediated by the ability of light to suppress melatonin activity. Further, Lewy has found that sufficiently bright light (1000–2000 lux) can suppress melatonin in humans, implying that circadian (and probably annual rhythms) in man are regulated by light just as in other mammals (1). Extensive basic knowledge about the effects of light on seasonal rhythms in animals, in addition to the discovery that bright lights (BL) suppress melatonin in man, spawned a number of experiments to test the antidepressant properties of bright light, primarily for seasonal affective disorder (SAD).

Mechanism of Action

Three major hypotheses have been advanced to explain the effects of light therapy:

- The *melatonin* hypothesis
- The circadian *rhythm phase shift* hypothesis
- The circadian *rhythm amplitude* hypothesis.

The *melatonin hypothesis* postulates that winter depression is triggered by alterations in nocturnal melatonin secretion, which acts as a chemical signal of darkness. Thus, by giving light therapy before dawn or after dusk, you can prolong the light period and diminish secretion of melatonin. Recent evidence that atenolol, which suppresses melatonin secretion, was not an effective therapy for SAD weakens this particular hypothesis (2).

The leading theory is the *circadian rhythm phase shift hypothesis*. Here, fall-onset seasonal affective disorder (FOSAD) develops when the normal circadian rhythm phases are delayed relative to sleep because dawn comes later. Since morning light advances (while evening light delays) the phase position of circadian rhythms, BL early in the day should theoretically improve winter depression. Indeed, there is some preliminary supportive evidence; however, benefit from evening BL therapy has been consistently noted as well. Lewy has hypothesized an energizing effect to explain this phenomenon (3).

The *circadian rhythm amplitude hypothesis* postulates that FOSAD is caused by a reduction in the amplitude of various rhythms, which are increased by light therapy. There is evidence that amplitudes of certain rhythms are abnormally low in depression, particularly in FOSAD. This hypothesis has yet to be tested under experimental conditions.

Also of interest is the recent report by Anderson and colleagues that found a reduction in the urinary output of NE and its metabolites in 9 female SAD patients treated with BL. They concluded that the results were compatible with changes seen after antidepressant (AD) drug therapy and recommended controlled trials to confirm this preliminary finding (4).

Therapeutic Factors

In an attempt to shed light on the critical therapeutic components of phototherapy, investigators have also evaluated several aspects, including:

- Intensity
- Duration
- Timing
- Spectral qualities
- Anatomical route of administration.

Studies of *light intensity* have established that BL treatment (i.e., 2,500 lux) is superior to dim light (i.e., 300 lux or less); and more recently Terman has shown that 10,000 lux was superior to the standard of 2,500 lux (5). *Duration of exposure* to light also appears to be an important factor and may be inversely related to the intensity, such that a half hour of 10,000 lux exposure may be as effective as 2 hours at 2,500 lux. The *timing of treatments* may be important as well for the beneficial effect. Thus, morning treatments appear to be relatively more effective than evening exposure, especially in patients with hypersomnia versus those with terminal insomnia. Further, some patients seem to respond only to morning therapy (6). The consideration of *spectral quality* is important since there is a potential for toxicity with long-term use of ultraviolet light. Results of preliminary studies have been mixed, with some indicating UV light was not necessary and others showing it was useful for a specific subset of depressive symptoms. This is an issue that clearly requires further investigation to avoid, if possible, any long-term potential eye or skin complications (7). Finally, almost all studies have used *eye exposure*, with one study by Wehr et al. indicating that this route of administration was significantly more effective than skin exposure (8).

Acute Management
Fall-Onset Seasonal Affective Disorder

In modern times, the first scientific report on the benefit of *phototherapy* for FOSAD was by Marx in 1946 (9). Since then there have been over 25 controlled trials of phototherapy. Rosenthal and colleagues recently reviewed this data and concluded that BL was a rapid and effective treatment for FOSAD, usually achieving statistically significant differences from control treatments (10). While dim light controls are technically acceptable, some patients who have read about SAD in the lay press may know they are receiving a placebo dose of light.

In reviewing the literature, Wehr and Rosenthal (11) summarized the findings for optimal phototherapy of FOSAD as follows:

- *Exposure to eyes* of diffuse visible light
- A light intensity of at least *2500 lux*
- Initial treatment duration of at least *2 hours*
- *Daily treatment* throughout the period of risk
- Preferably *morning treatment.*

Although quite limited, the data on drug therapy (with or without BL therapy) indicates that standard *antidepressants* may also benefit SAD, with agents such as imipramine reported to be comparable to phototherapy. One of the major drawbacks has been their unacceptable adverse effects. More recently, however, fluoxetine and bupropion have become the drugs of preference, primarily because of their less troublesome side-effect profiles. There is also case report data indicating benefit from the *atypical benzodiazepine* alprazolam and the *monoamine oxidase inhibitor* tranylcypromine (12, 13). Finally, the combination treatment of an *antidepressant plus phototherapy* may produce synergistic beneficial effects in patients who cannot tolerate adequate doses or who derive only partial benefit from either therapy alone.

Other Disorders

BL has been most studied as a treatment for SAD, and perhaps subsyndromal SAD, than for other types of depression (14). In reviewing the literature, however, Terman found that there is also evidence, albeit preliminary, that phototherapy may benefit:

- Jet lag
- Delayed sleep syndrome
- Chronobiologic disorders in shift workers (5).

Lewy and Sack recently reported on the beneficial effects of BL therapy for circadian phase disorders (15). They recommend BL (1–2 hours at 2500 lux) to be given 1 hour before bedtime in those with a phase advancement and immediately upon awakening in those who are phase delayed. Further, in attempting to help patients who are blind, they report that melatonin (0.5 mg orally) can also produce beneficial phase shifts but must be administered in the opposite manner to BL for phase advanced or delayed conditions.

Mood disorders. Levitt and colleagues found that augmentation with bright lights resulted in substantial improvement in 7 out of 10 patients who met Research Diagnostic Criteria (RDC) for recurrent nonpsychotic treatment-resistant major depression (16). All had been given adequate trials with antidepressants or had relapsed after a successful course of drug therapy. While 5 of these patients reported exacerbations of their depression in the winter months, none had experienced remissions during the summer.

Deltito and colleagues (1991) studied a group of 17 non-SAD, depressed patients to test the hypothesis that bipolar spectrum, depressed patients might preferentially respond to BL therapy (17). They randomly assigned subjects to either 400 or 2500 lux of phototherapy (2 hr/day for 7 days), and noted that the unipolar depressed group realized an overall mild improvement, consistent with the previous literature. Somewhat surprisingly, however, the bipolar spectrum, depressed patients improved dramatically on both 400 and 2500 lux of BL therapy. The authors were unsure why low intensity light also produced a beneficial effect, but speculated that the use of the light visor in this study may have been an important factor. It is also possible these patients may be particularly sensitive to light exposure. They concluded that light therapy may be a safe and effective treatment for non-SAD related, bipolar depressed patients. These findings were recently reaffirmed by Kripke and colleagues, who treated 51 major depressed and bipolar depressed patients randomly assigned to either BL therapy (2000–3000 lux) or dim, red light placebo. During a 1-week treatment trial there was a significantly greater improvement on global depression scores favoring the BL therapy group (18). Others, however, have not as much improved with BL therapy for classic, endogenous depression.

Maintenance and Prophylactic Therapy

There is virtually no controlled data addressing these issues for the treatment of SAD.

Conclusion

Bright light phototherapy may be a relatively safe and effective alternative to medication, primarily for SAD. It may also have an additive or synergistic effect when used in combination with antidepressants for SAD, as well as other nonseasonal depressive disorders. One major difficulty is the inconvenience (i.e., sitting in front of a bank of lights for extended periods of time daily), but recent experience with portable BL visors and dawn simulation may diminish this problem (19).

The major problems with defining the benefits of this therapy involve:

- Its utilization primarily for a *less ill group of outpatients*
- The difficulty in establishing an *adequate placebo control*
- The *lack of controlled trials* with adequate sample sizes comparing this approach to established alternatives.

As a result, we would presently characterize this treatment as experimental.

SLEEP DEPRIVATION THERAPY

There is a good rationale for associating sleep disturbances with the pathophysiology of mood disorders. Many depressed patients experience marked sleep disruption, usually insomnia, but also hypersomnia, and aberrant REM activity (e.g., earlier onset, increased density). Bipolar patients often convert to mania in the early morning hours (i.e., 2 to 3 AM), while many depressed patients feel worse in the morning, implicating a rhythmic disturbance. In this context, a striking clinical observation was that sleep deprivation produced a brief (e.g., about 24 hours) antidepressant effect (20). This phenomenon is supported by studies with varying degrees of experimental control, in addition to a substantial amount of uncontrolled evidence.

Thus, sleep deprivation may be an alternate somatic approach that holds promise for the treatment of certain depressive disorders, as well as an aid in elucidating the biological basis of mood disorders.

Literature Review: Efficacy

In 1990, Wu and Bunney cited 61 open reports encompassing over 1700 subjects (21). Sixty-seven percent of those who were diagnosed as having an endogenous depression demonstrated improvement after sleep deprivation. Eighty-three percent of those who were not on medication relapsed after only one night of sleep, compared to 59% of those on medication. They also report several cases where even a brief nap was able to induce a relapse. Wu and Bunney argue persuasively for the depressogenic property of sleep and how wakefulness may rapidly counteract this effect, albeit temporarily. They further postulate the possible existence of a depressive substance that is released by sleep but metabolized during the waking period, using diurnal variation in mood as evidence for this position.

Vogel reported that selective disruption of REM sleep, without interrupting slow wave sleep, produced a gradual but sustained antidepressant effect (22).

Reports of hypomania or mania after sleep deprivation led Wehr to hypothesize that sleep reduction may precipitate a manic phase in bipolar patients (23). As all effective antidepressant therapies may precipitate a manic episode, this observation strengthens the evidence for a commonality between sleep deprivation and antidepresssants.

Wu and colleagues reported on the results of a PET scan study of 15 depressed and 15 normal controls after a night of normal sleep and a night with sleep deprivation (24). They found evidence for overactive limbic system metabolism in a subset of depressed patients who subsequently experienced reduced activity in this area, as well as a lessening of their depression, after sleep deprivation.

Leibenluft and Wehr (1992) critically reviewed the literature on the clinical application of sleep deprivation for depressive disorders, focusing on six areas: *potentiation* of AD response; *hastening* the onset of response to ADs or mood stabilizers; preventing *recurrence* of mood cycling; as an *alternative* to ADs; as a *diag-*

nostic probe; and as a *predictor* of AD or ECT response (25).

They concluded that the use of sleep deprivation is counterintuitive (given that sleep disturbances typically accompany depression); that the literature to support its utility is largely uncontrolled; and that the transient and unpredictable response to this approach limits its value for most unmedicated depressed patients. They do, however, suggest that existing evidence supports the use of this modality:

- As a *possible potentiation strategy* in partial drug responders
- As a technique *to hasten drug response*
- In the treatment of *late luteal phase dysphoric disorder* (LLDD)
- In *differentiating depressive pseudodementia* from primary degenerative dementia with secondary depression.

Conclusion

As with BL phototherapy, the authors would emphasize that this approach is still at the experimental stage, but its noninvasive nature and preliminary positive results justify further controlled studies to attempt replication of these early findings.

REFERENCES

1. Lewy AJ, Sack RL, Miller S, Hoban TM. Antidepressant and circadian phase-shifting effects of light. Science 1987;235:352–54.
2. Rosenthal NE, Jacobsen FM, Sack DA, Arendt J, James SP, Parry BL, Wehr TA. Atenolol in seasonal affective disorder: a test of the melatonin hypothesis. Am J Psychiatry 1988;145:52–56.
3. Lewy AJ, Sack RL, Singer CM, White DM, Hoban TM. Winter depression and the phase shift hypothesis for bright light's therapeutic effect: history, theory, and experimental evidence. J Biol Rhythms 1988;3:121–134.

4. Anderson JL, Vasile RG, Mooney JJ, Bloomingdale KL, Samson JA, Schildkraut JJ. Changes in norepinephrine output following light therapy for fall/winter seasonal depression. Biol Psychiatry 1992;32:700–704.

5. Terman M. On the question of mechanism in phototherapy: considerations of clinical efficacy and epidemiology. J Biol Rhythms 1988;3:155–172.

6. Lam RW, Buchanan A, Mador JA, Corral MR. Hypersomnia and morning light therapy for winter depression. Biol Psychiatry 1992;31:1062–1064.

7. Remé CE, Terman M. Does light therapy present an ocular hazard? [Letter] Am J Psychiatry 1992;149:12:1762.

8. Wehr TA, Skwerer RG, Jacobsen FM, Sack DA, Rosenthal NE. Eye versus skin phototherapy of seasonal affective disorder. Am J Psychiatry 1987;144:753–757.

9. Marx H. "Hypophysäre Insuffizienz" bei Lichtmangel. Klin Wochenschr 1946;24/25:18–21.

10. Rosenthal NE, Sack DA, Skwerer RG, Jacobson FM, Wehr TA. Phototherapy for seasonal affective disorder. J Biol Rhythms 1988;3:101–120.

11. Wehr TA, Rosenthal NE. Seasonality and affective illness. Am J Psychiatry 1989;146(7):829–839.

12. Teicher MH, Glod CA. Seasonal affective disorder: rapid resolution by low-dose alprazolam. Psychopharmacol Bull 1990;26(2):197–202.

13. Dilsaver SC, Jaeckle RS. Winter depression responds to tranylcypromine. American College of Neuropsychopharmacology Abstracts 23rd Annual Meeting, 1984:199.

14. Kasper S, Roger SLB, Yancey A, Schulz PM, Skwerer RG, Rosenthal NE. Phototherapy in individuals with and without subsyndromal SAD. Arch Gen Psychiatry 1989;46:837–844.

15. Lewy AJ, Sack RL. Chronobiologic treatments for circadian phase disorders. Abstracts of the Annual ACNP Meeting, December 1992:8.

16. Levitt AJ, Joffe RT, Kennedy SH. Bright light augmentation in antidepressant nonresponders. J Clin Psychiatry 1991;52(8):336–337.

17. Deltito J, Moline M, Pollak C, Martin LY, Maremmani I. Effects of phototherapy on nonseasonal unipolar and bipolar depressive spectrum disorders. J Affective Disord 1991;23:231–237.

18. Kripke DF, Mullaney DJ, Klauber MR, Risch SC, Gillin JC. Controlled trial of bright light for nonseasonal major depressive disorders. Biol Psychiatry 1992;31:119–134.

19. Avery DH, Bolte MA, Dager SR, et al. Dawn simulation treatment of winter depression: a controlled study. Am J Psychiatry 1993;150:113–117.

20. Pflug B, Tolle R. Disturbances of the 24 hour rhythm in endogenous depression and the treatment of endogenous depression by sleep deprivation. International Pharmacopsychiatry 1971;6:187–196.

21. Wu JC, Bunney WE. The biological basis of an antidepressant response to sleep deprivation and relapse: review and hypothesis. Am J Psychiatry 1990;147:14–21.

22. Vogel GW, Vogel F, McAbee RS, Thurmond AJ. Improvement of depression by REM sleep deprivation. Arch Gen Psychiatry 1980;37:247–253.

23. Wehr TA, Sach DA, Rosenthal NE. Sleep reduction as a final common pathway in the genesis of mania. Am J Psychiatry 1987;144:201–204.

24. Wu JC, Gillin JC, Buchsbaum MS, Hershey T, Johnson JC, Bunney WE. Effect of sleep deprivation on brain metabolism of depressed patients. Am J Psychiatry 1992;149(4):538–543.

25. Leibenluft E, Wehr TA. Is sleep deprivation useful in the treatment of depression? Am J Psychiatry 1992;149:159–168.

CHAPTER 9

Indications for Mood Stabilizers/Antimanics

Bipolar Disorders

Bipolar disorder (manic-depressive illness) represents one of the most dramatic presentations in all of medicine and simultaneously poses one of the more difficult therapeutic challenges. It is characterized by mania and/or hypomania alternating irregularly with episodes of depression; however, a small group (approximately 1%) may only experience recurrent manic episodes (i.e., unipolar mania). The estimated risk of developing a bipolar disorder is 0.5 to 1%, and the incidence of new cases per year is in the range of 0.01% for men and from 0.01 to 0.03% for women (1). Onset usually occurs by the third decade, but the disorder can develop later in life. Recent information indicates that it may be more prevalent in adolescents as well as in children than previously believed (2).

Because the disorder consists of both manic and depressive episodes, it presents an organizational problem for any text. This is in part because the depressive phase is virtually identical to a unipolar depressive disorder, but discussion of its treatment is more complicated. Further, bipolar patients often present with one or two depressive episodes before experiencing a manic phase. Thus, initial depressive episodes in a young adult do not necessarily dictate the diagnosis of unipolar disorder, especially with a family history of bipolarity. We want to emphasize that bipolar disorder is a different disease than unipolar disorder, and its successful management, including the prevention of either phase, is best accomplished by mood stabilizers (e.g., lithium). The primary evidence that these disorders are distinct entities is their family histories (see also Mechanism of Action in Chapter 10).

Although the emphasis in this chapter will be on the manic phase, we underscore that the interplay between mania and depression is integral to an understanding of bipolar disorder. Thus, depression may:

- *Precede* an episode of hypomania/mania
- *Intermingle* with manic symptoms during the throes of an acute exacerbation
- *Succeed* a hypomanic/manic phase
- *Occur* as a *distinct episode* in an intermittent and irregularly alternating pattern with manic episodes.

These circumstances have important implications for management because drug treatment of the depressive phase may precipitate a manic swing or a more virulent course of the illness (3). We hasten to state that the existence of this phenomenon is controversial and by no means clearly established. Thus, if bipolar disorder is known or suspected, patients are best managed (acutely, as well as for maintenance/prophylaxis) with a mood stabilizer in addition to an antidepressant.

In this chapter we will focus on mania and hypomania, referring to the depressive phase when appropriate. A more detailed discussion of the phenomenology of a depressive phase is contained in Chapter 6.

THE MANIC SYNDROME

The essential feature of mania is a distinct period of an elevated, expansive, or irritable mood accompanied by several other symptoms (4). *Mania* is not synonymous with euphoria or elation, but is a syndrome that can occur in a wide variety of disorders and involves aberrations in mood, behavior, and thinking. Other clinical manifestations usually include:

- Hyperactivity
- Pressure of speech
- Flight of ideas
- Inflated self-esteem
- Decreased need for sleep
- Distractibility
- Excessive involvement in activities that have a high potential for painful consequences (5).

The estimated average length of an untreated acute episode is 4 to 13 months, with a range as brief as a day and as long as several years (6).

Hypomania is a less severe form of its manic counterpart, typically without many of the consequences experienced during an acute, full-blown episode. Subtle indicators of hypomania may include:

- Transition period in and out of depression
- Increased productivity
- Heightened perceptions
- Symptom overlap and fluctuation
- Altered view of spouse, friends, others.

Some have postulated a continuum from mild cognitive, perceptual, and behavioral disorganization to more severe presentations, ranging from hypomania to acute mania to manic delirium, occasionally culminating in a chronic manic state. Carlson and Goodwin described the various stages of mania using this model, and presented important differential diagnostic considerations at each stage (7) (see Table 9.1). This model may help to characterize the severity of an episode, as well as guide the level of treatment intervention.

Paralleling this continuum of severity in the manic phase, are the various levels of depression, which can range from nonpsychotic to psychotic, to delirious, to depressive stupor.

Primary Symptoms of the Manic Syndrome

The *elevated mood* may be initially experienced as feeling unusually good, happy, or cheerful, later as euphoric or elated. It often has an expansive quality, characterized by indiscriminate involvement with people and the environment. In this early period, manic patients can be playful and unaware of their changing mood, which is often recognized as excessive by those who know them well. In more severe episodes, thinking may develop into delusional notions about one's own power and self-importance.

Although an elevated mood is the pro-

Table 9.1.
Stages of Mania[a]

Stages	Differential Diagnosis
I Hypomania	Idealized norm
Energetic	Substance abuse
Extroverted	Borderline disorder
Assertive	
II Mania	Schizophrenia
Euphoric-grandiose	Substance abuse
Paranoid-irritable	Metabolic derangement
Hyperactive	
III Psychotic Mania	Schizophrenia
Paranoid	Substance abuse
Delusional	Metabolic derangement
Confused	

[a]Adapted from Carlson GA, Goodwin FK. The stages of mania: a longitudinal analysis of the manic episode. Arch Gen Psychiatry 1973;28:221.

totypical symptom, the predominant disturbance may be irritability, which is most evident when the individual's goal-directed behavior is thwarted. Indeed, the clinical picture can suddenly change, with the euphoric mood quickly replaced by anger and irritability. Inasmuch as these patients are acutely sensitive to criticism, they often become contentious and easily angered, even by seemingly harmless remarks. Verbal abuse is frequent, with physical violence occurring less commonly.

Goodwin and Jamison (1990) summarized the incidence of typical *mood symptoms* during a manic phase from 14 studies that included 751 patients as:

- Irritability 80%
- Depression 72%
- Euphoria 71%
- Lability 69%
- Expansiveness 60% (8).

We would note the incidence of depressive symptoms occurred in about three-quarters of these patients, again underscoring the interplay between the two mood states in bipolar disorder.

Psychomotor acceleration often accompanies the mood disturbance and is manifested by increased sociability, including efforts to renew old acquaintances; quick changes from one activity to another; and/or inappropriate increase in sexual activity. Because of inflated self-esteem, unwarranted optimism, and poor judgment, patients may engage in buying sprees, reckless driving, or foolish business investments. Such behavior may have a disorganized, flamboyant, or even bizarre quality (e.g., wearing brightly colored or strange garments or excessive, distasteful makeup); however, many also demonstrate a marked tendency to neglect themselves.

Speech can be loud, rapid, and often difficult to interrupt, frequently punctuated by jokes, puns, word play, rhymes, and witty, risqué, or droll irrelevancies. Euphoria often leads to speaking with a theatrical or dramatic flair. **As the activity level increases, associations may loosen, and speech can become totally incoherent, virtually indistinguishable from an acute schizophrenic exacerbation.** When mood is predominantly irritable, verbalizations can include complaints, hostile comments, and angry tirades.

Goodwin and Jamison calculated the incidence of *behavioral symptoms* per episode and found the following:

- Rapid speech 98%
- Overtalkativeness 89%
- Hyperactivity 87%
- Reduced sleep 81%
- Hypersexuality 57%
- Overspending 55% (9).

Although reduced sleep is often an early prodromal symptom, patients are usually brought for evaluation and treatment when their behaviors create the potential for more severe consequences (e.g., self-injurious behavior; atypical sexual behavior; significant financial indiscretions).

Associated Symptoms of the Manic Syndrome

Flight of ideas is an almost continuous flow of accelerated speech with abrupt changes from one topic to another, at times so pronounced that it becomes incomprehensible. These ideas are usually based on understandable associations, distracting stimuli, or plays on words.

Distractibility is common and characterized by rapid changes in speech or activity, resulting from a tendency to respond to irrelevant external stimuli, such as background noises or objects.

Inflated self-esteem may range from uncritical self-confidence to marked grandiosity, often reaching delusional proportions. Patients may give advice on matters for which they are untrained or about which they have no special knowledge. Despite average talents, they may unrealistically boast of extraordinary abilities (e.g., that they can compose music, write poetry, publish books, or design new inventions).

Lability of affect is characterized by rapid shifts from euphoria to anger or depression. **Depressive symptoms (e.g., tearfulness, suicidal threats, insomnia, etc.) may last moments, hours, or, more rarely, days, occasionally intermingled with or rapidly alternating with mania (e.g., mixed or dysphoric mania).**

A decreased need for sleep is a frequent prodromal sign, and is characterized by early awakening (sometimes by several hours), a significant reduction in total sleep time, and when severe, several sleepless days with no apparent fatigue.

Psychotic symptoms, such as delusions and hallucinations, may be present in more severe episodes (both manic and depressed phases) and are usually (but not always) mood-congruent. The delusions seen in mania often have a religious, sexual, or persecutory theme. Grandiose delusions can lead to convictions about a special relationship to God or some well-known figure from the political, religious, or entertainment world. Persecutory delusions may be based on the idea that the individual is singled out because of some special relationship or attribute (10). Hallucinations may be auditory or visual (e.g., seeing or hearing God) and usually consistent with the patient's mood (7).

Although the DSM-III-R distinguishes between psychotic features that are either mood-congruent or mood-incongruent, the usefulness of this distinction remains controversial. Pope and Lipinski found that "schizophrenic" symptoms were present in 20 to 50% of manic patients and that many of the delusions were mood-incongruent (i.e., delusions of persecution, catatonic symptoms, formal thought disorder, and auditory hallucinations not consistent with the mood state) (11). In addition, Schneiderian first-rank symptoms, once thought to be pathognomonic of schizophrenia, have been reported in 8 to 23% of manic cases (12, 13).

Blumenthal et al. reported that psychotic features in both unipolar and bipolar disorders were indicative of an earlier age of onset and first hospitalization in comparison with their nonpsychotic counterparts (14). Age of onset for the first episode was found to be earlier in the bipolar group regardless of psychotic categorization. Furthermore, the authors hypothesize that delusional depressions may be related to bipolar disorders, given a higher prevalence of bipolar disorder in relatives, and postulate a predictive relationship between psychoticism and bipolarity.

Secondary effects of bipolar disorder can include:

- Job changes
- Moves
- Repetitive marriages, divorces
- Bankruptcy
- Hypersexuality
- Altered self-concept (e.g., grandiosity; low self-esteem).

CRITERIA FOR AN ACUTE MANIC EPISODE

In the United States, the RDC and the DSM-III-R both provide clear inclusion and exclusion criteria for a current episode (15, 16) (see Table 9.2). Evaluation of past episodes can be made using the Schedule for Affective Disorders and Schizophrenia—Lifetime Version (SADS-L) (17). In other countries, the Present State Exam (PSE) can reliably distinguish mania from other disorders (18). Table 9.3 reviews the various clinical presentations of primary bipolar disorder and their related DSM-III-R diagnoses (19) (see also Appendices A, I, and J).

Bipolar I disorder is characterized by a history of one or more manic episodes and one or more major depressive episodes. This category can be further subclassified as either manic, depressed, or mixed in presentation.

Bipolar II (or NOS) disorder is defined by a history of at least one hypomanic episode and at least one major depressive phase but never meeting criteria for a manic episode or a cyclothymic disorder. Several recent family studies have indicated that in the American population there may be an increased risk for mania among relatives of Bipolar II patients. More importantly, the highest morbid risk for Bipolar II illness may occur in relatives of Bipolar II rather than Bipolar I or unipolar patients, suggesting that this illness breeds true in some families (20). Coryell supports this position, stating that the illness appears to be phenomenologically stable over time and across generations, despite its poor diagnostic reliability (21).

Rapid cyclers represent a more severe, treatment-resistant subgroup that is characterized by a minimum of four episodes (i.e., hypomanic, manic, or depressive) within a 12-month period (22). Bauer et al. assessed hypothyroidism as a risk factor and found that of 30 rapid cycling patients, 23% had grade I hypothyroidism, 27% grade II, and 10% grade III (23). Although approximately 63% of this cohort was taking lithium carbonate or carbamazepine, the percentage of grade I hypothyroidism was significantly greater than that reported in studies of unselected patients on long-term lithium treatment. **Their findings indicate that hypothyroidism in bipolar disorder may be a risk factor for the development of rapid cycling, and lends support to the hypothesis that a relative central thyroid hormonal deficiency predisposes to this course. Therefore, close**

Table 9.2.
Comparison of DSM-III-R and RDC Criteria for Mania

DSM-III-R (1987)	RDC (1985 Update)
A. Distinct period of elevated/irritable mood	A. Distinct period of elevated/irritable mood
B. At least three of the following for elevated mood, four for irritable mood: 1. Increased self-esteem/grandiosity 2. Decreased need for sleep 3. More talkative or pressure of speech 4. Flight of ideas or racing thoughts 5. Distractibility 6. Increased goal-directed activity/agitation 7. Excessive involvement in activities	B. At least three of the following for elevated mood, four for irritable mood: 1. More active or physically restless 2. More talkative or pressure of speech 3. Flight of ideas or racing thoughts 4. Inflated self-esteem/grandiosity 5. Decreased need for sleep 6. Distractibility 7. Excessive involvement in activities
C. Marked impairment in social/occupational functioning or hospitalization	C. At least one of the following: 1. Meaningful conversation not possible 2. Serious impairment at home, work, or socially 3. Hospitalization
D. Delusions and/or hallucinations have not been present for as long as 2 weeks in the absence of prominent mood symptoms	D. Duration of manic features at least 1 week
E. Not superimposed on schizophrenia, schizophreniform disorder, delusional disorder, or psychotic disorder	E. None of the following is present: 1. Delusions of thought control, insertion, withdrawal, broadcasting 2. Nonaffective hallucinations throughout the day or intermittently for 1 week 3. Auditory hallucinations commenting on person's thoughts/actions or two or more voices conversing with each other 4. Had delusions/hallucinations for 1 week in absence of manic/depressive symptoms 5. Had marked thought disorder with either blunted/inappropriate affect, delusions/hallucinations, or grossly disorganized behavior for at least 1 week in absence of manic symptoms
F. Not attributable to a known organic factor.	

Note: DSM-III-R also distinguishes between psychotic features that are mood-congruent or mood-incongruent.
Adapted from Altman E, Janicak PG, Davis JM. Mania, clinical manifestations and assessment. In: Howells JG, ed. Modern perspectives in the psychiatry of mood disorders. New York: Brunner/Magel, 1989.

attention to the early symptoms and signs of thyroid dysregulation should be a routine aspect of any evaluation.

Dysphoric mania is described by patients as feeling out of synch and is associated with complaints of malaise and a greater emphasis on feelings during the depressive rather than manic state. Post et al. found a high proportion of manic patients (46%) presented with marked to moderate dysphoria, as well as anger and anxiety (24). He also noted a positive correlation between dysphoric mania and rapid cycling. A substantial number of these episodes were correlated with two measures of severity, the peak intensity of

Table 9.3.
Primary Bipolar Disorders[a]

Disorder	Defining Characteristics	DSM-III-R Diagnosis
Bipolar I	Mania and depression	Bipolar disorder
Bipolar II	Hypomania and depression	Bipolar NOS
Bipolar III	Cyclothymic personality	Cyclothymia
Bipolar IV	Hypomania or mania precipitated by antidepressant drugs	Organic mood disorder
Bipolar V	Familial history of bipolar disorder	Major depression
Bipolar VI	Mania without depression	Bipolar disorder

[a]Adapted from Klerman G. The classification of bipolar disorders. Psychiatr Ann 1987;17:13–17.

an episode and a greater need for hospitalization, especially in females. CSF norepinephrine concentrations were positively correlated with ratings of anger, depression, and anxiety during an episode; however, this elevation was seen in other diagnostic conditions where anxiety was a major component.

Mixed manic states are characterized by the simultaneous presence of both depressive and manic symptoms. This may be a relatively common occurrence, as noted earlier in the data of Goodwin and Jamison (i.e., 71% present with euphoria and 72% with depression).

Cyclothymia is a milder version of the classic bipolar disorder, characterized by a chronic course, with swings between mild depressive and hypomanic traits that never reach the severity of a full manic or depressive episode. An interesting hypothesis raised by Akiskal is the concept of *subclinical or subsyndromal mood* disorders (25). These disorders are often missed in cross-sectional diagnoses and are characterized by milder bipolar conditions, often with abrupt biphasic shifts, at times precipitated by the introduction of an antidepressant. These patients have very stormy interpersonal relationships, are frequently misdiagnosed as having Axis II characterological disorders, and are recommended for long-term psychotherapy, which is usually ineffective. If these pa-

tients are properly diagnosed and managed with mood stabilizers, however, significant improvement in their overall functioning may be achieved.

Case Example. A 29-year-old female presented for consultation on referral from a psychiatrist who had seen her in psychodynamically oriented psychotherapy for approximately 10 years. The primary difficulty was intermittent interpersonal strife with fellow workers and supervisors. Thus, although quite competent, she had switched positions frequently because of these difficulties. Her history indicated that she had never experienced a full depressive, hypomanic, or manic episode, but that these problems seemed to coincide with intermittent periods of irritability. As a result, she was placed on a trial of lithium, with therapeutic blood levels. Within several weeks of treatment initiation, her difficulties with fellow coworkers and supervisors ceased, and up to 1 year follow-up, she had not had a recurrence of these problems.

Differential Diagnosis of an Acute Manic Episode

Bipolar disorder can be divided into *primary and secondary* types, with the latter developing as a consequence of various medical or organic processes that can alter brain structure. This categorization underscores the view of mania as a syndrome subsequent to various pathophysiologies.

It is important to consider explanatory

precipitants in a patient with no prior history of a mood disorder. Clearly, the diagnosis of bipolar mania should not be made if the syndrome can be explained by known organic factors, which vary widely and include:

- Stroke
- Neoplasms
- Epilepsy
- Infections (e.g., AIDS)
- Metabolic and endocrine disturbances
- Substance abuse.

Therefore, a careful medical evaluation is critical and appropriate referral for consultation mandatory if an underlying organic process is suspected.

Complicated mania is an elaboration on the theme of the secondary type and is defined as "the presence of antecedent or coexisting nonaffective psychiatric disorders and/or serious medical disorders." These patients can be grouped into psychiatric or medical cluster patients. The psychiatric cluster patients have had fewer prior psychiatric hospitalizations, an earlier onset of illness, and a history of prior suicide attempts. This contrasts with the medical cluster, which had a later age of onset, no prior history of suicide attempts, more organic features, and more deaths during the follow-up period.

Black et al. (1988) in a retrospective, chart review, case-controlled study of 57 manic patients assigned to one of four treatment groups (ECT, adequate or inadequate lithium therapy, or neither treatment), found complicated manics responded poorly in comparison to their uncomplicated counterparts (26). They concluded that adequate treatment was associated with recovery in the latter group, but the outcome was less clear for the complicated manics. Although there are always drawbacks to any chart review

study, it does suggest consideration of alternative strategies for this subgroup (see also Alternate Treatment Strategies in Chapter 10).

Because the coexistence of substance and/or alcohol abuse disorders is much higher in bipolar patients than in the general population, their importance as comorbid factors has become increasingly recognized (27). It is important to decide whether:

- An episode of mania/depression is drug- or alcohol-*induced*
- Concurrent drug or alcohol use is an attempt to *self-medicate*
- Such activity is *unrelated to the present exacerbation.*

Further, concurrent substance abuse may:

- *Complicate interpretation* of the presenting symptoms
- *Undermine* the beneficial effects of *treatment*
- Adversely effect the *long-term course.*

Finally, comorbid substance abuse, particularly with bipolar males, is a strong predictor of suicide-related lethality. It is critically important to recognize these complicating disorders and aggressively intervene. Referral to Alcoholics Anonymous (AA), Narcotics Anonymous (NA), and other related counseling support programs may also help to diminish the risk of serious morbidity.

Schizophrenia-related disorders, particularly schizophreniform disorder, can closely mimic an acute exacerbation of mania. Attention to premorbid personal and family history may help differentiate them from mood disorders. A definitive diagnosis may not be possible, however, until the course of the illness is followed for a period of time. Clinical clues include the propensity of bipolar manics (in contrast to schizophrenics) to demonstrate pressured speech, flight of ideas, grandiosity, and overinclusive thinking. Hallucinations are less common than delusions in both mania and depression, with delusions normally taking on the qualities of expansivity, hyperreligiosity, or grandiosity. Delusions are also relatively less fixed than in schizophrenia.

Schizoaffective disorder, characterized by symptoms of both schizophrenia and a mood disorder, but not meeting full criteria for either category, can also pose a difficult diagnostic dilemma. Schizoaffective probands tend to have family members with both affective and schizophrenic disorders. One family study indicated that the schizoaffective-manic type tended to aggregate with classic bipolar disorder, while the schizoaffective-depressive type seemed to be more closely related to schizophrenia (28).

A final major differential consideration is a *severe characterological (or Axis II) disturbance.* For example, five of the eight criteria for borderline personality disorder in the DSM-III-R overlap with symptoms for hypomania, including:

- Impulsivity
- Affective instability
- Inappropriate anger
- Recurrent suicidal behavior
- Unstable interpersonal relationships.

Some patients initially diagnosed as having borderline disorder and followed longitudinally will develop periodic exacerbations in their interpersonal relationships. At times they may even be reclassified as having either a classic bipolar disorder, a subsyndromal variant, or an atypical presentation.

Conversely, patients may also display certain *interpersonal styles* that fluctuate with the course of their illness. Janowsky et al. (1974) demonstrated that manic patients have a characteristic interactional style that clearly distinguishes them from schizoaffective and schizophrenic patients (29). Using their Manic Interpersonal Interaction Scale (MIIS) to assess changes in personality style, they found these patients more likely to:

- *Evoke anger* from treating personnel
- *Project responsibility* onto others
- Attempt to *divide treatment personnel* through manipulative behavior
- *Test limits*
- *Exploit or attack* others' vulnerabilities.

In Table 9.4, scores on each item are presented during the manic phase and again after recovery with lithium therapy. They concluded that such behaviors are not attributable to premorbid personality, but rather are as characteristic of a manic episode as classic symptom changes (e.g., euphoria, flight of ideas, overtalkativeness, and grandiosity). Further, the pattern of interpersonal interactions occurred only when a patient was in a manic phase, and disappeared with lithium therapy.

COURSE OF ILLNESS

Onset

Longitudinal observations indicate that early in the course of the illness various phases (depressive, hypomanic, manic) are often associated with identifiable external stressors. Over time, however, patients may begin to show spontaneous fluctuations in mood as well as increased frequency and severity of episodes.

Methods for accurately assessing the longitudinal course of mood disorders were first described by Adolph Meyer, and more recently illustrated by Post et al. (1988), who encourage retrospective and

Table 9.4.
Mean Item and Total Manic Interpersonal Interaction Scale Scores Before and After Clinical Remission[a]

Item	Acutely Ill	Remitted	Significance[b]
Testing of limits	8	1	$p < 0.0001$
Projection of responsibility	5	1	$p < 0.02$
Sensitivity to others' soft spots	5	1	$p < 0.01$
Attempts to divide staff	2	1	$p < 0.02$
Flattering behavior	3	1	$p < 0.002$
Ability to evoke anger	6	1	$p < 0.002$
MIIS total score	29	7	$p < 0.002$

[a]Adapted from Janowsky DS, El-Yousef M, Davis JM. Interpersonal maneuvers of manic patients. Am J Psychiatry 1974;131:250–254.
[b]From paired Student's t-test, one-tailed. (N = 5; all numbers are rounded.)

prospective historical graphing as an invaluable guide to the disorder's progression and response to therapy (30, 31). They recommend grading episodes by three levels of severity:

- *Nonfunctional,* indicating severe depression or mania
- *Moderate severity,* reflecting impairment in work or social function
- *Mild severity,* indicating no impairment but the presence of recognized mood or behavioral alterations.

The chart should also include important life events, mood, and behavior, as well as medication(s) (mg/day) or other treatment(s). Such methods can help the clinician:

- Supply data for *proper diagnosis*
- Plot psychological *stressors*
- Formulate *treatment* recommendations
- *Monitor* the effect of psychological and pharmacological *interventions.*

Sex differences in the age of onset of bipolar disorder were evaluated by Sibisi, who used the annual United Kingdom "Inpatient Statistics from the Mental Health Inquiry" (32). The cumulative inception rate was nearly equal for men and women, indicating that the liability is similar between the sexes. Results such as these imply that the observed excess of middle-aged, bipolar women may be attributable to life experiences, a greater willingness to seek treatment, and/or other demographic factors.

Recovery Phase

It appears that a number of complications await the recovering bipolar patient after an episode of mania. For example, Lucas et al. reported on a retrospective linear discriminant analysis of 100 manic episodes (1981–1985) during the recovery phase and found that the incidence of *subsequent depression* was 30% in the first month (33). Many episodes were transient, however, and did not necessarily require treatment. This phenomenon could be successfully predicted in 81% of cases in which there is a pre-morbid history of cyclothymia with either a personal or family history of depression. The highly significant association between family history and post-manic depression again supports the hypothesis of a genetic basis for bipolar disorder.

Keller and colleagues reported the *recovery rate* in 155 Bipolar I patients in an uncontrolled, naturalistic follow-up study

(34, 35). Patients were in the community and received different types of treatment after their index episode. He defined recovery as being either asymptomatic or manifesting only one or two symptoms of minimal severity for eight consecutive weeks. The different types of index episode (i.e., purely manic, purely depressed, or mixed/cycling) afforded significantly different rates of recovery, such that by 8 weeks, 61% of the purely manic patients had recovered, compared with 44% of the pure depressives, and only 33% of the mixed/cycling patients ($p = 0.05$). With a median follow-up of 1.5 years, they estimated that the probability of remaining ill for pure manics was about 7%, compared to 32% in patients who had mixed or cycling symptoms at the index episode. Pure depressed bipolar patients fell somewhere in the middle, with about a 22% probability of remaining ill. **They concluded that subtyping of episodes may be useful in terms of classifying the longitudinal course of bipolar disorders.**

Predictors of delayed recovery by subtype included:

- *Purely manic.* A long duration of the index manic episode, few previous major affective episodes, and the admitting research center
- *Purely depressed.* Longer previous episodes and earlier nonaffective psychiatric disorders
- *Mixed/cycling.* The presence of psychosis and endogenous features.

Keller et al. (1986) were also surprised to find that 75% of the nonrecovered patients had been treated with sustained, high levels of drug and/or somatic therapies (35). They concluded that mixed/cycling patients have a more pernicious course and require more effective therapies. In addition, to achieve earlier remission, clinicians should begin aggressive treatment in the initial symptomatic stages, because the purely manic and depressed groups also had severe episodes despite adequate treatment.

Long-Term Course and Prognosis

While biological and genetic factors are undoubtedly important, they may not explain all the variance in the course and prognosis of a bipolar disorder. Results from studies of life events and long-term course are mixed. Ellicott et al. (1990), in a 2-year prospective, longitudinal design, studied the *effect of life stress on course of illness* in 61 stable Bipolar I or II outpatients (36). Using survival analysis, they found a significant association (i.e., 4.53 times higher risk in patients with the highest levels of stress) between life event and relapse or recurrence. Further, this was not explained by other potential moderating variables such as levels of medication and treatment compliance. Improvements in their design over earlier studies, which found no association between life events and episodes of illness, included:

- A sufficient period of *time*
- *Prospective, systematic methods* appropriate for assessing symptoms and life stresses
- Careful attention to the appropriateness of *medication and compliance*
- The use of *sophisticated statistical models* to evaluate the association between probability of relapse and life events.

These results affirm the important impact of psychosocial factors on the course of a presumed biologically based disorder. Clinically, they imply that careful attention to and reduction of stressful life events may help prevent subsequent episodes.

Role of Psychotic Symptoms

Rosen and colleagues administered a structured interview based on the Schedule for Affective Disorders and Schizophrenia (SADS) to 89 Bipolar I patients, to compare psychotic and nonpsychotic manic patients on a number of clinical outcome and demographic variables (i.e., age, age at first treatment, and duration of illness). Overall, the psychotic manic group had a significantly poorer outcome in terms of social functioning (37).

Harrow et al. (1986) studied the *longitudinal course of thought disorder* in 34 manics, comparing them to 30 schizophrenics, 30 nonpsychotic patients, and 34 normal control subjects (38). During the acute hospitalization, both manic and schizophrenic patients demonstrated severe thought disorder, which was still evident at 1 year follow-up in both the schizophrenic patients and a subsample of manics, although significantly reduced in both groups. Although they found less thought pathology at follow-up for both disorders, the trend favored manic patients, who had a more stable reduction in symptoms.

Coryell et al. (1990) also conducted *a longitudinal study in patients with psychotic manic syndromes* (39). Fourteen patients with schizoaffective mania and 56 with psychotic mania completed a 5-year study. Mean time for recovery from the index episode for the former group was 58.6 weeks, compared with only 36.2 weeks for the latter. Schizoaffective manics also relapsed more quickly than the psychotic group, with respective means of 44.5 versus 61.8 weeks; however, the differences for the two groups did not persist into the second episode. Schizoaffective patients experienced more cumulative morbidity during follow-up, with the mean cumulative inpatient time double that for

the psychotic manics. Mean scores on the Global Assessment Scale (GAS) were significantly worse for the schizoaffective patients, who were four times as likely to have sustained psychotic outcomes. Those with chronic subtypes of schizoaffective mania were admitted five times as often as their nonchronic counterparts, had lower GAS scores, more persistent delusions, and greater impairment in interpersonal relationships.

When combining patients from this and an earlier study, Coryell et al. (1990) found that baseline variables that significantly and independently predicted a sustained delusional outcome were:

- A longer duration of the episode
- Temporal disassociation between psychotic features and affective syndrome
- Impaired adolescent friendship patterns (40).

Subsyndromal Affective Symptoms

Fichtner and colleagues followed 38 unipolar, 27 bipolar, 35 schizophrenic, and 27 other psychiatric patients for 4 years after hospital discharge, as well as 153 normal control subjects, to assess *cyclothymic mood swings and psychosocial adjustment* (41). Patients were significantly more cyclothymic at follow-up than normal controls, and those who demonstrated mood swings tended to have poorer posthospital outcomes than their noncycling counterparts. Although the authors commented that the presence of mood instability might reflect a greater vulnerability to persistent psychopathology, they could not distinguish significant differences among the diagnostic groups. **Monitoring for an increase in affective lability or reactivity may be useful in managing major mood disorders, as well as for predicting impending exacer-**

bations in nonaffective psychotic disorders.

Mortality Risk

Most recently, Tohen and colleagues investigated outcome by using a 4-year follow-up study of 75 bipolar patients who had recovered from an episode of mania and found the mortality risk during this period was 4% (42). They noted that *predictors of an unfavorable outcome* included:

- *Poor occupational status* before the index episode
- A history of *previous episodes*
- A history of *alcoholism*
- *Psychotic features*
- Symptoms of *depression* during the index manic episode (mixed mania)
- *Male* gender
- *Interepisode affective symptoms* (perhaps a reflection of incomplete remission) at 6 month follow-up.

Interventions that may improve prognosis include referrals for vocational testing and training; substance- and alcohol-abuse counseling; and aggressive management of depressive symptoms at any time point.

CONCLUSION

In summary, it is important to emphasize the syndrome of mania has symptoms that can overlap other illnesses, including organic affective, schizoaffective, and schizophreniform disorders. In addition, there is an ongoing and intimate relationship between the manic and the depressive phases, which has significant implications for diagnosis, treatment, and prognosis. The diagnosis of a bipolar disorder, manic phase, can usually be made by existing inclusion and exclusion criteria, as well as its distinctive personal and family histories. As our con-

cept of what constitutes the syndrome of mania evolves, elaboration and refinement should help improve diagnosis as well as assessment of response to present and future treatments for mania. Studies of the longitudinal course should clarify clinical presentation, as well as psychosocial factors that can alert the clinician to early, aggressive interventions to minimize the impact of this disorder.

To underscore the importance of adequate treatment for bipolar disorder, we note that it is estimated that one of every four or five untreated or inadequately treated patients commit suicide during the course of their illness. Further, an increase in deaths secondary to accidents or intercurrent illnesses contributes to the greater mortality rate seen in this disorder. Unfortunately, recent epidemiological studies have indicated that only one-third of bipolar patients are in active treatment despite the availability of effective therapies.

REFERENCES

1. Weissman M, Boyd J. The epidemiology of affective disorders: rate and risk factor. Psychiatry Update 1983;2:406–426.
2. Joyce PR. Age of onset in bipolar affective disorder and misdiagnosis as schizophrenia. Psychol Med 1984;14:145–149.
3. Solomon RL, Rich CL, Darko DF. Antidepressant treatment and the occurrence of mania in bipolar patients admitted for depression. J Affective Disord 1990;18:253–257.
4. Altman E, Janicak PG, Davis JM. Mania, clinical manifestations and assessment. In: Howells JG, ed. Modern perspectives in the psychiatry of mood disorders. New York: Brunner/Mazel, 1989;292–302.
5. Tyrer S, Shopsin B. Symptoms and assessment of mania. In: Paykel ES, ed. Handbook of affective disorders. New York: Guilford Press, 1982:2–23.
6. Goodwin FK, Jamison KR. Manic-depressive illness. New York: Oxford University Press, 1990:138.

7. Carlson GA, Goodwin FK. The stages of mania: a longitudinal analysis of the manic episode. Arch Gen Psychiatry 1973;28:221.

8. Goodwin FK, Jamison KR. Manic-depressive illness. New York: Oxford University Press, 1990:31.

9. Goodwin FK, Jamison KR. Manic-depressive illness. New York: Oxford University Press, 1990:36–37.

10. Taylor MA, Abrams R. Acute mania: clinical and genetic study of responders and nonresponders to treatments. Arch Gen Psychiatry 1975;32:863.

11. Pope H, Lipinski J. Differential diagnosis of schizophrenia and manic depressive illness: a reassessment of the specificity of schizophrenia symptoms in the light of current research. Arch Gen Psychiatry 1978;35:811–828.

12. Carpenter WT, Strauss JS, Muleh S. Are there pathognomonic symptoms in schizophrenia? An empiric investigation of Schneider's first-rank symptoms. Arch Gen Psychiatry 1973;28:847.

13. Taylor MA, Abrams R. The phenomenology of mania. A new look at some old patients. Arch Gen Psychiatry 1973;29:520.

14. Blumenthal RL, Egeland JA, Sharpe L, et al. Age of onset in bipolar and unipolar illness with and without delusions or hallucinations. Compr Psychiatry 1987;28:547–554.

15. Spitzer RL, Endicott J, Robins E. Research diagnostic criteria: rationale criteria: rationale and reliability. Arch Gen Psychiatry 1978;35:773.

16. American Psychiatric Association. Diagnostic and statistical manual of mental disorders, 3rd ed. Rev. Washington, DC: 1987.

17. Endicott J, Spitzer RL. A diagnostic interview: the schedule for affective disorders and schizophrenia. Arch Gen Psychiatry 1978;35:837.

18. Wing JK, Cooper JE, Sartorius N. Description and classification of psychiatric symptoms. Cambridge: Cambridge University Press, 1974.

19. Klerman G. The classification of bipolar disorders. Psychiatr Ann 1987;17:13–17.

20. Dunner EL. Stability of bipolar II affective disorder as a diagnostic entity. Psychiatr Ann 1987;17:18–20.

21. Coryell W. Outcome and family studies of bipolar II depression. Psychiatr Ann 1987;17:28–31.

22. Dunner DL, Vijayalakshmy P, Fieve RR. Rapid cycling in manic depressive patients. Compr Psychiatry 1977;18:561–566.

23. Bauer MS, Whybrow PC, Winokur A. Rapid cycling bipolar affective disorder. I. Association with grade I hypothyroidism. Arch Gen Psychiatry 1990;47:427–432.

24. Post RM, Rubinow DR, Uhde TW, et al. Dysphoric mania: clinical and biological correlates. Arch Gen Psychiatry 1989;46:353–358.

25. Akiskal HS. The milder spectrum of bipolar disorders: diagnostic, characterologic and pharmacologic aspects. Psychiatr Ann 1987;17:32–37.

26. Black DW, Winokur G, Bell S, et al. Complicated mania: comorbidity and immediate outcome in the treatment of mania. Arch Gen Psychiatry 1988;45:232–236.

27. Regier DA, Farmer ME, Rae DS, et al. Comorbidity of mental disorders with alcohol and other drug abuse. Results from the epidemiologic catchment area (ECA) study. JAMA 1990;264:2511–2518.

28. Mendlewicz J, Linkowski P, Wilmotte J. Relationship between shizoaffective illness and affective disorders or schizophrenia. J Affective Disord 1980;2:289–302.

29. Janowsky DS, El-Yousef M, Davis JM. Interpersonal maneuvers of manic patients. Am J Psychiatry 1974;131:250–254.

30. Meyer A. The life chart and the obligation of specifying positive data in psychopathological diagnosis. In: Winters E, ed. The collected papers of Adolph Meyer. Vol 3: Medical teachings. Baltimore: Johns Hopkins University Press, 1951.

31. Post RM, Roy-Bryne PP, Uhde TW. Graphic representation of the life course of illness in patients with affective disorder. Am J Psychiatry 1988;145:844–848.

32. Sibisi CDT. Sex differences in the age of onset of bipolar affective illness. Br J Psychiatry 1990;156:842–845.

33. Lucas CP, Rigby JC, Lucas SB. The occurrence of depression following mania: a method of predicting vulnerable cases. Br J Psychiatry 1989;154:705–708.

34. Keller MB. The course of manic-depressive illness. J Clin Psychiatry 1988;49:4–7.

35. Keller MB, Lavori PW, Coryell W, et al. Differential outcome of pure manic, mixed/cycling, and pure depressive episodes in patients with bipolar illness. JAMA 1986;255:3138–3142.

36. Ellicott A, Hammen C, Gitlin M, et al.

Life events and the course of bipolar disorder. Am J Psychiatry 1990;147:1194–1198.

37. Rosen LN, Rosenthal NE, Dunner DL, et al. Social outcome compared in psychotic and nonpsychotic bipolar I patients. J Nerv Ment Dis 1983;171:272–275.

38. Harrow M, Grossman LS, Silverstein ML, et al. A longitudinal study of thought disorder in manic patients. Arch Gen Psychiatry 1986;43:781–785.

39. Coryell W, Keller M, Lavori P, et al. Affective syndromes, psychotic features, and prognosis. II. Mania. Arch Gen Psychiatry 1990;47:658–662.

40. Coryell W, Keller M, Lavori P, et al. Affective syndromes, psychotic features, and prognosis. I. Depression. Arch Gen Psychiatry 1990;47:651–657.

41. Fichtner CG, Grossman LS, Harrow M, et al. Cyclothymic mood swings in the course of affective disorders and schizophrenia. Am J Psychiatry 1989;146:1149–1154.

42. Tohen M, Waternaux CM, Tsuang M. Outcome in mania. Arch Gen Psychiatry 1990;47:1106–1111.

CHAPTER 10

Treatment with Mood Stabilizers/Antimanics

History

Lithium has been utilized as a medicinal agent since the mid-19th century for such varied disorders as gout, diabetes, and rheumatism. With the seminal reports of Cade and Schou almost a century later, it emerged as the standard of treatment for bipolar disorders (1, 2). John Cade, an Australian physician, serendipitously discovered this agent's antimanic properties when he injected lithium urate into guinea pigs. Mistaking toxicity for sedation in the animals, he then used it successfully in an open trial with manic patients. Mogens Schou, following up on Cade's report, was the first European to use lithium in a series of trials employing increasing degrees of methodological rigor (2–4). The term "normothymic" was proposed by Schou to describe lithium's action against both phases of a bipolar disorder, as well as its ability to prevent recurrences of unipolar depressive disorder (3).

In another serendipitous finding, Cade noted that the first patient treated with lithium relapsed when medication was withdrawn (5). From this he inferred that lithium may also be effective for maintenance treatment. Baastrup, Schou's co-worker, carried out the first definitive study of its prophylactic properties (6). The ability of lithium to decrease the rate of recurrence in both unipolar and bipolar disorders was then confirmed in a series of studies by Hartigan and Baastrup (7–9).

Unfortunately, just as lithium had been toxic when used as a salt substitute in cardiac patients, it also caused problems when used for mania. Indeed, until its safe use was mastered, Cade is said to have banned lithium in his own hospital, regarding it as too dangerous for use in man.

Lithium was reintroduced in the United States by Gershon in the late 1960s, and since then has remained the standard therapy for bipolar disorder (10). More recently, there has been a growing recognition that a significant proportion of patients cannot tolerate or are not adequately helped by this therapy. This has led to the reexamination and clarification of alternate treatments.

One line of investigation has been the anticonvulsant strategy. This approach includes such varied therapies as electroconvulsive therapy (ECT), valproic acid

(VPA), and carbamazepine (CBZ). It is worthy to note that these treatments have a recent history, also dating back to the 1960s. The first empirical investigation of carbamazepine was performed by Dehing (1968) (11). While studying the behavioral effects of this anticonvulsant in epileptic patients, he noted that it had an antiaggressive effect. Interestingly, lithium also has antiaggressive properties, but its antimanic effect was discovered first, whereas the reverse is true for CBZ. Next, CBZ was used for mania by a series of investigators in Japan (12, 13). As Schou in Europe and Gershon in the United States are credited with the introduction of lithium, Post similarly deserves credit for introducing carbamazepine to the United States (14).

Valproic acid was first utilized as a mood stabilizer by Lambert and associates in 1966 (15). Their favorable results in a heterogeneous population of psychiatric patients were followed by several open and controlled trials both in the United States and elsewhere. Currently, this agent has been better studied than lithium as a mood stabilizer for acute mania (16).

In summary, while lithium has revolutionized the treatment of bipolar disorder, its narrow therapeutic index, numerous adverse effects, and relative ineffectiveness in a large proportion of bipolar patients has led to an expanding number of alternate approaches.

REFERENCES

1. Cade JFJ. Lithium salts in the treatment of psychotic excitement. Med J Aust 1949;36: 349–352.
2. Schou M, Juel-Neilson N, Stromgren E, et al. The treatment of manic psychosis by the administration of lithium salts. J Neurol Neurosurg Psychiatry 1954;17:250–260.
3. Schou M. Normothymotics, "mood normalizers": are lithium and the imipramine drugs specific for affective disorders? Br J Psychiatry 1963;109:803–804.
4. Baastrup PC, Schou M. Prophylactic lithium. Lancet 1968;i:1419–1422.
5. Cade JFJ. The story of lithium. In: Ayd FJ Jr, Blackwell B, eds. Discoveries in biological psychiatry. Philadelphia: JB Lippincott, 1970:218–229.
6. Baastrup P, Poulsen KS, Schou M, et al. Prophylactic lithium: double-blind discontinuation in manic-depressive and recurrent-depressive disorders. Lancet 1970;ii: 326–330.
7. Hartigan GP. The use of lithium salts in affective disorders. Br J Psychiatry 1963;109:810–814.
8. Baastrup PC. The use of lithium in manic-depressive psychosis. Compr Psychiatry 1964;5:396–408.
9. Baastrup PC. Lithium-behandling of manidepressiv psykose: en psykoseforebyggende behandlingsmade (Lithium treatment of manic-depressive psychosis: a procedure for preventing psychotic relapses). Nordisk Psykiatrisk Tiddskrift 1966;20:441–450.
10. Gershon S, Yuwiler A. Lithium ion: a specific psychopharmacological approach to the treatment of mania. J Neuropsychiatry 1960;1:229–241.
11. Dehing J. Studies on the psychotropic action of tegretol. Acta Neurol Belg 1968;68: 895–905.
12. Takezaki H, Hanaoka M. The use of carbamazepine (Tegretol) in the control of manic-depressive psychosis and other manic, depressive states (in Japanese). Sheishin-Igaku 1971;13:173–183.
13. Okuma T, Kishimoto A, Inoue K, et al. Anti-manic and prophylactic effects of carbamazepine on manic-depressive psychosis. Folia Psychiatr Neurol Jpn 1973;27:283–297.
14. Post RM, Ballenger JC, Reus VI, et al. Effects of carbamazepine in mania and depression. Paper presented at the Scientific Proceedings of the 131st Annual Meeting of the American Psychiatric Association, Atlanta, May 1978. New Research Abstracts, No. 7.
15. Lambert PA, Cavaz G, Barselli S, Carrel S. Action neuropsychotrope d'un novel antiepeliptique: le depamide. Ann Med Psychol 1966;1:707–710.
16. Janicak PG, Newman R, Davis JM. Advances in the treatment of mania and related disorders: a reappraisal. Psychiatric Annals 1992;22(2):92–103.

Mechanism of Action

Since the mid-1960s, when Schild-kraut, and Bunney and Davis, independently developed the *monoamine hypothesis* of mood disorders, a great wealth of data has been generated to test this theory (see also Mechanism of Action in Chapter 7) (1, 2). Since the early development of psychotropic agents was based on the concept that altering norepinephrine (NE) or serotonin (5-HT) activity could benefit depression or mania, it is not surprising that the action of these drugs would support the original concept. There is also a growing appreciation that receptor changes and neuromodulators (e.g., neurohormones, neuropeptides), which are slower and more sustained in their actions in comparison to neurotransmitters, may be more consistent with the time course of mood changes. Models to further clarify the underlying pathophysiology of bipolar disorder have also incorporated such factors as genetic vulnerability and cyclicity.

As we have already noted, the history of psychiatry contains numerous preliminary findings of biologic abnormalities attributed to a given diagnostic entity. Unfortunately, the great majority have not been replicated. More recently, the technology has been developed to measure blood flow and to image structural changes, as well as biological activity, through magnetic resonance imaging (MRI) or positron emission tomography (PET). All of these have the potential to better "localize" pathophysiologic processes. While there will be some false starts (i.e., unreplicated findings) with these methods, we anticipate a greater probability for meaningful replications. For now, however, before assuming that such findings are more than background noise and indeed represent findings with clear implications for etiology, a healthy degree of scepticism is appropriate in interpreting any early positive findings.

NEUROTRANSMITTER AND RELATED HYPOTHESES

While the therapeutic mechanism(s) of various mood stabilizers is unknown, studies have concentrated on:

- The classic neurotransmitters (NE, 5-HT) implicated in affective disturbances
- Cellular processes involving the classic ligand-receptor interaction and beyond (e.g., second messenger systems)
- The modulating interactive processes among various neurotransmitter systems, neuromodulators, and genetic influences
- The role of circadian rhythms.

Mood stabilizers have been shown to interact with several neurotransmitters, including the catecholaminergic, indolaminergic, cholinergic, and γ-aminobutyric acid systems. While the data is conflicting, it appears that they affect both the pre- and the post-neuronal receptors as well as the post-receptor activity (or second messenger system) of these neurotransmitters. Still, the exact mechanism(s) by which they relate to the biological substrates subserving mood disorders remains unclear.

Catecholamines

Research at the Illinois State Psychiatric Institute has shown that treatment with lithium decreases the β-adrenergic receptor number, consistent with the noradrenergic down-regulation hypothesis but difficult to reconcile with a complementary theory of mania (3). Lithium can also block dopamine receptor supersensitivity, and this is consistent with the postulate that mania is associated with an increased sensitivity of catecholamine receptors.

Lithium blocks the release of *thyroid hormones*, which are known to *potentiate β-noradrenergic receptor sensitivity*. This has led to the speculation that excessive thyroid activity may precipitate an episode of mania in susceptible patients, and that the antimanic effect of lithium is, at least in part, due to its anti-thyroid action. Carbamazepine can also decrease various thyroid indices.

Another approach has been the investigation of agents such as clonidine, which stimulates the α_2-noradrenergic, presynaptic receptors, setting into motion a short-loop, negative-feedback system. This culminates in a shutdown of tyrosine hydroxylase, the rate-limiting enzyme for the production of the catecholamines, thus slowing NE synthesis and release. Further, this drug acts in a rapid fashion and is highly specific for the locus coeruleus, the central nervous system (CNS) location with the richest concentration of NE-containing neurons. As a result, it can rapidly and effectively shut down norepinephrine production.

Indolamines

Lithium may facilitate the release of 5-HT, perhaps by increasing tryptophan uptake, as well as by increasing activity at postsynaptic 5-HT receptors (i.e., act as a 5-HT agonist). Recent data, however, question the long-term effect of lithium on 5-HT enhancement when studied in patients, as opposed to healthy controls (4).

Similar to lithium, clonazepam can increase 5-HT synthesis and cerebrospinal fluid (CSF) levels of its major metabolite 5-hydroxyindoleacetic acid (5-HIAA). Other agents known to enhance 5-HT activity by different mechanisms have also shown initial promise as potential antimanic treatments, including L-tryptophan (a precursor) and fenfluramine (which enhances release and blocks reuptake).

Cholinergic System

Lithium has been shown to increase red blood cell (RBC) levels of choline, but the significance of this finding is yet to be determined (5). This activity is consistent with the cholinergic-adrenergic balance hypothesis of mood disorders, which promulgates a lack of cholinergic relative to noradrenergic activity in the manic state and the reverse in the depressed phase (6). These findings have led to the administration of drugs with cholinomimetic effects, such as physostigmine, to treat acute mania. For example, a single i.v. dose of this agent reversed a manic state to a depressed phase for about 1 hour (6).

GABA Activity

GABA is a major CNS inhibitory neurotransmitter, which, among other effects, may attenuate catecholaminergic systems. VPA (through inhibition of this transmitter's degradation by GABA transaminase) as well as CBZ and lithium all enhance GABA activity (see also Mechanism of Action in Chapter 12).

Second Messenger Systems

Lithium's interactions with *second messenger systems*, particularly the phosphoinositide cycle, may deplete free inositol and alter intracellular calcium mobilization. Antagonists such as verapamil decrease calcium channel activity, diminishing intracellular Ca^{2+} concentrations, and have shown early promise as potential antimanics; however, the mechanistic significance of this is unclear.

Membrane/Cation Hypothesis

Electrolyte disturbances have been extensively studied, with disruptions in calcium and sodium activity the most consistently reported aberrations in mood disorders. In a series of studies, Dubovsky et al. have measured intracellular calcium ion concentrations in bipolar, manic and depressed patients (7). Most recently, they found decreases in mean intracellular calcium ion concentrations in four bipolar, manic, and five bipolar, depressed, patients, in comparison to seven normothymic subjects without personal or first-degree relative histories of psychiatric disorders. Their findings were consistent with a diffuse abnormality in the mechanisms modulating intracellular calcium homeostasis. Further, this phenomenon's presence in both platelets and lymphocytes lends credence to a disruption in the cell membrane, the G protein, or other mechanism involved in the homeostasis of intracellular calcium ion concentrations. This may also support an extension of their findings from peripheral to neuronal tissue.

Calcium antagonists (e.g., verapamil) can also block dopamine, serotonin, and endorphinergic activity; alter sodium activity via a sodium-calcium counterexchange; and act as anticonvulsants. Any or all of these actions could be involved in their putative antimanic effects.

Cellular ionic transport mechanisms have been another line of investigation into amine neurotransmitter and neuroendocrine function in affective disturbances.

Lithium and the calcium antagonists block the influx of Ca^{2+} as well as alter intracellular calcium mobilization, thus dampening neuroelectrical activity and enhancing stabilization of neuronal membranes. Meltzer postulated a specific macromolecular complex composed of at least the sodium/potassium and calcium pumps, the ion channel, and ankyrin, which may be abnormally constituted in bipolar illness (8). Further elucidation of this hypothesis might help identify a specific membrane fault in bipolar disorder as well as lead to new, more specific pharmacotherapy. For example, novel agents could possibly regulate insertion of specific proteins into the membrane or alter the linkage of integral membrane proteins to their underlying cytoskeleton.

NEUROANATOMIC/ NEUROPHYSIOLOGIC HYPOTHESES

Prior to the development of brain imaging techniques, *neuroanatomical correlates* were primarily related to structural lesions of the central nervous system. Despite the fact that abnormalities have been found in both schizophrenia and affective illness, interest in the neuropathology of mood disorders has not been as intense as for schizophrenia.

Recently, Jeste, Lohr, and Goodwin reviewed the neuroanatomical studies of major mood disorders, noting that several found no difference in abnormalities between schizophrenic and mood disorders (9). Swayze and colleagues, utilizing MRI, found a nonsignificant trend for ventricular enlargement in bipolar men, while bipolar women did not differ significantly from normal controls (10). Dupont et al. have reported on subcortical abnormalities (i.e., hyperintensities in some bipolar patients using MRI (10a). Recent studies of *cerebral blood flow* (CBF), however, found no significant correlation between symptoms of mania and overall CBF (11).

One of the more consistent findings is the apparent association between secondary mania and right frontal-temporal or left parietal-occipital lesions. Such data are also consistent with neuropsychological studies pointing to a right frontal lobe disturbance in these syndromes. Taken as a whole, these results suggest a differential pathophysiological origin for structural brain abnormalities underlying bipolar disorders. If confirmed, and not simply due to epiphenomena such as treatment, substance abuse, or associated medical conditions (e.g., hypertension), these findings can serve as an important way to differentiate the neuroanatomical and neurophysiological mechanisms subserving schizophrenia and bipolar disorder.

Central electrophysiological measures are also partially supportive, in that *evoked response* and *computer-assisted electroencephalogram (EEG) mapping* indicate bipolar-unipolar differences, with right-sided abnormalities more common in bipolar patients.

The efficacy of ECT for mania is intriguing, vis-à-vis the emerging anticonvulsant strategy, since it has many of the same antiseizure effects as clonazepam, CBZ, and VPA. Thus, over a course of ECT, the seizure threshold is usually raised, the duration of a given seizure episode decreases, neurometabolic response to a given seizure episode is diminished, and the phenomenon of amygdaloid kindling is attenuated. *Kindling* occurs in animals who are exposed to repeated, subthreshold seizurogenic, electrical stimuli and eventually develop spontaneous seizures. This is particularly interesting, in that kindling in the mesolimbic structures has been analogized to the course of some bipolar disorders. Post and colleagues

(1988) have also noted similarities between the increasing intensity of response to subthreshold stimulations and eventual spontaneous seizure activity and the natural course of certain bipolar patients whose illness progressively worsens, culminating in increasing vulnerability to more frequent, non–stress-induced episodes (e.g., behavioral sensitization) (12). In this context, Post and Weiss (1989) have argued for differing pharmacosensitivity as a function of the stage of illness (13). By implication, different treatments (e.g., lithium, antipsychotics, anticonvulsants) may interrupt this natural course at different phases, favorably altering the disorder's progression.

BIOLOGICAL RHYTHMS HYPOTHESIS

Chronobiological factors are important considerations, given the cyclic pattern of disturbances in bipolar disorders. Studies are hampered, however, by a dearth of longitudinal data and the masking of internal and external oscillator-driven rhythms that can alter rhythmic phase or amplitude.

One of the most consistent findings is the sleep disturbance that often precedes, and may even trigger a manic phase. Studies on *circadian rhythms* have demonstrated that many aspects of the sleep cycle are phase-advanced in mania (i.e., occur earlier than normal) and often these patterns resemble the free-running rhythms seen in normal individuals who are removed from any time cues. In addition, there is a blunting of amplitude and a doubling of the sleep-wake cycle up to 48 hours. Lithium is known to delay the sleep-wake cycle and often slow such free-running rhythms, which in turn are partly modulated by neurotransmitters such as NE, 5-HT, and acetylcholine (Ach). Further, manipulation of the sleep-wake cycle may prevent a manic episode or be used to treat the depressive phase (e.g., sleep deprivation therapy) (see also Experimental Somatic Therapies in Chapter 8).

The phenomenon of *seasonal variation* is discussed in the sections Seasonal Affective Disorders in Chapter 6 and Bright Light Phototherapy in Chapter 8. This is another chronobiological rhythm that is manifested by increases in depression and suicide in spring (with smaller peaks in autumn), as opposed to mania, which increases in the summer months. These observations have led to preliminary studies on the alteration of both light and temperature as potential therapies for the two seasonal patterns of affective disturbance.

NEUROENDOCRINE HYPOTHESIS

Lithium has several effects on the endocrine system. For example, it can interfere with the synthesis and the release of testosterone, leading to an increase in luteinizing hormone levels. The thyroid system has been most implicated in neuroendocrine theories of lithium's antimanic effects. In particular, thyroid hormones can potentiate β-NE activity and lithium's ability to block their release may subserve its mood stabilizing properties (i.e., the thyroid-catecholamine-receptor hypothesis) (14, 15). More recently, Dinan and colleagues (1991) found a significant blunting of desipramine-induced growth hormone (GH) stimulation in seven drug-free bipolar patients, in comparison to seven control subjects. They suggested that this phenomenon was consistent with a down-regulation of α_2-noradrenergic responses. Since a similar phenomenon has been reported for major depressive disorder (MDD), they feel this might provide an important marker to identify patients susceptible to clinically relevant mood fluctuations (16).

IMMUNOLOGICAL HYPOTHESIS

This line of investigation is based on evidence suggesting a close interaction between the immune and the central nervous systems. For example, immunological abnormalities have been reported in relation to psychological stress in patients with psychiatric disorders such as major depression. Kronfol and House looked at different immune variables in manic versus schizophrenic patients and normal controls (17). In general, they found no significant differences for most measures. Results of the mitogen stimulation assays, however, revealed significant reductions in lymphocyte responsivity to the mitogens phytohemagglutin-P (PHA) and concanavalin-A (Con-A) in bipolar patients when compared to schizophrenic patients and normal controls. They speculate that this may represent an impairment in cell-mediated immune response, as the mitogens in question stimulate mostly T cells. Potential confounds to the study include its small sample size and the effects of ongoing psychotropic drug treatment.

GENETIC HYPOTHESIS

Consistent with the dominant mode of transmission, it appears that first-degree relatives of bipolar patients have a 15–35% morbid risk for developing an affective disturbance. *Concordance rates* for mood disorders in twin studies demonstrate a strikingly higher incidence in monozygotic versus dizygotic twins (see Table 10.1) (18). Bipolar disorder occurs more often in families with a history of this illness; similarly, unipolar disorder occurs more often in families with a history of unipolar illness. Therefore, these two variants of affective disease appear to breed true. **In addition, bipolar patients seem to have a greater genetic loading for mood disorders than their**

Table 10.1.
Concordance (+) and Discordance (−) of Mood Disorder in Pairs of Twins

Study	Monozygotic		Dizygotic	
	(+)	(−)	(+)	(−)
Luxenburger (1928)	2	1	0	13
Rosanoff et al. (1934)	16	7	11	56
Essen-Moller (1941)	2	6	0	3
Slater and Shields (1953)	4	4	7	23
Kallmann (1954)	25	2	13	42
Da Fonseca (1959)	15	6	15	24
Kringlen (1967)	2	4	0	20
Allen et al. (1974)	5	10	0	34
Bertelsen et al. (1977)	32	23	9	43
TOTAL	103 (**62%**)	63 (38%)	55 (**18%**)	258 (82%)

Chi square = 98.7; $p < 0.0001$ (Mantel-Haenszel)
Davis, JM, Noll KM, Sharma R. Differential diagnosis and treatment of mania. In: Swann AC, ed. Mania: new research and treatment. Washington, D.C.: American Psychiatric Press, 1986:1–58. Copyright 1986, the American Psychiatric Association. Reprinted by permission.

unipolar counterparts (19, 20). Thus, the rate of this illness in relatives of bipolar probands is 4 to 10 times greater than in unipolar proband relatives. Furthermore, even while a large proportion of bipolar proband relatives develop only unipolar symptoms, unipolar proband relatives develop predominantly unipolar symptoms.

Other disorders that are reported to be cotransmitted with bipolar, and to a lesser extent unipolar, disorder(s) include:

- *Schizoaffective* disorder
- *Cyclothymic* personality
- *Hypomania* (without depression).

Another approach has been the study of *red blood cell:plasma lithium concentrations,* which is an expression of the relationship between intracellular and extracellular levels. The lithium-sodium counter-transport (an exchange diffusion process) mechanism is located in the cell membrane and determines the relative concentration of these ions (21). An abnormality in this transport function could represent an inheritable marker of susceptibility for the development of bipolar disorder (22). Clinical studies of lithium administration find that the RBC:plasma lithium ratio varies from 0.15 to 0.60 (average = 0.30) and remains constant for individuals, independent of change in symptoms (23). There is also evidence that bipolar patients have a higher mean ratio than the normal population or those with other psychiatric diagnoses, and that a greater proportion of their first-degree relatives have this elevation. This phenomenon has been demonstrated using both statistical and genetic models (24, 25).

Genetic linkage studies are particularly useful in resolving issues regarding the myriad of clinical presentations, while contributing to an increased understanding of the basis for vulnerability to various mood disorders. Many studies, however, have unequivocally established a genetic heritability for bipolar illness. For example, linkage to the genetic markers of color blindness, which is associated with a region of the X chromosome, was reported in some but not all pedigrees (26, 27). The association of bipolar disorder to chromosome 11 suggested to occur in the Amish pedigree did not replicate with a larger sample (28). A fascinating corollary to the chromosome 11 story is the nearby location of genes involved in tyrosine hydroxylase production, as well as a muscarinic cholinergic receptor gene. Similar discrepancies have plagued attempts at linkage to the human leukocyte antigen (HLA) region of chromosome 6 (29).

CONCLUSION

Whether any or all of these factors relate to the efficacy of mood stabilizers is still uncertain, but the final common pathway may well be the inhibition of neurotransmitter/receptor (e.g., NE and/or 5-HT) mediated processes. What is not clear is how these drugs alter neurotransmitter function or interactions, ultimately leading to their normothymic effects. A further complication stems from the combined antimanic and antidepressant properties of these therapies (e.g., ECT, lithium, CBZ, etc.), making it difficult to theorize how opposite clinical effects are mediated by biochemical changes in one direction.

REFERENCES

1. Schildkraut JJ. The catecholamine hypothesis of affective disorders (a review of supporting evidence). Am J Psychiatry 1965;122:509–522.
2. Bunney Jr WE, Davis JM. Norepinephrine in depressive reactions. Arch Gen Psychiatry 1965;13:483–494.
3. Pandey G, Davis JM. Treatment with antidepressants and down regulation of beta-adrenergic receptors. Drug Dev Research 1983;3:393–406.
4. Price LH, Charney DS, Delgado PL, Henenger GR. Lithium treatment and serotonergic function. Arch Gen Psychiatry 1989;46:13–19.
5. Hanin I, Mallinger AG, Kopp V, Hemmelhoch JM, Neil JF. Mechanism of lithium induced elevation in red blood cell choline content: an in vitro analysis. Comm in Psychopharmacol 1980;4:345–355.
6. Janowsky D, El Yousef MK, Davis JM, et al. A cholinergic-adrenergic hypothesis of mania and depression. Lancet 1972;2:6732–6735.
7. Dubovsky SL, Murphy J, Thomas M, Rademacher J. Abnormal intracellular calcium ion concentration in platelets and lymphocytes of bipolar patients. Am J Psychiatry 1992;149:118–120.
8. Meltzer HL. Is there a specific membrane defect in bipolar disorders? Biol Psychiatry 1991;30:1071–1074.
9. Jeste DV, Lohr JB, Goodwin FK. Neuroanatomical studies of major affective disorders. A review and suggestions for further research. Br J Psychiatry 1988;153:444–459.
10. Swayze VW, Andreasen NC, Alliger RJ, et al. Structural brain abnormalities in bipolar affective disorder: ventricular enlargement and focal signal hyperintensities. Arch Gen Psychiatry 1990;47:1054–1059.
10a. Dupont RM, Jernigan TL, Butler N, Delis D, Hesselink JR, Hundel W, Gillin C. Subcortical abnormalities detected in bipolar affective disorder using magnetic resonance imaging. Clinical and neuropsychological significance. Arch Gen Psychiatry 1990;47:55–59.
11. Silfverskiold P, Risberg J. Regional cerebral blood flow in depression and mania. Arch Gen Psychiatry 1989;46:253–259.
12. Post RN, Roy-Byrne PP, Uhde TW. Graphic representation of the life course of illness in patients with affective disorder. Am J Psychiatry 1988;145:844–848.
13. Post RM, Weiss SRB. Sensitization, kindling, and anticonvulsants in mania. J Clin Psychiatry 1989;50(12, suppl):23–30.
14. Whybrow PC, Prange AJ. A hypothesis of thyroid-catecholamine-receptor interaction: its relevance to affective illness. Arch Gen Psychiatry 1981;38:106–113.
15. Joffe RT, Roy-Byrne PP, Udhe TW, et al. Thyroid function and affective illness: a reappraisal. Biol Psychiatry 1984;19:1685–1691.
16. Dinan TG, Yatham LM, O'Keane V, Barry S. Am J Psychiatry 1991;148:936–938.
17. Kronfol Z, House DJ. Immune function in mania. Biol Psychiatry 1988;24:341–343.
18. Davis JM, Noll KM, Sharma R. Differential diagnosis and treatment of mania. In: Swann AC, ed. Mania: new research and treatment. Washington, D.C.: American Psychiatric Press, 1986:1–58.
19. Mendlewicz J, Fieve RR, Rainer JD, et al. Manic-depressive illness: a comparative study of patients with and without a family history. Br J Psychiatry 1972;120:523–530.
20. Mendlewicz J, Rainer JD. Adoption study supporting genetic transmission in manic-depressive illness. Nature 1977;268:327–329.

21. Dorus E, Paney GN, Davis JM. Genetic determinant of lithium ion distribution. Arch Gen Psychiatry 1975;32:1097–1102.
22. Dorus E, Pandey GN, Shaughnessy R, et al. Lithium abnormality across red cell membrane: a cell membrane abnormality in manic-depressive illness. Science 1979;205:932–934.
23. Garver DL, Hitzemann R, Hirschowitz J. Lithium ratio in vitro. Arch Gen Psychiatry 41;1984;41:497–505.
24. Dorus E, Cox NJ, Gibbons RD, et al. Lithium ion transport and affective disorders within families of bipolar patients. Arch Gen Psychiatry 1983;40:545–552.
25. Gibbons RD, Dorus E, Ostrow DG, et al. Mixture distributions in psychiatric research. Biol Psychiatry 1984;19:935–961.
26. Risch N, Baron M. X-linkage and genetic heterogeneity in bipolar-related major affective illness: reanalysis of linkage data. Ann Hum Genet 1982;46:153–166.
27. Baron M, Risch N, Hamburger R, et al. Genetic linkage between X-chromosome markers and bipolar affective disorders. Nature 1987;326:289–292.
28. Kelsoe JR, Ginns EI, Egeland JA, Gerhard DS, Goldstein AM, Bale SJ, Pauls DL, Long RT, Kidd KK, Conte G, Housman DE, Paul SM. Re-evaluation of the linkage relationship between chromosome 11p loci and the gene for bipolar affective disorder in the Old Order Amish. Nature 1989; 342:238–242.
29. Turner WJ, King S. Two genetically distinct forms of bipolar affective disorder. Biol Psychiatry 1981;16:417–439.

Management of an Acute Manic Episode

Data on the efficacy of mood stabilizers for bipolar disorder focuses on:

- Treatment of an *acute exacerbation*
- Prevention of *relapse* after an acute episode has been controlled
- Prevention of *future episodes*.

We reviewed the existing literature, emphasizing the controlled trials comparing these agents to either placebo or other standard treatments for acute, maintenance, and prophylactic purposes. When feasible, the results were combined using meta-analysis (see Statistical Summarization of Drug Studies in Chapter 2).

EFFICACY FOR ACUTE TREATMENT

Lithium

Approximately 60% of all acutely ill bipolar, manic patients benefit from lithium.

This agent's efficacy has been estab-lished within a well-defined therapeutic blood level range for optimal benefit and minimal adverse or toxic reactions. Optimism over lithium's impact has diminished, however, because of a significant proportion of patients who are nonresponders, insufficiently responsive, or intolerant to its adverse effects. Given the alarmingly high suicide rate for untreated or inadequately treated bipolar patients, the need for other effective therapies is clear. Lithium may also be utilized in the depressive phase of a bipolar disorder, alone or to augment other antidepressants; and/or in combination with divalproex sodium or carbamazepine (see Efficacy for Acute Treatment and Alternate Treatment Strategies in Chapter 7).

Lithium versus Placebo

Schou (1954), in a now classic study, charted the natural history of several bipolar patients and found that the introduction of lithium induced remissions, dramatically altering the course of the disorder (1). While some patients were also assigned to placebo, the data was not presented systematically, and therefore could not be included in our meta-analysis. Bunney, Goodwin, Davis, and Fawcett (1968) reported on a patient treated with lithium or placebo in a longitudinal ABA design who failed to respond to placebo, improved when switched to lithium, and then relapsed when lithium was discontinued (2). They also described a second patient who responded to lithium after failure to respond to a long, 10-day placebo lead-in period, and again relapsed when lithium was discontinued. A subsequent report by Goodwin et al. (1969) described two additional cases with an unequivocal response to lithium; four others with a probable response; one with an equivocal response; and three who deteriorated on lithium; however, there was no control group (3). While not as definitive as the Class I or II study designs, these naturalistic reports strongly support lithium's efficacy (see Evaluation of Drug Study Designs in Chapter 2).

Approximately 46 acutely manic patients have undergone some form of controlled trial comparing lithium to placebo, and the results indicate a significantly better effect with lithium; no investigators, however, have undertaken a definitive Class I or II study addressing this question. Maggs (1963) conducted the only double-blind, random-assignment, placebo-controlled, parallel trial of lithium without concomitant medications (4). While he found lithium clearly superior to placebo, he probably underestimated the true drug/placebo difference since he did not include the placebo, nonresponding dropouts. Stokes (1971) also conducted a 10-day double-blind, placebo-controlled, random-assignment trial of lithium using only a modest amount of adjunctive anti-

psychotics. He crossed over nonresponders every subsequent 10-day period to the opposite arm, for a total of four switches, and found lithium superior to placebo throughout the study (5). Again, he may have underestimated the true drug/placebo difference, however, since 10 days is often insufficient to achieve full benefit with lithium. In 1976, Stokes used the same crossover design, this time assigning patients to high or low doses of lithium (6). Combining the data from his two studies, he was able to demonstrate a dose- (and plasma level-) response relationship to remission.

While there have been no definitive placebo-controlled trials (i.e., Class I or II) with lithium for acute mania, its efficacy has clearly stood the test of time.

Lithium versus Antipsychotics

Lithium has also been systematically compared to antipsychotics for the management of acute mania. Most believe it produces a better qualitative response, but this observation is difficult to substantiate with controlled studies. A patient once analogized this difference to an automobile engine racing out of control, describing the effect of antipsychotics as similar to applying the brakes, while lithium was similar to adjusting the carburetor (7). Lithium has a more narrowly defined range of indications, primarily benefitting mania, while relatively ineffective for schizophrenia, particularly the more chronic subtypes. Given its narrow spectrum of efficacy, the inclusion of groups such as schizoaffective disorder and schizophrenia in studies comparing it to antipsychotics may bias the results against lithium. Also, since antipsychotics usually have a faster onset of action, a design that allows patients to drop out early may underestimate lithium's relative efficacy.

There have been five well-controlled, albeit small, trials comparing lithium to an antipsychotic in pure manic patients. Table 10.3 summarizes the results from four of these studies, which presented their data in a way that allowed for inclusion in a meta-analysis. **Each study was a well-controlled, double-blind design, finding lithium superior to an antipsychotic, and the meta-analysis of the combined studies demonstrated this difference to be highly statistically significant.**

Platman (1970) studied 13 patients on lithium and 10 on chlorpromazine (CPZ), finding lithium consistently superior overall, but not statistically significant on any individual rating scale (8). The general state of patients on lithium was markedly superior to those on CPZ since the majority were discharged with no other treatment, while all of the patients on CPZ required additional concurrent drugs. Since he did not present data on individual patients, these results could not be included in the meta-analysis, but his results

are also consistent with the outcome in Table 10.3. Due to the small number of studies and sample sizes, the results should be interpreted cautiously.

Prien et al. (1972) studied 255 Veteran's Administration (VA) patients diagnosed as bipolar, manic, or schizoaffective, and assigned to lithium or CPZ (9). They subdivided patients into highly versus mildly agitated categories based on the Inpatient Multidimensional Psychiatric Scale (IMPS), which describes patients as "exhibiting overactivity, restlessness, and/or accelerated body movement." Also, patients were categorized by the Brief Psychiatric Rating Scale (BPRS) for baseline levels of excitement, uncooperativeness, grandiosity, mannerisms, tension, and conceptual disorganization. Twenty-two percent of the lithium-treated and 14% of the chlorpromazine-treated patients dropped out, leaving approximately 60 in each of the four groups: highly active, lithium- or CPZ-treated; and mildly active, lithium- or CPZ-treated. They found

Table 10.2.
Lithium versus Placebo for *Bipolar Disorder*: Acute Treatment

Number of Subjects	Responders (%)		Difference (%)	Chi Square	p Value
	Lithium (%)	Placebo (%)			
28	91.7	43.8	47.8	NA	NA

Table 10.3.
Lithium versus Antipsychotics in the Treatment of Acute Mania

Study	Lithium		Antipsychotics	
	Responders (Number of Subjects)	Nonresponders (Number of Subjects)	Responders (Number of Subjects)	Nonresponders (Number of Subjects)
Johnson et al. (1968, 1971)	16	2	8	3
Spring et al. (1970)	8	1	3	3
Takahashi et al. (1975)	33	4	24	10
Shopsin et al. (1971)	7	3	3	17
Total	64 (89%)	10 (11%)	38 (54%)	33 (46%)

Chi square (MH) = 13.1; df = 1, p = 0.0003
Adapted from Janicak PG, Newman RH, Davis JM. Advances in the treatment of manic and related disorders: a reappraisal. Psychiatr Ann 1992;22(2):94.

substantially more dropouts in the highly active group receiving lithium, usually due to poor response or uncooperativeness, but the pre/post rating differences in all four groups were similar. An analysis of covariance found that the outcome for lithium completers did not differ from the CPZ completers. An endpoint analysis, however, found CPZ superior to lithium in the highly active group on such measures as conceptual disorganization, psychoticism, grandiosity, and suspiciousness. There were no significant differences between the two drugs in the mildly active group. When schizoaffective patients and many of the severely disturbed patients who did not receive lithium for a sufficient duration were included, the antipsychotics were found to be superior.

Garfinkel et al. (1980) compared haloperidol, lithium, and their combination for the treatment of mania, but did not present data on patients as individuals (10). Initially, there were 7 patients in each group. By day 15, 3 in the lithium group, 2 in the haloperidol group, and 1 in the combined drug group had dropped out. The two haloperidol groups improved slightly more than the lithium monotherapy group; however, considering the small sample and the high dropout rate, we would speculate that these patients were highly disturbed and could not be managed on lithium alone for a sufficient period of time.

Braden et al. (1982) did a similar study in *primarily schizophrenic or schizoaffective patients,* but the sample also included some affectively ill cases (i.e., 21% met Feighner criteria for mood disorder) (11). Of the 43 patients on lithium, 15 dropped out because they did not improve, worsened, or were unmanageable or confused. By comparison, only 1 of 35 treated with CPZ dropped out in the first 10 days. Chlorpromazine produced better results

in the overactive group, while both drugs were comparable in the non-overactive group. As with the VA study, the poor results with lithium in the overactive group may have been an artifact of insufficient duration due to the high dropout rate, or because of the inclusion of patients with a core schizophrenic illness.

Cookson et al. (1981) in a random-assignment design found 10 of 12 *manic patients* responded to pimozide and 11 of 12 patients to CPZ (12). This is consistent with the observation of Post et al. (1980), who, after a placebo lead-in period, found the time course of improvement with pimozide (N = 8) to be similar to lithium (N = 8) or a phenothiazine (N = 9) (13). Since pimozide is a more specific D_2 antagonist than CPZ, this outcome provides further support for a beneficial role with D_2 receptor blockers in the treatment of mania.

Johnstone et al. (1988) performed a random-assignment, double-blind trial comparing pimozide; lithium; a combination of these two; and placebo in 120 patients with a *variety of psychotic disorders* (e.g., psychotic mania, psychotic depression, schizoaffective disorder, schizophreniform disorder, schizophrenia, etc.) (14). Patients were classified as having an elevated or depressed mood or no consistent change in mood. Pimozide had a robust effect on positive symptoms across all categories (i.e., elevated mood, depressed mood, and no mood change); whereas lithium only had a modest beneficial effect ($p <$ 0.07) in affectively disordered patients with an elevated mood. Heterogeneity in the diagnostic categories, however, must temper interpretation of their results.

Thus, while lithium therapy of sufficient duration may be the treatment of choice in classic mania, the antipsychotics may be preferable in conditions such as schizoaffective disorder, given their faster onset of effect and broader spectrum of activity.

Table 10.4.
Laboratory Evaluation during Lithium Treatment

PRIOR TO INITIATION OF TREATMENT
  Renal function testing
    General screening—serum creatinine; BUN; urinalysis
    If further testing required:
      24-hour urine volume
      Creatinine clearance
      Test of renal concentrating ability
  Thyroid function
    T_3, T_3RU, and T_4
    TSH
  Cardiac
    ECG (if elderly or at risk for heart disease)
  General (if indicated)
    CBC and differential
    Serum electrolytes
    SMA-12
DURING MAINTENANCE TREATMENT
  Renal function
    Urinalysis; BUN (every 6–12 months)
    Serum creatinine (every 6–12 months when clinically indicated)
    Test of renal concentrating ability (when clinically indicated)
  Thyroid function
    TSH (every 6–12 months)
    Repeat full battery with elevated TSH and/or clinical signs/symptoms

ADMINISTRATION OF LITHIUM

As part of the standard pre-lithium workup, a thorough medical evaluation should be completed. Table 10.4 lists the various laboratory tests recommended to assess overall physical status, especially renal, thyroid, hematological, and cardiac function, prior to initiation of treatment. In particular, the renal and the thyroid systems require a baseline assessment and periodic reevaluation with long-term maintenance or prophylactic therapy.

Since lithium has a half-life of approximately 24 hours and it takes 4–5 half-lives to achieve steady-state, blood levels should be obtained every 5 days until an adequate therapeutic concentration is achieved or adverse effects preclude further increases. Attempts to develop dose prediction formulae to obtain therapeutic concentrations more rapidly have been promising, but they have not enjoyed widespread utilization (15, 16). While premature monitoring may lead to higher than necessary dosing, more frequent measuring of levels may be warranted in patients with known sensitivity to lithium, or if unexpected reactions occur. Once the initial treatment has begun, we recommend blood levels in the range of 0.8–1.2 mEq/liter for optimal efficacy. Some patients who do not benefit from these levels may respond at 1.2–1.5 mEq/liter, or even slightly higher. Conversely, a small number of patients who are unable to tolerate levels in the lower end of the usual therapeutic range (i.e., around 0.6, 0.7 mEq/liter) can acclimate to and benefit from concentrations at 0.3–0.6 mEq/liter. Blood samples for lithium levels should be drawn 10–12 hours after the last dose, to measure the concentration at its trough. Lithium saliva and RBC concentrations have also been promoted as more accessible or more accurate measures, respectively, but have not gained general acceptance.

Typical starting doses of lithium are 300 mg two or three times a day. The dose can vary from a low of 300 mg/day to as high as 3,000 mg/day, with the average range between 900 and 1,800 mg/day. An individual's age, renal function, and general physical condition are important associated determining factors for the ideal dose. Dosing schedules have traditionally been on a three or four times a day basis, but more recent data indicate once or twice a day regimens may enhance compliance and minimize certain adverse effects, while not compromising efficacy.

Lithium preparations include *lithium carbonate, sustained-release preparations,* and the liquid form, *lithium citrate.* The sustained-release preparations allow for a more gradual absorption of the drug, leading to blunted peak plasma levels. **Since lithium has a slow onset of action, it can take up to 3 weeks, and occasionally longer, to obtain a reasonable clinical response. Thus, it is important to avoid a premature abandonment in those who are simply slower to respond.**

Whenever possible, we prefer to treat with a mood stabilizer (e.g., LiCO$_3$; VPA) alone, because of their specificity for bipolar disorder and to minimize adverse effects. This is particularly true in mild to moderately severe episodes of acute mania. In addition, if the patient can benefit from a single drug during the acute episode, this would support its benefit for maintenance/prophylactic purposes.

LITHIUM PLUS OTHER PSYCHOTROPICS

From the perspective of clinical trial methodology, concurrent medications can create a dilemma for the investigator by complicating the interpretation of results.

Intermediate rescue medications are often required, however, since lithium, valproic acid, and carbamazepine are relatively slow in their onset of action. Further, if they are avoided, this usually introduces the confound of dropouts before the experimental drug can be fully effective. When feasible, a reasonable compromise is the use of modest amounts of a BZD, such as lorazepam, only when necessary and for no more than 1 week into the active trial. This reduces the number of nonresponding, highly active dropouts early in treatment. In a trial of several weeks, the initial lorazepam effect should have dissipated by the final assessments.

There are several studies that combined lithium with other treatments such as antipsychotics; anticonvulsants (e.g., carbamazepine, valproic acid); calcium channel blockers (e.g., verapamil); or benzodiazepines (e.g., lorazepam). Generally, in partial responders, the addition of these medications was beneficial and well tolerated.

Lithium Plus Antipsychotics

Many patients present in a very explosive, belligerent, and agitated manner, and waiting several days to weeks to gain control of an episode is not feasible. Thus, antipsychotics alone, or as adjuncts, are frequently required in the earliest phases of treatment, particularly with moderate to severe exacerbations, often associated with psychotic features. As a result, antipsychotics are the most commonly employed adjunctive agents, since more than half of all acutely ill bipolar patients present with psychotic symptoms. In addition, many require maintenance antipsychotics to prevent frequent relapses. Antipsychotics are usually initiated in conjunction with lithium because of their more rapid impact, then carefully tapered and discontinued, when possible, after the full effect of lithium is realized.

Unfortunately, manic patients may be exposed to higher than necessary acute antipsychotic doses, perhaps because of the explosivity often associated with an exacerbation. Baldessarini et al. (1984) conducted an epidemiological survey in the Boston area and found that antipsychotic dosing schedules of higher potency agents (e.g., haloperidol, fluphenazine) were 3–5 times greater than the chlorpromazine dose equivalents of lower potency drugs (e.g., chlorpromazine, thioridazine) (17). This was consistent across a number of different diagnostic categories, including the affectively disordered patients. He postulated that the different (and at least perceived as more benign) adverse effect profile of the higher-potency drugs encouraged aggressive increases in dose to control severe, acute psychotic exacerbations.

Addressing this issue in hospitalized acutely manic patients, Janicak et al. (1988) conducted a 2-week study of lithium plus random assignment to equivalent doses of chlorpromazine or thiothixene (18). The dose-equivalent ratio used was 5 mg of thiothixene to 100 mg of chlorpromazine (i.e., 1 to 20). During the waking hours, patients' antipsychotic doses were titrated on a 2-hourly basis so that response and adverse effects to the prior dose were the determinants for administering or holding the next dose. The aim was to compare the efficacy, side-effect profiles, and optimal dose required for either antipsychotic. Our hypothesis, based on the existing empirical dose-response literature, was that the effective dose would fall between 300 to 800 mg of chlorpromazine or a bioequivalent amount of thiothixene. After the first 4 days, patients receiving thiothixene averaged 30 mg/day and those receiving chlorpromazine averaged 380 mg/day. By the end of the 2-week trial, the mean dose in the thiothixene-treated group was 36 mg, and the mean dose of chlorpromazine was 480 mg (i.e., a ratio of 1:13). These amounts fell in the low-to-mid range of the

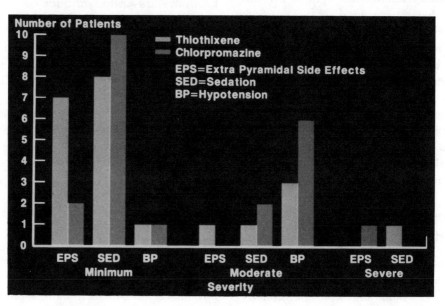

Figure 10.1. Adverse effects of thiothixene versus chlorpromazine.

dose-response curve previously reported. Secondly, the overall response rate was statistically significant for the entire group when baseline values were compared to day 14, but did not differ between the two antipsychotic groups. Finally, since relatively lower doses were used, adverse effect profiles, although typical and in the expected direction (i.e., slightly more EPS for those patients receiving thiothixene and slightly more sedation and hypotension in those receiving chlorpromazine), allowed for optimal and tolerable dosing regimens (see Fig. 10.1). The blood levels of lithium (i.e., approximately 1.0 mEq/liter) by the end of week 1 were adequate and almost identical for both groups. No other concomitant medications were employed.

We concluded that relatively low-to-moderate doses of either a high- or low-potency antipsychotic were sufficient to control acutely manic patients with associated psychotic features, and at these doses, adverse effects remained in the tolerable range.

Lithium plus Benzodiazepines

Unfortunately, a recent retrospective chart review found that a substantial number of manic patients started on an antipsychotic while hospitalized were still on these agents 6 months after discharge (19). **Its authors conclude that antipsychotic adjuncts to lithium should be reconsidered frequently and reduced whenever possible.** In this context, there has been an increasing interest in adjunctive antianxiety agents for acutely manic patients to avoid concomitant antipsychotics or at least to minimize their total amount (20). The literature is generally anecdotal and parallels a similar literature of adjunctive lorazepam use in treating acute psychosis,

but there have been some recent controlled trials (see Management of Acute Psychosis in Chapter 5). The most commonly studied drugs have been *lorazepam* and *clonazepam,* due to their rapidity of onset and duration of action. In addition, lorazepam can be administered intramuscularly with adequate absorption, in contrast to other benzodiazepines. *Alprazolam* and *diazepam* have also been studied.

The major benefit of this strategy may be in diminishing some of the secondary symptoms of an acute exacerbation (e.g., insomnia, agitation, panic, and other general anxiety symptoms) that are not necessarily specifically affected by lithium or antipsychotics. With this approach, exposure to antipsychotics may be precluded in some situations and kept to a minimum in others, thus avoiding the potential for more serious antipsychotic-induced adverse effects.

Relative contraindications to the use of BZDs involve patients with a history of:

- Alcohol or other substance abuse or dependency
- Paradoxical response to BZDs (i.e., behavioral disinhibition)
- Known sensitivity to this group of agents
- Acute narrow angle glaucoma
- Pregnancy.

Lorazepam

Lenox et al. (1992) found lorazepam and haloperidol comparable in efficacy when used as adjuncts to lithium in a double-blind study of 20 acutely manic patients (21). Interestingly, a recent report comparing lorazepam to clonazepam found a better outcome with lorazepam, using mean doses of 12–13 mg (22).

Clonazepam

Clonazepam is marketed primarily for petit mal variant, myoclonic, and akinetic seizures. It also has had wide psychiatric application, including the treatment of acute mania or other agitated psychotic conditions, usually in combination with lithium or antipsychotics. The literature on clonazepam's efficacy for acute mania is primarily based on the work of Chouinard (1987) and coworkers, who have compared this agent to placebo or standard treatments, primarily for acute mania (23). As noted earlier, a more recent study, also from Montreal, found that comparable doses of lorazepam were more effective than clonazepam for acute mania (22).

Typical doses of clonazepam have been in the range of 2–16 mg/day given on a once- or twice-a-day schedule due to its longer half-life. A major advantage of this anticonvulsant is its relative lack of adverse effects and freedom from laboratory monitoring, in comparison to CBZ and VPA. Clonazepam may be more useful when used in conjunction with lithium or CBZ rather than as a pure antimanic agent, perhaps supplanting the need for antipsychotics. In this sense, it can be viewed as a "behavioral suppressor," rather than a true "mood stabilizer."

LITHIUM PLUS THYROID SUPPLEMENTATION

Bauer et al. entered 11 rapid cycling, treatment-refractory patients into an open trial of high-dose levothyroxine sodium, added to their previously stabilized medication regimen (24). The dosage of the levothyroxine was increased by 0.05 to 0.1 mg/day every 1 to 2 weeks, as tolerated, until symptoms improved or adverse effects prevented further increases. Scores on both the depressive and the manic symptom rating scales decreased significantly, compared with baseline scores. This data indicates that levothyroxine, used in doses sufficient to produce supranormal circulating hormone levels, may induce remission of both depressive and manic symptoms in an otherwise refractory group of bipolar patients.

These results complement other reports suggesting that many treatment nonresponders may suffer from subclinical hypothyroidism and improve with the addition of thyroid supplementation. While this is an open case report on a small sample size, the promising results warrant further study under more controlled conditions.

CONCLUSION

In a highly disturbed hospitalized patient, we prefer to supplement lithium with an adjunctive BZD, such as lorazepam, adding an antipsychotic only if necessary. Caution must be exercised, however, due to the possible disinhibiting effects of BZDs. After a stabilization period, the adjunctive medication(s) may then be gradually withdrawn and the patient often managed successfully with lithium only. In resistant patients, assuring adequacy of the lithium dose/level, as well as duration; discontinuation of concurrent antidepressants; and supplemental thyroid medication (e.g., levothyroxine, 50–300 µg daily; triiodothyronine, 25–100 µg daily) may all improve outcome. Antipsychotics are utilized only when absolutely necessary and should be carefully titrated upward to avoid excessive exposure.

REFERENCES

1. Schou M, Juel-Nielson N, Stromgren E. The treatment of manic psychoses by the administration of lithium salts. J Neurol Neurosurg Psychiatry 1954;17:250–260.

2. Bunney WE, Goodwin FK, Davis JM, Fawcett JA. A behavioral-biochemical study of lithium treatment. Am J Psychiatry 1968;125:499–512.

3. Goodwin FK, Murphy DL, Bunney WE. Lithium. Lancet 1969;212–213.

4. Maggs R. Treatment of manic illness with lithium carbonate. Br J Psychiatry 1963; 109:562–565.

5. Stokes PE, Stoll PM, Shamoian CH. Efficacy of lithium as acute treatment of manic-depressive illness. Lancet 1971;i:1319–1325.

6. Stokes P, Kocsis J, Arcuni O. Relationship of lithium chloride dose to treatment response in acute mania. Arch Gen Psychiatry 1976;33:1080–1085.

7. Schou M. Lithium Treatment of manic-depressive illness: a practical guide. 3rd ed. Basel, Switzerland: Karger, 1986.

8. Platman SR. A comparison of lithium carbonate and chlorpromazine in mania. Am J Psychiatry 1970;127:351–353.

9. Prien RF, Caffey EM, Klett CJ. Comparison of lithium carbonate and chlorpromazine in the treatment of mania. Arch Gen Psychiatry 1972,26:146–153.

10. Garfinkel PE, Stancer HC, Persad E. A comparison of haloperidol, lithium carbonate, and their combination in the treatment of mania. J Affective Disord 1980;2:279–288.

11. Braden W, Fink EB, Qualls CB, Ho CK, Samuels WO. Lithium and chlorpromazine in psychotic inpatients. Psychiatry Res 1982;7:69–81.

12. Cookson J, Silverstone T, Wells B. Double-blind comparative clinical trial of pimozide and chlorpromazine in mania. Acta Psychiatr Scand 1981;64:381–397.

13. Post RM, Jimerson DC, Bunney WE, Goodwin FK. Dopamine and mania: behavioral and biochemical effects of the dopamine receptor blocker pimozide. Psychopharmacology 1980;67:297–305.

14. Johnstone EC, Crow TJ, Frith CD, Owens DGC. The Northwick Park "functional" psychosis study: diagnosis and treatment response. Lancet 1988;2:119–125.

15. Markoff RA, King Jr M. Does lithium dose prediction improve treatment efficiency? Prospective evaluation of a mathematical method. J Clin Psychopharmacol 1992; 12(5):305–308.

16. Zetin M, Garber D, De Antonio M, Schlegel A, Feureisen S, Fieve R, Jewett C, Reus V, Huey LY. Prediction of lithium dose: a mathematical alternative to the test-dose method. J Clin Psychiatry 1986; 47(4):175–178.

17. Baldessarini RJ, Katz B, Cotton P. Dissimilar dosing with high potency and low potency neuroleptics. Am J Psychiatry 1984;141:748–752.

18. Janicak PG, Bresnahan DB, Sharma RP, Davis JM, Comaty JE, Malinick C. A comparison of thiothixene with chlorpromazine in the treatment of mania. J Clin Psychopharmacol 1988;8:33–37.

19. Sernyak MJ, Johnson R, Griffin R, Pearsall HR, Woods SW. Neuroleptic exposure in lithium-treated mania. Presented at the annual APA meeting, May 1992.

20. Easton M, Janicak P. The use of benzodiazepines in psychotic disorders: a review of the literature. Psychiatric Annals 1990;20:535–544.

21. Lenox RH, Newhouse, PA, Creelman WL, Whitaker TM. Adjunctive treatment of manic agitation with lorazepam versus haloperidol: a double-blind study. J Clin Psychiatry 1992;53(2):47–52.

22. Bradwejn J, Shriqui C, Koszycki D, Meterissian G. Double-blind comparison of the effects of clonazepam and lorazepam in acute mania. J Clin Psychopharmacol 1990;10:403–408.

23. Chouinard G. Clonazepam in the acute and maintenance treatment of bipolar affective disorder. J Clin Psychiatry 1987;48(10, suppl):29–36.

24. Bauer MS, Whybrow PC. Rapid cycling bipolar affective disorder. II. Treatment of refractory rapid cycling with high-dose levothyroxine: a preliminary study. Arch Gen Psychiatry 1990;47:435–440.

Maintenance/Prophylaxis

It is estimated that as many as **90% of patients who have a manic episode will have one or more recurrences.** These episodes are disruptive, life threatening and often have a progressive deteriorating effect on the capacity to cope with life's activities. Therefore, it is of critical importance that we develop effective and safe long-term treatments. The ideal agent would be effective for both the manic and the depressed phases as an acute, maintenance, and prophylactic therapy. Unfortunately, this is not the case for any of the present agents.

LITHIUM

Interestingly, there are more studies comparing lithium to placebo for maintenance and prophylactic purposes than for acute treatment. It was apparent from the earliest observations that patients relapsed when lithium was discontinued and that indefinite treatment seemed to diminish recurrences. Baastrup and Schou (1967) were the first to clarify this phenomenon in a controlled, mirror-imaged trial with 88 bipolar patients, when they counted the number of episodes before and after lithium therapy (1). This was a large naturalistic study with objective, verifiable, and clinically important outcome measures, such as weeks in hospital or number of relapses; and a large sample size of typical, very ill patients. They found a highly significant decrease in relapses after initiation of treatment (i.e., every 60 months versus every 8 months), and that the average time in a severe episode decreased from 13 weeks per year before lithium, to 1 ½ weeks per year with active treatment. Thus, lithium led to a seven-fold decrease in the number of episodes or weeks ill, representing a substantial improvement in the natural history of the disease.

Time Course of Relapse

Schou et al. then studied the time course of relapse in both bipolar and unipolar patients (2). The plot of the natural log of the relapse rate versus time takes the form of a straight line, indicating an exponential distribution. In other words, the rate of relapse as a proportion of unrelapsed patients is fairly constant over time. Since approximately 15% receiving placebo relapsed each month (i.e., the rate constant for relapse = 0.15), the "half-life" of untreated remitted patients is approximately 4 ½ months. Generalizing from the population studied, this figure gives an indication of what would happen to those not treated with lithium. Although the number of relapses is modest during the first few weeks, the cumulative number is impressive several months to years later.

Schou et al. also compared the relapse rate of patients in their double-blind clinical trial to those in their naturalistic open study and found a similar rate (1).

Maintenance Strategies

The maintenance properties of lithium have since been verified in a large number of random-assignment, double-blind studies comparing this agent to placebo in the preventive treatment of unipolar and bipolar disorders. To summarize these studies, lithium was effective in preventing or attenuating recurrences (i.e., 50% fewer recurrences), with an average failure rate of approximately 37%.

Since lithium is superior to placebo in preventing a relapse once the acute episode has been controlled, duration of treatment, concurrent drug use, ideal blood levels, and method of discontinuation become critical issues.

Patients who have had more than one severe episode are probably best managed with continual, indefinite lithium prophylaxis. Even in patients who have experienced a single episode, there may be as high as a 50% chance for a recurrence within 5 months of stopping drug therapy

(3). In these patients, if lithium is tolerated without breakthrough symptoms, maintenance therapy can be reevaluated in 1 to 2 years; however, there is some data that initial responders to lithium who stop treatment may trigger a more virulent phase of the disease, or may experience a recurrence less likely to benefit from the drug's reinstitution (4). For this reason we advocate indefinite lithium therapy after one significant episode.

Since there is also some data that concurrent use of antidepressants can lead to rapid cycling in vulnerable patients, these agents may best be cautiously utilized on an as-needed basis or as adjuncts when there are early signs of breakthrough depressive, psychotic, or anxious symptoms. In particular, antidepressants do not prevent manic episodes, and may even precipitate them. The fact that many patients on antidepressants experience a manic phase, however, could be coincidental, rather than drug-induced. To answer this question, we would need to show that the number who switch to mania is higher on as opposed to off antidepressant therapy. Thus, a very large sample would have to be assigned to continued antidepressants or placebo and the number of switches counted. Unfortunately, such a study would deny treatment to a large number of patients and could not be done for ethical as well as practical reasons. Thus, while the common wisdom supports the "antidepressant conversion" hypothesis, we would caution that adequate studies have not been conducted to definitively answer this question. We advocate the use of lithium in a protective role to block a switch to mania in bipolar depressed patients placed on concurrent antidepressant therapy.

In regard to optimal blood levels, Gelenberg et al. (1989) found that patients maintained on standard concentrations of lithium (i.e., 0.8–1.0 mmol/liter) had a significantly lower risk of relapse (i.e., 13%) than those on lower dose/plasma level regimens (i.e., a 38% relapse rate with levels in the range of 0.4–0.6 mmol/liter) (5).

Finally, recent data indicate that more rapid lithium discontinuation may decrease the time to recurrence (6).

Compliance

Unfortunately, patient noncompliance may be as high as 50% within the first year of treatment, posing a serious public health issue (7). Sensitivity to *somatic adverse effects* (especially memory problems, impaired coordination, weight gain, and tremor); *unrealistic expectations*, leading to secondary depression; *cognitive and psychological adverse effects* on long-term lithium treatment without relapse; the positive reaction to *early euphoria and/or hypomania;* and *severity of illness* all may play a role. Further, *dual diagnosis disorders* (i.e., bipolar plus substance or alcohol abuse) appear to be much more common than previously thought and may contribute to more frequent exacerbations (8).

Strategies to improve compliance include:

- Intensive *educational efforts* at the onset of therapy
- *Dose reduction,* when feasible
- Supportive, individual, family, and when indicated, drug/alcohol abuse *counseling*
- Aggressive *intervention with early signs of relapse.*

In summary, there is evidence for a higher relapse rate in patients not maintained on adequate levels of lithium, the potential for concurrent drugs (e.g., antidepressants) to exacerbate the disorder, a more rapid recurrence with abrupt discontinuation, and possible compromised

future lithium responsiveness when it is stopped (4, 9). Compliance issues remain a major factor in providing adequate long-term treatment.

Longitudinal Course

Bipolar patients treated under typical clinical conditions may have a more difficult post-hospital course than has been generally appreciated. For example, Mander reported on 2745 bipolar patients initially admitted because of an episode of mania or depression, and found that lithium did not reduce the readmission rate within 3 months of discharge (10). As a result, he proposed that its full prophylactic effect may not occur for 6–12 months after the start of treatment, and that it should be reserved for long-term prophylaxis in those who have had a number of severe episodes in a defined period of time.

Harrow et al. followed 73 bipolar (BP) and 66 unipolar (UP) patients in a longitudinal naturalistic design for 1.7 years after hospital discharge (11). BP patients generally had poorer outcomes than their depressive counterparts, with more than 40% demonstrating a manic syndrome during follow-up. Surprisingly, BP patients complying with lithium maintenance fared no better than those who did not. The authors opine that using the "management trial" model (i.e., assessing treatment under routine clinical conditions), as opposed to the "exploratory trial" model (i.e., optimal controlled research conditions) reveals a less-positive outcome for these patients. Further, lithium prophylaxis was far less effective than the 70–80% response rate reported in earlier trials. They conclude that a significant proportion of BP patients may suffer from a severe, recurrent, and pernicious disorder. Shortcomings in their design, such as inadequate

monitoring of drug compliance or inadequate blood levels, however, limit the interpretability of their results.

Another way of assessing the long-term course is to monitor functional as well as symptomatic disability. To this end, Dion et al. followed 67 bipolar or atypical bipolar patients in a prospective 6-month follow-up study after discharge from the hospital (12). Forty-four of the original 67 were interviewed at 6 months and about one-third of the sample was found to be clearly disabled functionally, despite dramatic drops in their average symptom ratings in the Brief Psychiatric Rating Scale, the Mania Rating Scale, and the Hamilton Depression Rating Scale. Further, in those with a previous history of more than one psychiatric admission, the rate of functional disability was closer to 50%. They conclude that their findings belie the assumption that bipolar illness has a good prognosis and that appropriate rehabilitative interventions are crucial to meet the needs of these patients.

Literature Review

As noted earlier, lithium's efficacy as a maintenance therapy is one of the best-studied psychopharmacological effects. We have summarized all the placebo-controlled studies on the use of lithium to prevent relapse, including both unipolar and bipolar patients. We also performed a meta-analysis of these studies, separating out unipolar and bipolar patients (see Tables 10.5 and 10.6).

Baastrup and associates studied manic-depressive and recurrently depressed Danish patients who had been successfully stabilized on lithium for at least 1 year (13). This ensured that subjects had the type of illness that is helped by lithium, and that they could tolerate the treatment. Since it was a prospective, well-controlled, ran-

Table 10.5.
Lithium versus Placebo for _Unipolar Disorder:_ Maintenance Treatment

Number of Subjects	Relapsed (%)		Difference (%)	Chi Square	p Value
	Lithium (%)	Placebo (%)			
183	31.6	70.5	38.9	29.7	5×10^{-8}

Table 10.6.
Lithium versus Placebo for _Bipolar Disorder:_ Maintenance Treatment

Number of Subjects	Relapsed (%)		Difference (%)	Chi Square	p Value
	Lithium (%)	Placebo (%)			
739	37.3	79.3	21.3	65.3	$<10^{-33}$

dom-assignment, double-blind study (i.e., Class I), potential biases were effectively eliminated. They demonstrated a dramatic and positive effect for lithium when compared to placebo. None of the patients who received lithium over a 5-month period relapsed, whereas 55% of the bipolar and 53% of the unipolar patients on placebo did so.

In a multi-hospital collaborative design, Prien and associates studied patients in VA, public, and private hospitals to assess a 2-year maintenance therapy program (14, 15). They first examined the prophylactic value of lithium in hospitalized manic patients, and in a second study, compared prophylactic lithium, imipramine, and placebo in hospitalized depressed patients. These studies did not select known lithium responders, and therefore, included many who had not previously been exposed to this therapy. Hence, there was a greater base rate of relapse in their lithium groups than in the previous Danish studies, with the relapse rate even higher in the placebo groups (i.e., almost all patients relapsed). Despite these higher absolute rates, the difference in relapse between the lithium and the placebo groups in the two VA studies was comparable to the Danish studies. In the two VA studies, while nearly half on lith-

ium relapsed, almost all placebo patients (89%) did so (13–15). In Baastrup's study, no lithium patients relapsed, but 54% on placebo did (13). Similar results were obtained by Mendlewicz and associates in a study conducted in New York City (16, 17). Overall, when both the American and the European studies were combined, the drug/placebo difference was about 45%.

Coppen et al. performed a collaborative study at four separate centers, randomly assigning patients to lithium or placebo for up to 2 years (18, 19). This study used a slightly different design, in that patients who relapsed or became more symptomatic short of relapse, were treated with other medication(s) (excluding lithium) so they could remain in the study. Their results were consistent with earlier findings. Cundall and associates in the United Kingdom confirmed these earlier findings in a separate study (20).

We also included Persson's Swedish study, which used matched patients (21). Despite some methodological flaws, we feel it was a valid study and should be counted even though it only met criteria for a Class II design. Their findings were also consistent with the overall results.

More recently, Mander and Louden studied 14 patients with a history of mania (by DSM-III criteria) who entered a randomized, double-blind, placebo-controlled, crossover trial (22). These patients had been stable on lithium for at least 18 months and were not taking any other psychotropics. The protocol consisted of three phases, each lasting 4 weeks. During the first phase, patients were stabilized on lithium, with adequate levels, and baseline clinical ratings were obtained. During the second and the third phases, the patients were randomized under double-blind conditions to receive an additional 4 weeks of lithium followed by 4 weeks of placebo or vice versa, so that patients acted as their own control. Relapse was defined as meeting DSM-III criteria for mania, with an increase of at least five points from baseline on the symptom checklist, and a score over 20 on the modified Manic Rating Scale. Seven patients during the placebo phase and none during the lithium phase relapsed ($p = 0.006$). The authors conclude that the recognition of withdrawal relapse will lead to better use of lithium so that its proven prophylactic advantages can be translated into improved prognosis. Further, unnecessary relapses may be prevented by counseling patients about the risks of sudden lithium discontinuation.

Using data from a National Institute of Mental Health collaborative project, Shapiro et al. applied a survival analysis model to the reexamination of response to maintenance therapy in 117 patients who met Research Diagnostic Criteria (RDC) for a bipolar disorder (23). They divided the group according to whether the index admission was for a manic or a depressive episode. Patients were stabilized in the preliminary phase and maintained on adequate doses and blood levels of lithium and imipramine for 2 months. After this, they were randomized to receive a lithium-imipramine combination (N = 37), lithium only (N = 45), or imipramine only (N = 35), for a 24-month study period or until relapse. They found that imipramine alone was a poor prophylactic treatment for bipolar disorders and that the combination therapy was the most effective strategy, not appreciably increasing the risk of relapse in either group. The most striking difference between their analysis and the earlier report of Prien et al. (1984) was that the combination therapy appeared to be particularly effective after an index episode of depression (24). They attribute this difference in outcome to the use of the survival analysis model.

Finally, Strober et al. conducted an 18-month, prospective, naturalistic follow-up study of 37 BP-I adolescents (i.e., 13–17 years old) stabilized on lithium and found a relapse rate almost three times higher in those who discontinued prophylactic lithium (92%), as compared with those who complied (38%) (25). Further, they noted that earlier relapse in these patients predicted a greater risk of subsequent relapse; and that an early onset may be associated with a more virulent course, resistance to lithium, and the need to consider alternate mood stabilizers.

Methodological problems with this study included: small sample size; lack of assessment for personality disturbances and intrafamilial environment; only a 4-week initial drug stabilization period; and lack of precision in monitoring compliance to treatment.

Bipolar Manic Versus Bipolar Depressive Phases

It is important to make a conceptual distinction between lithium's relative prophylactic effect for the manic and the depressive phases of a bipolar disorder, and by extension, its ability to prevent recurrent depressions in unipolar disorder.

In reviewing these studies, it is useful

to distinguish statistical significance from magnitude of association, or effect size. A high correlation involving five subjects may be barely statistically significant, but a low correlation involving thousands of subjects may be highly significant. The percent of patients relapsing on lithium or placebo and the difference in their relapse rates are effect sizes, whose probability of being significant is determined by both the difference in relapse rates as well as the sample size. Since most studies noted here had more subjects in the bipolar than in the unipolar group, statistical significance does not provide an adequate comparison of the degree of lithium prophylaxis (effect size) in each subgroup (see Table 10.7).

Further, some of the studies did not report the number of manic versus depressive relapses. One exception is Coppen et al. (1963, 1971), who reported the mean affect morbidity score of patients receiving placebo (mean score = 0.33, standard deviation (SD) = 0.05) and lithium (mean = 0.09, SD = 0.05) for the manic phase, as well as placebo (mean = 0.31, SD = 0.06) and lithium (mean = 0.07, SD = 0.03) for the depressive phase (18, 19).

Thus, this study found very similar prophylactic effects. Baastrup and associates reported a comparable number of manic and depressed phase relapses in their bipolar patients (13). In 22 bipolar patients, 12 relapsed: six into a manic phase, five into a depressed phase, and one into a mixed phase. By contrast, Prien et al. and Cundall et al. found that lithium had a greater effect in preventing the manic than the depressed phase of bipolar disorder (20, 24). Overall, lithium was effective in preventing both phases of a bipolar disorder.

Bipolar versus Unipolar Disorder

An important body of evidence from descriptive, clinical, and genetic sources finds that bipolar mood disorder is a separate entity from unipolar disorder (i.e., genetically the two variants breed true; see also Mechanism of Action earlier in this chapter). When we pooled data from several studies that investigated bipolar or unipolar disorders, lithium was more effective than placebo in preventing relapse in bipolar disorders, as well as preventing

Table 10.7.
Effectiveness of Lithium in Preventing Recurrence of the Manic versus the Depressive Phase of Bipolar Disorder[a]

Study	Manic Phase		Depressive Phase	
	Placebo	Lithium	Placebo	Lithium
Coppen A et al. (1963, 1971)				
Mean affect morbidity score	0.33 ± 0.05	0.09 ± 0.05	0.31 ± 0.06	0.07 ± 0.03
Baastrup P et al. (1970)[b]				
Number relapsed	6	10	5	10
Number not relapsed	0	28	0	28
Cundall R et al. (1972)				
Number relapsed	9	1	5	3
Number not relapsed	3	11	7	9
Prien R et al. (1984)				
Number relapsed	76	34	35	20
Number not relapsed	41	85	82	99

[a]Adapted from Appleton WS, Davis JM. Practical clinical psychopharmacology. 2nd ed. Baltimore: Williams & Wilkins, 1980:125–126.
[b]In this study, 12 out of 22 bipolars relapsed. Of the 12 patients who relapsed, one relapsed to a mixed phase of bipolar illness.

unipolar episodes (see Tables 10.8 and 10.9).

Naturalistic Trials

We also reviewed a longitudinal naturalistic, collaborative study conducted in three European countries (26–28). Although not a Class I design, it does provide a large number of patients and supplements the evidence from double-blind comparisons. Workers from Denmark, Czechoslovakia, and Switzerland used a design similar to Baastrup and Schou's classic naturalistic study (with the addition of their multinational sampling), to compare the relative effect of lithium on the course of recurrent unipolar versus bipolar disorder. As an index of prophylactic effect, the investigators counted the number of episodes that occurred before and during lithium treatment, and utilized a linear regression to provide a quantitative estimate for lithium's effect. The major inde-

Table 10.8.
Lithium Maintenance versus Placebo in *Bipolar Depressed* Patients[a]

Study	Placebo	Lithium	Total
Baastrup P et al. (1970)			
Number relapsed	12	0	12
Number not relapsed	10	28	38
Coppen A et al. (1963, 1971)			
Number relapsed	21	3	24
Number not relapsed	0	14	14
Persson G (1972)			
Number relapsed	11	5	16
Number not relapsed	1	7	8
Prien R et al. (1984)			
Number relapsed	93	47	140
Number not relapsed	24	72	96

[a]Adapted from Appleton WS, Davis JM. Practical clinical psychopharmacology. 2nd ed. Baltimore: Williams & Wilkins, 1980:125–126.

Table 10.9.
Lithium Maintenance versus Placebo in *Unipolar Depressed* Patients[a]

Study	Placebo	Lithium	Total
Baastrup P et al. (1970)			
Number relapsed	9	0	9
Number not relapsed	8	17	25
Coppen A et al. (1963, 1971)			
Number relapsed	12	1	13
Number not relapsed	3	10	13
Persson G (1972)			
Number relapsed	14	6	20
Number not relapsed	7	15	22
Prien R et al. (1984)			
Number relapsed	14	13	27
Number not relapsed	2	14	16

[a]Adapted from Appleton WS, Davis JM. Practical clinical psychopharmacology. 2nd ed. Baltimore: Williams & Wilkins, 1980:125–126.

pendent variable was the length of time the patient was free from active disease. Lithium prevented the recurrence of both unipolar and bipolar illness equally well.

Aagaard and Vestergaard followed 133 consecutive affectively disordered patients (UP, BP, uncertain diagnosis) on lithium prophylaxis in a 2-year prospective, naturalistic design to identify predictors of outcome (29). The frequency of admissions prior to the index episode and substance abuse were the primary predictors of *nonadherence* (noncompliance), defined as stopping treatment against medical advice at least once in those 2 years. *Nonresponse* (defined as more than one readmission in 2 years) in compliant patients was predictable by sex (females did worse), age (younger did worse), and chronicity. It should be noted that lithium levels (0.5–0.8 mml/liter) tended to be in the lower end of the therapeutic range and could have contributed to the higher relapse rate. Disappointingly, the overall response rate (63%) was poor, with a mortality rate of 15.3% (i.e., seven patients). The authors suggest that patients with a history of substance abuse should not begin lithium prophylaxis unless intensive support and well-controlled management settings are available, and that alternative and/or supplementary treatment should be considered for those with frequent prior admissions and a chronic course.

Maj et al. studied the long-term outcome in 79 affectively disordered patients (43 BP; 36 UP) who had been successfully managed on lithium prophylaxis for 2 years (30). Their goal was to prospectively monitor the course of illness for an additional 5-year period. Forty-nine completed this phase, two died (of cancer), seven were lost to follow-up, and 21 interrupted their treatment. Twenty-five patients relapsed (10 BP, 15 UP) during this period, calling into question long-term prognosis, given a favorable initial 2-year response to lithium prophylaxis. The authors discussed several other notable issues, including:

- While lithium was *an effective prophylaxis in 44%* of these patients, the relapse rate was higher than that reported by earlier studies
- There was a *decrease in morbidity* in the 5-year follow-up period, as compared to the pre-lithium phase
- *Some patients,* despite adequate treatment with lithium, *relapsed after several years of successful prophylaxis,* returning to the same level of morbidity as during their pre-lithium period
- Some patients developed a *persistent mild dysphoria* while on prolonged maintenance lithium.

Attitudes and Adjustment during Remission

The *correlates of attitudes toward lithium compliance* in bipolar patients were studied by Cochran and Gitlin (31). This questionnaire study was part of a larger design looking at factors in lithium *prophylaxis*. The questionnaire packets were sent to 146 patients, 48 of whom were ultimately included in the analysis. This study evaluated the usefulness of Ajzen and Fishbein's "Theory of Reasoned Action" to explain the relationships among lithium-related beliefs and attitudes, normative beliefs, behavioral intentions, and self-reported compliance with treatment. According to the model, lithium patients' normative beliefs (i.e., beliefs that other relevant people such as family, friends, personal psychiatrist, and lithium experts want the patient to take lithium) predict their subjective norms, which is the expectation that others want them to take lithium. Subsequently, both the subjective norm and the evaluative behavioral attitudes (i.e., positive nature of treatment) were predictive of the patients' reported intent to take lithium. This, in turn, was predictive of concurrent self-reported compliance with the medication regimen. **These results underscore the importance of the patient-physician relationship in lithium compliance.**

The possibility of an adverse effect with prophylactic lithium or some sequelae of affective illness impacting on the *life satisfaction and adjustment of patients in remission*, was explored by Lepkifker et al. (32). Life satisfaction scores and adjustment scores in four areas were obtained for 100 remitted patients (50 bipolar and 50 unipolar patients) matched for sex and age, a control group of 50 healthy individuals, and a control group of patients with personality disorders. Each subject rated his feelings of satisfaction in life by indicating his position on a 10-point ladder device, which was based on a modification of Cantril's Self-Anchoring Striving Scale. A similar 10-point scale was used by patients to assess their levels of adjustment and overall functioning. In addition, the treating psychiatrist or therapist was asked to rate the same issues. Patients' life satisfaction and adjustment scores in the various areas investigated were significantly and positively correlated with the corresponding ratings given by the psychiatrist in the two scales of adjustment. Analysis of variance and the *post-hoc* Duncan test were conducted on the differences obtained from the four groups for life satisfaction, currently, 5 years previously, and 5 years in the future. Unipolar and bipolar patients did not differ from healthy controls for current life satisfaction, but the mean rating for psychiatric controls was significantly lower than in any other group (F = 7.92; $p = 0.001$).

Affective patients and healthy controls rated life as more satisfying at present than in the past, and they also rated themselves higher than most others on scores of life satisfaction at present. The authors concluded that neither lithium as a prophylactic agent nor the affective illness interfered with either the manifest functioning or the patients' feelings of satisfaction while in remission.

Long-Term Outcome of Bipolar and Unipolar Mood Disorders

Coppen et al. evaluated the status of 104 BP or UP, recurrent patients after 10 years of lithium maintenance to assess mortality rate, in part because of reports indicating unusually high rates, with many deaths attributed to suicide (33). Compliance was very high, with only 6% discontinuing lithium therapy, and patients also received adjunctive antipsychotic and/or antidepressants when clinically indicated. No patient died of suicide during this period, in contrast to the results in lithium non-compliant patients. They concluded that the absence of suicide resulted from the significant reduction in morbidity achieved by the careful administration of lithium.

Schou and Weeke reported on 92 Danish bipolar patients admitted between 1969 and 1983 with a first episode and who committed suicide before July 1, 1986 (34). Information was obtained on any prophylactic or continuation treatment at the time of the suicide, and the patients were divided into seven groups (A–G), based on the type of treatment and status of their illness. It appeared that 70% of the sample were receiving the best medical and prophylactic therapy available, however, 30% may have benefited from a more effective use of the available measures. They noted that previous suicide attempts, complicating alcoholism, and a mixture of neurotic or hypochondriacal features should heighten the clinician's suspicion of a potential to commit suicide. They further recommend:

- That a successful course of electroconvulsive therapy should be followed by at least 6–12 months, and often a lifetime, of prophylactic drug therapy
- That prophylactic antidepressants should be given in full therapeutic dosages
- That prophylactic lithium should be considered in unipolar patients when antidepressants are unsatisfactory
- That conscientious psychological support should be given to improve compliance and help patients to cope with emergent problems in living.

CARBAMAZEPINE

Although data is quite limited, Prien and Gelenberg reviewed the literature on drug treatment for the prevention of recurrences in bipolar disorder, emphasizing alternative therapies to lithium, especially *carbamazepine,* which was the most extensively studied (35). Prien and Gelenberg felt that the strongest evidence for the prophylactic efficacy of carbamazepine has, thus far, come from other design paradigms such as:

- Longitudinal trials in which the test drug is periodically discontinued and/or replaced by a placebo
- Mirror-image longitudinal trials in which the course of illness during treatment is compared with the course of illness during an equivalent time preceding the treatment
- Long-term open trials evaluating the test drug in patients who have failed to respond to traditional treatments or have a recent history of frequent recurrences.

They concluded that before carbamazepine can be viewed as a long-term treatment for bipolar disorders, carefully designed prospective, controlled trials with adequate sample sizes are needed to confirm its efficacy and safety and to establish its specific indications and range of clinical effects.

Literature Review

We reviewed seven *double-blind,* controlled trials comparing CBZ to lithium as a preventive treatment for bipolar disorder but note that the existing data does not constitute the strict demonstration of efficacy (i.e., in comparison to placebo) that is required for FDA approval (36–42) (see Table 10.10).

For example, Lusznat et al. studied 54 acutely manic patients who were allocated on a double-blind basis to either carbamazepine or lithium (38). The short-term effects of treatment were evaluated in an initial 6-week acute phase, and the prophylactic effects in 29 patients up to a year. Additional "rescue" medications consisted of antipsychotics, antidepressants, and sedatives. Nine of the patients in the CBZ group had a satisfactory result (i.e., did not relapse during the 12-month follow-up), compared with five in the lithium group. The authors speculated that insufficient doses may have contributed to the poor results in both treatment groups. No statistically significant differences were found, however, with carbamazepine slightly less effective than lithium for acute mania and slightly more effective as a prophylactic treatment.

VALPROIC ACID

While there is little data, currently, controlled studies are in progress on the maintenance/prophylactic properties of

Table 10.10.
Lithium versus Carbamazepine: Maintenance Treatment

Study	Number of Subjects	Relapsed (%)		Difference (%)
		Carbamazepine (%)	Lithium (%)	
Placidi (1986)	56	28	26	− 2
Watkins (1987)	37	68	56	− 13
Lusznat (1988)	29	64	80	16
Stoll (1989)	98	46	52	4
Cabrera (1990)	10	25	0	− 25
Small (1991)	16	100	88	− 13
Coxhead (1992)	28	46	53	7
Total	274	50%	50%	0.7%

VPA. Calabrese (1990), in an open trial monitored the prophylactic effect of divalproex sodium in 33 rapid-cycling patients over a 12-month period, and results were comparable to similar studies with lithium (42). This is an important issue to confirm, given the strong evidence supporting its acute antimanic effects (see also Alternate Treatment Strategies later in this chapter).

CONCLUSION

Maintenance/prophylaxis with lithium, and perhaps other mood stabilizers, favorably alters the longitudinal course of a bipolar disorder. Thus, efforts to enhance long-term compliance are a necessary part of any overall strategy. The incidence of adverse or toxic events is relatively low, and close attention to the more clinically relevant consequences can usually prevent serious sequelae (43). **An issue of critical importance for future research is the potential efficacy of alternate anti-manic maintenance medication for those who fail to respond adequately to acute and/or long-term lithium therapy.**

It is becoming increasingly evident that prevention of relapse, as well as adequate prophylactic strategies for patients with major mood disorders is much more com-plicated than was originally assumed. Factors that contribute to this situation include:

- *Personal and family histories* of psychiatric disorders
- *Type of presentation* at the index episode
- Subsequent symptomatic and functional *disability*
- *Inadequate or less than aggressive* use of combined medication and psychotherapeutic strategies
- Lack of effective drug *alternatives*.

On a slightly more positive note, combination treatments, such as lithium with imipramine, may decrease relapse rates; early, aggressive intervention may shorten subsequent episodes; and newer agents, such as divalproex sodium or carbamazepine, may benefit previously resistant subgroups of bipolar disorders. It is also encouraging that patients in good remission on lithium view themselves favorably compared with normal controls on life satisfaction and adjustment measures.

It is apparent that the task of generating a systematic body of knowledge to identify prognostic indicators and successful treatment strategies for patients with major mood disorders is complicated by a multitude of issues. Results of recent studies

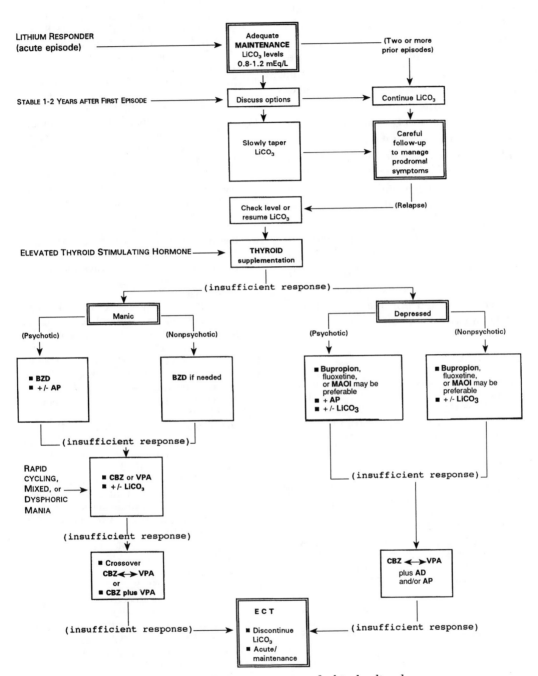

Figure 10.2.   Maintenance strategy for bipolar disorder.

investigating precipitating life events, thyroid status, lithium augmentation, diagnostic subtypes, and demographic variables have not yet led to reliable predictors. Similarly, the results of treatment studies with prophylactic and maintenance lithium therapy were also varied. It seems, however, that the overall response and mortality rates improved as compliance increased and adjunctive therapy with antipsychotics and/or antidepressants or levothyroxine was utilized. Additionally, careful attention to and reduction of stressful life events may prevent or attenuate subsequent episodes of the illness.

We have developed an approach to managing difficult-to-treat patients during the maintenance phase (see Figure 10.2). Another discussion on the management of bipolar, depressed episodes is contained in Chapter 7.

REFERENCES

1. Baastrup P, Schou M. Lithium as a prophylactic agent. Arch Gen Psychiatry 1967;16:162–172.
2. Schou M, Thomsen K, Baastrup PC. Studies on the course of recurrent endogenous affective disorders. International Pharmacopsychiatry 1970;5:100–106.
3. Suppes T, Baldessarini RJ, Faedda GL, Tohen M. Risk of recurrence following discontinuation of lithium treatment in bipolar disorder. Arch Gen Psychiatry 1991;48:1082–1088.
4. Post RM, Leverich GS, Altshuler L, Mikalauskas K. Lithium-discontinuation refractoriness: preliminary observations. Am J Psychiatry 1992;149:1727–1729.
5. Gelenberg AJ, Kane JM, Keller MB, et al. Comparison of standard and low levels of lithium for maintenance treatment of bipolar disorder. N Engl J Med 1989;321:1489–1493.
6. Faedda GL et al. Arch Gen Psychiatry (in press).
7. Shaw E. Lithium noncompliance. Psychiatric Annals 1986;16:583–587.
8. Regier, DA, Farmer ME, Rae DS, Locke BZ, Keith SJ, Judd LL, Goodwin FK. Comorbidity of mental disorders with alcohol and other drug abuse. Results from the epidemiologic catchment area (ECA) study. JAMA 1990;264(19):2511–2518.
9. Post RM, Weiss SRB. Sensitization, kindling, and anticonvulsants in mania. J Clin Psychiatry 1989;50(12, suppl)23–30.
10. Mander AJ. Use of lithium and early relapse in manic-depressive illness. Acta Psychiatr Scand 1988;78:198–200.
11. Harrow M, Goldberg JF, Grossman LS, Meltzer HY. Outcome in manic disorders. A naturalistic follow-up study. Arch Gen Psychiatry 1990;47:665–671.
12. Dion GL, Tohen M, Anthony WA, Waternaux CS. Symptoms and functioning of patients with bipolar disorder six months after hospitalization. Hosp Community Psychiatry 1988;39:652–657.
13. Baastrup P, Poulsen KS, Schou M, et al. Prophylactic lithium: double-blind discontinuation in manic-depressive and recurrent-depressive disorders. Lancet 1970;ii:326–330.
14. Prien RF, Caffey Jr EM, Klett CJ. Prophylactic efficacy of lithium carbonate in manic-depressive illness. Arch Gen Psychiatry 1973;28:337–341.
15. Prien RF, Caffey Jr EM, Klett CJ. Factors associated with lithium responses in the prophylactic treatment of bipolar manic-depressive illness. Arch Gen Psychiatry 1974;31:189–192.
16. Mendlewicz J, Fieve R, Stallone F. Relationship between effectiveness of lithium therapy and family history. Am J Psychiatry 1973;130:1011–1013.
17. Stallone F, Shelley E, Mendlewicz J, et al. The use of lithium in affective disorders: III. A double-blind study of prophylaxis in bipolar illness. Am J Psychiatry 1973;130:1006–1010.
18. Coppen A, Noguera R, Bailey J, et al. Prophylactic lithium in affective disorders. Lancet 1971;ii:275–279.
19. Coppen A, Peet M, Bailey J, et al. Double-blind and open prospective studies of lithium prophylaxis in affective disorders. Psychiatr Neurol Neurochir 1963;76:500–510.
20. Cundall RL, Brooks PW, Murray LG. A controlled evaluation of lithium prophylaxis in affective disorders. Psychol Med 1972;2:308–311.
21. Persson G. Lithium prophylaxis in affective disorders: an open trial with matched controls. Acta Psychiatr Scand 1972;48:462–479.

22. Mander AJ, Louden JB. Rapid recurrence of mania following abrupt discontinuation of lithium. Lancet 1988;ii:15–17.

23. Shapiro DR, Quitkin FM, Fleiss JL. Response to maintenance therapy in bipolar illness. Arch Gen Psychiatry 1989;46:401–405.

24. Prien RF, Kupfer DJ, Mansky PA, Small JG, Tuason VB, Voss CB, Johnson WE. Drug therapy in the prevention of recurrences in unipolar and bipolar affective disorders. Report of the NIMH Collaborative Study Group comparing lithium carbonate, imipramine, and a lithium carbonate-imipramine combination. Arch Gen Psychiatry 1984;41:1096–1104.

25. Strober M, Morrell W, Lampert C, Burroughts J. Relapse following discontinuation of lithium maintenance therapy in adolescents with Bipolar I illness: a naturalistic study. Am J Psychiatry 1990;147:457–461.

26. Angst J, Weiss P, Grof P, et al. Lithium prophylaxis in recurrent affective disorders. Br J Psychiatry 1970;116:604–614.

27. Schou M, Baastrup PC, Grof P, et al. Pharmacological and clinical problems of lithium prophylaxis. Br J Psychiatry 1970;116:615–619.

28. Grof P, Schou M, Angst J, et al. Methodological problems of prophylactic trials in recurrent affective disorders. Br J Psychiatry 1970;116:599–603.

29. Aagaard J, Vestergaard P. Predictors of outcome prophylactic lithium treatment: a 2 year prospective study. J Affective Disord 1990;18:259–266.

30. Maj M, Pirozzi R, Kemali D. Long-term outcome of lithium prophylaxis in patients initially classified as complete responders. Psychopharmacology 1989;98:535–538.

31. Cochran SD, Gitlin MJ. Attitudinal correlates of lithium compliance in bipolar affective disorders. J Nerv Ment Dis 1988;176:457–467.

32. Lepkifker E, Horesh N, Floru S. Life satisfaction and adjustment in lithium-treated affective patients in remission. Acta Psychiatr Scand 1988;78:391–395.

33. Coppen A, Standish-Barry H, Bailey J, Houston G, Silcocks P, Hermon C. Long-term lithium and mortality. Lancet 1990;335:1347.

34. Schou M, Weeke A. Did manic depressive patients who committed suicide receive prophylactic or continuation treatment at the time? Br J Psychiatry 1988;153:324–327.

35. Prien RF, Gelenberg AJ. Alternatives to lithium for preventive treatment of bipolar disorder. Am J Psychiatry 1989;146:840–848.

36. Placidi GF, Lenzi A, Lazzerini F, Cassano GB, Akiskal HS. The comparative efficacy and safety of carbamazepine versus lithium: a randomized, double-blind 3-year trial in 83 patients. J Clin Psychiatry 1986;47(10):490–494.

37. Watkins SE, Callender K, Thomas DR, Tidmarsh SF, Shaw DM. The effect of carbamazepine and lithium on remission from affective illness. Br J Psychiatry 1987;150:180–182.

38. Lusznat RM, Murphy DP, Nunn CMH. Carbamazepine vs lithium in the treatment and prophylaxis of mania. Br J Psychiatry 1988;153:198–204.

39. Stoll KD, Goncalves N, Krober HL, Demisch K, Bellaire W. Use of carbamazepine in affective illness. In: Lerer B, Gershon S, eds. New directions in affective disorders. New York: Springer-Verlag, 1989:540–544.

40. Small JG, Klapper MH, Milstein V, et al. Carbamazepine compared with lithium in the treatment of mania. Arch Gen Psychiatry 1991;48:915–921.

41. Coxhead N, Silverstone T, Cookson J. Carbamazepine versus lithium in the prophylaxis of bipolar affective disorder. Acta Psychiatr Scand 1992;85:114–118.

42. Calabrese JR, Delucchi GA. Spectrum of efficacy of valproate in 55 patients with rapid cycling bipolar disorder. Am J Psychiatry 1990;147:431–434.

43. Scou M. Lithium prophylaxis: myths and realities. Am J Psychiatry 1989;146:573–576.

Alternate Treatment Strategies

While lithium has been a major advance in the pharmacotherapy of severe mood disorders, a number of problems limit its usefulness, including:

- *Slow onset* of action in treating an acute episode
- *Diminished effectiveness* in severe manic exacerbations
- *Inadequate response* (20–40%)
  - Nonresponse
  - Partial response
  - Intolerance to lithium
- *Adverse effects*
  - Thyroid
  - Renal (e.g., excessive urination)
  - Troublesome adverse effects (e.g., mental dulling, tremor, edema, weight gain)
- *Noncompliance* (often due to adverse effects)

Further, certain subgroups of affectively disordered patients may be less likely to benefit from lithium, including:

- *Rapid-cyclers* (5–20% of all bipolar patients)
- *Dysphoric, mixed,* or *complex* mania (up to 40% of all episodes)
- *More severe episodes* (e.g., with associated psychosis)
- *Schizoaffective* disorder
- *Organic* mood syndromes
- The *elderly manic patient*
- Patients with coexisting *alcohol or substance abuse*
- *Personality disorders*
- *Mental retardation*

As a result, there are ongoing attempts to develop alternate strategies for these patients (1).

Since lithium has been the standard treatment for bipolar disorder, it is usually the drug of first choice. Patients who have only a partial or poor response are then often treated with carbamazapine or valproic acid; and some will respond to the latter two drugs. There has never been a controlled study, however, comparing the efficacy of lithium to carbamazapine or valproic acid in difficult-to-treat manic patients. It is also possible that if carbamazapine and/or valproic acid had been discovered first, they would have become the first line treatment(s) for bipolar disorder, and the difficult-to-treat patients may have then been treated with lithium, giving it the reputation of being the drug of choice for these subtypes.

ELECTROCONVULSIVE THERAPY

ECT is the only truly bimodal therapy, in that it is equally effective for both the acute depressed and manic phases of the disorder. While the primary indication for ECT is a severe, unremitting, or drug-nonresponsive depressive episode, there is also data from as early as the 1940s supporting its use for the treatment of acute mania, particularly manic delirium (2, 3). Based on clinical experience, we would expect mania to remit rapidly with ECT, whereas lithium can take weeks. Hence, there may be a superiority for ECT over lithium in the early phases of treatment. What the final outcome would be is more problematic, but clearly, there is a need for further studies on the efficacy of ECT in mania. In this light, Schnur and colleagues (1992) reported on the relationship between various pretreatment symptoms and therapeutic outcome to ECT in 18 manic patients. They found that while severity of mania was not predictive, anger, irritability, and suspiciousness were more characteristic of nonresponders to ECT (4).

Case Example. A 28 year-old female had been stable on lithium treatment for several years. When she became pregnant, her lithium was discontinued, and within a few weeks she was hospitalized for a severe exacerbation of mania unresponsive to CPZ in doses up to 1200 mg/day. After a course of ECT she became euthymic and was adequately maintained on lower doses of CPZ (i.e., 50–100 mg/day) for the remainder of her pregnancy. The delivery and immediate postpartum period went well, but lithium was not resumed since she opted to nurse her infant. Several weeks later she was rehospitalized for an episode of depression, which also responded to a course of ECT. She then agreed to discontinue nursing her child and resume lithium. The patient was doing well at follow-up 1 year later.

Since the issue of informed consent is often problematic in such emergencies, a court-appointed, partial conservator may be required to provide substituted permission for treatment (see Informed Consent in Chapter 2).

Literature Review

Uncontrolled studies since the mid-1970s (McCabe et al., 1977; Black et al., 1987) have reported on ECT's comparable or superior benefit to antipsychotics or lithium (5, 6). More recently, Small et al. (1988) found that both the bilateral ECT (BILAT-ECT) and lithium-treated groups improved from baseline levels (7). Further, at all time points the ECT-treated group showed a greater improvement, reaching statistical significance by weeks 6, 7, and 8. These patients were then followed for up to 2 years with maintenance therapy at the clinician's discretion. No differences in relapse rates, recurrence, or rehospitalization between the two groups were found. They concluded that BILAT-ECT was an effective and safe treatment for acute mania that could be used in patients unable to tolerate or benefit from lithium or who may pose an immediate danger to themselves because of the severity of their episode.

Small's study, however, has several methodological issues that complicate the interpretation of its results. First, most patients randomly assigned to lithium or ECT also received antipsychotics. Second, those initially assigned to receive lithium began ECT 2–6 weeks later, so that all had been receiving a course of ECT for 2–5 weeks before the final evaluation. Third, the authors note that "most of the patients who underwent ECT were also taking lithium by the fifth week and had plasma levels between 0.51 and 0.69 during weeks 4 to 8 of the study." Clearly, the most appropriate time to interpret the study would have been in the first 3 weeks, when only two of the patients receiving lithium had also received ECT and few ECT patients had begun lithium. When we looked at this period, there was no difference between the treatment groups. Again this could be artifactual because the majority of the patients were receiving antipsychotics as well.

Administration of ECT

The administration of ECT to treat acute mania generally follows the same guidelines as for depression (see also Chapter 8). There is some evidence that lithium should be discontinued during a course of treatments to avoid neurotoxicity. Recent data indicate that BILAT rather than UND electrode placement may be the procedure of choice, but this opinion is not universal (8). A controlled trial by Milstein et al. (1987) randomly assigned patients in a partially blinded design to receive lithium or ECT for an 8-week, acute treatment period (9). Initially, those patients assigned to the ECT group were given unilateral nondominant (UND) administration; however, they did not respond. The design was then altered, and all subsequent patients were administered BILAT-ECT. Statistical and clinical comparisons were then based on the BILAT-ECT versus the lithium-treated groups, with ECT demonstrating superior efficacy over the 2-month trial period.

Complications

The central and the peripheral effects of ECT, as well as associated complications, are discussed in detail in the sections on ECT for depression (see Electroconvulsive Therapy in Chapter 8).

ANTICONVULSANTS

Carbamazepine (CBZ) and *valproic acid* (VPA), marketed primarily as anticonvulsants, have also been studied for their mood stabilizing properties. *Clonazepam,* discussed earlier, appears to have nonspecific effects on hyperactivity and related anxiety features. *Phenytoin,* studied extensively in the 1940s, rendered results that were generally disappointing.

The rationale for the use of selected anticonvulsants in the treatment of bipolar disorder is based on the following factors:

* *Noncompliance* with lithium due to intolerable adverse effects
* *Only partial response* or *refractoriness* to lithium
* Possible improved efficacy for specific *subtypes*
* VPA and CBZ probably have the same acute and possibly the same maintenance actions
* *Lack of more serious complications,* such as tardive dyskinesia, neuroleptic malignant syndrome, other extrapyramidal reactions, or significant hypotension
* Combined CBZ and VPA may have beneficial *synergistic effects* in selected patients (10).

Of note, the FDA has only approved carbamazepine and valproic acid for certain seizure and paroxysmal pain disorders, but not for the treatment of mood disorders. While the use of drugs for other than FDA-labelled indications is a common and appropriate practice (e.g., antidepressants for panic disorder), this should always be discussed with patients as well as their families; and properly documented, including the discussion of the rationale and the potential complications (see also Informed Consent in Chapter 2).

Carbamazepine

Carbamazepine is labelled for the management of temporal lobe epilepsy and paroxysmal pain disorders. CBZ's anticonvulsant actions are apparently associated with its ability to reduce postsynaptic responses and to block post-tetanic potentiation. The initial half-life ranges from 25–65 hours, but due to CBZ's ability to induce its own metabolism (i.e., autometabolism), this may be reduced to 12–17 hours after several weeks of treatment. Its primary psychiatric application has been as a treatment for bipolar disorder, based on the initial work of two Japanese groups in the early 1970s (11, 12). Interestingly, CBZ has a chemical structure resembling imipramine and was originally synthesized as a possible antidepressant agent.

Our qualitative and quantitative analyses of CBZ's efficacy in acute mania find it to be a potential alternative therapy when lithium is unsuccessful. There is also an emerging argument for its preferential use in certain lithium-resistant subtypes; however, the amount and quality of the data thus far limit any firm conclusions.

Indications/Contraindications

Carbamazepine's spectrum of efficacy appears similar to that of lithium; however, as noted earlier, it may be superior to lithium in mixed or dysphoric mania, rapid cyclers, and *more severe episodes* (e.g., fulminant, aggressive, psychotic) (13). The number of patients treated with

CBZ for acute mania in some form of placebo-controlled design is very limited. In fact, we are not aware of any double-blind, placebo-controlled parallel design to address this question (i.e., Class I design). It should also be noted that the studies supporting CBZ's efficacy are based primarily on data from Japan and NIMH, whose subject populations may not allow for generalization to more typical patient groups.

Literature Review

Recent reviews of the literature comparing CBZ or oxcarbamazepine to placebo, lithium, or various antipsychotics for acute mania find a response rate approaching 70% (14, 15). One of the problems with this literature, however, is that most studies qualify for only a Class III design (see also Evaluation of Drug Study Designs in Chapter 2).

The first controlled empirical study of the effects of CBZ on behavior was done by Dehing (1968), who described its behavioral effects in epileptic patients (16). He noted that it made them more active and communicative; less egocentric and stubborn; improved dysphoria, emotional lability, aggressiveness, and outbursts of rage; and had a positive effect on apathy, depression, anxiety, and hypochondriasis. He then studied its effects in a mostly nonepileptic, chronic psychiatric population that suffered from such varied disorders as dementia, psychosis, mental deficiency, and psychopathy, but not bipolar disorder. In a double-blind, random-assignment design, he treated most of these patients for 1 month with placebo or CBZ. He continued the investigation after the double-blind phase on patients initially assigned to placebo and added others to the trial, for a total of 58 patients. Those receiving CBZ showed a marked improvement, in contrast to those on placebo, but

there were two patients on CBZ who developed either a slight or a marked aggravation of their disorder.

Dehing qualitatively identified aggressiveness and outbursts of rage as the symptoms most helped by CBZ. It is of interest that, in addition to lithium's antimanic effect, there is evidence it also exerts an antiaggressive effect. This raises the question of whether mood stabilizers impact at a more fundamental level than the specific disorder being treated. Thus, like anti-inflammatory agents, they may benefit various disorders that share phenomenological and pathophysiological similarities.

Carbamazepine/Oxcarbamazepine versus Placebo.   Post and Uhde (1985) studied nine manic patients using an ABA design. In our judgement, three patients had a good response to CBZ and relapsed when switched to placebo; one had an equivocal response but relapsed when CBZ was discontinued; one responded to CBZ but failed to relapse on placebo; and three did not demonstrate a clear-cut response to CBZ nor relapsed when administered placebo later (17). To some degree the placebo lead-in period in the ABA design controls for the placebo effect, but with no true control group, we cannot be sure improvement was not due to:

- Cycling
- Spontaneous remission
- Nonspecific effects of hospitalization
- An unrecognized carryover medication effect.

Emrich et al. (1985) treated six patients with oxcarbamazepine, the keto derivative of CBZ. Three showed a good response, with one improving during two separate episodes (18). Here again, the design was a Class III type, with no control group, and although the outcome was suggestive of efficacy, it is not definitive.

Goncalves and Stoll (1985) studied six patients on CBZ and six on placebo; however, substantial amounts of antipsychotic augmentation were used (19). Virtually every placebo patient had some additional haloperidol, and 2 of 3 also received other supplemental antipsychotics. In the CBZ group, 4 out of 6 received supplemental haloperidol, with none needing other antipsychotics. Despite the greater use of antipsychotics in the placebo group, the CBZ group was found statistically superior. Since significant amounts of concomitant antipsychotics were used, it is hard to draw any firm conclusion, but the outcome could be suggestive of the need for antipsychotic supplementation when CBZ is employed.

Carbamazepine versus Lithium. Other relevant evidence for carbamazepine comes from studies comparing it to standard treatments. Lerer et al. (1987) compared CBZ to *lithium* without concomitant medication (20). Fourteen patients were randomly assigned to lithium and 14 to CBZ. Lithium appeared superior, with 11 patients improving, in contrast to only four patients improving with CBZ. A second study, by Small and colleagues, found CBZ and lithium comparable in efficacy in a group of 52 hospitalized, treatment-refractory manic patients (21). This was a double-blind, randomized design that followed patients during both the acute (i.e., 8 weeks) and the maintenance phase (up to 2 years). There was a trend favoring the lithium group on the survival analysis ($p <$ 0.14).

Carbamazepine versus Antipsychotics

Since there is evidence that lithium is superior to *antipsychotics* in acute epi-

sodes of pure mania, it is relevant to review the data comparing carbamazepine to antipsychotics. There are four studies investigating acute mania (two with random-assignment, double-blind conditions and no concomitant drugs) (22–25). While the two Class I studies found no statistical difference between CBZ and chlorpromazine, one found a trend favoring CBZ and the other chlorpromazine. When a meta-analysis was done combining these two studies, the pooled data show the relative outcomes to be virtually equal. The effect size is 0.05 and the Z score 0.2, indicating that the two nonsignificant trends virtually cancel each other out. We note that the four well-controlled studies comparing lithium to antipsychotics found lithium significantly superior (see Table 10.2).

Carbamazepine Plus Other Psychotropics (Open Studies)

In an open study, Okuma et al. (1989) added *carbamazepine to the previous treatment* of 107 affective, 54 schizophrenic, and 26 schizoaffective patients (25). Improvement was 73%, 56%, and 62%, respectively. In an open design, Nolen (1984) added *CBZ to lithium* (and, when necessary, an antipsychotic and/or antidepressant) in a small group of treatment-resistant manic patients, who then showed further improvement (26). Kramlinger and Post (1989) added *lithium to CBZ* in seven patients with varying degrees of mania, noting that six improved and one worsened (27). Since there was no control group, we do not know whether the patients would have shown similar improvement had the CBZ alone been continued for a longer period of time. Indeed, one responder had been on CBZ 2 weeks, and another for 3, but the other four responders had been on treatment about a month, which is sufficient time for

CBZ's effects to peak. Thus, while the data is suggestive that lithium may augment carbamazepine's effect, the absence of a control group and the small sample size do not allow for a definitive conclusion.

Carbamazepine Plus Antipsychotics versus Antipsychotics Alone. Klein et al. (1984) augmented *haloperidol with carbamazepine* (CBZ) in a group of newly admitted, highly destructive psychotic patients (affectively disordered or schizophrenic) and found that 19 out of 23 carbamazepine-augmented patients improved, in contrast to 11 out of 20 of the placebo-augmented (28). Mueller and Stoll (1984) and Goncalves and Stoll (1985) using random-assignment, double-blind designs in small samples of 6–10 patients per group found that the *addition of carbamazepine to haloperidol* also produced some increased benefit over the antipsychotic alone (19, 29). Specifically, Mueller found less supplemental medication was needed when CBZ was added, and Goncalves found CBZ superior to placebo supplementation of haloperidol.

Carbamazepine Plus Antipsychotics versus Lithium Plus Antipsychotics. Lenzi et al. (1986) compared patients randomly assigned to *lithium or carbamazepine augmented by chlorpromazine* (30). During the first week every patient required chlorpromazine, in the second 14 out of 15, and in the third, 11 out of 15 in each group. The therapeutic result of the chlorpromazine-carbamazepine combination was equal to the chlorpromazine-lithium combination, and the only difference was that patients on CBZ required less chlorpromazine in the first week. Lusznat et al. also found the CBZ-antipsychotic combination equal to the lithium-antipsychotic combination (31). In studies where most but not all patients receive two active drugs, the design clouds the effectiveness of the drug alone versus an augmentation strategy. When every patient receives a basic drug that is then supplemented with another, one can more readily determine if the augmenting drug is helpful. All must receive the basic drug in a constant dose, however.

Administration of Carbamazepine

If CBZ is considered as an antimanic therapy, the routine pre-treatment workup includes assessment of baseline *hematological and hepatic functions,* since these two organ systems may be significantly affected by this agent. Once baseline medical status has been established, typical starting doses are 400–600 mg/day, given in divided doses. Increments of 200 mg/day are given every few days until adverse effects preclude higher dosing or desired clinical response is reached. Less aggressive titration and even dose reduction may be required early in the treatment until the patient develops tolerance to its adverse effects. In terms of adequate *blood levels,* 4–12 µg/ml is considered the accepted therapeutic range for CBZ when used as an anticonvulsant, but an ideal blood level of CBZ as an antimanic is unknown. Preliminary data, however, find a relationship with CSF levels of CBZ's principal epoxide metabolite and clinical response. Therefore, it is desirable to titrate the dose based on clinical response and adverse effects rather than rigidly relying on plasma levels. As we will discuss later, therapeutic drug monitoring (TDM) of CBZ, especially during the first several weeks of therapy, is crucial due to the phenomenon of autometabolism, and the potential for clinically significant drug interactions.

Case Example. A 23 year-old female with a long history of bipolar disorder resistant to lithium monotherapy and characterized by mixed episodes and rapid cycling, was hospitalized in a manic phase. She was on lithium, carbamazepine, and trifluoperazine, with a therapeutic lithium level but a carbamazepine level of only 5 μg/ml. The patient underwent a washout, during which she deteriorated, and was then placed on VPA. Because of increasing confusion, nausea and vomiting at therapeutic levels, she was then switched back to CBZ, plus low-dose trifluoperazine. She had minimal response to CBZ blood levels in the range of 6–10 μg/ml, but when levels were titrated up to a range of 12–14 μg/ml, she demonstrated marked stabilization in mood, with minimal adverse effects. When the antipsychotic was discontinued, the patient continued to do well and was discharged to outpatient follow-up.

While the sequence is strongly suggestive of a beneficial effect with higher CBZ levels, we cannot rule out the possibility of a spontaneous improvement due to her history of rapid cycling.

Valproic Acid

Reports on the benefit of this anticonvulsant (which include such various formulations as divalproex sodium, i.e., a compound comprised of sodium valproate and valproic acid; dipropylacetic acid; and a closely related form, valpromide or dipropylacetamide) for the management of mood disorders date back to the mid-1960s. In the early European experience, much of the interest focused on maintenance therapy of manic-depressive disease, with patients stabilized on valproate or valpromide for up to 10 years using the drug alone or in conjunction with other psychotropics. A few investigators also studied the drug in acute mania, usually in combination with antipsychotics, and found it to be beneficial, often allowing for substantial reductions in the antipsychotic dose (31a).

Valproic acid's anticonvulsant efficacy may be related to its ability to increase CNS levels of GABA. Due to its rapid absorption, blood levels peak in 1–4 hours after oral administration; and the half-life ranges from 6 to 16 hours. It is metabolized primarily through the liver, and is eliminated in the urine. **VPA is highly protein-bound and usually does not saturate binding sites with serum levels below 50 μg/ml. Thus, this level would be the expected minimal threshold for its psychotropic effects.**

Indications/Contraindications

VPA appears to be at least comparable to lithium and CBZ for the acute manic phase of bipolar disorder, and may also benefit some of the more lithium-resistant subtypes described earlier in the discussion of CBZ. Also, like lithium and CBZ, it does not appear to be as beneficial for the depressive phase of this illness. There is also limited data that nonresponsiveness to one anticonvulsant (e.g., CBZ) does not necessarily portend a poor response to another (e.g., VPA) (32, 33). The drug is contraindicated in patients with hepatic diseases, during pregnancy, and in those with a prior known hypersensitivity to VPA.

Literature Review

Lambert et al. (1966) first investigated VPA in a series of clinical trials including a wide variety of patients (34). More recently, 12 (mostly open) studies, representing 297 acutely ill patients, found an overall moderate to marked response rate to VPA of 56%. Only one, however, met more rigorous double-blind, placebo-controlled conditions, with a total of 17 patients on VPA (35).

Brennan et al. (1984) observed that six out of eight manic patients responded to valproate (36). All then had their medication discontinued for a few days, with one relapsing but again improving upon reinstatement of valproate.

Emrich et al. (1985) used a placebo lead-in period in five patients treated with VPA and found that four responded, but no subsequent placebo period was mentioned (18).

While the overall response rate to VPA was 61%, a number of methodological problems complicate the interpretation of these results, including: most patients were studied under *nonblind conditions;* VPA was often *used in combination* with other psychotropics; VPA *concentrations* were usually *not monitored;* and *formal diagnostic criteria* derived from standard clinical ratings *were typically not employed.*

Valproic Acid versus Placebo. Two Class I studies have now examined the efficacy of VPA in comparison to placebo for acute mania. The first is the investigation by Pope et al. (1991) in which 17 acutely manic patients were treated with divalproex sodium and 19 with placebo in a 3-week random-assignment, double-blind design (35). Supplemental lorazepam was used in the first 10 days; otherwise there was no additional rescue medication. The definitive assessment of most patients occurred in the second and the third weeks, when no adjunctive medication was used. VPA was found to be substantially more effective than placebo, with 12 of 17 patients responding, versus only 6 of 13 placebo responders. This difference might have even been greater if lorazepam was not used, since more was required in the placebo group. Further, only four patients in the VPA group had lack of improvement or worsening, whereas 12 in the placebo group were rated unimproved or worse. Pope also investigated possible correlates of a favorable outcome with VPA and found

that the only predictor of response was a high plasma level during the early phase of the study (i.e., days 2 to 6) (37). By contrast, rapid cycling, predominant euphoria or dysphoria, family history of mood disorder, increased severity of mania, or EEG abnormalities did not predict response.

The authors have recently participated in a multicentered investigation of divalproex sodium for acute mania that is the only parallel-design, double-blind, placebo-controlled trial including a lithium arm and placebo control (Bowden et al., submitted for publication). It included 179 intent-to-treat subjects, by far the largest sample of bipolar patients studied under these conditions. Both divalproex sodium and lithium (as a positive control) were compared to placebo for a 21-day treatment trial of acute mania. Concurrent rescue medications were limited to low doses of chloral hydrate and/or lorazepam, used only when absolutely necessary during the washout phase and the first 7 days of the double-blind trial. Both active drug therapies produced at least moderate improvement in about 50% of the patients. This effect was significantly better than for those patients on placebo. VPA was found to benefit such core manic symptoms as elevated mood, grandiosity, insomnia, hyperactivity, and psychosis. Finally, the lithium group had a significantly higher drop out rate due to adverse effects in comparison to those in the placebo group. The authors concluded that VPA was a safe and effective alternative to lithium for the treatment of acutely manic, bipolar patients.

Due to these two carefully controlled trials, the evidence that VPA is effective in acute mania is presently the best controlled data for any treatment, including lithium.

Valproic Acid versus Lithium. Freeman et al. (1992) conducted a 3-week double-blind, parallel-group comparison of VPA and lithium for acute mania (38). Both drugs demonstrated clinically significant efficacy (i.e., 9 of 14 responded to VPA and 12 of 13 to lithium), and there was no difference in the need for rescue medications (i.e., lorazepam or chloral hydrate) between the two treatment groups. Response to VPA was associated with high pretreatment depression scores.

Administration of Valproic Acid

Starting doses of VPA should be 250–500 mg twice a day, with doses titrated up to achieve blood levels in the range of 50–120 μg/ml. Most patients require 750–1250 mg/day to achieve these levels. Since VPA is highly protein-bound, minimal free drug is available until concentrations of 50 μg/ml are achieved, which in essence defines the lower end of a therapeutic range. A possible upper end is less clear, but most positive results reported occurred with levels about 70–90 μg/ml. Given the drug's relatively short half-life, blood levels should be checked in 3–5 days to monitor C_{SS}, with dosage increased until the optimal effect is achieved or intolerable adverse effects intervene.

> **Case Example.** A 34-year-old male was hospitalized on CBZ, chlorpromazine, Li_2CO_3, and lorazepam for an acute exacerbation of mania. Despite a history of rapid cycling, he responded to an initial trial of Li_2CO_3, thiothixene, and lorazepam, but then relapsed. Increasing the thiothixene (up to 120 mg/day) was unsuccessful and poorly tolerated. The patient then improved on a regimen of loxapine (up to 250 mg/day) and clonazepam (up to 20 mg/day), but doses of each had to be reduced because of intolerable adverse effects (i.e., excessive sedation, drooling, pseudoparkinsonism), and he suffered another relapse. He again received chlorpromazine (up to 900 mg/day) and VPA (plasma level stabilized at 80 μg/ml) while the clonazepam was tapered slowly and

discontinued. He gradually became euthymic and was able to leave the hospital after a 4-month stay, stabilized solely on chlorpromazine (600 mg/day) and VPA (1250 mg/day).

Conclusion

Currently, VPA is the best-studied of the mood stabilizers and is emerging as a highly effective alternate treatment to lithium for acute mania. It may also benefit the maintenance and the prophylactic phases as well, but there is only limited data in this regard, in contrast to lithium, which remains the best-studied maintenance therapy. VPA has a favorable and relatively safe side-effect profile compared to other agents and can be combined with other commonly employed psychotropics without significantly altering their metabolism or compromising adequacy of blood levels (39). There is also limited anecdotal data that this agent can be safe and effective in the elderly patient (40).

EXPERIMENTAL THERAPIES

Noradrenergic Agents

Clonidine

This α_2-noradrenergic presynaptic receptor agonist is approved by the FDA as an antihypertensive. The rationale for employing clonidine is based on the original catecholamine hypothesis (Bunney and Davis, 1965; Schildkraut, 1965), which postulates a *hyperfunctionality* of the noradrenergic system leading to mania (41, 42). Since the hypothesis suggests that increases in norepinephrine neurotransmission may underlie such symptomatology, drugs that decrease central NE activity might prove therapeutic in this condition. Limited, less well-controlled data indicated a possible benefit for this agent, either alone or as a substitute for antipsychotics, in the earliest phases of an acute manic exacerbation. Our own double-blind, placebo-controlled trial, however, did not support such efficacy when clonidine was used alone for moderate to severe exacerbations of an acute manic episode (43).

A similar line of reasoning has also generated some equivocal data for the β-blocking agent propranolol (44–46).

Literature Review. A number of open trials initially reported positive results with the use of clonidine for treating acute mania. For example, Jouvent et al. (1980) observed improvement in three of eight bipolar patients and partial improvement in three others in an open trial with doses of clonidine ranging from 0.15 to 0.45 mg/day (47). However, patients were also taking various concurrent drugs (i.e., droperidol, diazepam, chlorpromazine, and lithium). A subsequent study found that three bipolar patients experienced rapid and complete remission with the addition of clonidine in doses ranging from 0.4 to 0.8 mg/day (48). Hardy et al. (1986) treated 24 newly admitted acutely manic patients with doses ranging from 0.45 to 0.9 mg/day, in addition to droperidol (25–50 mg orally), if necessary, and some were also maintained on their previous lithium regimen (49). Thirteen patients showed either marked or partial improvement within 5 days of treatment. Four others, in the higher dose range (0.75–0.9 mg/day), did show some worsening, particularly in aggressiveness and hostility, that improved when the drug was discontinued. Another report stated three treatment-resistant manic patients demonstrated a rapid response with the addition of clonidine (0.2–0.4 mg/day) to their treatment regimens (50).

Three different partially controlled trials for acute mania have also been reported

(51–53). In the first study, 11 patients were administered clonidine in three divided doses of 17 μg/kg/day (or approximately 1.2 mg/day) under double-blind conditions. The blind consisted of telling patients and treating physicians that the capsules may or may not contain active medication, when in fact all patients received clonidine. No concurrent medications were given. After 25 days, patients showed significant reductions in their Biegel-Murphy Manic State Ratings, and all eight who discontinued the drug relapsed. Hypotension and sedation were present but tolerated. The second study was a double-blind crossover design comparing clonidine (17 μg/kg/day) with verapamil (80 mg p.o. q.i.d.) in 20 manic male patients for two 20-day periods separated by a 5-day placebo crossover phase. Verapamil demonstrated greater antimanic properties and caused no adverse effects, in contrast to clonidine, which also produced significant hypotension. The third study had a design similar to the second, but the comparison treatment was lithium and the two treatment phases were 30 days long, separated by a 15-day placebo crossover phase. The doses of clonidine were again 17 μg/kg/day, and the lithium dose was adjusted to maintain serum levels at 1.2 mEq/liter. Lithium was statistically superior to clonidine after the first 30-day period, while after the second 30 days, neither drug group was significantly better than the other, but the trend favored the lithium group. It is not clear whether these patients were in an acute exacerbation or on maintenance therapy. If the latter situation were true, the time period would be too short to adequately assess efficacy.

In the only double-blind, placebo-controlled parallel design of clonidine, Janicak et al. (1989) studied a group of acutely ill, hospitalized manic patients, many with associated psychotic features (43). After a washout period averaging 1 week, patients were randomly assigned to receive either clonidine or placebo for a 2-week trial. The intent was to ascertain if clonidine alone had any inherent antimanic properties, and therefore, no other concomitant psychotropics were allowed. Unfortunately, improvement in either group was minimal and did not differ, with some patients on clonidine developing problems with rash and hypotension. Doses of clonidine were comparable to those reported in prior positive studies, averaging 0.5 mg/day.

Other possible uses, not addressed in this study, are the potential benefit of clonidine as an adjunct to lithium or anticonvulsants, thus serving as a substitute for antipsychotics; or its benefit in less severe exacerbations of mania.

Calcium Channel Blockers

Calcium antagonists (channel blockers; influx inhibitors) have been used primarily for the treatment of cardiovascular disorders (e.g., supraventricular arrhythmias, angina, and hypertension). Calcium ion inhibitors, such as verapamil, exert their effects by modulating the influx of Ca^{2+} across the cell membrane, thus interfering with calcium-dependent functions. More recently, based partly on the common effects of lithium and this class of drugs (e.g., effects on Ca^{2+} activity), they have been studied as a potential treatment for mania. The evidence for efficacy rests on one very small study (i.e., six patients) and two partially controlled studies; but another (apparently controlled) study had a negative result. At present, we believe there is enough positive data to encourage further studies, but given the contradictory information, the hypothesis that verapamil helps mania remains unproven.

More recently, Post and colleagues have suggested that voltage-gated calcium antagonists, such as nimodipine, may be more effective, especially in ultra rapid and ultradian cycling patients (i.e., cycles every several weeks or hours, respectively) (54).

Literature Review

Verapamil versus Placebo. Dubovsky demonstrated a reduction of mania with verapamil in three patients, and later included four more in a random-assignment, crossover study *comparing verapamil to placebo* (55). Unfortunately, one of the seven patients did not undergo the placebo arm of the study. Five showed a relatively dramatic response to verapamil, and the sixth a slight trend toward improvement. The patient who failed to undergo the placebo arm also showed some improvement with verapamil. Given the degree of improvement these data suggest efficacy.

In a single-blind, crossover design *comparing verapamil, lithium, and placebo* in 12 manic patients, Giannini et al. (1984) found no difference between lithium and verapamil (56). The study is inconclusive, however, since it is not clear whether these patients were in an acute manic episode; and if not, a month's trial would be insufficient to evaluate the maintenance properties of either. The predominant symptoms, as measured by the Brief Psychiatric Rating Scale (BPRS), were mild depression, anxiety, tension, and guilt, with only a slight degree of excitement or grandiosity (i.e., a rating of 2.5 and 1.7 on a 7-point scale, respectively, at the beginning of the study), and virtually no patients had hallucinations or delusions. While this was an AB paradigm, and not a random-assignment, crossover design with a control group, it did support the benefit of verapamil. Thus, patients went from mildly symptomatic to remission over a 30-day treatment period, worsened during the 10-day placebo period, and then improved again when they received lithium for 30 days.

Dose and coworkers compared *verapamil to placebo* in eight patients employing an ABA design (57). Seven showed some degree of response, five with symptoms reemerging to a minor extent with placebo, and two showing no relapse on placebo. A concomitant antipsychotic was used in two, and lithium in one.

Verapamil versus Other Psychotropics. Garza-Trevino et al. (1992) recently conducted a 4-week, randomized double-blind study *comparing verapamil to lithium* for acute mania and found no clinical or statistically significant differences between the two treatments (58). These results are difficult to interpret, however, because data about the amount and timing of rescue medication (i.e., haloperidol and lorazepam) were not presented. Further, more patients on verapamil required these agents.

Arkonac and his coworkers investigated *verapamil in comparison to lithium* in a random-assignment, double-blind, crossover study of 15 manics (four weeks of lithium or verapamil, 10 days of placebo, then followed by a crossover to the other agent) (59). Patients improved on lithium but unexpectedly worsened with verapamil. This was a well-controlled study of verapamil, but unfortunately did not confirm the previous results. Further, it is only available in abstract form, and the complete publication is needed to evaluate the study critically. However, its outcome suggests caution in interpretation of earlier positive results.

Giannini studied 24 patients in a random-assignment crossover design, finding *verapamil superior to clonidine;* but quantitative measures of change, such as the BPRS scores, were not provided (52).

Hoschl and Kozeny reported that the degree of improvement was comparable in 12 manic patients treated with *verapamil,* 24 with *antipsychotics,* and 11 with *antipsychotics plus lithium* (60).

Currently, the evidence for this agent's effectiveness rests with six patients in a double-blind study and eight patients in a Class III, ABA design trial. The authors are completing a prospective, double-blind, placebo-controlled trial to clarify the usefulness of verapamil for acute mania (Janicak et al., unpublished data).

Verapamil Case Report Literature. Several case reports in the literature have not supported verapamil's potential antimanic properties. For example, Barton and Gitlin (1987) found that none of eight acutely manic or hypomanic patients treated openly improved on verapamil (61). By contrast, there are several case reports of hypomania (some MAOI-induced) improving with verapamil. Dubovsky notes that in his experience with spontaneous mania, he has been unimpressed with verapamil in patients who had previously been unresponsive to lithium.

Administration of Verapamil

Doses of verapamil reported to have antimanic effects have ranged from 80 mg b.i.d. to 160 mg t.i.d. Typically, the initial dose is 80 mg two or three times daily, with rapid escalation up to, but not exceeding, 480 mg/day. (Personal communication with Dubovsky and Giannini indicates some patients may require and safely tolerate doses up to 640 mg/day.) The drug is usually well tolerated and no specific laboratory monitoring is required.

Other Treatment Strategies

A number of other theoretically interesting, as well as potentially clinically relevant treatments, have also been studied, including:

- *Cholinomimetic* agents
- Drugs that enhance *serotonin* functioning (e.g., precursors such as L-tryptophan)
- *Psychostimulants* (such as amphetamines or methylphenidate)
- *Atypical antipsychotics* (i.e., clozapine).

We would emphasize that while all of these approaches are theoretically important and may possess clinical applicability, none are presently employed routinely.

Cholinomimetic Agents

Earlier data indicated that physostigmine may enhance cholinergic activity as well as bring about temporary improvement in manic symptoms. The beneficial effect of *precursors* (e.g., lecithin), *cholinesterase inhibitors* (e.g., physostigmine), or *drugs with cholinomimetic effects* (e.g., bethanechol) was discovered in part from the work of Janowsky et al. (1972), leading to their *cholinergic/ noradrenergic balance hypothesis* (62). Interestingly, lithium is also able to raise RBC choline concentrations and CNS cholinergic activity (63).

Serotonin Agents

There is limited evidence that the amino acid precursor of serotonin, L-tryptophan, may be useful, alone or in combination with other antimanic agents to enhance overall efficacy. Unfortunately, contaminants in the production of this agent have led to several cases of the Eosinophilia Myalgia Syndrome (EMS)

and its removal from the market, for at least the time being.

The possible antimanic effect of this 5-HT precursor was postulated based on the *permissive hypothesis* concept of diminished 5-HT activity. When oral doses of L-tryptophan (1–4 g) are administered, there is evidence of increased 5-HT synthesis. Three of four double-blind studies have yielded positive results, holding up the promise of an effective treatment if the issue of EMS can be resolved (64). A major advantage to this drug was its relative lack of adverse effects before the complication of EMS.

Fenfluramine, which has serotonergic agonist properties, has also been considered, but data is lacking to support or refute any antimanic properties (65).

Psychostimulants

Anecdotal case reports and small sample size trials have shown some benefit for the use of psychostimulants to manage episodes of excitability in mania. This counterintuitive, paradoxical effect parallels their beneficial use in children with hyperactivity (66). The theoretical basis may be related to an indirect effect of these agents that leads to *enhancement of serotonin functioning.*

Clozapine

Two intriguing reports have found this atypical antipsychotic to benefit a small number of affectively disordered patients (e.g., bipolar, schizoaffective). This group had previously been treatment-refractory, but improved rapidly and significantly on clozapine (67, 68). Further, most sustained their early gains in psychosocial functioning over a 3- to 5-year period. Obviously, these preliminary results should be followed up with controlled prospective trials. Given this agent's life-threatening adverse effects, a careful risk/benefit assessment would be a prerequisite to its use for these patients. We caution against the combined use of clozapine plus CBZ, given the former's propensity toward agranulocytosis and the latter's ability to suppress bone marrow production.

CONCLUSION

Figure 10.3 depicts an updated treatment strategy for acute mania that the authors first recommended in an earlier report (1). Patients presenting with mild to moderate symptoms should first have an adequate trial of lithium, with blood level ranges of 0.8–1.5 mEq/liter, if tolerated. Adjunctive BZDs may be beneficial if:

- The presentation is complicated by continued marked agitation, insomnia, anxiety
- There is concern about adverse effects from antipsychotics
- Response is still unsatisfactory.

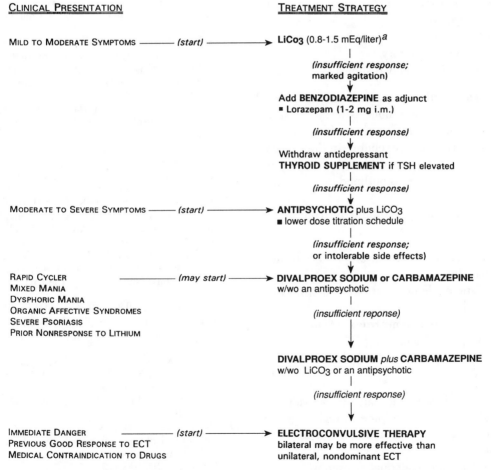

<u>CLINICAL PRESENTATION</u>

<u>TREATMENT STRATEGY</u>

MILD TO MODERATE SYMPTOMS ——— (start) ———→ **LiCo3** (0.8-1.5 mEq/liter)[a]

(insufficient response; marked agitation)

Add **BENZODIAZEPINE** as adjunct
- Lorazepam (1-2 mg i.m.)

(insufficient response)

Withdraw antidepressant
THYROID SUPPLEMENT if TSH elevated

(insufficient response)

MODERATE TO SEVERE SYMPTOMS ——— (start) ———→ **ANTIPSYCHOTIC** plus LiCO3
- lower dose titration schedule

(insufficient response; or intolerable side effects)

RAPID CYCLER ——— (may start) ———→ **DIVALPROEX SODIUM or CARBAMAZEPINE**
MIXED MANIA   w/wo an antipsychotic
DYSPHORIC MANIA
ORGANIC AFFECTIVE SYNDROMES
SEVERE PSORIASIS
PRIOR NONRESPONSE TO LITHIUM

(insufficient reponse)

DIVALPROEX SODIUM *plus* **CARBAMAZEPINE**
w/wo LiCO3 or an antipsychotic

(insufficient response)

IMMEDIATE DANGER ——— (start) ———→ **ELECTROCONVULSIVE THERAPY**
PREVIOUS GOOD RESPONSE TO ECT   bilateral may be more effective than
MEDICAL CONTRAINDICATION TO DRUGS   unilateral, nondominant ECT

[a] If VPA is demonstrated to have prophylactic properties, it may be a viable alternative to LiCO3.

Figure 10.3. Strategy for the management of acute mania. Adapted from Janicak PG, Newman RH, Davis JM. Advances in the treatment of mania and related disorders: a reappraisal. Psychiatr Ann 1992;22(2):92–103.

The discontinuation of concurrent antidepressants and/or the use of supplemental thyroid agents may benefit the treatment-resistant patient and perhaps preclude rapid cycling.

Lorazepam (1–2 mg) given every 4 hours, with doses up to 12 mg/day, has shown promise, or alternatively, clonazepam, up to 24 mg/day. In fact, short-term aggressive dosing with BZDs may preclude the need for antipsychotics.

Antipsychotics may be warranted if patients:

- Demonstrate associated psychotic symptoms
- Suffer from severe agitation
- Remain refractory
- Are only partially responsive.

In fact, with more moderate to severe episodes, lithium alone is usually insufficient, and initial treatment often requires a concurrent antipsychotic. In these situations, we advocate using a lower-dose titration schedule, as outlined in our earlier discussion.

Anticonvulsants should be considered if:

- Initial treatment attempts are unsuccessful
- Patients demonstrate a history of rapid cycling
- There are symptoms of mixed or dysphoric mania
- An organic mood syndrome is suspected.

The two best-studied agents are valproic acid and carbamazepine, which may be used with or without lithium or antipsychotics.

Given an inadequate response, or in patients with manic delirium who pose an immediate risk to themselves or others, we would recommend ECT. While BILAT stimulus electrode placement may be more effective than either the UD or UND placement, this conclusion is currently only tentative, given the small number of patients involved.

REFERENCES

1. Janicak PG, Newman RH, Davis JM. Advances in the treatment of mania and related disorders: a reappraisal. Psychiatric Annals 1992;22(2):92–103.
2. Rennie TAC. Manic-depressive disease: prognosis following shock treatment. Psychiatr Q 1943;17:642–654.
3. Thorpe FT. Intensive electrical convulsive therapy in acute mania. J Mental Science 1947;93:89–92.
4. Schnur DB, Mukherjee S, Sackeim HA, Lee C, Roth SD. Symptomatic predictors of ECT response in medication-nonresponsive manic patients. J Clin Psychiatry 1992;53:63–66.
5. McCabe MS. ECT in the treatment of mania: a controlled study. Am J Psychiatry 1976;133:688–691.
6. Black DW, Winokur G, Nasrallah H. Treatment of mania: a naturalistic study of ECT versus lithium in 438 patients. J Clin Psychiatry 1987;48:132–139.
7. Small JG, Klapper MH, Kellams JJ, et al. ECT compared with lithium in the management of manic states. Arch Gen Psychiatry 1988;45:727–732.
8. Mukherjee S, Sackeim HA, Lee C. Unilateral ECT in the treatment of manic episodes. Convulsive Therapy 1988;4(1):74–80.
9. Milstein V, Small JG, Klapper MH, et al. Uni- versus bilateral ECT in the treatment of mania. Convulsive Therapy 1987;3(1):1–9.
10. Ketter TA, Pazzaglia PJ, Post RM. Synergy of carbamazepine and valproic acid in affective illness: case report and review of the literature. J Clin Psychopharmacol 1992;12(4):276–281.
11. Takezaki H, Hanaoka N. The use of CBZ in the control of manic-depressive psychosis and other manic-depressive states. Clin Psychiatry 1971;13:173–183.
12. Okuma T, Kishimoto A, Inoue K, et al. Antimanic and prophylactic effects of CBZ on manic-depressive psychosis. Folia Psychiatr Neurol JPN 1973;27:283–297.

13. Post RM. Non-lithium treatment for bipolar disorder. J Clin Psychiatry 1990; 51(suppl 8):9–16.
14. Post RM. Alternatives to lithium for bipolar affective illness. In: Tasman A, Goldfinger S, Kaufman C, eds. American Psychiatric Press review of psychiatry, vol 9. Washington D.C.: APA Press 1990:170–202.
15. Chou JCY. Recent advances in the treatment of acute mania. J Clin Psychopharmacol 1990;11:3–21.
16. Dehing J. Studies on the psychotropic action of Tegretol. Acta Neurol Belg 1968;68:895–905.
17. Post RM, Uhde TW. Carbamazepine in bipolar illness. Psychopharmacol Bull 1985;21:10–17.
18. Emrich HM, Dose M, Zerssen DV. The use of sodium valproate, carbamazepine, and oxcarbazepine in patients with affective disorders. J Affective Disord 1985; 8:243–250.
19. Goncalves N, Stoll KD. Carbamazepin bei manischen Syndromen. Nervenarzt 1985; 56:43–47.
20. Lerer B, Moore M, Meyendorff E, Cho SR, Gershon S. Carbamazepine versus lithium in mania: a double-blind study. J Clin Psychiatry 1987;48:89–93.
21. Small JG, Klapper MH, Milstein V, et al. Carbamazepine compared with lithium in the treatment of mania. Arch Gen Psychiatry 1991;48:915–921.
22. Okuma T, Inanaga K, Otsuki S, Sarai K, Takahashi R, Hazama H. Comparison of the antimanic efficacy of carbamazepine and chlorpromazine: a double-blind controlled study. Psychopharmacology 1979; 66:211–217.
23. Grossi E, Sacchetti E, Vita A, et al. Carbamazepine versus chlorpromazine in mania: a double-blind trial. In: Emrich HM, Okuma T, Muller AA, eds. Anticonvulsants in affective disorders. Amsterdam, Netherlands: Excerpta Medica; 1984:177–187.
24. Sethi BB, Tiwari SC. Carbamazepine in affective disorders. In: Emrich HM, Okuma T, Muller AA, eds. Anticonvulsants in affective disorders. Amsterdam, Netherlands: Excerpta Medica; 1984:167–177.
25. Okuma T, Yamashita I, Takahashi R, et al. A double-blind study of adjunctive carbamazepine versus placebo on excited states of schizophrenia and schizoaffective disorder. Acta Psychiatr Scand 1989; 80:250–259.
26. Nolen WA. Carbamazepine: an alternative in lithium-resistant bipolar disorder. In: Emrich HM, Okuma T, Muller AA, eds. Anticonvulsants in affective disorders. Amsterdam, Netherlands: Excerpta Medica, 1984.
27. Kramlinger KG, Post RM. Adding lithium carbonate to carbamazepine: antimanic efficacy in treatment-resistant mania. Acta Psychiatr Scand 1989;79:378–385.
28. Klein E, Bental E, Lerer B, Belmaker RH. Carbamazepine and haloperidol versus placebo and haloperidol in excited psychoses. Arch Gen Psychiatry 1984;41:165–170.
29. Mueller AA, Stoll KD. Carbamazepine and oxcarbazepine in the treatment of manic syndromes: studies in Germany. In: Emrich HM, Okuma T, Muller AA, eds. Anticonvulsants in affective disorders. Amsterdam, Netherlands: Excerpta Medica, 1984:139–147.
30. Lenzi A, Grossi E, Massimetti G, Placidi GF. Use of carbamazepine in acute psychosis: a controlled study. J Int Med Res 1986;14:78–84.
31. Lusznat RM, Murphy DP, Nunn CMH. Carbamazepine vs lithium in the treatment and prophylaxis of mania. Br J Psychiatry 1988;153:198–204.
31a. Ballinger JC. The use of anticonvulsants in manic-depressive illness. J Clin Psychiatry 1988;49(Suppl 11):21–25.
32. Post RM. Introduction: emerging perspectives on valproate in affective disorders. J Clin Psychiatry 1989;50(3, suppl):3–9.
33. Post RM, Berrettini W, Uhde TW. Selective response to the anticonvulsant carbamazepine in manic-depressive illness: a case study. J Clin Psychopharmacol 1984; 4:178–185.
34. Lambert PA, Cavaz G, Borselli S, Carrel S. Action neuro-psychotrope d'un novel anti-epileptique: le depamide. Ann Med Psychol 1966;1:707–710.
35. Pope HG Jr, McElroy SL, Keck PE, Hudson JL. A placebo-controlled study of valproate in mania. Arch Gen Psychiatry 1991;48:62–68.
36. Brennan MJW, Sandyk R, Borsook D. Use of sodium valproate in the management of affective disorders: basic and clinical aspects. In: Emrich HM, Okuma T, Muller AA, eds. Anticonvulsants in affective disorders. Amsterdam, Netherlands: Excerpta Medica, 1984:56–65.

37. McElroy SL, Keck PE, Pope HG, et al. Correlates of antimanic response to valproate. Psychopharmacol Bull 1991;27:127–133.

38. Freeman TW, Clothier JL, Pazzaglia P, Lesem MC, Swann AC. A double-blind comparison of valproate and lithium in the treatment of acute mania. Am J Psychiatry 1992;149:108–111.

39. Wassef A, Watson DJ, Morrison P, Bryant S, Flack J. Neuroleptic-valproic acid combination in treatment of psychotic symptoms: a three-case report. J Clin Psychopharmacol 1989;9(1):45–48.

40. McFarland BH, Miller MR, Straumfjord AA. Valproate use in the older manic patient. J Clin Psychiatry 1990;51(11):479–481.

41. Bunney WE and Davis JM. Norepinephrine in depressive reactions. Arch Gen Psychiatry 1965;13:483–494.

42. Schildkraut JJ. The catecholamine hypothesis of affective disorders: a review of supporting evidence. Am J Psychiatry 1965;122:509–522.

43. Janicak PG, Sharma RP, Easton M, Comaty JE, Davis JM. A double-blind, placebo-controlled trial of clonidine in the treatment of acute mania. Psychopharmacol Bull 1989;25:243–245.

44. von Zerssen D. Beta-adrenergic blocking agents in the treatment of psychoses. A report on 17 cases. Advances in Clinical Pharmacology 1976;12:105–114.

45. Emrich HM, von Zerssen D, Mller H-J, Kissling W, Cording C, Schietsch HJ, Riedel E. Action of propranolol in mania: comparison of effects of the d- and the l-stereoisomer. Pharmakopsychiat 1979;12:295–304.

46. Mäoller H-J, von Zerssen D, Emrich HM, Kissling W, Cording C, Schietsch HJ, Riedel E. Action of d-propranolol in manic psychoses. Archives of Psychiatry and Neurological Sciences 1979;227:301–317.

47. Jouvent R, Lecrubier Y, Puesh AJ, Simon P, Widlocker D. Antimanic effect of clonidine. Am J Psychiatry 1980;137:1275–1276.

48. Zubenko GS, Cohen BM, Lipinski JF, Jones JM. Clonidine in the treatment of mania and mixed bipolar disorder. Am J Psychiatry 1984;141:1617–1618.

49. Hardy C, Lecrubier Y, Widlocker D. Efficacy of clonidine in 24 patients with acute mania. Am J Psychiatry 1986;143:1450–1453.

50. Maguire J and Singh AN. Clonidine: an effective antimanic agent? Br J Psychiatry 1987;150:863–864.

51. Giannini AJ, Extein I, Gold MS, Pottash ALC, Castellani S. Clonidine in mania. Drug Dev Res 1983;3:101–103.

52. Giannini, AJ, Loiselle RH, Price WA, Giannini JD. Comparison of antimanic efficacy of clonidine and verapamil. J Clin Pharmacol 1985;25:307–308.

53. Giannini AJ, Pascarzi GA, Loiselle RH, Price WA, Giannini JD. Comparison of clonidine and lithium in the treatment of mania. Am J Psychiatry 1986;143:1608–1609.

54. Post RM, Ketter TA, Pazzaglia PJ, George MS, Marangell L, Weiss SRB. Receptor, ion channel, and neuropeptide targets for drug development: implications from the anticonvulsant model. American College of Neuropsychopharmacology Abstracts of Panels and Posters, December, 1992:9.

55. Dubovsky SL, Franks RD, Allen S, et al. Calcium antagonists in mania: a double blind study of verapamil. Psychiatry Res 1986;18:309–320.

56. Giannini AJ, Houser WL, Loiselle RH, Giannini MC, Price WA. Antimanic effects of verapamil. Am J Psychiatry 1984;141:1602–1603.

57. Dose M, Emrich HM, Cording-Tommel C, Zerssen DV. Use of calcium antagonists in mania. Psychoneuroendocrinology 1986;11:241–243.

58. Garza-Trevino ES, Overall JE, Hollister LE. Verapamil versus lithium in acute mania. Am J Psychiatry 1992;149:121–122.

59. Arkonaç O, Kantarci E, Eradamlar N, Algäur T. Verapamil vs. lithium in acute manics. Biol Psychiatry 1991;29:376S.

60. Hoschl C, Kozeny J. Verapamil in affective disorders: a controlled, double-blind study. Biol Psychiatry 1989;25:128–140.

61. Barton BM, Gitlin MJ. Verapamil in treatment-resistant mania: an open trial. J Clin Psychopharmacol 1987;7:101–103.

62. Janowsky D, El Yousef MK, Davis JM. A cholinergic-adrenergic hypothesis of mania and depression. Lancet 1972;ii:6732–6735.

63. Stall AL, Cohen BM, Hanin I. Erythrocyte choline concentrations in psychiatric disorders. Biol Psychiatry 1991;29(4):309–320.

64. Chouinard G, Young SN, Annable L. A controlled clinical trial of L-tryptophan in acute mania. Biol Psychiatry 1985;20:546–557.

65. Pearce JB. Fenfluramine in mania. Lancet 1973;i(7800):427.
66. Chiarello RJ, Cole JO. The use of psycho-stimulants in general psychiatry. Arch Gen Psychiatry 1987;44:286–295.
67. Suppes T, McElroy SL, Gilbert J, Dessain EC, Cole JO. Clozapine in the treatment of dysphoric mania. Biol Psychiatry 1992;32:270–280.
68. McElroy SL, Dessain EC, Pope HG Jr, et al. Clozapine in the treatment of psychotic mood disorders, schizoaffective disorder, and schizophrenia. J Clin Psychiatry 1991;52:411–414.

Adverse Effects of Lithium

Lithium is an alkali metal in Group IA and shares many properties with similar elements such as sodium and potassium. It is rapidly absorbed and reaches peak blood levels in approximately 1–3 hours (6–8 hours with sustained release preparations), with absorption being completed in approximately 8 hours. Unlike other psychotropics, it is not protein-bound, and steady-state levels are usually achieved after 4–6 days on a fixed dose.

There are a number of significant complications that may develop with either acute or chronic lithium treatment, and they are listed in Table 10.11. The most common systems involved are the:

• Renal
• Central nervous system
• Gastrointestinal
• Endocrine (e.g., thyroid)
• Cardiovascular.

While renal, thyroid, and cardiovascular complications pose the most potentially serious problems, careful monitoring of these systems during long-term treatment can prevent most adverse sequelae (1).

Contraindications to lithium are primarily based on the presence of medical disorders involving electrolyte balance and the cardiovascular and the renal systems. Thus, patients with unstable fluid and electrolyte states, azotemia, or who require diuretics must be monitored very closely. Since lithium can impair sinus node function and aggravate the sick sinus node syndrome (SSNS), it should not be used in such conditions (2). When feasible, hypertensive patients on diuretics should be switched to β-blockers so that lithium can be prescribed. If lithium is used in patients on diuretics, plasma levels must be monitored more closely and doses usually adjusted downward. Any renal disorder that impedes the filtration of lithium can lead to increased retention and possible intoxication. While contraindicated with acute renal failure, lithium may be used in chronic but stable states or in patients on hemodialysis, but careful monitoring and lower doses are mandatory. Alternative drugs that are metabolized by the liver (e.g., VPA, CBZ) or ECT should be considered where appropriate.

In addition, special problems posed by *pregnancy* and *toxicity* must be considered. Adverse events can generally be managed by adjusting the lithium dose, adding supplements, such as L-thyroxine, in patients who develop hypothyroidism, or considering an alternate drug strategy.

RENAL SYSTEM

It is important to note that the proximal reabsorption of sodium and lithium in the kidneys is similar; therefore, states of sodium depletion, such as salt restriction,

Table 10.11.
Lithium: Adverse Effects

Organ System	Clinical Presentation	Comments
Cardiovascular	ECG changes	T-wave suppression, delayed or irregular rhythm, increase in PVCs
		Sick sinus node syndrome (SSNS)
		Myocarditis
Dermatological	Acne	Worsens
	Psoriasis	Treatment refractory worsening
	Rashes	Maculopapular and follicular
Endocrine	Hypothyroid state	about 5% goiter; about 4% clinically significant hypothyroidism
	Hyperparathyroid state	Clinically nonsignificant
Fetus (teratogenic)	Tricuspid valve malformation	Ebstein's anomaly (as yet unproven)
	Atrial septal defect	
Gastrointestinal	Anorexia	Usually early in treatment and usually transient; may be early sign of toxicity
	Nausea (10–30%), Vomiting	
	Diarrhea (5–20%)	Slow-release preparations may help
Hematological	Granulocytosis	May be useful in disorders such as Felty's syndrome, iatrogenic neutropenia. May counter CBZ-induced leukopenia
Neurological	Tremor	Propranolol may help
Renal	Polyuria-polydipsia (Nephrogenic diabetes insipidus)	May be an indication of morphologic changes
		Requires adequate hydration

may increase retention of lithium and increase the chance for toxicity. Excretion is almost entirely through the kidneys, with a biphasic elimination half-life. The half-life of lithium varies with age, taking 18–20 hours in the young adult and as long as 36 hours or more in the elderly or uremic patient. Conversely, someone with a high sodium intake may also require a higher dose of lithium. This constitutes a narrow margin of safety and requires repeated monitoring of blood levels and precise instructions to the patient regarding changes in diet, exercise patterns, or other medications that may alter this drug's serum concentration.

Lithium's effects on renal function have engendered much interest over the past 20 years, since it may induce certain minor morphological changes (e.g., interstitial fibrosis, tubular atrophy, glomerular sclerosis) in the kidneys of about 10% of patients. In a review of the literature we concluded that unless there are extremely toxic levels from an overdose or sustained or excessively high treatment levels, lithium's impact on the kidney does not appear to translate into clinically relevant renal dysfunction (3). An interesting study by Coppen in 1980 found no significant differences in several areas of renal function between lithium- and nonlithium-treated patients with a history of bipolar illness (4). He concluded that the similarity between these two groups requires controlled studies of lithium toxicity with age- and sex-matched controls suffering from the same disorders, since mood disorders themselves may have adverse effects on renal morphology. The authors are only aware of a single questionable case report demonstrating renal failure in the absence of either acute or sustained lithium toxicity (5). Hetmar et al. (1986) concluded that lithium-related impairment in renal function (i.e., tubular and glomerular) is related to age, episodes of toxicity, pre-existing renal disease, and treatment schedule (i.e., multiple versus single daily doses) rather than duration of therapy (6). **In summary, while morphological changes occur secondary to chronic lithium exposure, clinically relevant nephrotoxicity is unlikely.**

At one time sustained-release preparations were thought to reduce renal toxicity, but recent evidence has cast doubt on this assumption. A patient on long-term maintenance lithium should have renal function periodically monitored (i.e., every 12 months) with a urinalysis, BUN, and creatinine. If abnormal, a more intensive evaluation should include 24-hour urine osmolality, and creatinine clearance. It is advisable to reduce maintenance lithium to optimum minimal dose/blood levels and, if possible, to avoid concomitant antipsychotics, which may enhance toxicity. **Recent information supports the use of a once-a-day dose schedule to minimize peak lithium concentrations over a 24-hour period** (7).

The syndrome of *polyuria-polydipsia* occurs in about 60% of lithium patients, leading to the abandonment of an otherwise effective treatment in some. Polyuria, usually resulting in urine volumes in excess of 3,000 ml/24 hours, may imply kidney damage and should be prevented or corrected when possible. Strategies to manage this complication include:

- Adequate *fluid replacement*
- *Dose or schedule adjustments* (e.g., reduce dose or switch to a single daily dose schedule)
- The use of *diuretics*, such as a thiazide or amiloride, with careful attention paid to lithium and potassium levels
- *Switching preparations* from a standard to a sustained-release form, or vice versa
- *Indomethacin* may also be helpful, but lithium dose reduction would be required (8).

The *nephrotic syndrome,* characterized clinically by proteinuria, is a rare and idiosyncratic reaction to lithium. As with other uncommon adverse effects, the issue of causation versus coincidence must be considered. Treatment includes cessation of the drug and, when necessary, corticosteroids, such as prednisone (9).

GASTROINTESTINAL SYSTEM

The most frequent early complaints involve this organ system. Nausea, which typically occurs shortly after a dose, can be controlled by taking the drug with meals, and while sustained-release preparations can also help in this regard, they may lead to diarrhea because of the unabsorbed drug's local irritation to the bowel.

ENDOCRINE SYSTEM

Lithium appears to exert its primary antithyroid effect by preventing the release of thyroid hormones (i.e., T_3, thyroxine) (10). In addition, it inhibits iodine uptake into the thyroid gland and the iodination of tyrosine. While it has several antithyroid effects, significant clinical sequelae are relatively few. It is estimated that approximately 5% of patients taking lithium for 18 months or more will develop *hypothyroidism* or diffuse nontender goiter, with females at much greater risk (11).

Some extra precautions should be exercised in patients with pre-existing thyroid disease or those taking other drugs that may interfere with thyroid function. During maintenance therapy, physiological monitoring at baseline and on at least a yearly basis is generally recommended (e.g., thyrotropin-stimulating hormone (TSH), T_3, T_4, T_3 resin uptake, free thyroxin index) but careful attention to early signs and symptoms of hypofunction (e.g., weight gain, cold intolerance, hair loss) may be more productive. TSH is sensitive to early thyroid changes, and if elevated, should prompt treatment with thyroid supplements to avoid goiter or hypothyroidism.

Ironically, this adverse effect may at times be heralded by the onset of depression and can be mistaken for a recurrence of the original disorder. An early warning may be an increase in TSH levels at or slightly above the upper limits of normal. Further, this situation may render a patient less responsive to lithium and/or precipitate a phase of rapid cycling (12). If it is necessary to continue lithium despite clinical hypothyroidism, thyroid supplements (i.e., T_3 or T_4) should be instituted. Once lithium is stopped, in almost all cases the hypothyroid condition is reversible.

The effect of long-term lithium prophylaxis (up to 22 years) on thyroid function was examined by ultrasonic evaluation in 100 BP and UP patients by Perrild et al. (13). Goiter was more common in those patients on lithium for 1–5 years (40%), as well as in those on treatment for more than 10 years (50%), when compared with those who had never received lithium previously (i.e., 16%). Smoking also appeared to contribute significantly to goiter and thyroid size. Subclinical or overt hypothyroidism was found in 4% and 21% of patients (mostly female) treated with lithium for 1 to 5 and for more than 10 years,

respectively. Interestingly, more than half had no signs of autoimmune thyroid disease, indicating a direct effect by lithium on the thyroid gland. The authors noted that earlier reported discrepancies in the frequency of goiter (i.e., 3.6–48%) may be due to reliance on palpation only, an inaccurate and irreproducible method of assessment.

CARDIOVASCULAR SYSTEM

The effects of lithium on the cardiovascular system are usually tolerated at both therapeutic and toxic plasma levels. Common changes include:

- T-wave flattening or inversion
- U-waves
- Conduction delays, such as first-degree atrioventricular (AV) block.

As noted earlier, lithium is contraindicated in patients with unstable congestive heart failure (CHF) or the SSNS (2). In older patients or those with prior cardiac histories, a pretreatment electrocardiogram (ECG) should be obtained. Except for the potential adverse interactions with diuretics, the concomitant use of other cardiac drugs is generally safe. Since verapamil may lower serum levels of lithium, however, more careful monitoring may be required to assure continued therapeutic effects (14). There is also some data that verapamil may predispose to lithium neurotoxicity. Conversely, increased lithium levels leading to toxicity may occur with methyldopa and enalapril. When antihypertensive therapy is necessary, β-blockers may be the agents of choice when lithium is coadministered.

OTHER ADVERSE EFFECTS

Patients also experience miscellaneous complications such as:

- *Edema*
- *Weight gain*
- *Tremors*
- *Psychological complaints* (15, 16).

While most of these adverse effects can be readily managed by the tincture of time, dose adjustment, or alternative preparations, they may precipitate noncompliance in patients particularly sensitive to such complications. *Edema* is probably related to secondary sodium retention and is usually more troublesome than significant. *Tremor,* also a frequent complaint, is the benign essential type and can usually be managed with propranolol (30–120 mg) taken 2 hours prior to the need for steadier hands. Caution about self-medicating with diuretics to manage *weight gain* should be given. These and other effects, while not posing a serious threat, are potentially significant in terms of compliance (see Table 10.12).

Complications of Pregnancy

When clinically possible, lithium treatment should be discontinued during pregnancy and nursing (see also The Pregnant Patient in Chapter 14). Prophylactic lithium is often given to female BP patients of child-bearing age, but there are questions about potential teratogenicity, with the greatest concern centering on the possibility of cardiac malformations (e.g., Ebstein's anomaly). A recent, prospective study of first trimester exposure to lithium by Jacobsen et al. (1992), however, found no differences in overall teratogenesis between pregnant women on lithium and a matched control group not exposed to this agent (17).

Schou has recently reviewed and sum-

Table 10.12.
Lithium: Other Common Adverse Effects

Adverse Effect	Estimated Incidence	Comments
Edema	10–15%	Primarily ankles and feet Transient or intermittent Secondary to effects on sodium/carbohydrate metabolism Caution about diuretics and sodium restriction to avoid lithium toxicity
Weight gain	Approximately 75%	Mean = 4 kg 2% over 20 kg 20% over 10 kg Worse with ADs or APs
Tremor	10–65%	Dose-related Worse with ADs or APs Men > women Incidence greater with increasing age Reduce dose or use β-blocker
Psychological complaints Poor concentration/memory Fatigue/weakness Diminished sex drive "Greyness of life" or mental dulling	Approximately 10%	Often leads to noncompliance with treatment May be early sign of toxicity May mimic depressive phase of disorder Check for hypothyroidism Patients may miss the euphoria or "high"

marized five important questions in this area, including:

- The risk of *malformations* in the unborn child
- The potential for *later developmental anomalies*
- Changes in lithium *pharmacokinetics during pregnancy*
- The possibility of lithium exerting *"other effects"* during pregnancy
- The inadvisability of lithium therapy if the mother is *breast-feeding* her newborn (18).

Because of the possible, but as yet unproven, increased risk of cardiovascular malformation (i.e., Ebstein's anomaly, a tricuspid valve malformation), Schou suggests that fertile women treated with lithium should use contraceptive methods and that the drug be stopped before a planned pregnancy or immediately upon recognition of an unplanned event. In a woman known to experience severe exacerbations on discontinuation of lithium, however, the risk/benefit ratio of continuing lithium must be carefully weighed, especially in light of the more recent data of Jacobsen and colleagues (17). Unfortunately, potential alternate treatments, such as carbamazepine and valproic acid, also have teratogenic potential, particularly neural tube defects (19).

Considering the potential interaction between pregnancy and the course of a bipolar disorder, Schou notes that one study found:

- A *decrease in admission frequency* for BP patients *during pregnancy* (i.e., about three-quarters normal rate)
- An *eight-fold increase* in admissions during the *first month postpartum*
- *Twice the admission rate* between the *second and twelfth month postpartum.*

Finally, when given in large doses, lithium may increase the risk of fetal macrosomia, premature delivery, and perinatal mortality (based on unpublished data on 241 infants).

Newborn infants of mothers on lithium have also shown transient CNS depression, reduced feeding activity, as well as goiter and hypothyroidism, which generally resolve spontaneously in a few months postpartum. Since lithium can produce goiter in the newborn, the thyroid status of the mother should be carefully monitored during pregnancy. Lithium concentrations one-tenth to one-half of the mother's have been found in nursing infants, and this fact must be balanced by an increasing awareness of the beneficial mental and physical effects of nursing for both mother and child.

The issue of later "behavioral teratogenesis" was studied in 60 "lithium" children (whose mothers took lithium when pregnant) as compared with 57 normal siblings. Reassuringly, the incidence of anomalous developmental disorders was essentially equal (20).

The renal clearance of lithium can become altered during the various phases of pregnancy, usually requiring:

- *Increased doses* late in pregnancy
- The *cessation* of lithium 2–3 days before delivery
- *Restarting* lithium a few days postpartum at an appropriately lowered dose.

Another issue, yet to be adequately addressed, are the risks posed by a father on lithium therapy at the time of conception.

Toxicity

Lithium toxicity (chronic, subacute, or acute) can be secondary to any factor that reduces body clearance, or secondary to acute or sustained elevated doses (and therefore plasma levels) (21). The degree of toxicity can be classified as:

- *Early signs*—ataxia, dysarthria, lack of coordination (22)
- *Mild*—usually occurring in the range of 1.5–2.0 mEq/liter and most often characterized by listlessness, nausea, slurring of speech, diarrhea, and coarse tremors
- *Moderate*—usually occurring in the range of 2.0–2.5 mEq/liter and most often characterized by coarse tremors and other central nervous system (CNS) reactions, confusion or delirium, and pronounced ataxia
- *Severe*—beginning with levels at 2.5–3.0 mEq/liter and above, most often characterized by significant alterations in consciousness, spontaneous attacks of hyperextension of the extremities, choreoathetosis, seizures, coma, or death.

The EEG will often show diffuse slow-wave activity in the 5–7 cps range. The more severe episodes usually occur in patients who accidentally or purposely overdose on lithium, and this may lead to other medical complications, such as pulmonary edema, pneumonia, and cardiac arrhythmias.

With an acute overdose, treatment includes discontinuation of lithium and use of various supportive measures, since no antidote is available. Initial steps recommended by Ayd (1988) include:

- *Serum measurements* of lithium, creatinine, electrolytes, and plasma osmolality
- *Gastric lavage*
- *Monitoring of fluid* intake and output
- Obtaining a history about the *timing and amount of lithium* taken
- A *neurological exam*, including a mental status examination (MSE) and a baseline EEG (23).

With normal renal function, all that may be necessary is watchful waiting, careful monitoring of the clinical status, and repeated serum lithium determinations.

The goal is to remove lithium from the system and correct any electrolyte imbalance. Emesis or gastric lavage is often helpful, with forced diuresis, peritoneal dialysis, and hemodialysis utilized only in more moderate to severe cases (e.g., levels exceeding 2.5 mEq/liter). Generally, the outcome even with severe lithium toxicity is recovery; however, there is the possibility of irreversible neurological or renal damage in a small percentage of patients. When death occurs, it is usually secondary to circulatory or respiratory collapse.

Drug Interactions

There are several clinically significant drug interactions with lithium, including:

- Many *nonsteroidal anti-inflammatory agents* (indomethacin, phenylbutazone, sudinlac, naproxen, diclofenac), ibuprofen can raise lithium levels
- *Thiazide diuretics* can raise lithium levels
- *Indapamide,* a nonthiazide sulfonamide diuretic, can raise lithium levels
- *Certain antibiotics* (e.g., oral tetracyclines), which may diminish lithium's clearance through the kidneys, leading to increases in plasma levels and possible intoxication (24, 25).
- Other drugs, such as *verapamil, caffeine, theophylline, osmotic diuretics, carbonic anhydrase inhibitors,* or *aminophylline,* which can increase lithium excretion, possibly dropping plasma levels below the therapeutic threshold (14). Further, if doses are increased to compensate for this effect, care must be

taken to readjust the lithium downward when these concomitant agents are reduced or discontinued.

Analgesics such as *aspirin* or *acetaminophen,* and *furosemide,* a loop diuretic, are better choices since they apparently do not interfere with lithium's reabsorption.

Neurotoxic reactions have been periodically reported with lithium alone or in combination with *antipsychotics, carbamazepine, verapamil,* and *methyldopa,* with the elderly probably at much greater risk for such events (see Table 10.13). While such drug combinations are often necessary and usually well tolerated, common clinical sense dictates that only the minimally effective dose(s) be prescribed. It is also advised that patients carry or wear some form of identification indicating they are receiving lithium treatment.

The question of increased neurotoxic reactions with the combination of lithium and an antipsychotic (especially haloperidol) has been vigorously debated since the report of Cohen and Cohen (26–29). Possible explanations have included:

- The use of *increased doses* of high potency antipsychotics
- *Toxic blood levels* of lithium
- *An additive or synergistic effect* with the combination, thus increasing the chances of neurotoxicity
- Misdiagnosed *neuroleptic malignant syndrome* (NMS).

Table 10.13.
Lithium: Neurotoxicity

Cerebellar symptoms are the most common neurological sequelae (including tremors, cogwheeling, drowsiness, confusion, disorientation, muscle fasciculation, ataxia, EPS, and seizures)
Risk factors include:
  Fever
  Major surgery
  Renal failure
  Low food/salt intake
  Age
  Acute overdose
Concurrent medications that may predispose
  Neuroleptics
  Carbamazepine
  Calcium channel blockers
  Diuretics
  Methyldopa
May correspond more closely to CSF lithium levels

Adverse Effects of Other Drugs

ANTIPSYCHOTICS

These agents possess an adverse effect profile that poses significant and potentially serious complications (see also Adverse Effects in Chapter 5). In particular, patients suffering from mood disorders and associated psychosis who are exposed to antipsychotics may be at greater risk for *tardive dyskinesia* (TD), and perhaps the *neuroleptic malignant syndrome* (NMS) (30). While lower potency agents are likely to induce less severe *extrapyramidal reactions,* they are more likely to produce significant *anticholinergic effects, excessive sedation,* and *orthostasis,* as well as a *mental dulling,* which many consider a major impediment to compliance. As noted earlier, the lithium-antipsychotic combination has also been associated with an increased risk for *neurotoxic reactions,* but debate continues as to the most critical factor(s) involved with this complication.

BENZODIAZEPINES

Significant adverse effects include *excessive drowsiness, ataxia, possible withdrawal syndrome* with abrupt discontinuation, and complaints of *behavioral* and *dysphoric mood* changes (see also Chapter 12). Common adverse drug interactions include the potentiation of alcohol and other sedative-hypnotics, issues of concern especially with outpatients, given the large percentage of bipolar patients who abuse these drugs (see Tables 10.11, 10.12, 10.13, 10.14, 10.15, and 10.16 for comparison to lithium, as well as other non-BZD anticonvulsants) (31).

CARBAMAZEPINE

CBZ is contraindicated in patients with a history of drug-induced adverse hematological reactions; a previous history of bone marrow suppression; known hypersensitivity to this agent or other tricyclics; and/or the presence of hepatic dysfunction.

Aplastic anemia associated with CBZ treatment occurs in about 1 out of 125,000 cases, and is characterized by a reduction in all cellular blood elements secondary to a hypocellularity of the bone marrow (32, 33). Agranulocytosis is even less common and usually occurs within the first 2–3 months of treatment, but can occur at any time. While

Table 10.14.
Anticonvulsants: Adverse Effects

Clonazepam	Carbamazepine	Valproic Acid
GI upset	GI upset	GI upset
Nausea	Nausea, anorexia	Nausea
Vomiting	Vomiting	Vomiting
Diarrhea		Diarrhea
Sedation	Sedation	Sedation
Ataxia	Ataxia/ clumsiness	
Tremor	Dizziness	Tremor
	Blurred vision/diplopia	
Weight loss/gain		Weight gain/loss
Alopecia		Transient alopecia
Polydipsia/polyuria	Inappropriate antidiuretic hormone syndrome	Edema

Note: Adverse reactions are usually dose-related and subside with time. It is recommended to begin with low doses and gradually increase as clinically indicated to avoid premature discontinuation of medication trial.

Table 10.15.
Anticonvulsants: Behavioral and Cognitive Effects

Clonazepam	Carbamazepine	Valproic Acid
Lethargy	Lethargy	
	Impaired task performance	Impaired task performance
Behavioral disinhibition		
Irritability	Irritability	Hyperactivity
	Dysomnia	
Aggression		Aggression
Depression	Depression	Depression
Confusion	Confusion	Psychosis
Sexual dysfunction		

Table 10.16.
Anticonvulsants: Idiosyncratic Effects

Clonazepam	Carbamazepine	Valproic Acid
Elevated SGOT, SGPT, alkaline phosphatase	Elevated SGOT, SGPT, alkaline phosphatase Hepatic failure	Elevated LDH/SGOT, SGPT Hepatotoxicity or failure (1/40,000) Reye-like syndrome
Anemia	Pancreatitis Aplastic anemia/ agranulocytosis	Pancreatitis
Leukopenia Thrombocytopenia Eosinophilia	Leukopenia Thrombocytopenia	Thrombocytopenia
	Cardiovascular CHF Edema AV block	
Rash	Rash Allergic dermatitis Stevens-Johnson syndrome (severe form of erythema multiforme) Lyell's syndrome	Rash Allergic dermatitis

the development of *aplastic anemia* or *agranulocytosis* is rare, they must be distinguished from the more frequent occurrence of *leukopenia*, which is a benign and self-limiting phenomenon. While it is important to obtain hematological parameters initially, the optimal frequency for repeated measures during treatment is controversial. More important than repeated complete blood counts (CBCs) is instruction to patients about signs and symptoms of *hematological dysfunction*, such as fever, sore throat, malaise, and petechiae. Emergence of such symptoms should prompt patients to immediately stop the medication, contact their physician, or present to the emergency room.

Carbamazepine may also have deleterious *hepatic effects*, and liver function tests (LFTs) should be obtained initially and monitored during treatment at 6–12 month intervals.

Other common adverse effects associated with CBZ are listed in Tables 10.14, 10.15, and 10.16. These problems include *gastrointestinal symptoms, rash, sedation, dizzines, ataxia,* and *hyponatremia.* Severe dermatological reactions (i.e., Stevens-Johnson Syndrome, Lyell's Syndrome) have also been reported and may require aggressive intervention, including hospitalization.

Drug Interactions

A major concern with carbamazepine is its numerous, clinically significant, drug-drug interactions, primarily due to stimulation of the hepatic P-450 microsomal oxidative enzyme system, which culminates in an accelerated metabolism of various drugs (34). Interestingly, CBZ also has the ability to *autometabolize*, so that within the first several weeks of treatment with good compliance, as well as initially adequate doses and blood levels, there can be a reduction in concentrations below the therapeutic range, which may lead to a recrudescence of symptoms (35). As a result, close monitoring of serum levels during this phase and increased doses are usually required.

Further, carbamazepine interacts with many other agents that are often used concurrently. Thus:

- CBZ can *lower antipsychotic (e.g., haloperidol) and oral contraceptive plasma levels*
- Certain anticonvulsants (e.g., valproic acid), erythromycin, propoxyphene, cimetidine, isoniazid, and calcium channel blockers (e.g., verapamil, diltiazem) can *raise CBZ levels* to toxic ranges
- Other anticonvulsants, such as phenytoin; barbiturates; and primidone, can *lower CBZ levels*.

Patients stabilized on haloperidol (and perhaps other antipsychotics) may demonstrate worsening of their symptoms when CBZ is added, necessitating an increase in the antipsychotic dose (36, 37). Conversely, if CBZ is discontinued, the antipsychotic level will rise, perhaps precipitating significant adverse effects.

Since carbamazepine may induce *teratogenicity* (e.g., developmental delay, minor craniofacial abnormalities, spina bifida), levels of oral contraceptives need to be monitored and the dose probably increased to prevent an accidental pregnancy.

Acute *overdoses* are potentially lethal and range from:

- Early symptoms of drowsiness and ataxia (11–15 μg/ml)
- Combativeness, psychosis, and choreiform movements (15–25 μg/ml)
- Seizures and coma (25 μg/ml) (38).

VALPROIC ACID

The most serious adverse effect of VPA involves the *hepatic system*, with reported deaths due to liver failure; however, this has only been reported in patients under the age of 10 (the majority were under the age of 2) receiving more than one anticonvulsant concurrently for seizure control (39). Recent surveys indicate that the overall incidence is about 1 in 40,000 cases (40). We know of no reported deaths due to liver failure in adults receiving VPA monotherapy. After baseline values, treatment-phase LFTs should be obtained during the first several weeks and every 3–6 months subsequently. Again, there is debate over the usefulness of monitoring these values, and patient education about early symptoms of hepatotoxicity may be more productive. These include:

- Decreased *appetite*
- *Gastrointestinal distress* (nausea, vomiting, abdominal pain)
- Periorbital and dependent *edema*
- *Malaise* and/or lethargy
- Easy *bruising*.

Common adverse effects experienced by patients include *tremors, nausea,* and *weight gain* (see also Tables 10.14, 10.15, and 10.16). The tremors are benign and similar to those resulting from treatment with lithium. Gastrointestinal symptoms can be minimized or avoided by use of the enteric coated formulation (i.e., divalproex sodium) (41). Patients should be encouraged to initiate a weight maintenance program at the onset of therapy.

Women of child-bearing age exposed to VPA should be counseled as to its *possible teratogenic effects* (e.g., a 1–2% incidence of spina bifida) (42, 43).

Unlike carbamazepine, VPA does not enhance its own metabolism or that of other drugs; however, it may inhibit enzyme systems responsible for the metabolism of other agents (e.g., CBZ), leading to possible increases in their blood levels. The clinical significance of these changes is not clear, however (44). In *acute overdoses*, coma and death can occur, but hemodialysis and naloxone may reverse or prevent these serious complications (45, 46).

CALCIUM CHANNEL BLOCKERS

The most common adverse effects are *hypotension* and *bradycardia*, which are usually easily managed, unless there is preexisting heart disease. Dubovsky et al. reported severe cardiotoxicity when verapamil was combined with lithium in two elderly patients (47). One had a profound bradycardia with a heart rate of 36 beats/min; another, who had a sinus bradycardia and AV ectopy, then developed an acute myocardial infarction and died.

Other reported potentially significant *drug interactions* include the combination of verapamil or nifedipine with CBZ, which at times can lead to toxicity secondary to increases in CBZ levels; and neurotoxic reactions when verapamil or diltiazem are combined with lithium.

CLONIDINE

The most common adverse effects with clonidine are *hypotension, dry mouth, drowsiness*, and *dermatological reactions*. These are usually mild, but hypotensive effects may be significant in normotensive manic patients. Higher doses (e.g., 0.8–1.2 mg) have also been reported to induce a *paradoxical excitement* in some patients (48).

CONCLUSION

While the adverse effects of mood stabilizers are typically mild and readily managed, the increasing number of potential drug therapies for bipolar disorder must necessarily complicate the issue of adverse effects. Of particular importance are problems associated with:

- The *hepatic* system
- The *hematopoietic* system
- The *thyroid* gland
- *Pregnancy.*

Further, since these agents are frequently used in combination with each other, as well as with antipsychotics, drug interactional issues have become increasingly relevant.

REFERENCES

1. Reisberg B, Gershon S. Side effects associated with lithium therapy. Arch Gen Psychiatry 1979;36:879–887.
2. Mitchell JE, Mackenzie TB. Cardiac effects of lithium therapy in man: a review. J Clin Psychiatry 1982;43:47–51.
3. Janicak PG, Davis JM. Clinical usage of lithium in mania. In: Burrows GD, Norman TR, Davies B, eds. Antimanics, anticonvulsants and other drugs in psychiatry. Amsterdam: Elsevier Science Publishers, 1987:21–34.
4. Coppen A, Bishop ME, Bailey JE, Cattell, Price RG. Renal function in lithium and non-lithium treated patients with affective disorders. Acta Psychiatr Scand 1980;62:343–355.
5. Ausiello DA. Case records of the Massachusetts General Hospital—Case 17-1981. N Engl J Med 1981;304:1025–1032.
6. Hetmar O, Bolwig TG, Brun C, Ladefoged J, Larsen S, Rafaelsen OJ. Lithium: long-term effects on the kidney: I. Renal function in retrospect. Acta Psychiatr Scand 1986;73:574–581.
7. Bowen RC, Grof P, Grof E. Less frequent lithium administration and lower urine volume. Am J Psychiatry 1991;148:189–192.
8. Jefferson JW, Greist JH, Ackerman DL, Carroll JA. Lithium encyclopedia for clinical practice. 2nd ed. Washington DC: American Psychiatric Press, 1987.
9. Wood IK, Parmelee DX, Foreman JW. Lithium-induced nephrotic syndrome. Am J Psychiatry 1989;146:84–87.
10. Shopsin B. Effects of lithium on thyroid

function; a review. Dis Nerv Sys 1970;31: 237–244.

11. Jefferson JW. Lithium carbonate-induced hypothyroidism. Its many faces. JAMA 1979;242(3):271–272.

12. Bauer M, Whybrow P. The effect of changing thyroid function on cyclic affective illness in a human subject. Am J Psychiatry 1986;143:633–636.

13. Perrild H, Hegedäus L, Baastrup PC, Kayser L, Kastberg S. Thyroid function and ultrasonically determined thyroid size in patients receiving long-term lithium treatment. Am J Psychiatry 1990;147:1518–1521.

14. Weinrauch LA, Beloh S, d'Elia JA. Decreased lithium during verapamil therapy. Am Heart J 1984;108:1378–1380.

15. Vestergaard P, Poulstrup I, Schou M. Prospective studies on a lithium cohort. 3. Tremor, weight gain, diarrhea, psychological complaints. Acta Psychiatr Scand 1988;78(4):434–441.

16. Garland EJ, Remick RA, Zis AP. Weight gain with antidepressants and lithium. J Clin Psychopharmacol 1988;8:323–330.

17. Jacobsen SJ, Jones K, Johnson K, Ceolin L, Kaur P, Sahn D, et al. Prospective multicentre study of pregnancy outcome after lithium exposure during first trimester. Lancet 1992;339(8792):530–533.

18. Schou M. Lithium treatment during pregnancy, delivery, and lactation: an update. J Clin Psychiatry 1990;51:410–412.

19. Rosa FW. Spina bifida in infants of women treated with carbamazepine during pregnancy. New Engl J Med 1991;324(10): 674–677.

20. Schou M. What happened later to the lithium babies? Acta Psychiatr Scand 1976; 54:193–197.

21. Simard M, Gumbiner B, Lee A, et al. Lithium carbonate intoxication. Arch Intern Med 1989;149:36–46.

22. Colgate R. The ranking of therapeutic and toxic side effects of lithium carbonate. Psychiatric Bull 1992;16(8):473–475.

23. Ayd FJ. Acute self-poisoning with lithium. International Drug Therapy Newsletter 1988;23:1–2.

24. Ragheb M. The clinical significance of lithium-nonsteroidal anti-inflammatory drug interactions. J Clin Psychopharamacol 1990;10:350–354.

25. Gelenberg AJ. Lithium and antibiotics. Biological Therapies in Psychiatry 1985;8: 46.

26. Kahn EM et al. Change in haloperidol level due to carbamazepine—a complicating factor in combined medication for schizophrenia. J Clin Psychopharmacol 1990;10(2):54–57.

27. Cohen WJ, Cohen NH. Lithium carbonate, haloperidol and irreversible brain damage. JAMA 1974;230:1283–1287.

28. Karki SD, Holden JMC. Combined use of haloperidol and lithium. Psychiatric Annals 1990;20(3):154–161.

29. Goldney RD, Spence ND. Safety of the combination of lithium and neuroleptic drugs. Am J Psychiatry 1986;143:882–884.

30. Wolf ME, De Wolfe AS, Ryan JJ et al. Vulnerability to tardive dyskinesia. J Clin Psychiatry 1985;46:367–368.

31. Regier, DA, Farmer ME, Rae DS, Locke BZ, Keith SJ, Judd LL, Goodwin FK. Comorbidity of mental disorders with alcohol and other drug abuse. Results from the Epidemiologic Catchment Area (ECA) study. JAMA 1990;264(19):2511–2518.

32. Hart RG, Easton JD. Carbamazepine and hematological monitoring. Ann Neurol 1982;11:309–312.

33. Joffe RT, Post RM, Roy-Byrne PP, et al. Hematological effects of carbamazepine in patients with affective illness. Am J Psychiatry 1985;142:1196–1199.

34. Baciewicz AM. Carbamazepine drug interactions. Ther Drug Monitor 1986;8:305–317.

35. Bertilsson L, Tomson T. Clinical pharmacokinetics and pharmacological effects of carbamazepine and carbamazepine-10,11-epoxide. Clin Pharmacokinet 1986;11:177–198.

36. Arana GW, Goff DC, Freedman H, et al. Does carbamazepine- induced reduction of plasma haloperidol-levels worsen psychotic symptoms? Am J Psychiatry 1986;143:650–651.

37. Jann MW, Ereshesfsky L, Saklad SR, et al. Effects of carbamazepine on plasma haloperidol levels. J Clin Psychopharmacol 1985;5:106–109.

38. Masland RL. Carbamazepine: neurotoxicity. In: Woodbury DM, Perry JK, Pippinger CE, eds. Antiepileptic drugs. New York: Raven Press, 1982:521–531.

39. Dreifuss FE, Santilli N, Langer DH, Sweeney KP, Moline KA, Menander KB. Valproic acid hepatic fatalities: a retrospective review. Neurology 1987;37:379–385.

40. Dreifuss FE, Langer DH, Moline KA,

Maxwell JE. Valproic acid hepatic fatalities. II. U.S. experience since 1984. Neurology 1989;39:201–207.

41. Wilder BJ et al. Gastrointestinal tolerance of divalproex sodium. Neurology 1983;33:808–811.

42. Jeavons PM. Sodium valproate and neural tube defects. Lancet 1982;ii:1282–1283.

43. Centers for Disease Control: Valproate: a new cause of birth defects—Report from Italy and follow-up from France. MMWR 1983;32:438–439.

44. Schnabel R, Rainbeck B, Janssen F. Fatal intoxication with sodium valproate. Lancet 1984;ii:221–222.

45. Mortensen PB, Hansen HE, Pedersen B, et al. Acute valproate intoxication: biochemical investigations and haemodialysis treatment. Int J Clin Pharmacol Ther Toxicol 1983;21:64–68.

46. Stelman GS, Woerpel RW, Sherard ES. Treatment of accidental sodium valproate overdose with an opiate antagonist [Letter]. Ann Neurol 1979;6:274.

47. Dubovsky SL, Franks RD, Allen S. Verapamil: a new antimanic drug with potential interactions with lithium. J Clin Psychiatry 1987;48:371–372.

48. Hardy C, Lecrubier Y, Widlocker D. Efficacy of clonidine in 24 patients with acute mania. Am J Psychiatry 1986;143:1450–1453.

CHAPTER 11

Indications for Antianxiety/ Sedative-Hypnotic Agents

From time immemorial, human beings have sought ways and means of achieving surcease from subjectively distressing and disabling anxiety, and of inducing sleep to counteract debilitating insomnia. Early recorded history documents that the anxiolytic and soporific effects of alcohol were discovered centuries ago, and ever since, people have imbibed to ease anxiety, tension, and agitation, and lull them into a somnolent state. It was not until the 19th century, however, that chemists synthesized the bromides and the barbiturates, thereby inaugurating an era of relentless attempts to manufacture safer and more effective alternatives to alcohol, bromides, and barbiturates.

The harvest of these efforts has been the advent of meprobamate, the benzodiazepines, and more recently, such nonbenzodiazepine anxiolytics as buspirone and nonbarbiturate, nonbenzodiazepine hypnotics, such as zopiclone and zolpidem. The more recent anxiolytics and hypnotics offer equiefficacy, fewer serious adverse effects, and less risk of a fatal consequence due to accidental or intentional overdose. Unfortunately, they have not entirely eliminated the hazards of tolerance, dependency, and withdrawal syndromes, although they have a lower abuse potential than their predecessors.

These assets, however, do not justify cavalier dispensing of these newer agents, which must also be prescribed judiciously. Failure to monitor their usage may endanger the patient, invite governmental restrictions, and possibly become the basis for a malpractice suit or the revocation of one's medical license. For these reasons, it is imperative for clinicians to become knowledgeable about the basic pharmacology of these drugs, along with their appropriate clinical indications, dosages, and duration of usage. **Most importantly, their limitations must receive as much attention as their assets.**

Generalized Anxiety Disorder

Anxiety is a common reaction to significant life stress. It is characterized by fear and apprehension that may or may not be associated with a clearly identifiable stimulus. It is almost invariably accompanied by physical symptoms such as:

- Tachycardia, palpitations, chest tightness; diaphoresis
- Breathing difficulties
- Nausea, diarrhea, intestinal cramping
- Dry mouth.

Anxiety accompanies almost every psychiatric disorder and is a common component of numerous organic disorders as well (e.g., hyperthyroidism, hypoglycemia, pheochromocytoma, complex partial seizures, pulmonary disorders, acute myocardial infarction, caffeine intoxication, substance abuse).

According to the Epidemiologic Catchment Area (ECA) Study (1990), anxiety disorders are the most prevalent psychiatric conditions in America (1–6). Of the nine categories listed in the Diagnostic and Statistical Manual of Mental Disorders, 3rd edition, revised (DSM-III-R), Generalized Anxiety Disorder (GAD) may be the most commonly diagnosed, although its true incidence may actually be lower than that of phobic and obsessive-compulsive disorders (See Appendices A, K, L, M, N, P, and S also).

Before 1980, the term *anxiety neurosis* was used to describe a syndrome that included both chronic generalized anxiety and panic attacks. GAD and panic were first listed as discrete diagnoses in the DSM-III, in part because of observed differences in their response to available drug treatments (i.e., the former to benzodiazepines, the latter to antidepressants).

To differentiate it from transient anxiety, the DSM-III-R defines GAD as unrealistic or excessive anxiety or worry for 6 months or longer about two or more life circumstances. In addition, the patient must have at least 6 of a list of 18 symptoms involving:

- Motor tension
- Autonomic hyperactivity
- Vigilance and scanning.

GAD may be diagnosed along with another Axis I disorder (including another anxiety disorder) provided GAD symptoms are at least sometimes present without symptoms of the other disorder and the anxiety is not focused on the symptoms of the other disorder.

Few long-term follow-up studies of GAD have been conducted, but available evidence indicates it may last for many years, with waxing and waning symptoms, often complicated by other, intercurrent physical and/or psychiatric disorders (7). Although a DSM-III-R-derived diagnosis requires an anxiety duration of at least 6 months, clinicians frequently encounter very symptomatic patients who do not meet this criterion (8). **Thus, in addition to formalized diagnostic criteria, clinical judgment and experience are critical in deciding when anxiety is a discrete disorder requiring primary treatment, and when it is a manifestation of another disorder.**

Differential psychiatric diagnosis includes organic mental disorders (such as caffeine intoxication); adjustment disorder with anxious mood (characterized by lack of full symptom criteria for GAD and the presence of a recognized psychosocial stressor); and psychotic, eating, and depressive disorders in which the anxiety is related to the underlying condition.

Phobic Disorders

AGORAPHOBIA

Agoraphobia (literally, fear of the marketplace) is the dread of being in places or situations from which escape might be difficult. It also includes worry about suddenly developing embarrassing or incapacitating symptoms (e.g., loss of bladder control, dizziness) for which help might not be available. The agoraphobic patient often:

- *Restricts travel*
- *Needs a companion* when away from home
- *Endures intense anxiety* when confronted with a feared situation.

Although agoraphobia may accompany panic disorder, ECA data indicate that the majority of agoraphobic patients either fail to meet lifetime criteria for panic disorder or have no history of panic symptoms (3).

SOCIAL PHOBIA

Social phobia is the fear of being judged by others and/or of embarrassing oneself in public (e.g., being unable to answer questions in social situations, fear of choking when eating in front of others). Exposure to the feared situation provokes an immediate anxiety response. The phobic situation is avoided or endured with intense anxiety; and secondarily, the avoidant behavior interferes with occupational or social functioning (but need not be incapacitating); or there is marked distress about having the fear. Typically, the person is aware of the excessive and/or unreasonable nature of these concerns. The diagnosis is not made if one simply avoids social situations that normally provoke some distress, such as public speaking. If an Axis III or another Axis I disorder is present, social phobia is diagnosed only if the fear is unrelated to these condition(s). **Social phobia is one of the least studied of the major psychiatric disorders, and hence, there are significant gaps in our knowledge con-**cerning **definition, prevalence, etiology, pathophysiology, assessment, and treatment.** Differential diagnosis includes:

- *Avoidant personality* disorder, characterized by marked anxiety and avoidance of most social situations
- *Simple phobia,* characterized by fear of a specific object or situation other than fear of social embarrassment or humiliation
- *Panic disorder* with agoraphobia, characterized by avoidance of certain social situations because of fear of having a panic attack.

SIMPLE PHOBIA

Simple phobia is an unrealistic and persistent fear of a specific object or situation, such as snakes, heights, or thunderstorms. Exposure to the phobic stimulus provokes immediate and intense anxiety that the individual recognizes as excessive or unreasonable. The degree of impairment frequently depends on whether the feared object or situation is commonly encountered or can be easily avoided. The diagnosis should only be made if avoidant behavior interferes with the person's normal routine, social activities, or relationships; or there is marked distress about having the fear. Differential diagnosis includes:

- *Schizophrenia,* characterized by avoidance behavior in response to delusions
- *Post-traumatic stress disorder,* characterized by avoidance of stimuli associated with the trauma
- *Obsessive-compulsive disorder,* characterized by avoidance of situations associated with dirt or contamination.

Psychological Factors Affecting Physical Condition

Formerly referred to as psychosomatic (DSM-I) or psychophysiological (DSM-II) disorders, this category was revised in the DSM-III and the DSM-III-R. The diagnosis is made when psychologically meaningful environmental stimuli are temporally related to the initiation or exacerbation of a physical condition with demonstrable organic pathology (e.g, rheumatoid arthritis) or a known pathophysiological process (e.g,

migraine). Further, the condition should not meet criteria for somatoform disorders, which are characterized by physical symptoms suggesting medical disease, but for which no demonstrable pathology or known pathophysiological process can be found.

Sleep Disorders

Like anxiety, disturbances of sleep affect nearly all of us at one time or another. Also like anxiety, disordered sleep may present as:

- *A transient phenomenon* that may or may not be related to an identifiable stimulus
- *Secondary* to numerous medical and/or psychiatric conditions
- *A primary*, discrete disorder.

The International Classification of Sleep Disorders lists 88 types, with insomnia the most prominent symptom for many of these (9). The DSM-III-R divides these disorders into two major groups, the *dyssomnias* (in which the predominant disturbance is the amount, quality, or timing of sleep) and the *parasomnias* (in which the predominant disturbance is an abnormal event occurring during sleep).

DYSSOMNIAS

Insomnia Disorders

Insomnia is the most common sleep problem, but is not classified as a disorder unless it occurs at least three times a week for at least a month. There are three general types:

- *Primary insomnia*
- Insomnia related to a known *organic factor*
- Insomnia related to a *mental disorder*.

All are characterized by difficulty initiating or maintaining sleep or by not feeling rested after an apparently adequate amount of sleep.

Primary insomnia may represent a lifelong pattern of poor sleep or it may develop as a result of distressing events but then persists after the stressor resolves. It is characterized by excessive daytime worry about being able to fall or stay asleep. Anxiety tends to perpetuate a vicious cycle of sleeplessness that is aggravated by worry about sleeplessness. Patients with primary insomnia, however, may fall asleep when they are not trying and may experience little or no difficulty sleeping away from their normal environment. The diagnosis is made only if this condition is not symptomatic of another mental disorder or known organic factor.

Insomnia related to a known organic factor occurs in conjunction with a physical illness (but not the person's emotional reaction to the illness), psychoactive substance abuse, or certain medications. Insomnia related to another mental disorder is judged to be due to an Axis I or Axis II disorder, or when the insomnia is apparently due to an emotional reaction secondary to a life-threatening physical disorder.

Hypersomnia Disorders

These disorders are characterized by excessive daytime sleepiness, sleep attacks, or sleep drunkenness. The *daytime sleepiness* (falling asleep easily and unintentionally) is not accounted for by an inadequate amount of sleep. *Sleep attacks* involve sudden periods of irresistible sleep, also not due to inadequate rest. *Sleep drunkenness* is difficulty making the transition to the fully awake state upon arising and may include ataxia and disorientation. Another criteria is the presence of hypersomnia nearly every day for at least a month or episodically for longer periods of time, resulting in occupational or social impairment.

As with the insomnia disorders, hypersomnias may be categorized as primary; secondary to another mental disorder (mood disorders, schizophrenia, somatoform disorder, borderline personality disorder); or secondary to a known organic factor such as:

- Psychoactive substance abuse
- Prolonged use of medications with sleep-inducing properties, such as sedatives or antihypertensives
- Sleep apnea, sleep myoclonus
- Restless legs syndrome
- Narcolepsy
- Kleine-Levin syndrome
- Epilepsy
- Hypothyroidism
- Hypoglycemia
- Multiple sclerosis
- Organic mental disorders.

The diagnosis is not made if hypersomnia occurs only during the course of a sleep-wake schedule disorder.

Two hypersomnia disorders, narcolepsy and sleep apnea syndrome, are relatively easy to diagnose using appropriate somnographic evaluations.

Narcolepsy is a relative uncommon condition that may be either idiopathic or, more rarely, secondary to organic brain damage. It is characterized by irresistible

sleep attacks lasting from 30 seconds to 20 minutes and the speedy appearance of rapid eye movement (REM) sleep, usually within 10 minutes of sleep onset. Additional symptoms may include cataplexy (brief weakness in isolated muscle groups or paralysis of almost all skeletal muscles) triggered by intense emotion, with or without a concomitant sleep attack; sleep paralysis; and hypnagogic or hypnopompic hallucinations.

Sleep apnea syndrome is a potentially life-threatening respiratory disorder characterized by cessation of both nasal and oral airflow for at least 30 periods of 10 seconds or more during a 7 hour sleep phase. In some patients, apneic periods may last up to 2 minutes. **The most prominent sign is loud snoring.** There are three types of sleep apnea:

- The *central type,* involving lack of diaphragmatic effort
- The *obstructive type,* involving blockage of the oropharynx
- The *mixed type,* which begins with a central episode followed by an obstructive episode.

Typical complications include disorientation; hypnagogic hallucinations; periods of automatic behavior; and excessive daytime sleepiness, due to frequent nighttime awakenings. Sleep EEG reveals absent or decreased slow wave sleep and in some patients, early-onset REM sleep.

Sleep-Wake Schedule Disorders

Sleep-wake schedule disorders occur when there is a mismatch between the normal rest-activity schedule for a person's environment and his or her circadian sleep-wake pattern. Transient disturbances may occur as a result of rapid time zone changes (as in transoceanic flights) or staying up late for a few days. Diagnosis of a sleep-wake schedule disorder, however, is made only if complaints meet criteria for an insomnia or a hypersomnia disorder. These disorders often improve when the person is able to resume a normal pattern. The differential diagnosis includes depression, psychosis, and personality disorders.

PARASOMNIAS

This group of disorders is characterized by an abnormal event that occurs during sleep or the threshold between sleep and wakefulness, and includes:

- *Dream anxiety disorder*
- *Sleep terror* disorder
- *Sleepwalking* disorder.

They usually involve complaints focused on the abnormal occurrence itself rather than any effect it might have on sleep.

Dream Anxiety Disorder

Also known as *nightmares,* this disorder involves vivid dreams, often characterized by recurring themes of threats to survival, security, or self-esteem. Because the dreams are most likely to occur during REM sleep, autonomic agitation is minimal during the dream but may occur upon awakening. The repeated awakenings associated with the dreams, as well as the dreams themselves, are accompanied by significant anxiety and difficulty returning to sleep. Upon awakening, however, the person is alert, fully oriented, and able to give a detailed account of the dream. The diagnosis is not made if the dreams are attributable to a known organic factor, such as the use of antipsychotics, antidepressants, or benzodiazepines, which may cause nightmares; or the abrupt withdrawal from REM-suppressant agents (e.g., tricyclic antidepressants) that may result in REM rebound and associated nightmares.

Sleep Terror Disorder

This disorder (also known as pavor nocturnus) is characterized by recurrent episodes of abrupt awakening from sleep, usually during nonrapid eye movement (NREM) periods that are characterized by EEG delta wave activity. The episode can be dramatic and is likely to begin with a panicky scream. The person often sits up in bed exhibiting signs of intense anxiety and autonomic arousal (e.g., tachycardia, rapid breathing and pulse, dilated pupils, sweating, etc.) and may be confused, disoriented, and unresponsive to comforting gestures. Patients may describe a sense of terror and fragmentary images, but are usually unable to recount a complete dream. Interestingly, morning amnesia for the episode usually occurs. An organic factor (e.g., brain tumor, epileptic seizures during sleep) responsible for these disturbances precludes the diagnosis of sleep terrors.

Sleepwalking Disorder

Like sleep terrors, sleepwalking disorder (or somnambulism) usually occurs during NREM sleep in association with EEG delta wave activity. It is characterized by episodes of complex behaviors that initially include sitting up and performing perseverative movements (e.g., picking at the sheet). It often proceeds to such activities as leaving the bed, walking, dressing, and opening or closing windows and doors. During an episode the person usually has a blank stare, is unresponsive to others, and is very difficult to awaken. With the exception of a brief period of confusion or disorientation, there is no impairment of mental activity or behavior upon awakening, although amnesia for the episode is typical. The diagnosis is not made if an organic factor such as epilepsy is responsible for the disturbance. Differential diagnosis includes psychogenic fugue and sleep drunkenness.

OTHER MEDICAL CONDITIONS

Sedative-hypnotics may be useful as primary or adjunctive treatments in various medical conditions. Selected benzodiazepines are also used in the treatment of some seizure disorders (e.g., clonazepam) and to induce general anesthesia (e.g, midazolam) (see also The Seizure-Prone Patient in Chapter 14).

CONCLUSION

In the attempt to manage anxiety-related phenomena, as well as sleep disturbances, various treatments (both drug and nondrug) have been employed over the course of history. Today, our understanding of the basis for such conditions is becoming more refined, allowing identification of differentiating qualities that will ultimately dictate more specific and effective remedies.

REFERENCES

1. Myers JR, Weissman MM, Tischler GL, et al. Six month prevalence of psychiatric disorders in three communities. Arch Gen Psychiatry 1984;41:959–970.
2. Robins LN, Helzer JE, Weissman MM, et al. Lifetime prevalence of specific psychiatric disorders in three sites. Arch Gen Psychiatry 1984;41:949–958.
3. Regier DA, Narron WE, Rae DS. The epidemiology of anxiety disorders: The Epidemiologic Catchment Area (ECA) experience. J Psychiatr Res 1990;24(2,Suppl):3–14.
4. Regier DA, Farmer ME, Rae DS, et al. Comorbidity of mental disorders with alcohol and other drug abuse. JAMA 1990;264:2511–2518.
5. Blazer D, Hughes D, George U. Stressful life events and the onset of generalized anxiety syndrome. Am J Psychiatry 1987;144:1178–1183.
6. Helzer JE, Robins LN, McEvoy L. Posttraumatic stress disorder in the general population: findings of the Epidemiologic Catchment Area Survey. N Engl J Med 1987;317:1630–1634.
7. Rickels K, Schweizer E. The clinical course and long-term management of generalized anxiety disorder. J Clin Psychopharmacol 1990;10:101s–110s.
8. Barlow DH, Blanchard EB, Vermilyea JA, et al. Generalized anxiety and generalized anxiety disorder: description and reconceptualization. Am J Psychiatry 1986;143:40–44.
9. Diagnostic Classification Steering Committee: International classification of sleep disorders: diagnostic and coding manual. Rochester, MN: American Sleep Disorders Association, 1990.

CHAPTER 12

Treatment with Antianxiety/Sedative-Hypnotic Agents

History

Humanity's centuries-old, avid search for substances that would relieve subjectively distressing anxiety and sleep disorders has resulted in a progression from alcohol to opiates to the synthesis of bromides and later, barbiturates. Each of these, however, shares treatment-limiting and potentially life-threatening disadvantages, including:

- Rapid development of *tolerance* to their therapeutic effects
- Serious *adverse effects*
- High risk of *dependence*
- *Lethality* in overdose.

Meprobamate, first marketed in the early 1950s, was originally considered an improvement over the barbiturates, but soon was recognized to have essentially the same liabilities as its predecessors.

Introduced nearly 30 years ago, the benzodiazepines (BZDs) were hailed as a breakthrough because they have fewer of the drawbacks of prior sedatives and hypnotics; are effective in a range of disorders; safe in combination with most drugs (except other sedatives), as well as alone in overdose; and generally mild in

terms of side effects. For these reasons they quickly became, and remain, among the most widely prescribed drugs worldwide.

Nevertheless, BZDs have become the subject of heated debate that tends to center on issues related to overuse, misuse, and abuse. Indeed, many BZD-treated patients, their families and their physicians now wonder if one should be considered an abuser after taking these drugs for longer than a few weeks. Recent reviews, however, generally support earlier conclusions that even long-term therapeutic use is rarely accompanied by inappropriate drug-taking or drug-seeking behavior (e.g., high and sustained dosage escalation; trying to obtain the drug from several physicians or illicitly) (1–6). Although this may occur, there appears to be a clear distinction between BZD abusers and therapeutic dose users. Almost exclusively, the former are reported to also abuse other prescription or street drugs and/or alcohol; take BZDs in large doses for euphoriant effects or to potentiate other drugs; and prefer drugs other than BZDs when available. By contrast, even long-term BZD users usually report taking therapeutic or only slightly higher doses; often report taking doses even lower than those prescribed; or attempt to discontinue the BZD altogether (see Table 12.1).

These distinctions are important because the advantages and disadvantages of the therapeutic use of BZDs should not be confused with their abuse.

REFERENCES

1. Ayd Jr FJ. Benzodiazepines: dependence and withdrawal. JAMA 1979;242:1401–1402.
2. Woods JH, Katz JL, Winger G. Abuse liability of benzodiazepines. Pharmacol Rev 1987;39:251–413.
3. American Psychiatric Association. Benzodiazepine dependence, toxicity, and abuse. Washington, DC: American Psychiatric Association, 1990.
4. Uhlenhuth EH, DeWit H, Balter MB, et

Table 12.1.
Medical Users versus Nonmedical Users/Abusers of Benzodiazepines

Medical Users	Nonmedical Users/Abusers
Are more likely to be females over age 50.	Are more likely to be males between the ages of 20 and 35.
Take a BZD prescribed and supervised by a physician for a recognized medical indication.	Take a BZD that may or may not have been obtained from a physician, but not for a recognized medical indication; self-administer the drug without physician supervision for "kicks" or to "get high."
Usually take the prescribed dose or less.	Usually take doses in excess of established therapeutic doses.
Take only the BZD.	Usually abuse a number of drugs. Abuse BZDs infrequently compared to other drugs. BZDs frequently abused with a wide variety of other drugs such as alcohol, illegal drugs (marijuana, cocaine), and controlled prescription drugs (methadone).
Do not usually develop tolerance and a need to progressively escalate the dose.	Often quickly develop tolerance and have to escalate the dose to obtain the desired effect.
Dislike BZD sedative effects.	Like and seek BZD sedative effects.
Prefer a placebo to a BZD.	Prefer a BZD to a placebo.
Seldom take more than diazepam, 40 mg/day, or its equivalent.	Frequently take diazepam, 80 to 120+ mg/day, or its equivalent.
Seldom at high risk of a severe withdrawal reaction.	Often at high risk of a severe withdrawal reaction.
Do not constitute a serious medical or social problem.	Constitute a serious medical and/or social problem.
Usually do not obtain a BZD from a "script doctor" who sells prescriptions for a fee.	Usually obtain a BZD from a "script doctor" or some other illegal source.

al. Risks and benefits of long-term benzodiazepine use. J Clin Psychopharmacol
1988;8:161–167.

5. Garvey MJ, Tollefson GD. Prevalence of
misuse of prescribed benzodiazepines in
patients with primary anxiety disorder or

major depression. Am J Psychiatry
1986;143:1601–1603.

6. Gelenberg AJ, ed. The use of benzodiazepine hypnotics: a scientific examination of
the clinical controversy. J Clin Psychiatry
1992;53(Suppl):1–87.

Mechanism of Action

In 1977, benzodiazepine receptors were identified when it became possible to map their location within the central nervous system (CNS). They were found to be intimately related to γ-aminobutyric acid (GABA), the most prevalent inhibitory neurotransmitter system in the brain, which acts in the:

• *Stellate inhibitory interneurons* in cortex
• *Striatal afferents* to globus pallidus and substantia nigra
• *Purkinje cells* in the cerebellum.

Further, the recognition sites for GABA receptors were found to be coupled to chloride ion channels. When GABA binds to its receptors, these channels open and allow chloride ions to flow into the neuron, making it more resistant to excitation. GABA exerts its actions at two physiologically and pharmacologically distinct classes of receptors, $GABA_A$ and $GABA_B$. Although $GABA_B$ receptors are insensitive to BZDs or barbiturates, these drugs do bind to a site on $GABA_A$ receptors, which are linked to, but distinct from, the GABA recognition site. BZDs enhance the affinity of the recognition site for GABA, ultimately potentiating its inhibitory action. Barbiturates apparently interact with sites directly related to the chloride channel, prolonging the duration of its opening by as much as four- to five-fold. There is

evidence that alcohol's effects are also due in part to enhancement of $GABA_A$ receptor function (1).

Current evidence indicates BZDs act at two different $GABA_A$ receptor subtypes (I and II). *Type I receptors* are predominant, with type II concentrated in the hippocampus, striatum superior colliculus, and neocortex. A number of compounds (CL 218872, quazepam, zolpidem) have been used to distinguish the two receptor types on the basis of binding affinities. In animals, CL 218872 exerts effects indicating anxiolytic action, but is much less sedating than nonspecific BZDs, such as diazepam. This suggests that different BZD receptors may be responsible for the sedative and anxiolytic effects of these agents, raising the possibility of more selective compounds.

Although an endogenous BZD ligand has not been identified, research indicates the BZD receptor in fact has three types of ligands:

• BZD agonists (e.g., BZD drugs)
• BZD antagonists (e.g., flumazenil)
• BZD inverse agonists (e.g., β-carboline-3-carboxylic acid ethyl ester).

Whereas BZD agonists have antianxiety and anticonvulsant effects, BZD inverse agonists are anxiogenic, convulsant, and capable of antagonizing GABA's effects. In one study an inverse agonist was administered to human subjects, producing anxiety, terror, cold sweats, tremor, agitation, fear of impending death, and "intense inner strain" (2). BZD antagonists apparently lack intrinsic activity, but may have both agonist and inverse agonist effects (3). BZD antagonists, for example, are reported to reverse the increased anxiety that may occur after withdrawal of chronic BZD or alcohol use and to reverse BZD-caused amnestic effects (4–7).

These and other findings related to manipulation of the benzodiazepine–GABA-receptor complex indicate it is an important substrate in the neurobiological regulation of anxiety. Other systems also may play a role, however, including the noradrenergic and serotonergic systems, as well as a number of peptides and hormones (1).

REFERENCES

1. Zorumski CF, Isenberg KE. Insights into the structure and function of GABA-benzodiazepine receptors: ion channels and psychiatry. Am J Psychiatry 1991;148:162–163.
2. Dorow R, Horowski R, Paschelke G, et al. Severe anxiety induced by FG-7142, a beta-carboline ligand for benzodiazepine receptors. Lancet 1983;2:98–99.
3. Handley SL. New directions in benzodiazepine research. Curr Opinion Psychiatry 1989;2:59–62.
4. File SE. Chronic diazepam treatment: effect of dose on development of tolerance and incidence of withdrawal in an animal test of anxiety. Hum Psychopharmacol 1989;4:59–63.
5. File SE. Zharkovsky A, Hitchcott PK. Effects of nitrendepine, chlordiazepoxide, flumazenil and baclofen on the increased anxiety resulting from alcohol withdrawal. Prog Neuropsychopharmacol Biol Psychiatry 1992;16:87–93.
6. Dorow R, Berenberg D, Duka T, et al. Amnestic effects of lormetazepam and their reversal by the benzodiazepine antagonist Ro 15-1788. Psychopharmacology 1987;93:507–514.
7. Gentil V, Gorenstein C, Camargo CHP, et al. Effects of flunitrazepam on memory and their reversal by two antagonists. J Clin Psychopharmacol 1989;9:191–197.

Treatment of Generalized Anxiety Disorder

Benzodiazepines are the drugs most commonly used in the treatment of anxiety symptoms, generalized anxiety disorder (GAD), and insomnia. Although other drugs exert anxiolytic effects, the BZDs are considered to be the primary pharmacological treatment, thus they are the primary focus of this chapter. Alternate treatment strategies, as well as disorders in which BZDs have demonstrated little or no efficacy, will also be discussed. Figure 12.1 overviews the differential diagnosis and related treatment strategies for various anxiety disorders.

ACUTE TREATMENT

Innumerable studies have examined the efficacy of BZDs in the acute treatment of anxiety and GAD. Almost all indicate that these anxiolytics quickly reduce symptoms in many patients, with most improvement occurring in the first week of treatment (1). Nevertheless, they may not be universally effective, with some investigators finding no difference between BZDs and placebo (2). Overall, Rickels (1978) has reported that about 35% of patients show marked improvement, 40%

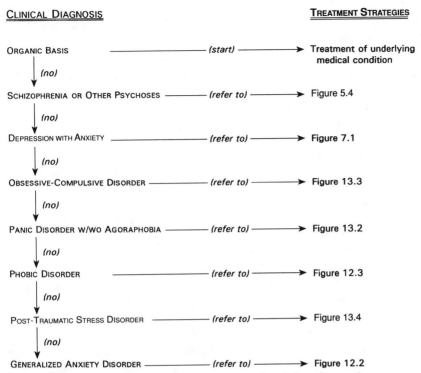

CLINICAL DIAGNOSIS   TREATMENT STRATEGIES

ORGANIC BASIS ————————— (start) ————————→ Treatment of underlying
                                                                    medical condition
   ↓ (no)

SCHIZOPHRENIA OR OTHER PSYCHOSES ——— (refer to) ————→ Figure 5.4
   ↓ (no)

DEPRESSION WITH ANXIETY ——————— (refer to) ————→ Figure 7.1
   ↓ (no)

OBSESSIVE-COMPULSIVE DISORDER ——— (refer to) ————→ Figure 13.3
   ↓ (no)

PANIC DISORDER W/WO AGORAPHOBIA ——— (refer to) ————→ Figure 13.2
   ↓ (no)

PHOBIC DISORDER ——————————— (refer to) ————→ Figure 12.3
   ↓ (no)

POST-TRAUMATIC STRESS DISORDER ——— (refer to) ————→ Figure 13.4
   ↓ (no)

GENERALIZED ANXIETY DISORDER ——— (refer to) ————→ Figure 12.2

Figure 12.1. Differential diagnosis of various anxiety-related disorders and treatment strategies (see specified figures in this and other chapters).

show moderate improvement, and 25% remain unchanged (3).

Patients most likely to respond to a BZD have been reported to have the following characteristics:

- Acute, severe anxiety
- Precipitating stress(es)
- Low level of depression; or interpersonal problems
- No previous treatment or good response to previous treatment
- Expectation of recovery
- Desire to use medication
- Awareness that symptoms are psychological
- Some improvement in the first treatment week (4, 5).

There is also evidence that many of these patients derive benefit from short-term BZD therapy only. In one study 50% of those treated with diazepam (15–40 mg/day) for 6 weeks maintained their improvement during placebo therapy for an additional 18 weeks (6). In another study, 70% treated for 4 weeks with either lorazepam or clorazepate maintained improvement during 2 weeks on placebo (7). Even the chronically anxious may benefit from brief (4–6 weeks) treatment (8). In many cases, although discontinuation of medication may eventually lead to a reemergence of anxiety, symptoms may not always be continuous, functionally significant, or cause patients to seek further treatment (9).

Most now agree that BZD treatment of acute anxiety, as well as GAD, should be with the lowest possible dose for the shortest possible time. Dosages should be flexible rather than arbitrary and taken intermittently at a time of increased symptoms rather than on a fixed daily schedule. In general, 1 to 7 days of BZD treatment is recommended for a reaction to an acute situational stress, although 1 to 6 weeks of treatment may be needed for short-term anxiety due to specific life events (10).

LONG-TERM TREATMENT

Clinical judgment plays a major role in the decision to continue BZD anxiolytic treatment beyond 4 to 6 weeks. Although long-term administration may maintain initial improvement, it is unlikely to result in further gains (11). To lessen the likelihood of adverse effects and withdrawal phenomena (discussed below), many American investigators now recommend limiting BZD use to 4 months or less, and British guidelines are even more stringent, indicating use should not exceed 2 to 4 weeks (12). The chronic nature of anxiety disorders and the frequency of eventual relapse after treatment discontinuation, however, suggest that in some patients long-term treatment may be indicated (6, 9, 10, 13).

Unfortunately, there is only limited controlled data on the efficacy of chronic BZD administration. In one double-blind study, the effectiveness of continuous treatment with diazepam (15–40 mg/day) for up to 22 weeks was assessed in chronically anxious subjects diagnosed according to the DSM-III (13). Half of all patients switched to placebo experienced a slow return of their original symptoms, indicating diazepam continues to be effective for at least 22 weeks. In a study involving clorazepate, investigators also found continuing efficacy for up to 6 months (14). Although no controlled studies have been conducted on the efficacy of BZD therapy beyond 6 months' duration, the fact that long-term therapeutic use is rarely accom-

panied by dosage escalation suggests anxiolytic efficacy is retained even after prolonged use (15–20).

Many long-term users, however, report high levels of baseline anxiety or "psychic distress" (15, 20, 21–26). This may represent:

- *Undertreatment*
- *Partial responsiveness* that would worsen without treatment
- Presence of symptoms *more responsive to a different class* of drug (e.g., an antidepressant)
- Development of some degree of *tolerance* to the anxiolytic effect of the BZD
- Development of a *chronic state of withdrawal.*

In two recent studies Rickels and coinvestigators found that baseline measures taken before BZD discontinuation showed significant anxiety and depressive symptomatology despite long-term drug therapy (25, 26). In addition, patients who successfully completed either abrupt or gradual drug withdrawal achieved lower anxiety and depression levels than they had while receiving medication. This is not an unexpected finding, since this process selects patients with a good prognosis.

In her study of 50 consecutive patients attempting withdrawal from BZDs taken for 1 to 22 years, Ashton reported that all patients had a variety of anxiety/depressive symptoms that had been gradually increasing over several years despite continuous BZD use (24). Ten had become agoraphobic, and several (number not given) had also received unsuccessful behavioral therapy. Twelve had undergone extensive gastroenterological or neurological investigations, for which various treatments had been ineffective. Ashton notes that it is arguable whether these patients would have developed their symptoms without BZD treatment; however, their symptoms:

- Were not present prior to initiation of the BZD
- Were not amenable to other treatments during BZD use
- Largely disappeared when the BZD was discontinued.

Conclusion

The diagnosis of all patients on long-term BZD therapy should be reassessed on a regular, intermittent basis because GAD's high rate of comorbidity for other psychiatric disorders suggests that an alternate approach (such as an antidepressant or BZD discontinuation) may be more appropriate in certain patients. In addition, regular treatment monitoring; use of the lowest possible dosages compatible with achieving the desired therapeutic effect; use of intermittent and flexible dosing schedules rather than a fixed regimen; and gradual dosage reduction offer the best means of avoiding the dependence and withdrawal associated with long-term use.

Summarizing their study of 119 long-term BZD users, Rickels et al. reported, "one hard-earned lesson is that [they] are in need of much more intensive psychiatric and social support than other anxious or depressed patients" (20). Nevertheless, the quality of life of certain patients may depend on long-term, therapeutic use of a BZD (27). Although periodic attempts to discontinue the medication should be made to determine whether return of anxiety represents a withdrawal reaction or reemergence of the original anxiety disorder, categorical withholding of BZDs may do more harm than good. For example, some may turn to more dangerous drugs in an effort to obtain relief, while others may seek a more permanent solution through suicide.

ALTERNATE TREATMENT STRATEGIES

In some patients, careful listening, astute questioning, and appropriate advice may be the best form of intervention. Bereavement-induced acute anxiety and insomnia should not be considered a disorder requiring drug therapy, although such patients may benefit from grief counseling and/or very brief use of a BZD if the disturbance is severe. Some psychotherapies have been reported effective to teach techniques for coping with and/or reducing anxiety. If drug therapy is indicated, some non-BZDs may be useful alternatives.

Buspirone

Buspirone, in contrast to the BZDs, has no immediate effect on the anxiety seen in patients undergoing medical procedures (e.g., endoscopy, cardioversion). Further, it cannot be given parenterally, since the drug is not available in an i.v. or i.m. formulation. It does not produce disinhibition euphoria; and even in high doses, has not been found to have antipsychotic activity.

The absence of adverse effects of the benzodiazepine type, and its lack of abuse potential are major advantages. The lack of sedative properties may be very important, since many dislike this feeling and find it interferes with various activities, such as problem solving, driving, and overall work function.

While this azaspirone anxiolytic does not interact with brain BZD receptors, it has been shown to be as effective as BZDs for GAD (28–31). In a long-term follow-up study of chronic GAD patients who participated in a 6-month trial comparing clorazepate and buspirone, Rickels and Schweizer found a nonsignificant trend for former buspirone-treated patients to report less anxiety than former clorazepate-treated patients (13). In addition, whereas 65% of the former clorazepate-treated group were still taking anxiolytic medication at 40-month follow-up, no former buspirone patient was taking a psychotropic.

The side-effect profile of this agent is different from BZDs in that there is:

• No sedation
• No memory or psychomotor impairment
• No interaction with alcohol
• No abuse potential
• No disinhibition phenomenon (32).

Buspirone differs clinically in four important ways from the benzodiazepines. First, it is only useful when taken regularly for several weeks, since it has no immediate effect after a single tablet, and is not helpful in treating an acute episode. Many patients who have taken BZDs expect relief after a single tablet, but buspirone cannot be used on such a prn basis. Secondly, it has demonstrated antidepressant properties in double-blind studies. Third, it has not been shown effective for panic attacks in several small studies. Finally, it does not block BZD withdrawal symptoms. This is often a critical consideration since many patients have previously been on and/or are presently taking a BZD. One cannot, however, expect an antianxiety agent without BZD-like habituation to alleviate abstinence symptoms.

Clinical studies have also found that anxious patients treated for up to 12 months are able to stop treatment abruptly without withdrawal symptoms (14, 33).

Buspirone has a slower onset of anxiolytic action (1–2 weeks) than the BZDs, however, and requires tid dosing. Increased antianxiety effects have been observed in some patients treated concurrently with low doses of buspirone and a BZD (34). Although this agent may not be as effective in patients who have previously used a BZD, some can be successfully switched (35). In such cases, a 2–4 week period of concurrent use before BZD tapering may help alleviate the return of anxiety.

We think that buspirone may be the drug of choice for many patients with generalized anxiety disorder who have not taken benzodiazepines previously. There may also be an advantage in patients who have problems with BZD withdrawal symptoms (see Table 12.2).

Table 12.2.
Clinical Differences between Buspirone and the Benzodiazepines

	Buspirone	BZD
Acute effect on anxiety	—[a]	+[b]
Acute effect on psychotic agitation	0	+
Anticonvulsant effects	0	+
Chronic effect on anxiety	+	+
Effect on depression	+	0[b]
Effect on acute panic attack	0	Alprazolam
Augment SRI for OCD	+	0
Sedation	0	+
Potentiate alcohol	0	+
Disinhibition euphoria	0	+
Potential for abuse	0	+
Alleviate BZD abstinence syndrome	0	+
Available i.v. or i.m.	0	+

[a]Not studied.
[b]+ = present; 0 = absent.
[c]Most BZD's do not have an antidepressant effect, with the possible exception of alprazolam.

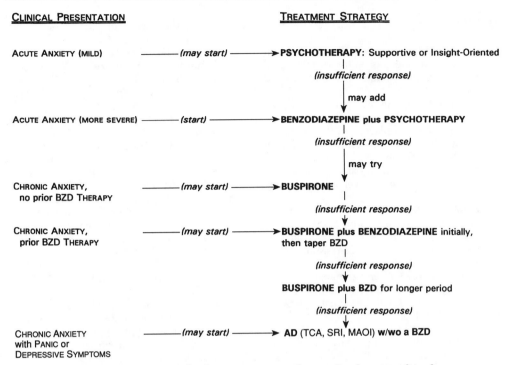

Figure 12.2. Strategy for the management of generalized anxiety disorder.

Imipramine

Two studies have indicated that the tricyclic antidepressant, imipramine may be as effective as BZDs in the treatment of GAD (36, 37). No studies beyond 8 weeks' duration have been conducted, however, and imipramine's onset of anxiolytic action may be even slower than that of buspirone. Although adverse effects also may limit usefulness, its lack of dependence liability may make it an appropriate alternative in chronically anxious patients who also suffer from panic and depression.

β-Blockers and Antihistamines

Despite very limited efficacy in most anxious patients, β-blockers may be useful for highly somatic individuals, such as those with performance anxiety. Antihistamines are quite sedating, have little dependence potential, and are generally safe in terms of other complications, except their anticholinergic effects, which are common.

CONCLUSION

It is not yet clear how useful, or how detrimental, chronic BZD therapy may be for patients with GAD. Whenever possible, BZD discontinuation (using a gradual tapering schedule) should be attempted to clarify persistence of anxiety or drug-induced adverse effects. Alternate strategies include:

- Nondrug interpretations
- The azaspirone buspirone
- ADs, such as imipramine
- β-Blockers or antihistamines, in selected cases.

Figure 12.2 summarizes the strategy we would recommend for the management of acute and chronic generalized anxiety.

REFERENCES

1. Downing RW, Rickels K. Early treatment response in anxious outpatients treated with diazepam. Acta Psychiatr Scand 1985;72:522–528.
2. Meibach RC, Dunner D, Wilson LG, et al. Comparative efficacy of propranolol, chlordiazepoxide, and placebo in the treatment of anxiety. A double blind trial. J Clin Psychiatry 1987;48:355–358.
3. Rickels K. Use of antianxiety agents in anxious outpatients. Psychopharmacology 1978;58:1–17.
4. Rickels K. Benzodiazepines in the treatment of anxiety. In: Usdin E, Skolnick P, Tallman JF, et al., eds. Pharmacology of benzodiazepines. London: Macmillan, 1982:37–44.
5. Dubovsky SL. Generalized anxiety disorder: new concepts and psychopharmacologic therapies. J Clin Psychiatry 1990;51 (1,Suppl):3–10.
6. Rickels K, Case G, Downing RW, et al. Long-term diazepam therapy and clinical-outcome. JAMA 1983;250:767–771.
7. Rickels K, Fox IL, Greenblatt DJ. Clorazepate and lorazepam: clinical improvement and rebound anxiety. Am J Psychiatry 1988;145:312–317.
8. Rickels K, Case WG, Downing RS, et al. Indications and contraindications for chronic anxiolytic treatment: is there tolerance to the anxiolytic effect? In: Kemali D, Racagni G, eds. Chronic treatments in neuropsychiatry. New York: Raven Press, 1985;193–204.
9. Rickels K, Case G, Downing R, et al. One-year follow-up of anxious patients treated with diazepam. J Clin Psychopharmacol 1986;6:32–36.
10. Rickels K, Case WG, Diamond L. Relapse after short-term drug therapy in neurotic outpatients. Int Pharmacopsychiatr 1980; 15:186–192.
11. Rickels K. Antianxiety therapy: potential value of long-term treatment. J Clin Psychiatry 1987;48:7–11.
12. Committee on Safety of Medicines: Benzodiazepines, dependence and withdrawal symptoms. Number 21, January 1988.
13. Rickels K, Schweizer E. The clinical course and long-term management of generalized anxiety disorder. J Clin Psychopharmacol 1990;10:101s–110s.
14. Rickels K. Buspirone, clorazepate and withdrawal. Presented at the Annual Meeting of the American Psychiatric Association, Dallas, TX, 1985.
15. Woods JH, Katz JL, Winger G. Abuse liability of benzodiazepines. Pharmacol Rev 1987;39:251–413.
16. American Psychiatric Association. Benzodiazepine dependence, toxicity, and abuse. Washington, DC: American Psychiatric Association, 1990.
17. Uhlenhuth EH, DeWit H, Balter MB, et al. Risks and benefits of long-term benzodiazepine use. J Clin Psychopharmacol 1988;8:161–167.
18. Garvey MJ, Tollefson GD. Prevalence of misuse of prescribed benzodiazepines in patients with primary anxiety disorder or major depression. Am J Psychiatry 1986;143:1601–1603.
19. Ayd Jr FJ. Benzodiazepines: dependence and withdrawal. JAMA 1979;242:1401–1402.
20. Rickels K, Case WG, Schweizer EE, et al. Low-dose dependence in chronic benzodiazepine users: a preliminary report on 119 patients. Psychopharmacol Bull 1986;22:407–15.
21. Rodrigo EK, King MB, Williams P. Health of long-term benzodiazepine users. Br Med J 1988;296:603–606.
22. Mellinger GD, Balter MB, Uhlenhuth EH. Prevalence and correlates of the long-term use of anxiolytics. JAMA 1984;251:375–379.
23. Le Goc I, Feline A, Frebault D, et al. Caracteristiques de la consommation de benzodiazepines chez des patients hospitalises dans un service de medicine interne. Encephale 1985;2:1–6.
24. Ashton H. Benzodiazepine withdrawal: outcome in 50 patients. Br J Addiction 1987;82:665–671.
25. Rickels K, Schweizer E, Case WG, et al. Long-term therapeutic use of benzodiazepines. I. Effects of abrupt discontinuation. Arch Gen Psychiatry 1990;47:899–907.
26. Schweizer E, Rickels K, Case WG, et al. Long-term therapeutic use of benzodiazepines. II. Effects of gradual taper. Arch Gen Psychiatry 1990;47:908–915.
27. Markowitz JS, Weissman MH, Ouellette R, et al. Quality of life in panic disorder. Arch Gen Psychiatry 1989;46:984–992.
28. Goldberg HL, Finnerty RJ. The comparative efficacy of buspirone and diazepam in the treatment of anxiety. Am J Psychiatry 1979;136:1184–1187.
29. Kastenholz KV, Crimson ML. Buspirone,

a novel nonbenzodiazepine anxiolytic. Clin Pharm 1984;3:600–607.

30. Rickels K, Weisman K, Norstad N, et al. Buspirone and diazepam in anxiety: a controlled study. J Clin Psychiatry 1982;43:81–86.

31. Sussman N. Treatment of anxiety with buspirone. Psychiatric Ann 1987;17:114–120.

32. Lucki I, Rickels K, Giesecki MA, et al. Differential effects of the anxiolytic drugs diazepam and buspirone on memory function. Br J Clin Pharmacology 1987;23:207–211.

33. Goa KL, Ward A. Buspirone: a preliminary review of its pharmacological properties and therapeutic efficacy as an anxiolytic. Drugs 1986;32:114–129.

34. Sussman N, Chou CY. Current issues in benzodiazepine use for anxiety disorders. Psychiatric Ann 1988;18:139–205.

35. Schweitzer E, Rickels K. Failure of buspirone to manage benzodiazepine withdrawal. Am J Psychiatry 1986;258:204–205.

36. Kahn RJ, McNair DM, Lipman RS, et al. Imipramine and chlordiazepoxide in depressive and anxiety disorders: 2. Efficacy in anxious outpatients. Arch Gen Psychiatry 1986;43:79–85.

37. Rickels K, Downing RW, Schweizer E. Antidepressants in generalized anxiety disorder. Presented at the Annual Meeting of the American Psychiatric Association, Chicago, May 1987.

Treatment of Phobic Disorders

AGORAPHOBIA

As noted in Chapter 11, agoraphobia may be associated with panic disorder (see also Panic Disorder in Chapter 13), although it also occurs as a discrete entity without panic attacks. Inasmuch as most drug treatment studies have involved agoraphobic patients with panic disorder, there is relatively little evidence to suggest any agent is more than minimally effective for agoraphobia alone. In vivo exposure therapy, however, may be very useful in those willing to tolerate the distress associated with confronting the feared situation (1, 2).

SOCIAL PHOBIA

Although behavioral treatments for social phobia have been well studied, there are very limited data on its pharmacologic management. β-*Blockers* (propranolol, atenolol) have been recommended, but available evidence indicates their effect may be no different than that of placebo (3). In a controlled study the *monoamine oxidase inhibitor* (MAOI) phenelzine has

been shown to be more effective than placebo (3, 4). Anecdotal reports have also described efficacy with *alprazolam, clonidine,* and *fluoxetine,* but systematic data are lacking (5–8).

SIMPLE PHOBIA

Available evidence indicates that *systematic desensitization* and *in vivo exposure* are the most effective treatment methods available for simple phobia. Pharmacologic treatment of simple phobia has not been well investigated, but studies involving antidepressants suggest tricyclics and MAOIs are ineffective (9–11). In addition, three studies suggest that sedative-hypnotic anxiolytics may have adverse effects on the behavioral treatment of simple phobias (12–14). In other studies, volunteers with simple animal phobias were exposed to their phobic object 1.5 hours after administration of either tolamolol, diazepam, or placebo in a double-blind crossover design. Tolamolol abolished the stress-induced tachycardia, but had no beneficial behavioral or subjective effects (15).

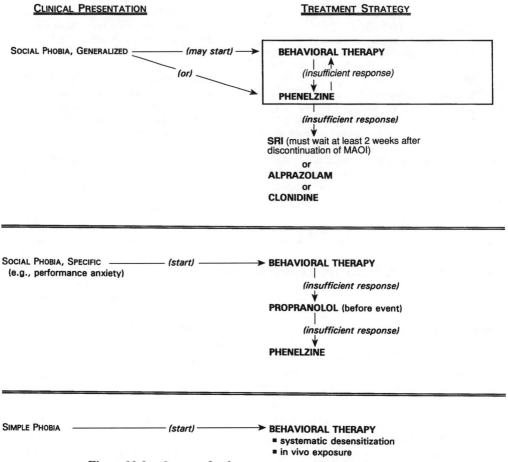

Figure 12.3.   Strategy for the management of phobic disorders.

CONCLUSION

There is a lack of data to support drug management in these disorders. Behavioral techniques, especially for simple phobic conditions, are the treatment of choice, presently. MAOIs, SRIs, clonidine, and alprazolam may benefit some patients. Figure 12.3 summarizes the management strategy we would recommend.

REFERENCES

1. Marks I, O'Sullivan G. Drugs and psychological treatments for agoraphobia/panic and obsessive-compulsive disorders: a review. Br J Psychiatry 1988;153:650–658.
2. Noyes R, Chaudry DR, Domingo DV. Pharmacologic treatment of phobic disorders. J Clin Psychiatry 1986;47:445–452.
3. Liebowitz MR, Fyer AJ, Gorman JM, et al. Phenelzine in social phobia. J Clin Psychopharmacol 1986;6:93–98.
4. Liebowitz MR, Gorman JM, Fyer AJ, et al. Pharmacotherapy of social phobia: an interim report of a placebo-controlled comparison of phenelzine and atenolol. J Clin Psychiatry 1988;49:252–258.
5. Lydiard RB, Laraia MT, Howell EF, et al. Alprazolam in social phobia. J Clin Psychiatry 1988;49:17–19.
6. Goldstein S. Treatment of social phobia with clonidine. Biol Psychiatry 1987;22: 369–372.
7. Sternbach H. Fluoxetine treatment of social phobia. J Affect Disord 1987;13:183–192.
8. Schneier FR, Chin SJ, Hollander E, et al. Fluoxetine in social phobia. J Clin Psychopharmacol 1992;12:62–64.

9. Zitrin CM, Klein DF, Woerner MG, et al. Treatment of phobias. I: Comparison of imipramine hydrochloride and placebo. Arch Gen Psychiatry 1983;40:125–138.
10. Ballenger JC, Sheehan DV, Jacobson G. Antidepressant treatment of severe phobic anxiety. Presented at the Annual Meeting of the American Psychiatric Association, Toronto, May 1977.
11. Sheehan DV, Ballenger JC, Jacobsen G. Treatment of endogenous anxiety with phobic, hysterical, and hypochondriacal symptoms. Arch Gen Psychiatry 1980;37:51–59.
12. Cameron OG, Liepman MR, Curtis GC, et al. Ethanol retards desensitization of simple phobias in non-alcoholics. Br J Psychiatry 1987;150:845–849.
13. Marks IM. Cure and care of neuroses: theory and practice of behavioral psychotherapy. New York: Wiley, 1981.
14. Hunt D, Adams R, Egan K, et al. Opioids: mediators of fear or mania. Biol Psychiatry 1988;23:426–428.
15. Bernadt MW, Silverstone T, Singleton W. β-Adrenergic blockers in phobic disorder. Br J Psychiatry 1980;137:452–457.

Treatment of Sleep Disorders

ACUTE TREATMENT

BZDs may offer temporary symptomatic relief for transient and short-term insomnia. They generally are not recommended for long-term treatment, as a primary treatment for chronic insomnia, or in patients with sleep apnea. Five of these agents are currently marketed in the United States for use as hypnotics (see Table 12.3), but other BZDs can also serve the same purpose.

Sleep onset latency generally is improved (i.e., shortened) with all BZD hypnotics, although this may vary considerably with individual patients. Those with relatively rapid onset of hypnotic activity include flurazepam, diazepam, and clorazepate. Somewhat slower onset occurs with triazolam, estazolam, quazepam, alprazolam, lorazepam, chlordiazepoxide, clonazepam, and temazepam, in the newer formulations. Early observations that temazepam was ineffective in improving sleep onset latency may be the result of the formulation initially used in the United States, which was slowly absorbed (1–3). Reformulation, however, has improved this agent's absorption rate and onset of hypnotic activity (4) (see also Chapter 3). In contrast, oxazepam, halazepam, and prazepam tend to have a *delayed onset*,

Table 12.3.
Benzodiazepine Hypnotics Available in the United States

Name (Proprietary Name)	Metabolism	Half-Life Including Metabolites (hours)	Lipophilicity	Active Metabolites
Estazolam (Prosom)	Oxidation	8–24	Low	No
Flurazepam (Dalmane)	Oxidation	48–120	Moderate	Yes
Quazepam (Doral)	Oxidation	48–120	High	Yes
Temazepam (Restoril)	Conjugation	8–20	Moderate	No
Triazolam (Halcion)	Oxidation	2–6	Moderate	No

requiring administration at least 30 to 60 minutes before bedtime (5).

Whereas long-acting BZDs usually maintain sleep throughout the night and tend to decrease daytime anxiety, short-acting drugs may result in early morning awakening.

Long-acting compounds, such as quazepam and flurazepam, have been demonstrated in sleep laboratory studies to maintain their hypnotic efficacy when given nightly for 4 weeks, although they were somewhat less effective toward the end of this period (6–13). Estazolam, a triazolobenzodiazepine with an intermediate half-life, was reported in one study to retain its hypnotic efficacy for up to 6 weeks. (14). Although triazolam in the 0.5 mg dose has been studied extensively and findings indicate a high degree of initial efficacy, there is evidence that the shorter-acting, high-potency BZDs such as triazolam and lorazepam may lose their sleep-promoting property within 3 to 14 days of continuous use (9, 15–21).

Whether hypnotic efficacy is retained with lower recommended doses of many BZDs is unclear. The efficacy of lower doses of triazolam (0.25 mg and 0.125 mg) has not been well established (22–27). Flurazepam (15 mg) may be effective for 1 week but not for 2 weeks (28–30). Temazepam (15 mg) was reported effective for 2 weeks in one study but not in another (2, 31). Estazolam (1.0 mg and 2.0 mg) has been reported effective for 1 week, but longer-term efficacy with the lower dose has not been reported (32).

LONG-TERM TREATMENT

No studies have demonstrated the hypnotic efficacy of BZDs beyond 12 weeks. Further, in studies involving a parallel placebo group, there was no difference between active medication and place-bo after 2 to 3 weeks of treatment (22, 29, 33).

A sleep laboratory study involving middle-aged and elderly chronic insomniacs indicated that tolerance develops with continuous use. Thus, Schneider-Helmert (1988) investigated the effects of continuous, long-term BZD use (6 months to years) in dosages ranging from 0.25 to 2 times the recommended dose (34). Compared to drug-free insomniacs, BZD users were found to have loss of hypnotic effectiveness and substantial suppression of delta and REM sleep. Abrupt drug discontinuation resulted in recovery from this suppression with no increase in insomnia. Although drugs with short, intermediate, and long half-lives were all represented, only small differences were found among BZDs. Subjectively perceived hypnotic efficacy was not confirmed by objective measurement (i.e., those on BZDs showed a 72-minute overestimation of sleep and upon drug withdrawal a 61-minute overestimation of sleep onset latency). Schneider-Helmert concluded that long-term users' overestimation of sleep while taking a BZD coupled with awareness of their sleep disturbance on discontinuation may explain why such patients develop "low-dose dependence." Citing the findings of Lucki et al. that with continuous use there were still BZD-impaired memory functions shortly after taking the drug, Schneider-Helmert also speculated that overestimation of time asleep may be the result of drug-induced anterograde amnesia (35).

ALTERNATE DRUG TREATMENTS

Low doses of a *sedative antidepressant*, such as amitriptyline, doxepin, or trazodone, have hypnotic efficacy and may be less likely to evoke the adverse effects associated with higher doses.

Antihistamines, such as diphenhydramine and doxylamine, may be effective for up to 1 week, but controlled data on longer use are lacking (36, 37). These drugs may produce excessive anticholinergic adverse effects.

Barbiturates and *barbiturate-like drugs,* such as chloral hydrate, although effective hypnotics, are considered far less safe than BZDs in terms of tolerance, interaction with alcohol, and lethality in overdose. Therefore, their use is not generally recommended. The safety of *tryptophan,* an essential amino acid with weak hypnotic effects, has been questioned recently, and it also should be avoided, at least until further data are available.

Nonbenzodiazepine hypnotics, such as zopiclone and zolpidem, are currently available in Europe. They have been found to be superior to placebo and equally effective as various BZD hypnotics in several well-controlled trials (38, 39).

Their low side-effect profiles make them attractive alternatives.

ALTERNATE NON-DRUG TREATMENTS

Sleep Hygiene Techniques

Patients should be encouraged to:

- Reduce or avoid the use of alcohol, nicotine, caffeine, or hypnotics (including over-the-counter preparations)
- Avoid daytime naps
- Get regular exercise
- Go to bed and wake up at the same time every day
- Use the bedroom only for sleep (not for reading, watching television, or working).

If sleep onset does not occur within 30 minutes, patients should get out of bed and not return until they are sleepy (5).

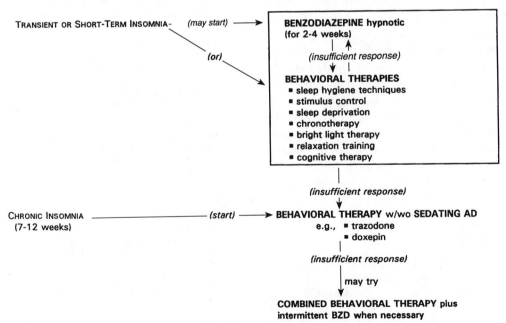

Figure 12.4.   Strategy for the management of sleep disorders.

Sleep Deprivation

Noting that chronic insomniacs often underestimate their actual sleep time, Spielman et al. (1987) conducted a study in which subjects initially were allowed to stay in bed only as long as their own estimate of time spent asleep (40). Results indicated that the mild sleep deprivation produced tended to improve sleep onset latency and efficiency.

Behavior Therapies

Although several behavioral approaches have been investigated, including biofeedback, progressive relaxation, hypnosis, and others, results have been mixed and there is little consensus regarding their use (41).

CONCLUSION

The BZDs will usually shorten sleep onset latency with brief (1–2 week) periods of treatment, and the use of longer acting agents (e.g., flurazepam) tends to avoid rebound insomnia. Lower dose strategies may also be effective for some patients, requiring only 1 to 2 weeks of therapy. No studies have demonstrated hypnotic efficacy beyond 3 months. Alternate strategies that may be effective for chronic insomnia include the use of sleep hygiene techniques and/or low doses of sedating antidepressants, such as trazodone (42). Figure 12.4 outlines the treatment strategy we would recommend.

REFERENCES

1. Mitler MM. Evaluation of temazepam as a hypnotic. Pharmacotherapy 1981;1:3–13.
2. Bixler EO, Kales A, Soldatos CR, et al. Effectiveness of temazepam with short-, intermediate-, and long-term use: sleep laboratory evaluation. J Clin Pharmacol 1978;18:110–118.
3. Mitler MM, Seidel WF, van den Hoed J, et al. Comparative efficacy of temazepam: a long-term sleep laboratory evaluation. Br J Clin Pharmacol 1979;8:63s–68s.
4. Greenblatt DJ. Benzodiazepine hypnotics: sorting the pharmacokinetic facts. J Clin Psychiatry 1991;52(9, Suppl):4–10.
5. Gillin JC, Byerley WF. The diagnosis and management of insomnia. N Engl J Med 1990;322:239–248.
6. Dement WC, Carskadon MA, Mitler MM, et al. Prolonged use of flurazepam: a sleep laboratory study. Behav Med 1978;5:25–31.
7. Kales A, Bixler EO, Scharf M, et al. Sleep laboratory studies of flurazepam: a model for evaluating hypnotic drugs. Clin Pharmacol Ther 1976;19:576–583.
8. Kales A, Bixler EO, Soldatos CR, et al. Quazepam and flurazepam: long-term use and extended withdrawal. Clin Pharmacol Ther 1982;32:781–788.
9. Mamelak M, Csima A, Price V. A comparative 25-night sleep laboratory study on the effects of quazepam and triazolam on the sleep of chronic insomniacs. J Clin Pharmacol·1984;24:65–75.
10. Oswald L, Adam K, Borrow S, et al. The effects of two hypnotics on sleep, subjective feelings and skilled performance. In: Passouant P, Oswald I, eds. Pharmacology of the states of alertness. Elmsford, NY: Pergamon Press, 1979.
11. Kales A, Allen C, Scharf MB, et al. Hypnotic drugs and their effectiveness. All night EEG studies of insomniac subjects. Arch Gen Psychiatry 1970;23:226–232.
12. Kales A, Kales JD, Bixler EO, et al. Effectiveness of hypnotic drugs with prolonged use: flurazepam and pentobarbital. Clin Pharmacol Ther 1975;18:356–363.
13. Kales J, Kales A, Bixler EO, et al. Effects of placebo and flurazepam on sleep patterns in insomniac subjects. Clin Pharmacol Ther 1971;12:691–697.
14. Lamphere J, Roehrs T, Zorick F, et al. Chronic hypnotic efficacy of estazolam. Drugs Exp Clin Res 1986;12:687–691.
15. Kales A, Kales JD, Bixler EO, et al. Hypnotic efficacy of triazolam: sleep laboratory evaluation of intermediate-term effectiveness. J Clin Pharmacol 1976;16:399–406.
16. Kales A, Bixler EO, Soldatos CR, Mitsky

DJ, Kales JD. Dose-response studies of lormetazepam: efficacy, side effects, and rebound insomnia. J Clin Pharmacol 1982;22:520–530.

17. Kales A, Soldatos CR, Bixler EO, et al. Midazolam: dose-response studies of effectiveness and rebound insomnia. Pharmacology 1983;26:138–149.

18. Kales A, Soldatos CR, Vela-Bueno A. Clinical comparison of benzodiazepine hypnotics with short and long elimination of half-lives. In: Smith DE, Wesson DR, eds. The benzodiazepines. Current standards for medical practice. Lancaster: MTP Press Limited, 1986.

19. Kales A, Bixler EO, Vela-Bueno A, et al. Comparison of short and long half-life benzodiazepine hypnotics: triazolam and quazepam. Clin Pharmacol Ther 1986;40:378–386.

20. Kales A, Bixler EO, Vela-Bueno A, et al. Alprazolam: effects on sleep and withdrawal phenomena. J Clin Pharmacol 1987;27:508–515.

21. Committee on the Review of Medicines. Systematic review of the benzodiazepines. Br Med J 1980;280:910–912.

22. Roth T, Kramer M, Lutz T. The effects of triazolam (0.25 mg) on the sleep of insomnia subjects. Drugs Exp Clin Res 1977;1:279–285.

23. Kales A, Bixler EO, Vela-Bueno A, et al. Comparison of short and long half-life benzodiazepine hypnotics: triazolam and oxazepam. Clin Pharmacol Ther 1986;40:378–386.

24. Mamelak M, Csima A, Price V. The effects of a single night's dosing with triazolam on sleep the following night. J Clin Pharmacol 1990;30:549–555.

25. Fernandez Guardiola A, Jurado JL. The effect of triazolam on insomniac patients using a laboratory sleep evaluation. Curr Ther Res 1981;29:950–958.

26. Seidel W, Cohen SA, Bliwise NG, et al. Dose-related effects of triazolam on a circadian rhythm insomnia. Clin Pharmacol Ther 1986;40:314–320.

27. O'Donnell VM, Balkin TJ, Andrade JR, et al. Effects of triazolam on performance and sleep in a model of transient insomnia. Hum Perform 1988;1:145–160.

28. Roehrs T, Zorick F, Kaffeman M, et al. Flurazepam for short-term treatment of complaints of insomnia. J Clin Pharmacol 1982;22:290–296.

29. Mamelak M, Adele C, Buck L, et al. A comparative study of the effects of brotizolam and flurazepam on sleep and performance in the elderly. J Clin Psychopharmacol 1989;9:260–267.

30. Bonnet MH. Effect of sleep disruption on sleep, performance, and mood. Sleep 1985;8:11–19.

31. Kales A, Bixler EO, Soldatos CR, et al. Quazepam and temazepam: effects of short- and intermediate-term use and withdrawal. Clin Pharmacol Ther 1986;39:345–352.

32. Pierce MW, Shu VS. Efficacy of estazolam: the United States clinical experience. Am J Med 1990;88(Suppl 3A):6s–11s.

33. Kripke DF, Hauri P, Roth T. Sleep evaluation in chronic insomnia during short- and long-term use of two benzodiazepines, flurazepam and midazolam. Sleep Res 1987;16:99.

34. Schneider-Helmert D. Why low-dose benzodiazepine-dependent insomniacs can't escape their sleeping pills. Acta Psychiatr Scand 1988;78:706–711.

35. Lucki I, Rickels K, Geller AM. Chronic use of benzodiazepines and psychomotor and cognitive test performance. Psychopharmacology 1986;88:416–433.

36. Rickels K, Morris RJ, Newman H, et al. Diphenhydramine in insomniac family practice patients: a double-blind study. J Clin Pharmacol 1983;23:235–242.

37. Rickels K, Ginsberg J, Morris RJ, et al. Doxylamine succinate in insomniac family practice patients: a double-blind study. Curr Ther Res 1984;35:532–540.

38. Scharf MB, Mayleben DW, Kaffeman M. Dose response effects of zolpidem in normal geriatric subjects. J Clin Psychiatry 1991;52:77–83.

39. Hindmarch I, Musch B, eds. Zopiclone in clinical practice. Int Clin Psychopharmacol 1990;5(Suppl 2):1–158.

40. Spielman AJ, Saskin P, Thorpy MJ. Treatment of chronic insomnia by restriction of time in bed. Sleep 1987;10:45–56.

41. Hauri P, Sataia MJ. Nonpharmacologic treatment of sleep disorders. In: Hales RE, Frances AJ, eds. Psychiatry update. American Psychiatric Association annual review. Washington, DC: American Psychiatric Press, 1985;4:361–378.

42. Mendelson WB, ed. Current strategies in the treatment of insomnia. J Clin Psychiatry 1992;53(Suppl 6):1–45.

Physiochemical and Pharmacokinetic Properties

It is sometimes said that all BZDs are essentially the same, with no major differences among them. This is misleading, however, because variations in chemical structure and pharmacokinetics profoundly influence:

- *Potency*
- *Onset and duration* of clinical activity
- Type and frequency of *adverse effects* after both single and multiple doses
- *Withdrawal* phenomena.

These differences often make it possible to select a specific drug most likely to benefit an individual patient, while minimizing the risk.

CHEMICAL STRUCTURE

Structurally, BZDs belong to one of three major subgroups:

- *1,4 BZDs* contain nitrogen atoms at positions 1 and 4 in the diazepine ring. This grouping accounts for most therapeutically important agents: bromazepam, chlordiazepoxide, clonazepam, chlorazepate, diazepam, flunitrazepam, flurazepam, lorazepam, lormetazepam, medazolam, nitrazepam, oxazepam, prazepam, quazepam, and temazepam.
- *1,5 BZDs* contain nitrogen atoms at positions 1 and 5 in the diazepam ring. Clobazam is a member of this subgroup.
- *Tricyclic BZDs* often consist of the 1,4 BZD nucleus with an additional ring fused at positions 1 and 2. Members of this subgroup are alprazolam, lorprazolam, midazolam, and triazolam.

In addition to these BZDs, another group of diazepines features replacement of the fused benzene ring with other heteroaromatic systems, such as thieno or pyrazolo. Most compounds of this type are under investigation, with the thienodiazepine brotizolam a currently available example. Because pharmacologic effects of this group are comparable to the BZDs, both classes of diazepines are considered "benzodiazepines" from a clinical standpoint.

PHARMACOKINETICS

Lipid Solubility

The more lipid-soluble the BZD, the more readily it passes from the plasma through the lipophilic blood-brain barrier, and thus the more rapid its onset of action. BZDs can be subdivided on the basis of lipophilicity—a factor that plays an important role in absorption. Midazolam, quazepam, and diazepam are among the more lipophilic of the BZDs. Because increasing lipophilicity also increases the rate of redistribution from blood and brain into adipose tissue, BZDs that are less lipophilic may have more persistent brain concentrations due to reduced peripheral distribution (1, 2).

Absorption

BZDs with rapid absorption produce a more rapid onset of clinical activity than those with slower absorption. BZDs given orally differ in their speed of absorption from the gastrointestinal tract. For example, absorption time is 0.5 hour for clorazepate, 1 hour for diazepam, 1.3 hours for triazolam, 2 hours for alprazolam and lorazepam, 2 to 3 hours for oxazepam, and

3.6 hours for flurazepam. Absorption, however, may be influenced by the presence or absence of food in the gastrointestinal tract. Thus, patients who take a BZD hypnotic with a bedtime snack may experience a slower onset of hypnotic activity than if the same drug were taken several hours after a meal.

Metabolism/Elimination

BZDs biotransformed by hepatic oxidation have relatively long half-lives and usually have active metabolites (see Table 12.4). Those biotransformed by glucuronide conjugation have relatively short half-lives and no active metabolites. Only a few BZDs (e.g., clonazepam) are biotransformed by nitroreduction. Although oxidized BZDs and their metabolites may be more likely to accumulate due to age, liver disease, or concomitant use of estrogens or cimetidine, clinical data substantiating this theory are incomplete.

Based on elimination half-life, BZDs can be divided into three groups:

- *Ultrashort-acting* (< 5 hours), such as midazolam, triazolam, and brotizolam
- *Short-to-intermediate* acting (6–12

hours), such as oxazepam, bromazepam, lorazepam, loprazolam, temazepam, lormetazepam, and alprazolam
- *Long-acting* (>12 hrs), such as flunitrazepam, clobazam, flurazepam, clorazepate, ketazolam, chlordiazepoxide, and diazepam.

Onset and duration of BZD clinical activity are not necessarily related to elimination half-life. When given in single doses, BZDs with long half-lives may have a shorter duration of action than BZDs with short(er) half-lives because of extensive distribution. During multiple dosing, however, BZDs with longer half-lives accumulate slowly, and after termination of treatment disappear slowly; whereas BZDs with short half-lives have minimal accumulation and disappear rapidly when treatment stops (3).

Potency

BZDs differ considerably in potency, which refers to the milligram dose needed to produce a given clinical effect. These differences are in part due to differences in receptor site affinity. If given in the appropriate dose, any BZD may exert anxiolytic, hypnotic, and anticonvulsant effects. For

Table 12.4.
Benzodiazepine Anxiolytics

Name (Proprietary Name)	Metabolism	Half-Life Including Metabolites (hours)	Lipid Solubility	Active Metabolites
Alprazolam (Xanax)	Oxidation	8–15	Moderate	No
Bromazepam[a]	Oxidation	20–30	Low	No
Chlordiazepoxide (Librium)	Oxidation	10–20	Moderate	Yes
Clobazam[a]	Oxidation	20–30	Moderate	Yes
Clorazepate (Tranxene)	Oxidation	40–100	—	Yes
Diazepam (Valium)	Oxidation	20–70	High	Yes
Halazepam (Paxipam)	Oxidation	40–100	Low	Yes
Lorazepam (Ativan)	Conjugation	10–20	Moderate	No
Oxazepam (Serax)	Conjugation	5–15	Moderate	No
Prazepam (Centrax)	Oxidation	40–100	Low	Yes

[a]Not available in the United States.

example, anxiolytic benzodiazepines, such as clorazepate and diazepam, are often used as hypnotics when anxiety is a prominent symptom associated with insomnia.

DRUG INTERACTIONS

With the important exception of additive effects when combined with other CNS depressants, including alcohol, BZDs interact with very few drugs. Disulfiram (see The Alcoholic Patient in Chapter 14) and cimetidine may increase BZD blood levels, and diazepam may increase blood levels of digoxin and phenytoin. Antacids may reduce the clinical effects of clorazepate by hindering its biotransformation to desmethyldiazepam. There is also a possibility that coadministration of a BZD and another drug known to induce seizures may increase seizure risk, especially if the BZD is abruptly withdrawn.

CONCLUSION

As reviewed and emphasized in Chapter 3, the physical and pharmacokinetic properties of various psychotropics, including the BZDs, often have clinically relevant implications. This realization can serve to enhance efficacy and/or minimize adverse effects. Thus, while ignorance of these properties may put patients at unnecessary risk, a working knowledge of these issues can often produce an ideal clinical outcome.

REFERENCES

1. Greenblatt DJ, Shader RI, Abernethy DR. Current status of benzodiazepines (1). N Engl J Med 1983;309:354–358.
2. Greenblatt DJ. Benzodiazepine hypnotics. Sorting the pharmacokinetic facts. J Clin Psychiatry 1991;52(9, Suppl):4–10.
3. Greenblatt DJ, Shader RI. Pharmacokinetics of antianxiety agents. In: Meltzer HY, ed. Psychopharmacology: the third generation of progress. New York: Raven Press, 1987:1377–1386.

Adverse Effects of Anxiolytics

Relative to other psychotropics, acute BZD treatment is associated with fewer unwanted effects. Sedation is usually the most prominent initial complication, subsiding in about a week as anxiolytic action emerges (1). Confusion, ataxia, excitement, agitation, transient hypotension, vertigo, and gastrointestinal distress may also occur in a small number of patients.

BEHAVIORAL DISINHIBITION

A possible association between the clinical use of a BZD and aggressive behavior was reported not long after chlordiazepoxide first became available for prescription (2). Since then, numerous case reports and studies have suggested that some BZD-treated patients experience increased hostility and aggressiveness, ranging from feelings to overt behavior. A recent literature review found that the phenomenon is difficult to characterize because it may include various manifestations, including:

- Hostility
- Aggressiveness
- Rage reactions
- Paroxysmal excitement
- Irritability
- Behavioral dyscontrol (3).

Nevertheless, the reviewers reported that no variable (e.g., pretreatment hostility, severity of anxiety, length of treatment, dose) was consistently predictive of hostility/aggressiveness. In addition, patients with a history of character disorder, aggressive behavior, or substance abuse are not more likely to experience aggressive dyscontrol during BZD treatment; and indeed, there are numerous reports of such patients experiencing no adverse consequences (4, 5). **Based on BZD efficacy studies that reported adverse effects, the reviewers estimated the incidence of aggressive dyscontrol to be less than 1%—comparable to that of placebo. The incidence of overt rage reactions appears to be even lower.**

OVERDOSE

Fatalities due to acute BZD overdose alone are extremely rare. Even with ingestion of massive doses, recovery appears to be rapid and without serious complications or aftereffects (6–9). Combined ingestion of BZDs with other CNS depressants (alcohol, barbiturates, narcotics, or tricyclic antidepressants), however, may result in severe CNS and respiratory depression or hypotension (6–8). Severity of symptoms appears to depend more on the type and quantity of the other drug(s) than on the BZD plasma level (6, 8).

PSYCHOMOTOR IMPAIRMENT

Numerous studies of acute and chronic dosing in normal volunteers and anxious patients indicate that BZDs may impair certain types of psychomotor functioning, such as coordination and sustained attention. These studies have produced conflicting results however, particularly in anxious subjects or those on chronic dosing. Some patients have exhibited few or no decrements, and it has been postulated that by reducing anxiety (which itself can

impair functioning), a BZD may paradoxically improve performance. Several studies have found, however, that drivers taking a BZD are at increased risk for a serious automobile accident (10–13). In addition, the combination of therapeutic doses of a BZD and even a small amount of alcohol may produce significant psychomotor decrements that are greater than would be expected with either substance alone (i.e., a synergistic effect).

COGNITIVE IMPAIRMENT

It has been known for almost three decades that even single doses of BZDs impair cognitive function. It also has been demonstrated that psychological impairment occurs in normal subjects and after short courses of treatment in anxious patients (14). In a study designed to establish whether ability is impaired in long-term BZD users, as well as to determine the nature and extent of any deficit, investigators assessed a wide range of cognitive functions using a battery of neuropsychological tests (15). **They found that patients taking high therapeutic doses for long periods of time performed poorly on tasks involving visual-spatial ability and sustained attention, implying that these individuals may not be functioning well in everyday life. Test results also indicated that subjects were not aware of their reduced ability.** This is consistent with clinical evidence provided by patients who after discontinuing a BZD often report improved concentration and increased sensory perception. Further, it was only after stopping the drug that they realized their functioning was below par (16).

Case Example. A 44-year-old tenured graduate school professor, after several years of analytically oriented psychotherapy, became dissatisfied with the persistence of his GAD symptoms. He persuaded his therapist to prescribe an anxiolytic for him, beginning with diazepam, 2 mg twice daily. Because of only minimal relief the diazepam dose was increased first to 5 mg bid and ultimately to 10 mg tid. This daily dose effectively alleviated the patient's more distressing GAD symptoms. For the next year and a half the patient took between 25 and 35 mg daily, as he attempted to adjust dose commensurate with his perceived need to be symptom-controlled. During this time his wife observed that he seemed "slowed down" at times, even though he worked regularly and was otherwise "the same as ever, only less anxious." His therapist, who saw him once monthly during this period, also thought that he was less anxious and improved and "doing well" on his maintenance diazepam regimen. The therapist's monitoring of the patient's diazepam prescriptions and refills did not suggest any overuse of this drug.

Everyone was surprised when school officials informed the patient of student complaints about a decline in his teaching performance. The patient indignantly challenged these allegations, insisting that he was not aware of any change in his teaching. Upon the insistence of school officials, however, the patient saw a second psychiatrist in consultation. Although the patient did not seem "drugged," various performance tests were ordered. These disclosed some cognitive impairment that the psychologist considered drug-induced. A tapered discontinuation of diazepam over a 3-month period to a maintenance dose of 5 mg bid resulted in a marked change in the patient. He became more alert and more active, and his teaching more dynamic and effective. His family was pleased with the transformation to his "old self." The patient acknowledged the change in himself, but continued to insist that he was unaware of the adverse drug-induced effects on his cognitive functions.

Similar findings were reported in a study of elderly patients, in whom the onset of cognitive impairment was often insidious, became evident only after years of treatment, and improved with drug discontinuation (17). In a study comparing chronic pain patients receiving no medica-

tion, narcotics alone, or BZDs alone, the last group was significantly more likely to exhibit signs of cognitive impairment and concomitant EEG changes than those treated with narcotics (18).

CT Studies

The demonstration of structural brain abnormalities in conjunction with cognitive impairment in those who have abused alcohol for prolonged periods prompted Lader et al. to ascertain if this could be true in long-term BZD users, some of whom had detectable cognitive impairment during drug withdrawal (19, 20). Brain CT scans were done on 20 patients, none of whom abused alcohol or took other drugs but were receiving or had recently discontinued long-term (2–20 year) BZD treatment. Their scans were then compared with those of age- and sex-matched normal controls, as well as chronic alcoholics. In some of the BZD patients the mean ventricular to brain ratio measured by planimetry was increased over the mean values of the control subjects, although it was less than that in the alcoholics. There was no significant relationship between CT scan appearance, age, or the duration of BZD therapy.

Schmauss and Krieg subsequently confirmed these findings in 17 BZD-dependent inpatients who reported no history of other types of chemical dependency, including abuse of alcohol (21). Brain CT scans before drug withdrawal revealed a significantly higher ventricular to brain ratio (VBR) in those dependent on high *and* low doses compared to matched controls. Further, the mean VBR was significantly higher in the high- than in the low-dose-dependent patients, suggesting a dose-dependent effect. Neither age nor duration of use accounted for the observed differences in the VBR values.

Uhde and Kellner reported a positive correlation between duration of BZD exposure and VBR in their study of panic patients, 19 of whom reported being treated with a BZD for a mean of 3.6 years (range was 0.5–12 years) (22). Noting that 70% of their sample was composed of subjects with less than 2.5 years of BZD treatment, they speculated that the lack of association between VBR and duration of BZD use in the Lader et al. study might be related to exclusion of subjects within the lower range of drug exposure.

The clinical significance of these CT scan alterations is unknown, and it is important to note that two similar studies found no statistically significant differences between the CT scans of long-term BZD users and matched controls (23, 24). Poser et al. did find, however, that patients with combined BZD-alcohol dependence showed some degree of cerebral atrophy (23). Uhde and Kellner also observed that the apparent association between VBR and duration of BZD exposure may be secondary to alcohol consumption, because long-term BZD users also may be more frequent users, but not necessarily abusers, of alcohol (22).

WITHDRAWAL PHENOMENA

During the past decade awareness of the capacity of all BZDs to produce dependence and evoke withdrawal symptoms has increased markedly. Although some studies have found little or no evidence, there is now a large body of data indicating that continuous use of a BZD, even at therapeutic doses, will result in withdrawal symptoms in some patients (25, 26). **It also has been reasonably well established that the longer a BZD is taken, even in therapeutic doses, the greater the likelihood of withdrawal reactions when it is discontinued, especially abruptly** (27).

The most commonly reported withdrawal symptoms include:

- Various *gastrointestinal* symptoms
- *Diaphoresis*
- Tremor; lethargy; dizziness; *headaches*
- Increased *acuity* for sound and smell
- *Restlessness;* insomnia; irritability; anxiety
- *Tinnitus*
- Feelings of *depersonalization.*

These are usually described as mild in intensity and fairly short in duration (i.e., a few days to a few weeks). None are considered life-threatening or permanently debilitating and, with the exception of the relatively rare occurrence of seizures, delirium, and/or psychosis, are thought to be readily managed.

In some patients, however, discontinuation, whether abrupt or gradual, may evoke highly distressing symptoms, including:

- Severe and prolonged *depression* (28, 29)
- *Hallucinations* (28, 30–32)
- Protracted *tinnitus* (30, 33)
- Opisthotonos, choreoathetosis, myoclonus, and bizarre *involuntary muscular movements* (34–36)
- *Delirium* with catatonic features (37)
- *Panic* and agoraphobia (28, 30, 38).

There are also reports indicating that in some patients withdrawal may be painful and protracted, possibly lasting 6 months to 1 year (28, 30, 39). Ashton, noting that her withdrawal patients were usually frightened, often in intense pain, and genuinely prostrated, stated, "The severity and duration of the illness are easily underestimated by medical and nursing staff, who tend to dismiss the symptoms as 'neurotic.' " (30). Chouinard has observed that rebound anxiety can be so severe the patient believes he or she is going to die (40).

Withdrawal symptoms are unlikely to occur before 3 to 4 months of continuous use of a BZD. Early indications of dependence have been noted, however, with reports of withdrawal symptoms after only 6 weeks of continuous use, particularly with the short-acting agents such as alprazolam (41–47).

Recent evidence also supports a clinically significant rebound/withdrawal phenomena between doses of alprazolam, sometimes referred to as "interdose" or "breakthrough" symptoms (48, 49). Mellor and Jain raised the possibility that some long-term diazepam users may be subject to a similar phenomenon:

> Patients receiving long-term diazepam treatment who complain of episodes of anxiety may be suffering from intermittent withdrawal symptoms. Characteristically, such patients have reduced their dose of diazepam after being symptom-free for a period. A week or so later their condition apparently recurs, so the previous dose is resumed and they obtain relief. Sometimes the dose of the drug has not changed, yet the symptoms reappear, causing the dose to be raised until they disappear (31).

SEIZURES

Although rare, seizures may occur after the abrupt discontinuation of both high and therapeutic doses of any BZD. Some researchers have suggested that short-acting drugs are associated with increased seizure risk when compared to longer-acting compounds, but this is difficult to evaluate due to the relatively small number of published case reports and inherent problems in assessing anecdotal data. A review of the reports on lorazepam and oxazepam, however, found that in almost all cases patients had stopped the drug abruptly and that at least one (and often more than one) of the following factors was present:

- *High dose*
- *Extended duration* of use (4 months to years)
- Concomitant or immediately subsequent ingestion of *other drugs associated with seizure* induction
- *History of seizures* (50).

Published case reports on alprazolam show a slightly different profile (51–54). Four patients had taken the drug for 4.5 months or less; one had also taken chlorpromazine and trazodone; and a fifth patient had taken alprazolam (3 mg/day for 26 weeks) and phenelzine (45 mg/day for 13 weeks), abruptly stopping both. According to the Food and Drug Administration's Spontaneous Adverse Event Reporting System, more seizures have been reported with alprazolam than with all other BZDs combined (55). The next highest incidence was reported for lorazepam. The Food and Drug Administration report stated that:

- Most alprazolam seizures were in connection with *high-dose therapy*
- Dose/duration data suggest occurrence at therapeutic doses with *chronic therapy* and a *shortened time* until risk when higher doses are used
- Although some seizures occurred during stable alprazolam therapy, they often occurred with *concomitant administration* of a drug that may also lower seizure threshold, such as maprotiline (see also The Seizure-Prone Patient in Chapter 14).
- With intentional taper, most seizures occurred *at or near the end.*

According to the report, reasons for excess seizure reports for alprazolam may include specific drug effect, higher degree of manufacturer surveillance, and higher doses used. This last issue may be due to this agent's reported efficacy and increasing use in panic disorder, which usually requires higher doses for longer periods.

DISCONTINUING TREATMENT

Short-Term Treatment

Although gradual discontinuation is generally thought to lessen the occurrence and/or intensity of withdrawal symptoms, rebound/withdrawal phenomena may still occur with slow tapering, even in patients who have taken a BZD for only a few weeks. **Rickels et al., reporting on a study of clorazepate and lorazepam, warned physicians not to mistakenly attribute a substantial return of symptoms that occurs early after BZD discontinuation as a recurrence of original symptoms necessitating further treatment** (42). They added, "Such guidelines are important for clinical practice because the few patients who experience rebound anxiety after only weeks of therapy and who resume medication needlessly may represent the very patients who become chronic users."

Long-Term Treatment

Abrupt discontinuation of long-term use of therapeutic doses is likely to result in withdrawal symptoms (42a). In a study of the effects of abrupt discontinuation of short and long half-life BZDs in long-term users, Rickels et al. found that:

- A withdrawal syndrome *occurred in the majority* of patients
- The withdrawal syndrome *occurred earlier and was more severe for short half-life* (alprazolam, lorazepam) than for long half-life drugs (diazepam, clorazepate)
- *Factors contributing* to greater withdrawal severity included short half-life,

higher daily dose, greater state and trait psychopathology, and lower educational level

- Only 73% of long half-life and 43% of short half-life BZD-treated patients were *able to remain drug-free for 1 week*
- At 5 weeks, only 45% of long half-life and 38% of short half-life BZD-treated patients were still *drug-free* (56).

Although gradual dose reduction may ameliorate the intensity of withdrawal symptoms after long-term therapeutic use of BZDs, mild to moderate symptoms are still likely to occur. In a companion study to the one just cited, the same group of investigators reported that almost 90% of short and long half-life BZD-treated patients experienced some withdrawal symptoms despite gradual dosage taper (25% per week) (57). They also reported that:

- 32% of long half-life and 42% of short half-life BZD-patients were *unable to tolerate taper* and either continued or resumed daily drug use
- Unlike the abrupt discontinuation study, *severity and time course of withdrawal symptoms were similar* for both short and long half-life agents
- Factors contributing to greater withdrawal severity included female sex, higher Eysenck *neuroticism*, and higher *alcohol* intake
- At 5 weeks, 56% of long half-life and 53% of short half-life BZD-treated patients were still *BZD-free*.

These findings indicate that, despite the likelihood of withdrawal symptoms with both abrupt and gradual discontinuation, gradual taper may lessen the incidence and intensity of symptoms, particularly in patients taking a short half-life compound.

Nevertheless, gradual withdrawal may

still be difficult. Schweizer et al. found that although the initial 50% dose reduction was characterized by minimal withdrawal severity and could be accomplished fairly rapidly, the majority of symptoms occurred during the last half of tapering process (57). Tyrer made a similar observation, stating that "withdrawal symptoms may develop only when patients have reduced to what many clinicians would regard as subtherapeutic doses, and the difficulty that patients have in withdrawing from this dose cannot be explained only by psychological dependence" (58). Schweizer et al. also concluded that dose reduction of 25% per week may be too rapid for many long-term users (57). In their study, 51% of patients were unable to tolerate that schedule and required an even more gradual taper.

Thus, with most BZDs, the rate of reduction may be fairly rapid down to about 50% of the original dose. Subsequent decreases should be slower (e.g., 10–20% of the new dose at 3- to 5-day intervals). For patients who become increasingly anxious as their dose is being decreased, **use of a plateau period** in which no further tapering occurs may allow them to relax, adjust to the lower dose, and then resume the gradual discontinuation process. Plateau periods also allow clinicians to assess whether anxiety that emerges during dose reduction is due to withdrawal or a recrudescence of an underlying anxiety disorder. Withdrawal anxiety lessens over time, whereas symptoms of an anxiety disorder worsen.

Alprazolam requires a very extended and gradual taper (49, 59, 60). The package insert suggests that "the daily dose be decreased not more than 0.5 mg every three days." According to this recommendation, if a patient has been treated with alprazolam 10 mg daily (a dose not uncommon for severe panic disorders), it would take at least 60 days to wean the patient off alprazolam. Some long-term alprazolam users, however, may require 0.25 mg decrements as far apart as every 4 to 7 days. Following this schedule, the patient taking alprazolam 10 mg daily would require up to 6 months to discontinue the drug (see Figure 13.1 in Chapter 13 for a suggested tapering schedule).

Lorazepam, also reported difficult to discontinue in some patients, has been associated with higher dropout rates and more severe withdrawal phenomena than longer-acting BZDs (61, 62). Ashton noted that patients taking lorazepam experienced drug-craving (feeling they could not get through the day without their tablets) before being switched to diazepam for BZD discontinuation (30).

Other than slow taper, no consistently effective treatment to alleviate withdrawal symptoms has been reported. Although several compounds have been studied (e.g., β-blockers, clonidine, carbamazepine), results have been contradictory. **Carbamazepine, however, may be useful in seizure-prone patients** (63). Valproic acid has also been reported to benefit patients with BZD discontinuation after long-term dependence (63a). This may be related to VPA's potential anxiolytic properties, its ability to alleviate withdrawal phenomena, or both. The azaspirone anxiolytic buspirone has been reported ineffective in suppressing withdrawal symptoms, particularly in long-term BZD users (64, 65).

To manage withdrawal insomnia, Rickels et al. recommend the supplemental use of hypnotics, such as diphenhydramine, doxylamine, chloral hydrate, or a sedating tricyclic antidepressant such as doxepin (63). These investigators also recommend that chronic BZD users with evidence of depression or panic be treated with adequate doses of an appropriate antidepressant, a management technique that may help patients succeed in discontinuation.

Conclusion

All patients should be instructed to adhere to their physician's gradual discontinuation program and not be swayed by well-meaning but ill-informed friends or relatives who may urge a "cold turkey" approach. The clinician also must recognize the particular susceptibilities of each patient and be willing to provide reassurance, encouragement, and information about symptoms, both in the early stages of discontinuation and for a prolonged follow-up period. As Farid and Bulto have observed: "Patients who have been on these drugs for longer periods need more sensitive handling, and with some of them it may take months if not years to wean them off their benzodiazepines.... The difficulty we face is not long-term prescribing of benzodiazepines but rather too quick a reduction of the prescribed dose with little other form of help being offered" (66).

Adverse Effects of Sedative-Hypnotics

Miscellaneous adverse effects reported with the various BZD hypnotics are listed in Table 12.5.

SEDATION AND CNS DEPRESSION

Although some studies have reported that sleep-deprived people are impaired in their daytime functioning, others have found that in patients with chronic insomnia sleep loss is actually slight, excessive daytime sleepiness is rare, and daytime performance is normal (67–71). Whether BZDs enhance daytime performance by reducing loss of sleep is in fact unknown. Many studies, however, indicate that they impair rather than improve next-day performance, and a review of those studies using performance and vigilance tests concluded that BZDs with short half-lives induce longer-lasting impairment than those with long half-lives due to the extensive distribution of the latter (72). **In general, the adverse effects of BZD hypnotics are dose-dependent, with higher doses tending to produce greater decrements than lower doses (73–79).**

BZDs with active metabolites and slow elimination, such as diazepam, flurazepam, and quazepam, are well known for producing unwanted daytime sedation (80–82). Nevertheless, other studies have found no or inconsistent residual impairment with lower doses of flurazepam and quazepam (73, 79, 80, 82–86). There is some evidence that quazepam (15 mg or 30 mg) may have a lower potential than the same dosages of flurazepam for producing daytime somnolence and residual impairment (79). Excessive daytime CNS depression, however, may occur with all BZDs, including those with short and intermediate half-lives (74, 81, 87). In a review of 45 double-blind, controlled trials, CNS depression (drowsiness, dizziness, fatigue, light-headedness, and incoordination) was the most frequent adverse effect of triazolam, occurring in 14.2% of patients receiving 0.25 mg and in 19.5% of those receiving 0.5 mg. (74). CNS effects also

Table 12.5.
Miscellaneous Adverse Effects Reported with Benzodiazepine Hypnotics

Estazolam	Flurazepam	Quazepam	Temazepam	Triazolam
Hypokinesia	Headache	Headache	GI disturbances	Headache
Headache	Paresthesias	Fatigue	Sleep disturbances	Paresthesias
Asthenia	Dizziness	Dry mouth	Visual	Visual
Nausea	Tinnitus	Dyspepsia	disturbances	disturbances
Nervousness	Bad taste in mouth		Weakness	Visual
Dizziness	Dry mouth		Lack of	disturbances
Lethargy	GI disturbances		concentration	Tinnitus
Dysphoria	Sleep disturbances		Loss of	GI disturbances
	Dermatologic		equilibrium	
	problems		Falling	

may be frequent with temazepam and estazolam (88–92).

CNS STIMULATION

With short-acting agents, such as triazolam, there have been numerous reports of increased daytime anxiety and early morning insomnia (93–101). Because these are the opposite of the intended therapeutic effect, they may not be attributed to the drug and may actually reinforce its use. CNS stimulation has been reported in 2.8% of patients given flurazepam, 30 mg (74).

BEHAVIORAL EFFECTS

Short-term use of triazolam has been associated with serious behavioral adverse effects, including:

- Confusion
- Psychotic-like symptoms
- Disinhibition
- Amnesia (81, 93, 94, 98, 102–109).

Memory impairment or entire periods of amnesia and automatic behavior have been reported with single doses of triazolam the day after its nighttime use (110–114). Amnesia has been reported with lorazepam and

other BZDs, but appears to be considerably more problematic with triazolam (87, 115–121). In a recent controlled study, for example, triazolam produced a 40% rate of next-day memory impairment/amnesia, although no episodes occurred with temazepam (114). Although behavioral adverse effects also have been reported for temazepam, FDA statistics indicate that for hostility reactions reported on 329 drugs, triazolam ranks first (109, 122). Analysis of individual cases reported to the Spontaneous Reporting System of the United States Food and Drug Administration for such symptoms as amnesia, confusion, bizarre behavior, agitation and hallucinations found that rates for triazolam were 22 to 99 times higher than those for temazepam (123). Even when reports involving triazolam dosages above 0.5 mg or other contributing factors were excluded, reporting rates for triazolam were still 4 to 26 times greater. This could, however, be partly due to the publicity in the media regarding this phenemenon.

Case History. A 56-year-old engineer consulted his family physician because of progressive fatigue of 3 months' duration. Aside from moderate obesity (176 pounds) and slight hypertension (145/90), the physical examination was negative. Urinalysis detected 2+ glycosuria. Blood chemistries were normal except for 285 blood glucose level. Further workup confirmed early adult onset diabetes. After being informed of his diagnosis, the patient developed distressing middle insomnia and a worsening of his fatigue. His physician advised a tropical vacation and prescribed triazolam (0.25 mg) at bedtime. On the first night of his vacation the patient took his first dose and retired early. Two days later he "woke up," that is, "I became aware of myself and my surroundings but I couldn't remember what I had done since I arrived in the Bahamas and took that sleeping pill."

Frightened by his amnesia, the patient returned home worried that he might have a more serious problem than "just diabetes." He told his physician he was afraid of "losing my mind." A complete physical, neurological, and psychiatric evaluation only confirmed the patient's diabetes. He was therefore diagnosed as having a triazolam-induced anterograde amnesia. The patient was reassured that he had an iatrogenic reaction and advised not to take triazolam.

DISCONTINUING TREATMENT

Rebound Insomnia

Even after relatively short periods of administration, discontinuation of short and intermediate half-life BZDs such as triazolam and temazepam may result in marked worsening of sleep, even worse than baseline levels (i.e., rebound insomnia) (80, 96, 115, 124–142). Gradual dose reduction may attenuate the incidence of rebound, and with flurazepam and quazepam, there is little sleep disturbance following even abrupt drug withdrawal (73, 75, 125, 126, 143–151).

Although one study of long-term BZD hypnotic use found no increase in insomnia after abrupt discontinuation of a variety of BZDs, a withdrawal syndrome consisting of inability to fall asleep and disruption of sleep may occur (132, 152, 153). Time of

onset may vary according to the drug's rate of elimination (154).

Syncope and Inflammatory Reactions

Triazolobenzodiazepines differ from other BZDs in being potent and specific inhibitors of the binding of platelet-activating factor (PAF) to its receptor (155). Noting that initial reports of serious adverse effects associated with triazolam included blistering of hands, feet, and tongue, some authors have speculated that effects on PAF mechanisms may account for the higher incidence of certain unusual withdrawal symptoms noted with these drugs (156, 157). They state that disturbance of PAF (a potent hypotensive agent) mechanisms could explain the association of triazolam with syncope, and added this problem to the United States package insert for 1990. In addition, they counted all adverse reactions suggesting inflammation or altered micropermeability reported to the United States Food and Drug Administration's Spontaneous Reporting System since the introduction of temazepam, flurazepam, and triazolam. Reactions including pharyngitis, glossitis, vasculitis, asthma, and facial edema totaled 31 for temazepam, 78 for flurazepam, and 673 for triazolam.

Seizures, Psychotic Reactions

Seizures have been reported after withdrawal of high doses of triazolam or relatively low doses combined with alcohol (158–160). The United States Food and Drug Administration has reported "a signal of an association" for withdrawal seizures associated with triazolam (161). In a chart review of 150 consecutive patients withdrawn from BZDs, 3 of 25 triazolam patients experienced seizures, compared to 2 of 125 given other BZDs (162). Psychosis with delirium also has been reported after discontinuation of high triazolam doses (163).

CONCLUSION

Although the BZD hypnotics are a significant advance over their predecessors in terms of safety, they also carry their own risks (164). In particular, the shorter acting agents may predispose patients to such complications as rebound anxiety, insomnia, amnesia, paradoxical disinhibition, and seizures with abrupt discontinuation. Coupled with the evidence that long-term benefit beyond 12 weeks is unproven, careful, time-limited, intermittent prescribing is the only reasonable management strategy.

REFERENCES

1. File SE, Pellow S. Behavioral pharmacology of minor tranquilizers. Pharmacol Ther 1987;35:265–290.
2. Ingram IM, Timbury GC. Side effects of librium. Lancet 1960;ii:766.
3. Dietch JT, Jennings RK. Aggressive dyscontrol in patients treated with benzodiazepines. J Clin Psychiatry 1988;49:184–188.
4. Lion JR. Benzodiazepines in the treatment of aggressive patients. J Clin Psychiatry 1979;40:70–71.
5. Kalina RK. Diazepam: its role in the prison setting. Dis Nerv Sys 1964;25:101–107.
6. Greenblatt DJ, Allen MD, Noel BJ, Shader RI. Special article: Acute overdosage with benzodiazepine derivatives. Clin Pharmacol Ther 1977;21:497.
7. Jatlow P, Dobular K, Bailey D. Serum diazepam concentrations in overdose. Their significance. Am J Clin Pathol 1979;72(4):571–577.
8. Divoll M, Greenblatt DJ, Lacasse Y, Shader RI. Benzodiazepine overdosage: plasma concentrations and clinical outcome. Psychopharmacology (Berlin) 1981;73:381–383.
9. Greenblatt DJ, Woo E, Allen MD, Orsulak PJ, Shader RI. Rapid recovery from massive diazepam overdose. JAMA 1978;240(17):1872–1874.
10. Bo O, Hafner O, Langard O, Trumpy JH, Bredesen J, Lunde PKM. Ethanol and diazepam as causative agents in road accidents. In: Iraelstam S, Lambert S, eds. Alcohol, drugs, and traffic safety. Toronto: Addiction Research Foundation of Ontario, 1975.
11. Skegg DCG, Richards SM, Doll R. Minor tranquilizers and road accidents. Br Med J 1979;i:917–919.
12. Warren R. Drugs detected in fatally injured drivers in the province of Ontario. In: Goldberg L, ed. Alcohol, drugs, and traffic safety. Vol 1. Stockholm: Almquist and Wiksell, 1981.
13. O'Hanlon JF, Haak TW, Blaauw GJ, Riemersma JBJ. Diazepam impairs lateral position control in highway driving. Science 1982;217:79–81.
14. McNair DM. Anti-anxiety drugs and human performance. Arch Gen Psychiatry 1973;29:609–617.
15. Golombok S, Moodley P, Lader M. Cognitive impairment in long-term benzodiazepine users. Psychol Med 1988;18:365–374.
16. Petursson H, Gudjonsson GH, Lader MH. Psychosomatic performance during withdrawal from long-term benzodiazepine treatment. Psychopharmacology 1983;81:345–349.
17. Larson E, Kukull WA, Buchner D, Reifler BV. Adverse drug reactions associated with global cognitive impairment in elderly persons. Ann Intern Med 1987;107:169–173.
18. Hendler N, Cimini C, Ma T, Long D. A comparison of cognitive impairment due to benzodiazepines and to narcotics. Am J Psychiatry 1980;137:828–830.
19. Ron M. The alcoholic brain: CT scan and psychological findings. Psychol Med Monograph (suppl 3). Cambridge: Cambridge University Press, 1983.
20. Lader MH, Ron M, Petursson H. Computed axial brain tomography in long-term benzodiazepine users. Psychol Med 1984;14:203–206.
21. Schmauss C, Krieg JC. Enlargement of cerebrospinal fluid spaces in long-term benzodiazepine users. Psychol Med 1987;17:869–873.
22. Uhde TW, Kellner CH. Cerebral ventricular size in panic disorder. J Affective Disord 1987;12:175–178.
23. Poser W, Poser S, Roscher D, Argyrakis A. Do benzodiazepines cause cerebral atrophy [Letter]. Lancet 1983;i:715.

24. Perera KMH, Powell T, Jenner FA. Computerized axial tomographic studies following long-term use of benzodiazepines. Psychol Med 1987;17:775–777.

25. Bowden CL, Fisher JG. Safety and efficacy of long-term diazepam therapy. South Med J 1980;73:1581–1584.

26. Laughren TP, Battey Y, Greenblatt DJ, Harrop DS III. A controlled trial of diazepam withdrawal in chronically anxious outpatients. Acta Psychiatr Scand 1982;65:171–179.

27. American Psychiatric Association. Benzodiazepine dependence, toxicity, and abuse. Washington, D.C.: American Psychiatric Association, 1990.

28. Ashton H. Benzodiazepine withdrawal: outcome in 50 patients. Br J Addiction 1987;82:665–671.

29. Olajide D, Lader M. Depression following withdrawal from long-term benzodiazepine use: a report of four cases. Psychol Med 1984;14:937–940.

30. Ashton H. Benzodiazepine withdrawal: an unfinished story. Br Med J 1984;288:1135–1140.

31. Mellor CS, Jain VK, Diazepam withdrawal syndrome. Its prolonged and changing nature. Can Med Assoc J 1982;127:1093–1096.

32. Schmauss C, Apelt S, Emrich HM. Characterization of benzodiazepine withdrawal in high- and low-dose dependent psychiatric inpatients. Brain Res Bull 1987;19:393–400.

33. Busto U, Fornazzari L, Naranjo CA. Protracted tinnitus after discontinuation of long-term therapeutic use of benzodiazepines. J Clin Psychopharmacol 1988;5:359–362.

34. Speirs CJ, Navey FL, Brooks DJ, Impallomeni MG. Opisthotonos and benzodiazepine withdrawal in the elderly. Lancet 1986;ii:1101.

35. O'Flaherty S, Evans M, Epps A, Buchanan N. Choreoathetosis and clonazepam [Letter]. Med J Australia 1985;142(8):453.

36. Rapport DJ, Covington EG. Motor phenomena in benzodiazepine withdrawal. Hosp Comm Psychiatry 1989;40:1277–1279.

37. Hauser P, Devinsky O, De Bellis M, Theodore WH, Post RM. Benzodiazepine withdrawal delirium with catatonic features. Occurrence in patients with partial seizure disorder. Arch Neurol 1989;46:696–699.

38. Arana GW, Epstein S, Molloy M, Greenblatt DJ. Carbamazepine-induced reduction of plasma alprazolam concentrations: a clinical case report. J Clin Psychiatry 1988;49:448–449.

39. Higgitt AC, Lader MH, Fonagy P. Clinical management of benzodiazepine dependence. Br Med J 1985;291:688–690.

40. Chouinard G. Additional comments on benzodiazepine withdrawal. Can Med Assoc J 1988;139:119–120.

41. Rickels K, Case G, Downing RW, Winokur A. Long-term diazepam therapy and clinical outcome. JAMA 1983;250:767–771.

42. Rickels K, Fox IL, Greenblatt DJ. Clorazepate and lorazepam: clinical improvement and rebound anxiety. Am J Psychiatry 1988;145:312–317.

42a. Busto V, Sellers EM, Naranjo CA, et al. Withdrawal reaction after long-term therapeutic use of benzodiazepines. N Engl J Med 1986;315:854–859.

43. Murphy SM, Owen RT, Tyrer PJ. Withdrawal symptoms after six weeks' treatment with diazepam [Letter]. Lancet 1984;ii:1389.

44. Pecknold JC, McClure DJ, Fleury D, Chang D. Benzodiazepine withdrawal effects. Prog Neuropsychopharmacol Biol Psychiatry 1982;6:517–522.

45. Power KG, Jerrom DWA, Simpson RJ, Mitchell M. Controlled study of withdrawal symptoms and rebound anxiety after six week course of diazepam for generalized anxiety. Br Med J 1985;290:1246–1248.

46. Fontaine R, Chouinard G, Annable L. Rebound anxiety in anxious patients after abrupt withdrawal of benzodiazepine treatment. Am J Psychiatry 1984;141:848–852.

47. Wells BG, Evans RL, Ereshefsky L, et al. Clinical outcome and adverse effect profile associated with concurrent administration of alprazolam and imipramine. J Clin Psychiatry 1988;49:394–399.

48. Herman JB, Rosenbaum JF, Brotman AW. The alprazolam to clonazepam switch for the treatment of panic disorder. J Clin Psychopharmacol 1987;7:175–178.

49. Rashid K, Patrissi G, Cook B. Multiple serious symptom formation with alprazolam. Presented at the Annual Meeting of the American Psychiatric Association, Montreal, 1988.

50. Ayd Jr FJ. Oxazepam: update 1989. Int Clin Psychopharmacol 1990;5:1–15.

51. Breier A, Charney DS, Nelson CJ. Seizures induced by abrupt discontinuation of

alprazolam. Am J Psychiatry 1984;141: 1606–1607.

52. Levy AB. Delirium and seizures due to abrupt alprazolam withdrawal: case report. J Clin Psychiatry 1984;45:38–39.

53. Noyes R, Perry PJ, Crowe RR, et al. Single case study: seizures following the withdrawal of alprazolam. J Nerv Ment Dis 1986;174:50–52.

54. Naylor MW, Grunhaus L, Cameron O. Single case study: myoclonic seizures after abrupt withdrawal from phenelzine and alprazolam. J Nerv Ment Dis 1987;175: 111–114.

55. Department of Health and Human Services, Public Health Service, Food and Drug Administration Center for Drugs and Biologics. Seizures associated with alprazolam. 1986.

56. Rickels K, Schweizer E, Case WG, Greenblatt DJ. Long-term therapeutic use of benzodiazepines. I. Effects of abrupt discontinuation. Arch Gen Psychiatry 1990;47:899–907.

57. Schweizer E, Rickels K, Case WG, Greenblatt DJ. Long-term therapeutic use of benzodiazepines. II. Effects of gradual taper. Arch Gen Psychiatry 1990;47:908–915.

58. Tyrer P. Dependence as a limiting factor in the clinical use of minor tranquilisers. Pharmacol Ther 1988;36:173–188.

59. Mellman TA, Uhde TW. Withdrawal syndrome with gradual tapering of alprazolam. Am J Psychiatry 1986;143:1464–1466.

60. Ayd Jr FJ. Benzodiazepine prescribing. Int Drug Ther Newsl 1989;24:41–42.

61. Kemper N, Poser W, Poser S. Benzodiazepin-abhaengigkeit. Dtsch Med Wochenschr 1980;105:1707–1712.

62. Tyrer PJ, Seivewright N. Identification and management of benzodiazepine dependence. Postgrad Med 1984;60:41–44.

63. Rickels K, Case WG, Schweizer E. Withdrawal from benzodiazepines. In: Hindmarch I, Beaumont G, Brandon S, Leonard BE, eds. Benzodiazepines: current concepts—biological, clinical and social perspectives. West Sussex: John Wiley & Sons, 1990:199–210.

63a. Apelt S, Emrich HM. Sodium valproate in benzodiazepine withdrawal. Am J Psychiatry 1990;147:950–951.

64. Schweizer E, Rickels K. Failure of buspirone to manage benzodiazepine withdrawal. Am J Psychiatry 1986;143(12): 1590–1592.

65. Jerkovich GS, Preskorn SH. Failure of buspirone to protect against lorazepam withdrawal symptoms [Letter]. JAMA 1987;258:204–205.

66. Farid BT, Bulto M. Benzodiazepine prescribing [Letter]. Lancet 1989;ii:917.

67. Linnoila M, Erwin CW, Logue PE. Efficacy and side effects of flurazepam and a combination of amobarbital and secobarbital in insomniac patients. J Clin Pharmacol 1980;20:117–123.

68. Balter MB, Uhlenhuth EH. The beneficial and adverse effects of hypnotics. J Clin Psychiatry 1991;52(suppl 7):16–23.

69. Hindmarch I. Residual effects of hypnotics: an update. J Clin Psychiatry 1991; 52(suppl 7):14–15.

70. Church MW, Johnson LC. Mood and performance of poor sleepers during repeated use of flurazepam. Psychopharmacology 1979;61:309–316.

71. Drugs and insomnia. The use of medications to promote sleep. JAMA 1984; 251:2410–2414.

72. Kaolega S. Benzodiazepines and vigilance performance: a review. Psychopharmacology 1989;91:143–156.

73. Kales A, Bixler EO, Soldatos CR, Vela-Bueno A, Jacoby J, Kales JD. Quazepam and flurazepam: long-term use and extended withdrawal. Clin Pharmacol Ther 1982;32:781–788.

74. Greenblatt DJ, Shader RI, Divoll M, Harmatz JS. Adverse reactions to triazolam, flurazepam, and placebo in controlled clinical trials. J Clin Psychiatry 1984;45:192–195.

75. Greenblatt DJ, Divoll M, Harmatz JS, MacLaughlin DS, Shader RI. Kinetics and clinical effects of flurazepam in young and elderly noninsomniacs. Clin Pharmacol Ther 1981;30:475–486.

76. Salkind MR, Silverstone T. A clinical and psychometric evaluation of flurazepam. Br J Clin Pharmacol 1975;2:223–226.

77. Johnson L, Chernik D. Sedative hypnotics and human performance. Psychopharmacology (Berlin) 1982;72:101–113.

78. Greenblatt DJ, Divoll M, Abernethy DR, Ochs HR, Shader RI. Benzodiazepine kinetics: implications for therapeutics and pharmacogeriatrics. Drug Metab Rev 1983;14:251–292.

79. Dement WC. Objective measurements of daytime sleepiness and performance comparing quazepam with flurazepam in two adult populations using the multiple sleep

latency test. J Clin Psychiatry 1991; 52(suppl 9):31–37.

80. Mitler MM, Seidel WF, van den Hoed J, Greenblatt DJ, Dement WC. Comparative hypnotic effects of flurazepam, triazolam, and placebo. A long-term simultaneous nighttime and daytime study. J Clin Psychopharmacol 1984;4:2–13.

81. Kales A, Soldatos CR, Vela-Bueno A. Clinical comparison of benzodiazepine hypnotics with short and long elimination half-lives. In: Smith DE, Wesson DR, eds. The benzodiazepines. Current standards for medical practice. Lancaster: MTP Press Ltd, 1986.

82. Bliwise D, Seidel WF, Karacan I, et al. Daytime sleepiness as a criterion in hypnotic medication trials: comparison of triazolam and flurazepam. Sleep 1983;6:156–165.

83. Ellinwood E, Linnoila M, Marsh G. Plasma concentrations in chronic insomniacs of flurazepam and midazolam during fourteen-day use and their relationship to therapeutic effects and next-day performance and mood. J Clin Psychopharmacol 1990;10(suppl):68s–75s.

84. Nikaido AM, Ellinwood EH. Comparison of the effects of quazepam and triazolam on cognitive-neuromotor performance. Psychopharmacology 1987;92:459–464.

85. Wickstrom E, Godtlibssen OB. The effects of quazepam, triazolam, flunitrazepam and placebo, alone and in combination with ethanol, on daytime sleep, memory, mood and performance. Human Psychopharmacol 1988;3:101–110.

86. Lee A, Lader M. Tolerance and rebound during and after short-term administration of quazepam, triazolam and placebo to healthy volunteers. Int J Clin Psychopharmacol 1988;3:31–47.

87. Bixler EO, Kales A, Brubaker BH, Kales JD. Adverse reactions to benzodiazepine hypnotics: spontaneous reporting systems. Pharmacology 1987;35:286–300.

88. Lamphere J, Roehrs T, Zorick F, Koshorek G, Roth T. Chronic hypnotic efficacy of estazolam. Drugs Exptl Clin Res 1986;12:687–691.

89. Heel RC, Brogden RN, Speight TM, et al. Temazepam: a review of its pharmacological properties and therapeutic efficacy as an hypnotic. Drugs 1981;21:321–340.

90. Walsh JK, Targum SD, Pegram V, et al. A multi-center clinical investigation of estazolam: short-term efficacy. Curr Ther Res 1984;36:866–874.

91. Dominguez RO, Goldstein BJ, Jacobson AF, Steinbook RM. Comparative efficacy of estazolam, flurazepam, and placebo in outpatients with insomnia. J Clin Psychiatry 1986;47:362–365.

92. Scharf MB, Roth PB, Dominguez RA, Catesby Ware J. Estazolam and flurazepam: a multi-center, placebo-controlled comparative study in outpatients with insomnia. J Clin Pharmacol 1990;40:461–467.

93. Kales A, Kales JD, Bixler EO, Scharf MB, Russek E. Hypnotic efficacy of triazolam: sleep laboratory evaluation of intermediate term effectiveness. J Clin Pharmacol 1976;16:399–406.

94. Kales A, Bixler EO, Vela-Bueno A, Soldatos CR, Niklaus DE, Manfredi RL. Comparison of short and long half-life benzodiazepine hypnotics: triazolam and quazepam. Clin Pharmacol Ther 1986;40:378–386.

95. Morgan K, Oswald I. Anxiety caused by a short-life hypnotic. Br Med J 1982; 284(6320):942.

96. Kales A, Soldatos CR, Bixler EO, Kales JD. Early morning insomnia with rapidly eliminated benzodiazepines. Science 1983;220:95–97.

97. Carskadon MA, Seidel WF, Greenblatt DJ, Dement WC. Daytime carryover of triazolam and flurazepam in elderly insomniacs. Sleep 1982;5:361–371.

98. Tan TL, Bixler EO, Kales A, Cadieux RJ, Goodman AL. Early morning insomnia, daytime anxiety, and organic mental disorder associated with triazolam. J Fam Pract 1985;20:592–594.

99. Adam K, Oswald I. Can a rapidly-eliminated hypnotic cause daytime anxiety? Pharmacopsychiatry 1989;22:115–119.

100. Moon CAL, Ankier SI, Hayes G. Early morning insomnia and daytime anxiety— a multicentre general practice study comparing loprazolam and triazolam. Br J Clin Pract 1985;Sept:352–358.

101. DeTullio PL, Kirking DM, Zacardelli DK, Kwee P. Evaluation of long-term triazolam use in an ambulatory veterans administration medical center population. DICP, The Annals of Pharmacotherapy 1989;23:290–293.

102. Poitras R. A propos d'episodes d'amnesies anterogrades associes a l'utilisation du triazolam. Union Med Can 1980;109:427–429.

103. Shader RI, Greenblatt DJ. Triazolam and anterograde amnesia: all is not well in the Z-zone [Editorial]. J Clin Psychopharmacol 1983;3:273.

104. Huff JS, Plunkett HG. Anterograde amnesia following triazolam use by two emergency room physicians. J Emer Med 1989;7:153–155.

105. Einarson TR, Yoder ES. Triazolam psychosis—a syndrome? Drug Intell Clin Pharmacol 1982;16(4):330.

106. Schogt B, Cohn D. Paranoid symptoms associated with triazolam. Can J Psychiatry 1985;30:462–463.

107. Soldatos CR, Sakkas PN, Bergiannaki JD, Stefanis CN. Behavioural side effects of triazolam in psychiatric inpatients: report of five cases. Drug Intell Clin Pharmacol 1986;20:294–297.

108. Kirk T, Roache JD, Griffiths RR. Dose-response evaluation of the amnestic effects of triazolam and pentobarbital in normal subjects. J Clin Psychopharmacol 1990;10:161–168.

109. Regestein QR, Reich P. Agitation observed during treatment with newer hypnotic drugs. J Clin Psychiatry 1985;46:280–283.

110. Morris HH, Estes ML. Traveler's amnesia: transient global amnesia secondary to triazolam. JAMA 1987;258:945–946.

111. Morris HH, Estes ML. in Letters to the Editor. JAMA 1988;259:351–352.

112. Bixler EO, Kales A, Manfredi RL, Vgontzas AN. Triazolam-induced brain impairment: frequent memory disturbances. Eur J Clin Pharmacol 1989;36:A171.

113. Kales A, Vgontzas AN. Not all benzodiazepines are alike. In: Stefanis CN, Rabavilas AD, Soldatos CR, eds. Psychiatry: a world perspective. Vol 3. Amsterdam: Elsevier Science Publishers, 1990.

114. Bixler EO, Kales A, Manfredi RL, et al. Next-day memory impairment with triazolam use. Lancet 1991;337:827–831.

115. Kales A, Bixler EO, Soldatos CR, Jacoby JA, Kales JD. Lorazepam: effects on sleep and withdrawal phenomena. Pharmacology 1986;32:121–130.

116. Healy M, Pickens R, Meisch R, et al. Effects of clorazepate, diazepam, lorazepam, and placebo on human memory. J Clin Psychiatry 1983;44:436–439.

117. Lister RG, File SE. The nature of lorazepam-induced amnesia. Psychopharmacology 1984;83:183–187.

118. Mac DS, Kumar R, Goodwin DW. Anterograde amnesia with oral lorazepam. J Clin Psychiatry 1985;46:137–138.

119. Sandyk R. Transient global amnesia induced by lorazepam. Clin Neuropharmacol 1985;8:297–298.

120. Lister RG. The amnesic action of benzodiazepines in man. Neurosci Biobehav Rev 1985;9:87–94.

121. Roth T, Hartse KM, Saab PG, Piccione PM, Kramer M. The effects of flurazepam, lorazepam, and triazolam on sleep and memory. Psychopharmacology 1980;70:231–237.

122. Kowley G, Springen K, Iarovice D, Hager M. Sweet dreams or a nightmare? Newsweek 1991;(Aug.19):38–44.

123. Wysowski DK, Barash D. Adverse behavioral reactions attributed to triazolam in the Food and Drug Administration's Spontaneous Reporting System. Arch Intern Med 1991;151:2003–2008.

124. Bixler EO, Kales A, Soldatos CR, Scharf MB, Kales JD. Effectiveness of temazepam with short- intermediate-, and long-term use: sleep laboratory evaluation. J Clin Pharmacol 1978;18:110–118.

125. Mamelak M, Csima A, Price V. A comparative 25-night sleep laboratory study on the effects of quazepam and triazolam on the sleep of chronic insomniacs. J Clin Pharmacol 1984;24:65–75.

126. Oswald L, Adam K, Borrow S, Odzikowski C. The effects of two hypnotics on sleep, subjective feelings and skilled performance. In: Passouant P, Oswald I, eds. Pharmacology of the states of alertness. Elmsford, N.Y.: Pergamon Press, 1979.

127. Adam K, Oswald I, Shapiro C. Effects of loprazolam and of triazolam on sleep and overnight urinary cortisol. Psychopharmacology (Berlin) 1984;82:389–394.

128. Kales A, Bixler EO, Soldatos CR, Mitsky DJ, Kales JD: Dose-response studies of lormetazepam: efficacy, side effects, and rebound insomnia. J Clin Pharmacol 1982;22:520–530.

129. Kales A, Soldatos CR, Bixler EO, Goff PJ, Vela-Bueno A. Midazolam: dose-response studies of effectiveness and rebound insomnia. Pharmacology 1983;26:138–149.

130. Kales A, Bixler EO, Vela-Bueno A, Soldatos CR, Manfredi RL. Alprazolam: effects on sleep and withdrawal phenomena. J Clin Pharmacol 1987;27:508–515.

131. Bixler EO, Kales A, Soldatos CR, Kales

JD. Flunitrazepam. An investigational hypnotic drug: sleep laboratory evaluations. J Clin Pharmacol 1977;17:569–578.

132. Kales A, Soldatos CR, Bixler EO, Kales JD. Rebound insomnia and rebound anxiety: a review. Pharmacology 1983;26:121–137.

133. Scharf MB, Bixler EO, Kales A, Soldatos CR. Long-term sleep laboratory evaluation of flunitrazepam. Pharmacology 1979;19:173–181.

134. Mamelak M, Csima A, Price V. The effects of brotizolam on the sleep of chronic insomniacs. Br J Clin Pharmacol 1983;16(suppl):377–382.

135. Monti JM. Sleep laboratory and clinical studies of the effects of triazolam, flunitrazepam and flurazepam in insomniac patients. Methods Find Exp Clin Pharmacol 1981;3:303–326.

136. Monti JM, Debellis J, Gratadoux E, et al. Sleep laboratory study of the effects of midazolam in insomniac patients. Eur J Clin Pharmacol 1982;21:479–484.

137. Roth T, Kramer M, Lutz T. Intermediate use of triazolam: a sleep laboratory study. J Int Med Res 1976;4:59–62.

138. Scharf MB, Kales A, Bixler EO, Jacoby JA, Schweitzer PK. Lorazepam—efficacy, side effects and rebound phenomena. Clin Pharmacol Ther 1982;31:175–179.

139. Vela-Bueno A, Oliveros JC, Dobladez-Blanco B, et al. Brotizolam: a sleep laboratory evaluation. Eur J Clin Pharmacol 1983;25:53–56.

140. Vogel GW, Thurmond A, Gibbons P, et al. The effect of triazolam on the sleep of insomniacs. Psychopharmacology 1975;41:65–69.

141. Vogel GW, Barker K, Gibbons P, Thurmond A. A comparison of the effects of flurazepam 30 mg and triazolam 0.5 mg on the sleep of insomniacs. Psychopharmacology 1987;47:81–86.

142. Gillin JC, Spinweber CH, Johnson LC. Rebound insomnia: a critical review. J Clin Psychopharmacol 1989;9:161–172.

143. Dement WC, Carskadon MA, Mitler MM, Phillips RL, Zarcone VP. Prolonged use of flurazepam: a sleep laboratory study. Behav Med 1978;5:25–31.

144. Kales A, Bixler EO, Scharf M, Kales JD. Sleep laboratory studies of flurazepam: a model for evaluating hypnotic drugs. Clin Pharmacol Ther 1976;19:576–583.

145. Kales A, Allen C, Scharf MB, Kales JD.

Hypnotic drugs and their effectiveness. All night EEG studies of insomniac subjects. Arch Gen Psychiatry 1970;23:226–232.

146. Kales A, Kales JD, Bixler EO, Scharf MB. Effectiveness of hypnotic drugs with prolonged use: flurazepam and pentobarbital. Clin Pharmacol Ther 1975;18:356–363.

147. Kales J, Kales A, Bixler EO, Slye ES. Effects of placebo and flurazepam on sleep patterns in insomniac subjects. Clin Pharmacol Ther 1971;12:691–697.

148. Greenblatt DJ, Harmatz JS, Zinny MA, Shader RI. Effect of gradual withdrawal on the rebound sleep disorder after discontinuation of triazolam. N Engl J Med 1987;317:722–728.

149. Bliwise D, Seidel W, Greenblatt DJ, Dement W. Nighttime and daytime efficacy of flurazepam and oxazepam in chronic insomnia. Am J Psychiatry 1984;141:191–195.

150. Mendelson WB, Weingartner H, Greenblatt DJ, Garnett D, Gillin JC. A clinical study of flurazepam. Sleep 1982;5:350–360.

151. Berlin RM, Conell LJ. Withdrawal symptoms after long-term treatment with therapeutic doses of flurazepam: a case report. Am J Psychiatry 1983;140:488–490.

152. Schnieder-Helmert D. Why low-dose benzodiazepine-dependent insomniacs can't escape their sleeping pills. Acta Psychiatr Scand 1988;78:706–711.

153. Lagier G. Troubles possible apres arret d'un traitement prolonge par les benzodiazepines chez l'homme (toxicomanies exclues). Therapie 1985;40:51–57.

154. Busto U, Sellers EM, Naranjo CA, et al. Withdrawal reaction after long-term therapeutic use of benzodiazepines. N Engl J Med 1986;315:854–859.

155. Kornecki E, Lenox RH, Hardwick DH, Bergdahl JA, Ehrlich YH. Interactions of the alkyl-ether-phospholipid, platelet activating factor (PAF) with platelets, neural cells, and the psychotropic drugs triazolobenzodiazepines. Adv Exp Med Biol 1987;221:477–488.

156. van der Kroef C. Het Halcion-syndroom-een iatrogene epidiemie in Nederland. Tijdschr Alcohol Drugs 1982;8:156–162.

157. Adam K, Oswald I. Possible mechanism for adverse reactions to triazolam [Letter]. Lancet 1991;338(8775):1157.

158. Tien Y, Gujavarty KS. Seizure following

withdrawal from triazolam. Am J Psychiatry 1985;142:1516–1517.

159. Schneider LS, Syapin PJ, Pawluczyk S. Seizures following triazolam withdrawal despite benzodiazepine treatment. J Clin Psychiatry 1987;48:418–419.

160. Laplane D, Baulac M, Lacombley L. Convulsions douze heures apres la prise d'une benzodiazepine a demi-vie courte. La Press Medicale 1988;17:439.

161. Anello C. Adverse behavior reactions attributed to triazolam in the FDA's Spontaneous Reporting System. Presentation to Pharmacological Drugs Advisory Committee Meeting, Washington, D.C., September 1989.

162. Martinez-Cano H, Vela-Bueno A. Triazolam [Letter]. Lancet 1991;337:1483.

163. Heritch AJ, Capwell R, Roy-Byrne PP. A case of psychosis and delirium following withdrawal from triazolam. J Clin Psychiatry 1987;48:168–169.

164. Gelenberg AJ, ed. The use of benzodiazepine hypnotics: a scientific examination of a clinical controversy. J Clin Psychiatry 1992;53(12 Suppl):1–87.

CHAPTER 13

Assessment and Treatment
of Other Disorders

Panic Disorder

CLINICAL PRESENTATION

In 1964 Klein described a syndrome characterized by:

- Sudden, spontaneous, unexpected feelings of *terror and anxiety*
- The *autonomic* equivalence of anxiety
- The *desire to flee* the situation and return to a safe place
- A *phobic avoidance* of the places where such attacks occur (1).

These attacks typically occur in public places, such as supermarkets on buses, in restaurants, elevators, and crowded stores. These patients in essence may develop three disorders: the *panic attack* itself; a secondary *anticipatory anxiety* that they will have another episode in certain places; and lastly, a *phobic avoidance* of the feared situation.

Many patients will have a few symptoms during an attack, but not every possible symptom. There is also a group of patients (perhaps 25%) who have these attacks without the subjective sense of anxiety or who experience insufficient symptoms to meet diagnostic criteria (i.e., limited symptom attacks). Thus, these pa-

tients may have a rapid heartbeat, diaphoresis, and tremors; but do not feel acutely anxious. This last point is important since they often develop the physiological symptoms of anxiety in public places or in situations that are unexpected or unprovoked. Although it may be in a public place, the patients are not under any specific stress nor in a highly emotional situation. When it occurs for the first time, patients frequently seek help in an emergency room or from a family physician. Typically, they receive a thorough medical workup and are then told that there is nothing wrong with them, that it is just stress. What is interesting is that the attacks occur in nonstressful situations, so the psychiatric stress-diathesis model is not appropriate. In other words, the explanation given by the medical personnel is obviously incorrect, because it is not consistent with what has happened to the patient. Thus, patients often assume the existence of a medical condition which has gone unrecognized.

Patients often develop this syndrome in their twenties, and some, with the more severe form, rarely leave home for periods of many years, or until they are effectively treated by medication. Family studies of panic disorder find an increased occurrence of attacks in first-degree relatives (2).

A serious complication of this syndrome is the abuse of sedatives and alcohol, through attempts at self-medication. In several studies, those who did well on antidepressants did not return to alcohol or drug abuse; but those in the control groups, not maintained on medication, often returned to a level of drug abuse that eventually necessitated rehospitalization. **As noted earlier, another complication is the risk of suicide, which may be as high in panic disorder patients as those suffering from a major depressive disorder (3–5a).**

Mitral Valve Prolapse Syndrome

Mitral valve prolapse syndrome occurs more frequently in panic disorder than in controls, but there is also a high incidence in the general population. It is often referred to as the click-murmur or Reed Barlow syndrome, and is characterized by a nonejection click with or without a late-systolic, high-pitched heart murmur, best heard at the apex. The syndrome also includes such symptoms as cardiac awareness, atypical chest pain, palpitations, shortness of breath, weakness, fatigue, dizziness, as well as musculoskeletal abnormalities (e.g., a double-jointed pectus excavatum, kyphoscoliosis, straight back and a tall-thin body habitus). The diagnosis can be confirmed by echocardiography.

DaCosta's Syndrome

Irritable heart, cardiac neurosis, or DaCosta's syndrome, has been described since the Civil War. It is associated with cardiac symptoms and autonomic adrenergic predominance (excess levels of or su-

persensitivity to peripheral catecholamines). Lactate-induced panic attacks in patients are also correlated with elevated epinephrine excretion in comparison to normal controls. Finally, symptomatic mitral valve prolapse patients excrete elevated urinary epinephrine and norepinephrine.

How panic disorder, mitral valve prolapse, DaCosta's syndrome, and a hyperadrenergic predominance might relate to each other is unknown at this time.

Provocative Tests for Panic Disorder

In 1951, Cohen and White observed that patients suffering from what they called "effort syndrome," developed abnormally high lactic acids levels after running (6). This led Pitts and McClure to show that lactate infusions can precipitate anxiety attacks in patients with this disorder, but not in controls (7). Further, Kelly observed that effective drug treatment resulted in a cessation of lactate-induced panic attacks (8). By contrast, unsuccessful treatment did not prevent reinfusion-produced panic attacks. Liebowitz et al. also noted that these patients often responded to lactate with a panic attack, but reinfusion after successful drug treatment failed to reproduce such episodes (9). Panic attacks have also been induced by such diverse compounds as CO_2, isoproterenol, mCPP, and flumazenil. The various mechanisms by which these agents produce symptoms provides fertile ground for elucidating the biological basis of panic disorder (10).

DRUG THERAPY FOR PANIC DISORDER

Like GAD, panic disorder (PD) with or without phobic avoidance is a chronic, debilitating illness (11–15). Although there is little consensus about the most effective drug treatments, options include:

- Selected *benzodiazepines*
- *Antidepressants*
  - Heterocyclic
  - Serotonin reuptake inhibitors
  - Monoamine oxidase inhibitors
- *Behavioral and/or cognitive therapy,* alone or in combination with pharmacotherapy.

Although drugs often prevent the panic attack, they may not alter the anticipatory anxiety. Thus, patients continue to expect the attacks, not realizing that with drug treatment they usually will not recur. Patients may insist that there is no improvement in their condition because they have not gone to public places to test the benefit of the medication. After imipramine, phenelzine, or alprazolam have blocked the panic attack, patients must then learn that they may never have another episode. Thus, drug response can dissociate the syndrome into its two pathopsychophysiological processes: panic attack and anticipatory anxiety. Psychological treatment is sometimes useful for overcoming the anticipatory anxiety and for helping patients return to the situations in which attacks were experienced.

Benzodiazepines

Until the 1980s, the BZDs were considered ineffective in the treatment of PD. Early controlled studies with the triazolobenzodiazepine *alprazolam,* however, demonstrated its antipanic properties, but this agent must usually be used in higher doses (4 to 10 mg/day) than when given as an anxiolytic. Although alpra-

zolam usually produces its therapeutic effect during the first week, phenelzine may take several weeks. This finding is particularly interesting because alprazolam may also have antidepressant properties. The observation that alprazolam prevents panic attacks and benefits depression implies that different classes of drugs (i.e., alprazolam, imipramine, serotonin reuptake inhibitors (SRIs), phenelzine) help both disorders.

Another high-potency BZD, *clonazepam,* also has been shown to be effective. In addition, there is evidence that higher than usual doses of *diazepam, lorazepam, bromazepam,* and *clobazam* may also block panic attacks (16).

Alprazolam

Short-Term Efficacy. Although at least one study found no difference between alprazolam and placebo, several short-term studies have reported that alprazolam reduces the frequency and intensity of panic attacks (17–25) (see also Table 13.1). In phase I of a cross-national collaborative study, including approximately 500 patients at 8 sites, alprazolam was superior to placebo at the end of week 1 in improving spontaneous and situational panic attacks, anxiety, and secondary disability (21). At week 4, 50% of alprazolam patients and 28% of placebo patients were free of panic attacks. At week 8, however, 50% of those on placebo were also free of panic attacks, compared to 59% of those receiving alprazolam. Investigators noted their data reflected group efficacy, not individual responses over time. Further, there was considerable variability and, at times, instability of response in individual patients. Explanations offered for the high rate of placebo response in this and other studies include:

Table 13.1.
Alprazolam versus *Placebo:* Treatment of Panic Disorder

Number of Studies	Number of Subjects	Responders (%)		Difference (%)	Chi Square	*p* Value
		Alprazolam (%)	Placebo (%)			
7	1486	72	45	26	122.7	2×10^{-28}

- The surreptitious use of antianxiety and antidepressant medication
- Consistently normal dexamethasone suppression tests
- Lower anxiety ratings at the start of treatment
- Behavioral benefits derived from inclusion in the study (26–28).

Long-Term Efficacy. The question of long-term benefit with alprazolam remains largely unanswered. Although improvement appears to be sustained in many patients as long as the medication is continued, several researchers have reported high rates of relapse when the drug is discontinued within 14 months (29–31).

Nagy et al. did a 2.5-year follow-up study of 60 patients with PD or agoraphobia with panic attacks who completed a 4-month combined drug and behavioral group treatment program and were discharged on a regimen of alprazolam (32). They found that the short-term improvement on alprazolam and behavior therapy was maintained during alprazolam maintenance, indicating tolerance to alprazolam did not develop. Further, many patients who decreased or discontinued the drug also sustained improvement. The ability to discontinue alprazolam was associated with lower initial frequency of panic attacks. Those receiving nonpharmacologic therapy in the follow-up period tended to have greater symptom severity. Finally, current or past depression was related to greater illness severity; episodes of depression after treatment were common;

and depression was not prevented by low-dose alprazolam and behavioral therapy. Because of the naturalistic design of the study and the use of both pharmacologic and nonpharmacological interventions, the investigators cautioned that their results did not differentiate among the relative contributions of alprazolam, behavioral therapy, or their combination.

Dose. Due to its relatively short duration of effect (2–6 hours), alprazolam must be given in divided doses, as frequently as four to five times daily. In the treatment of PD, effective doses range from 2 to 10 mg/day, which is considerably higher than those recommended for GAD. One acute fixed dose study found that about 60% of patients respond to 2 mg and 75% respond to 6 mg, whereas in another study 6 mg was more effective than 2 mg (33, 34).

There is some evidence that patients maintained on alprazolam therapy may require lower doses than those used initially. As noted above, Nagy et al. found that many patients sustained their improvement with lower dosages, and others have reported similar findings (29, 32, 35). By contrast, Rashid et al. found an increase in alprazolam dose over time (36).

Adverse Effects. *Sedation, ataxia,* and *fatigue* are the most common adverse effects reported with acute use of alprazolam in PD (37). Although tolerance to the sedative effect may develop within a few days of treatment initiation, this adaptation may be only partial. At weeks 4 and

8 in the cross-national collaborative study, many patients still showed signs of sedation (48 and 39%), ataxia (25 and 16%), and fatigue (19 and 16%, respectively) (21).

In an open study of outpatients who took alprazolam for a mean of 13.3 months, Rashid et al. reported the occurrence of the following symptoms:

- Bone or joint *stiffness* or lancinating *pain*
- Excessive *lacrimation* without accompanying affect
- *Tightness in the chest* intercostal muscles
- Labored *respirations* and/or air hunger
- Frequent *changes in accommodation;* visual clouding
- Brief bursts of *profuse sweating* unrelated to exertion
- Rapidly alternating *mood swings* (36).

Some of the symptoms were withdrawal-like, occurring within a 4-hour time frame of any given dose. Other "interdose" symptoms, including irritability, increased anxiety and panic, also have been reported with alprazolam (38).

The use of alprazolam in PD patients has been associated with the emergence of *depressive symptoms,* a phenomenon also reported with clonazepam and lorazepam (31, 32, 39–41). *Aggressive behavior* and *assaultiveness* also has been reported in panic patients with and without histories of major depression (42, 43). Although emergence of *behavioral dyscontrol* has been reported with a variety of BZDs and appears to be idiosyncratic, a question raised in recent years is whether there is an increased incidence with alprazolam. Rosenbaum et al. described extreme anger or hostility in eight of 80 private practice patients, one of whom had a history of aggressive behavior (44). Gardner and Cowdry reported that seven of 12 patients

with borderline personality disorder and histories of dyscontrol treated with alprazolam (1 to 6 mg/day) had serious recurrent episodes of dyscontrol (45). Finally, FDA statistics indicate that alprazolam ranks second (behind triazolam) for hostility reactions reported in 329 drugs (46).

Discontinuation Effects. Alprazolam requires an extended and very gradual taper, even when given for only a few weeks. Despite very slow dosage reduction, however, a substantial number of patients may experience worsening of symptoms, including severe rebound panic and increased anxiety (29, 31, 47–49a). Other reported symptoms are listed in Table 13.2. In some patients symptoms may not occur in the initial phases of taper, but appear when the dose reaches lower

Table 13.2.
Symptoms Reported with Discontinuation of Alprazolam Treatment of Panic Disorder

Confusion
Clouded sensorium
Heightened sensory perception
Dysosmia
Paresthesias
Muscle cramps
Muscle twitch
Blurred vision
Diarrhea
Decreased appetite
Weight loss
Malaise
Weakness
Insomnia
Tachycardia
Dizziness
Lightheadedness
Faintness
Confusion
Excessive sweating
Depression
Irritability
Increased plasma cortisol levels
Headache
Muscle tension
Motor restlessness

levels (47, 48, 50). Withdrawal symptoms have been reported to last as long as 4 weeks, although in many patients they subside within 1 to 2 weeks (31, 47). Abrupt taper or sudden discontinuation may increase the risk of delirium and seizures (51–53). A guide to properly tapering alprazolam is provided in Figure 13.1.

Clonazepam

Short-Term Efficacy. Several open trials have reported significant improvement or remission of panic attacks in patients treated with clonazepam (54–60). One double-blind, placebo-controlled study comparing the efficacy of alprazolam, clonazepam, and placebo found both drugs superior to placebo and comparable to each other (61). Because favorable response to clonazepam usually occurs early in treatment, lack of initial improvement may predict treatment failure (40, 55, 62). Interdose and morning rebound anxiety have not been reported.

Long-Term Efficacy.   In a 1-year follow-up study of clonazepam for PD or agoraphobia with panic attacks, Pollack et al. reported that 18 of 20 (90%) patients, many of whom had failed to respond to or tolerate other BZDs or antidepressants, maintained a good response (40). One patient was in complete remission at 44 weeks and remained well even off medication at 56 weeks. Tolerance to therapeutic efficacy did not appear to develop, although 40% required a dose increase (0.25 to 4.5 mg) to maintain initial improvement. Interestingly, ten patients (or 50%) had discontinued clonazepam at follow-up because of adverse effects, inadequate response, or preference for a previously used treatment.

Dose.   Effective daily doses of clonazepam have ranged from 0.25 mg to 9 mg. In a review of open trials, Pollack et al. reported that most patients were maintained on 2 to 3 mg/day (62). In the comparison between alprazolam and clonazepam, av-

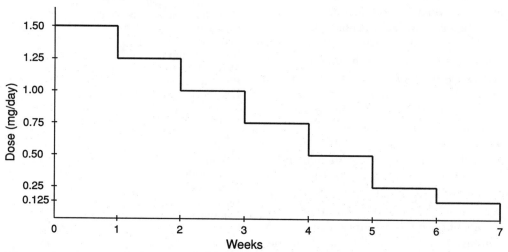

Figure 13.1.   Suggested alprazolam tapering schedule. To discontinue therapy with alprazolam, patients who have been taking more than 2.0 mg/day should reduce their daily dose by not more than 0.5 mg and they should maintain that daily dose for 1 week before further reduction. When the total daily dose is reduced to 2.0 mg or when a patient is taking less than 2.0 mg/day, the daily dose should be reduced by not more than 0.25 mg/day each week until complete discontinuation is achieved.

erage therapeutic doses were 5.2 mg/day and 2.4 mg/day, respectively (61). Due to its long half-life, clonazepam may be given twice daily, in the morning and at bedtime. Initially, lower doses should be given in the morning to allow for the development of tolerance to this agent's significant sedative effect.

Switching from Alprazolam. In an open trial, Herman et al. recruited 48 PD patients successfully treated with alprazolam but distressed by interdose or morning rebound (38). Using a standard protocol, 41 patients completed a transition to clonazepam treatment, and 39 continued on this drug for a mean duration of 40 weeks at an average dose of 1.5 mg/day (range, 0.125 to 3 mg/day). Panic was as well controlled with clonazepam as with alprazolam. Two patients reported mild sedation but did not discontinue the medication. Although two others rated clonazepam as "worse" than alprazolam and switched back successfully to the latter, 34 rated clonazepam better than, and five considered it the same as, alprazolam.

Adverse Effects. *Sedation* is the most prominent initial effect of clonazepam, usually subsiding in 2 to 3 days, but may persist in some patients. Other reported effects include:

- Ataxia
- Irritability
- Nausea
- Dysthymia.

In their long-term follow-up study, Pollack et al. found that five patients had stopped clonazepam due to adverse effects (dysthymia, one; irritability, two; nausea and sedation, two); and four patients required dose reductions because of adverse effects (predominantly sedation) (40).

Like alprazolam, clonazepam may cause treatment-emergent *depression* in some patients. Pollack et al. reported that only 10% of their patients who remained on clonazepam had a history of depression; although 47% lost to follow-up and 30% who eventually required alternate treatment had histories of dysthymia or depression (40). Of 31 patients without a prior history of affective illness, three developed depression on low daily dosages (0.75 mg, 1.5 mg, and 2 mg, respectively); one was switched to alprazolam; and the others responded to the addition of desipramine or imipramine. These investigators recommend that until further data are available, PD patients with chronic or concurrent depression should not be given clonazepam alone, and that those who develop depression during clonazepam therapy should have their dose lowered or an adjunctive antidepressant added.

There is some evidence that clonazepam may induce depression more often than alprazolam. In a review of 177 patients treated with clonazepam and a matched number treated with alprazolam, Cohen and Rosenbaum reported that 5.5% of the clonazepam patients developed depression, compared to only 0.7% of those on alprazolam (63).

An earlier review found a high incidence of *aggressive dyscontrol* in neurological patients treated with clonazepam, most of whom were children (64). This has led to speculation that this agent may be associated with an increased incidence of aggressivity in psychiatric patients. In this context, there have been reports of irritability in two of 50 panic patients and threatening or assaultive behavior in four of 13 schizophrenic patients on clonazepam (40, 65). Other investigators using this drug in panic patients, however, have not reported such adverse effects (54, 57).

Discontinuation Effects. There has been speculation that clonazepam's longer duration of action may provide better protection against withdrawal symptoms and rapid reemergence of panic. Limited data, however, are available on specific discontinuation effects associated with this treatment for PD, although mild rebound anxiety has been observed (57). A number of patients with a variety of psychiatric disorders have been switched successfully from high daily doses of alprazolam to clonazepam (66, 67). Subsequent gradual discontinuation of the latter produced no major withdrawal phenomena, although two patients experienced mild reemergence of panic symptoms that subsided with small dose increases, which did not recur during further dose tapering and discontinuation. Like all other BZDs, clonazepam should be reduced gradually, because abrupt cessation may lead to withdrawal symptoms ranging from mild to severe (68, 69).

Other Benzodiazepines

There is some evidence that higher than usual doses of lower potency BZDs may also be effective in treating PD (16, 23, 41, 70–73). For example, studies comparing alprazolam to lorazepam or diazepam indicate approximately equal efficacy (23, 41, 73, 74).

Two studies have also compared discontinuation effects in PD patients treated with either alprazolam or diazepam. Burrows et al. reported severe difficulties in 20 to 30% of patients discontinuing either drug, with those on diazepam having slightly more difficulty than those on alprazolam (50). Roy-Byrne et al. found greater increases in anxiety 1 week after abrupt discontinuation of medication in patients taking alprazolam compared to those taking diazepam (48). Although there were no significant differ-

ences in frequency of panic attacks during drug taper, at discontinuation the frequency of increased panic attacks was 50% higher in the alprazolam than in the diazepam group and three times greater in the diazepam versus placebo group.

Conclusion

In summary, many patients may require long-term, indefinite BZD therapy for their panic disorder. Fortunately, most naturalistic follow-up studies indicate an absence of tolerance to the antipanic/antiphobic effects of these drugs. Indeed, many patients appear to derive comparable efficacy at lower maintenance doses of BZDs (75). If discontinuation is appropriate or necessary, a gradual tapering and careful evaluation of withdrawal symptoms versus reemergence of the disorder itself will be required. Discontinuation is probably easier with the longer acting, high potency BZD (76).

Antidepressants

Tricyclics

Results from studies comparing TCAs, SRIs, and MAOIs to placebo in the treatment of panic disorder are summarized in Tables 13.3, 13.4, and 13.5. The results of studies comparing alprazolam or SRIs to standard TCAs are summarized in Tables 13.6 and 13.7. Here no significant differences in efficacy were noted.

Imipramine is the most widely studied tricyclic for the treatment of PD and agoraphobia, and is generally considered an effective antipanic agent (77, 78). Other tricyclics reported to have therapeutic efficacy in PD include:

- Desipramine
- Nortriptyline
- Amitriptyline
- Doxepin (77, 79).

Table 13.3.
Tricyclic Antidepressant versus *Placebo*: Treatment of Panic Disorder

Number of Studies	Number of Subjects	Responders (%)		Difference (%)	Chi Square	p Value
		TCA (%)	Placebo (%)			
7	1072	72	51	21	51.4	7×10^{-13}

Table 13.4.
Serotonin Reuptake Inhibitor versus *Placebo*: Treatment of Panic Disorder

Number of Studies	Number of Subjects	Responders (%)		Difference (%)	Chi Square	p Value
		SRI (%)	Placebo (%)			
4	148	80	30	50	35.5	3×10^{-9}

Table 13.5.
Monoamine Oxidase Inhibitor versus *Placebo*: Treatment of Panic Disorder

Number of Studies	Number of Subjects	Responders (%)		Difference (%)	Chi Square	p Value
		MAOI (%)	Placebo (%)			
3	92	90	34	56	29.3	6×10^{-8}

Table 13.6.
Alprazolam versus *Tricyclic Antidepressant*: Treatment of Panic Disorder

Number of Studies	Number of Subjects	Responders (%)		Difference (%)	Chi Square	p Value
		Alprazolam (%)	TCA (%)			
3	868	71	68	3	0.5	NS

Table 13.7.
Serotonin Reuptake Inhibitor versus *Tricyclic Antidepressant*:
 Treatment of Panic Disorder

Number of Studies	Number of Subjects	Responders (%)		Difference (%)	Chi Square	p Value
		SRI (%)	TCA (%)			
3	133	73	63	10	1.3	NS

Most, but not all, studies comparing imipramine and alprazolam indicate both drugs produce a comparable reduction of symptoms, although onset of action is considerably slower with the tricyclic, requiring two, to as long as 12 weeks (19, 22, 24, 34, 74, 74a).

In addition to producing anticholinergic effects and hypotension, tricyclics may actually worsen the patient's condition early in treatment by increasing anxiety, jitteriness, and dysphoria (overstimulation) (80). A patient's inability to tolerate these adverse effects may be the most treatment-limiting factor with these drugs. Use of very low initial doses (e.g., 10 mg) and gradual dosage increases may facilitate patient acceptance.

Data on recurrence after tricyclic discontinuation are sparse and inconsistent, in part due to varying definitions of relapse. Existing controlled and open trials note that patients do relapse after discontinuance of antidepressants. For example, Sheehan and Paj found that most of his panic disorder patients had a recurrence when medication was stopped (81). Rates have ranged from less than 33% to more than 90% (19, 77, 80, 82–86a).

Gittleman-Klein and Klein conducted a double-blind, placebo-controlled study of 35 nonpsychotic, school-phobic children (87). They found a good response in all children treated with imipramine but in only 21% of those on placebo. Because panic disorder patients often experienced separation anxiety as children, this suggests that some cases of school phobia may be the childhood equivalent of panic disorder, for which imipramine is effective.

Serotonin Reuptake Inhibitors

Preliminary evidence indicates that agents such as fluoxetine, sertraline, paroxetine, fluvoxamine, (as well as clomipramine, and trazodone) all possess antipanic efficacy, although the last may be less effective than imipramine (22, 88–91a). Because of more acceptable side-effect profiles, the SRIs may become the ADs of choice if initial positive results are confirmed.

Monoamine Oxidase Inhibitors

At about the same time that Klein was investigating imipramine in the United States, investigators in England noted that some patients with hysteria responded positively to monoamine oxidase inhibitors (MAOIs). Subsequently, researchers in England and Canada showed MAOIs to be superior to placebo in hysterics with phobic symptoms, a subcategorization that may be similar to the patients described by Klein.

Although clinical experience indicates *tranylcypromine* may be an effective antipanic agent, there are no controlled trials confirming this observation. *Phenelzine*, however, has been found very effective in both open and controlled designs (19, 92, 93). Onset of action is similar to that of other ADs, and although adverse effects tend to be less troublesome than with tricyclics, dietary restrictions may limit the usefulness of MAOIs in some patients. Unfortunately, relapse rate may be comparable to that seen with BZDs and tricyclics. For example, Kelly, in a follow-up of 246 patients, found that 50% who had discontinued MAOIs relapsed within 1 year (94).

Other Drug Therapies

There has been an emerging data base supporting the use of anticonvulsants (particularly valproic acid) for the management of panic disorder (95–97). Given this agent's effect on the GABA neurotransmitter system, its use alone or in combination with other GABA-ergic agents (e.g., clonazepam) may be particularly helpful in treatment-resistant panic disorders (98). Ongoing controlled investigations should soon clarify the value of this drug for panic disorder.

NON-DRUG THERAPIES FOR PANIC DISORDER

Non-drug approaches found to be beneficial include:

- Exposure therapy
- Cognitive therapy
- Applied relaxation (99–103).

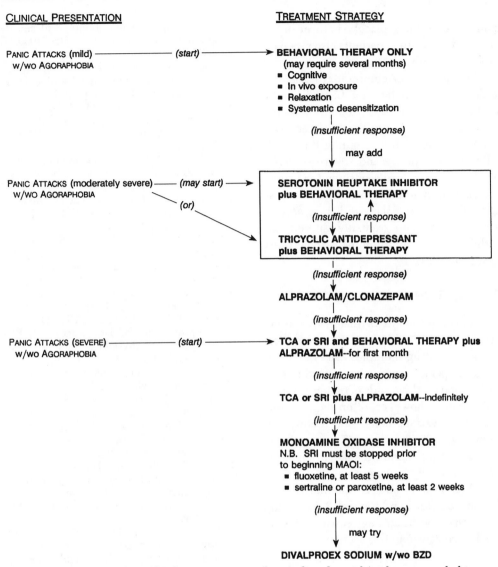

CLINICAL PRESENTATION   TREATMENT STRATEGY

PANIC ATTACKS (mild) ——————— *(start)* ————→ **BEHAVIORAL THERAPY ONLY**
w/wo AGORAPHOBIA   (may require several months)
                                               ▪ Cognitive
                                               ▪ In vivo exposure
                                               ▪ Relaxation
                                               ▪ Systematic desensitization

                                               (insufficient response)

                                                       may add

PANIC ATTACKS (moderately severe) —— *(may start)* —→ **SEROTONIN REUPTAKE INHIBITOR**
w/wo AGORAPHOBIA   **plus BEHAVIORAL THERAPY**

                                     (or)   *(insufficient response)*

                                               TRICYCLIC ANTIDEPRESSANT
                                               plus BEHAVIORAL THERAPY

                                               (insufficient response)

                                               ALPRAZOLAM/CLONAZEPAM

                                               (insufficient response)

PANIC ATTACKS (SEVERE) ——————— *(start)* ————→ **TCA or SRI and BEHAVIORAL THERAPY plus**
w/wo AGORAPHOBIA   **ALPRAZOLAM--for first month**

                                               (insufficient response)

                                               TCA or SRI plus ALPRAZOLAM--indefinitely

                                               (insufficient response)

                                               MONOAMINE OXIDASE INHIBITOR
                                               N.B. SRI must be stopped prior
                                               to beginning MAOI:
                                               ▪ fluoxetine, at least 5 weeks
                                               ▪ sertraline or paroxetine, at least 2 weeks

                                               (insufficient response)

                                                       may try

                                               DIVALPROEX SODIUM w/wo BZD

Figure 13.2.   Strategy for the management of panic disorder with/without agoraphobia.

According to Marks, however, non-exposure therapies usually fail to achieve reliable fear reduction (99). Although exposure may produce intense temporary discomfort, gains usually begin within a few hours of treatment; however, several weeks or months may be required to obtain maximum benefit. Long-term effect has been reported to range from 4 to 8 years, even with drug discontinuation (104).

COMBINATION THERAPIES

Although several studies have found that the combination of *imipramine and behavioral therapy* may be superior to either treatment alone, no studies have specifically examined the effects of combining the *behavioral techniques with BZDs* (105–108). In a review of the literature, however, Wardle found that diazepam was superior to placebo in three out of four studies in which patients also received exposure therapy (109).

The question of combining a *tricyclic with a BZD* also has not been formally studied. Nevertheless, to help patients achieve the rapid results associated with BZD treatment while avoiding the possibility of dependence and severe rebound that may occur on discontinuation, some clinicians initiate treatment with low dosages of both alprazolam and imipramine. Alprazolam is then gradually tapered and withdrawn when imipramine reaches therapeutic levels (110).

CONCLUSION

Panic disorder and its related symptoms can be quite disabling. The recognition that specific drug therapies can effectively block the panic episodes has brought newfound hope for thousands of patients. Optimal outcome, however, often requires the addition of various behavioral techniques to manage all related components of the disorder (e.g., panic attack, anticipatory anxiety, phobic avoidance).

Appendices K and L summarize the diagnostic criteria and Figure 13.2 summarizes a therapeutic strategy consistent with the data reviewed in this section.

REFERENCES

1. Klein DF. Delineation of two drug-responsive anxiety syndromes. Psychopharmacologia 1964;5:397–408.
2. Carey G, Gottesman II. Twin and family studies of anxiety, phobic and obsessive disorders. In: Klein DF, Rabkin J, eds. Anxiety: new research and changing concepts. New York: Raven Press, 1981.
3. Weissman MM, Klerman GL, Markowitz JS, et al. Suicidal ideation and suicide attempts in panic disorder and attacks. N Engl J Med 1989;321:1209–1214.
4. Johnson J, Weissman MM, Klerman GL. Panic disorder, comorbidity, and suicide attempts. Arch Gen Psychiatry 1990;47:805–808.
5. Fawcett J. Suicide risk factors in depressive disorders and in panic disorder. J Clin Psychiatry 1992;53(3, suppl):9–13.
5a. Lepine JP, Chignon JM, Teherani MS. Suicide attempts in patients with panic disorder. Arch Gen Psychiatry 1993;50:144–149.
6. Cohen M, White P. Life situations, emotions and neurocirculatory asthenia. Psychosomatic Medicine 1951;13:335–357.
7. Pitts FN, McClure JN. Lactate metabolism in anxiety neurosis. N Engl J Med 1967;277:132–136.
8. Kelly D, Mitchell-Heggs N, Sherman D. Anxiety and the effects of sodium lactate assessed clinically and physiologically. Br J Psychiatry 1971;119:129–41.
9. Liebowitz RR, Gorman JM, Fyer A, Levitt M, Dillon D, Levy G, Appleby I, Anderson S, Palij M, Davies S, Klein DF. Lactate provocation of panic attacks. II. Biochemical and physiologic findings. Arch Gen Psychiatry 1985;42:709–719.
10. Nutt D, Lawson C. Panic attacks. A neurochemical overview of models and mechanisms. Br J Psychiatry 1992;160:165–178.
11. Coryell W, Noyes R, Clancy J. Panic disorder and primary unipolar depression. A comparison of background and outcome. J Affective Disord 1983;5:311–317.
12. Uhde TW, Boulenger JP, Roy-Byrne PP, et al. Longitudinal course of panic disorder: clinical and biological considerations. Prog Neuropsychopharmacol Biol Psychiatry 1985;9:39–51.
13. Breier A, Charney DS, Heninger GR. Agoraphobia with panic attacks: development, diagnostic stability and course of illness. Arch Gen Psychiatry 1986;43:1029–1036.
14. Markowitz JS, Weissman MM, Ouellette R, et al. Quality of life in panic disorder. Arch Gen Psychiatry 1989;46:984–992.
15. Weissman MM. Impact of panic disorder on the quality of life. Presented at the Annual Meeting of the American Psychiatric Association, New York, May 1990.
16. Judd FK, Norman TR, Burrows GD. Pharmacotherapy of panic disorder. Int Rev Psychiatry 1990;2:287–298.
17. Klosko JS, Barlow DH, Tassinari RB, Cerny JA. Alprazolam vs cognitive behavior therapy for panic disorder: a preliminary report. In: Hand I, Witchen HU, eds.

Panic and phobias. New York: Springer Verlag, 1988:54–65.

18. Chouinard G, Annable L, Fontaine R, Solyom L. Alprazolam in the treatment of generalized anxiety and panic disorders: a double-blind, placebo-controlled study. Psychopharmacology 1982;77:229–233.

19. Sheehan DV, Claycomb JB, Surnam OS. The relative efficacy of alprazolam, phenelzine, and imipramine in treating panic attacks and phobias. Presented at the Annual Meeting of the American Psychiatric Association, Los Angeles, May 1984.

20. Sheehan DV, Coleman JH, Greenblatt DJ, et al. Some biochemical correlates of panic attacks with agoraphobia and their response to a new treatment. J Clin Psychopharmacol 1984;4:66–75.

21. Charney DS, Heninger GR. Noradrenergic function and the mechanism of action of antianxiety treatment. I. The effect of long term alprazolam treatment. Arch Gen Psychiatry 1985;42:458–467.

22. Charney DS, Woods SW, Goodman WK, et al. Drug treatment of panic disorder: the comparative efficacy of imipramine, alprazolam, and trazodone. J Clin Psychiatry 1986;47:580–586.

23. Dunner DL, Ishiki D, Avery DH, Wilson LG, Hyde TS. Effect of alprazolam and diazepam on anxiety and panic attacks and panic disorder: a controlled study. J Clin Psychiatry 1986;47:458–460.

24. Rizley R, Kahn RJ, McNair DM, Frankenthaler LM. A comparison of alprazolam and imipramine in the treatment of agoraphobia and panic disorder. Psychopharmacol Bull 1986;22:167–172.

25. Ballenger JC, Burrows GD, DuPont RL, et al. Alprazolam in panic disorder and agoraphobia: results from a multicenter trial. I. Efficacy in short-term treatment. Arch Gen Psychiatry 1988;45:413–422.

26. Clark DB, Taylor CB, Roth WT, et al. Surreptitious drug use by patients in a panic disorder study. Am J Psychiatry 1990;147:507–509.

27. Coryell W, Noyes R. Placebo response in panic disorder. Am J Psychiatry 1988;145:1138–1140.

28. Marks IM, De Albuquerque A, Cottraux J, et al. The "efficacy" of alprazolam in panic disorder and agoraphobia: a critique of recent reports. Arch Gen Psychiatry 1989;46:668–670.

29. DuPont RL, Pecknold JC. Alprazolam withdrawal in panic disorder patients. Presented at the Annual Meeting of the American Psychiatric Association, Dallas, Texas, May 1985.

30. Sheehan DV. One-year follow-up of patients with panic disorder and withdrawal from long-term antipanic medications. In: Program and Abstracts of the Panic Disorder Biological Research Workshop, April 16, 1986, Washington, D.C.:35.

31. Fyer AJ, Liebowitz MR, Gorman JM, et al. Discontinuation of alprazolam in panic patients. Am J Psychiatry 1987;144:303–308.

32. Nagy LM, Krystal JH, Woods SW, Charney DS. Clinical and medication outcome after short-term alprazolam and behavioral group treatment in panic disorder. 2.5-year naturalistic follow-up study. Arch Gen Psychiatry 1989;46:993–999.

33. Ballenger JC, Lydiard RB, Lesser IM, Rubin RT, DuPont RL. Acute fixed dose alprazolam study in panic disorder patients. Presented at the Pharmacology/Pharmacokinetic Studies Workshop at the Panic Disorder Biological Research Workshop, Washington, D.C., April 1986.

34. Uhlenhuth EH, Matuzas W, Glass RM, et al. Response of panic disorder to fixed doses of alprazolam or imipramine. J Affective Disord 1989;17:261–270.

35. Sheehan DV. Benzodiazepines in panic disorder and agoraphobia. J Affective Disord 1987;13:169–181.

36. Rashid K, Patrisi G, Cook B. Multiple serious symptom formation with alprazolam. Presented at the Annual Meeting of the American Psychiatric Association, Montreal Canada, May 1988.

37. Noyes R, DuPont RL, Pecknold JC, et al. Alprazolam in panic disorder and agoraphobia: patient acceptance, side effects, and safety. Arch Gen Psychiatry 1988;45:423–428.

38. Herman JB, Rosenbaum JF, Brotman AW. The alprazolam to clonazepam switch for the treatment of panic disorder. J Clin Psychopharmacol 1987;7:175–178.

39. Lydiard BR, Laraia MT, Ballenger JC, Howell EF. Emergence of depressive symptoms in patients receiving alprazolam for panic disorder. Am J Psychiatry 1987;144:664–665.

40. Pollack MH, Tesar GE, Rosenbaum JF, et al. Clonazepam in the treatment of panic disorder and agoraphobia: a one-year follow-up. J Clin Psychopharmacol 1986;6:302–304.

41. Charney DS, Woods SW, Goodman WK,

et al. The efficacy of lorazepam in panic disorders. Presented at the Annual Meeting of the American Psychiatric Association, Chicago, Illinois, May 1987.

42. Noyes R, DuPont RL, Pecknold J, et al. Alprazolam in panic disorder and agoraphobia: results from a multicenter trial. Arch Gen Psychiatry 1988;45:423–428.

43. Pyke RE, Kraus M. Alprazolam in the treatment of panic attack patients with and without major depression. J Clin Psychiatry 1988;49:66–68.

44. Rosenbaum JE, Woods SW, Groves JE, et al. Emergence of hostility during alprazolam treatment. Am J Psychiatry 1984; 141:792–793.

45. Gardner DL, Cowdry RW. Alprazolam-induced dyscontrol in borderline personality disorder. Am J Psychiatry 1985;142:98–100.

46. Kowley G, Springen K, Iarovice D, Hager M. Sweet dreams or a nightmare? Newsweek 1991;(Aug.19):38–44.

47. Pecknold JC, Swinson RP, Kuch K, Lewis CP. Alprazolam in panic disorder and agoraphobia: results from a multicenter trial. III. Discontinuation effects. Arch Gen Psychiatry 1988;45:429–436.

48. Roy-Byrne PP, Dager SR, Cowley DS, Vitaliano P, Dunner DL. Relapse and rebound following discontinuation of benzodiazepine treatment of panic attacks: alprazolam versus diazepam. Am J Psychiatry 1989;146:860–865.

49. Mellman TA, Uhde TW. Withdrawal syndrome with gradual tapering of alprazolam. Am J Psychiatry 1986;143:1464–1466.

49a. Rickels K, Schweizer E, Weiss S, Zavodnick S. Maintenance drug treatment for panic disorder. II. Short- and long-term outcome after drug taper. Arch Gen Psychiatry 1993;50:61–68.

50. Burrows GD, Norman TR, Judd FK, Marriott PF. Short-acting versus long-acting benzodiazepines: discontinuation effects in panic disorders. J Psychiatr Res 1990; 24(suppl 2):65–72.

51. Levy AB. Delirium and seizures due to abrupt alprazolam withdrawal: case report. J Clin Psychiatry 1984;45:38–39.

52. Noyes Jr R, Chaudhry DR, Domingo DV. Pharmacologic treatment of phobic disorders. J Clin Psychiatry 1986;47:455–452.

53. Brown JL, Hauge KJ. A review of alprazolam withdrawal. Drug Intell Clin Pharm 1986;20:837–884.

54. Spier SA, Tesar GE, Rosenbaum JF, et al.

Treatment of panic disorder and agoraphobia with clonazepam. J Clin Psychiatry 1986;47:238–242.

55. Tesar GE, Rosenbaum JF. Successful use of clonazepam in patients with treatment resistant panic. J Nerv Ment Dis 1986;174:477–482.

56. Fontaine R, Chouinard G. Antipanic effect of clonazepam. Am J Psychiatry 1984;141:149.

57. Fontaine R. Clonazepam for panic disorders and agitation. Psychosomatics 1985;26(suppl 12):13–16.

58. Beaudry P, Fontaine R, Chouinard G, Annable L. Clonazepam in the treatment of patients with recurrent panic attacks. J Clin Psychiatry 1986;47:83–85.

59. Beckett A, Fishman SM, Rosenbaum JF. Clonazepam blockade of spontaneous and CO_2 inhalation-provoked panic in a patient with panic disorder. J Clin Psychiatry 1986;47:475–476.

60. Judd FK, Burrows GD. Clonazepam in the treatment of panic disorder [Letter]. Med J Aust 1986;145(1):59.

61. Tesar GE, Rosenbaum JE, Pollack MH, et al. Clonazepam versus alprazolam in the treatment of panic disorder: interim analysis of data from a prospective, double-blind, placebo-controlled trial. J Clin Psychiatry 1987;48(suppl):16–19.

62. Pollack MH, Rosenbaum JE, Tesar GE, et al. Clonazepam in the treatment of panic disorder and agoraphobia. Psychopharmacol Bull 1987;23:141–144.

63. Cohen LS, Rosenbaum JF. Clonazepam: new uses and potential problems. J Clin Psychiatry 1987;48(suppl 10):50–55.

64. Browne TR. Clonazepam. N Engl J Med 1978;299:812–816.

65. Karson CN, Weinberger DR, Bigelow L, et al. Clonazepam treatment of chronic schizophrenia: negative results in a double-blind, placebo-controlled trial. Am J Psychiatry 1982;139:1627–1628.

66. Albeck JH. Withdrawal and detoxification from benzodiazepine dependence: a potential role for clonazepam. J Clin Psychiatry 1987;48(suppl 10):43–48.

67. Patterson JF. Withdrawal from alprazolam dependency using clonazepam: clinical observations. J Clin Psychiatry 1990;5(suppl 5):47–49.

68. Jaffe R, Gibson E. Clonazepam withdrawal psychosis [Letter]. J Clin Psychopharmacol 1986;6:193.

69. Ghadirian AM, Gauthier S, Wong T. Con-

vulsions in patients abruptly withdrawn from clonazepam while receiving neuroleptic medication [Letter]. Am J Psychiatry 1987;144:686.

70. Noyes Jr R, Anderson DJ, Clancy J, et al. Diazepam and propranolol in panic disorder and agoraphobia. Arch Gen Psychiatry 1984;41:287–292.

71. Rickels K, Schweizer EE. Benzodiazepines for treatment of panic attacks: a new look. Psychopharmacol Bull 1986;22:93–99.

72. Howell EF, Laraia M, Ballenger JC, Lydiard RB. Lorazepam treatment of panic disorder. Presented at the Annual Meeting of the American Psychiatric Association, Chicago, Illinois, May 1987.

73. Schweizer E, Fox I, Case WG, Rickels K. Alprazolam versus lorazepam in the treatment of panic disorder. Presented at the Annual NCDEU Meeting, Key Biscayne, Florida, May 1987.

74. Ballenger JC, Howell EF, Laraia MT, et al. Comparison of four medications in panic disorder. Presented at the Annual Meeting of the American Psychiatric Association, Chicago, Illinois, May 1987.

74a. Schweizer E, Rickels K, Weiss S, Zavodnick S. Maintenance drug treatment of panic disorder. I. Results of a prospective, placebo-controlled comparison of alprazolam and imipramine. Arch Gen Psychiatry 1993;50:51–60.

75. Davidson JRT. Continuation treatment of panic disorder with high-potency benzodiazepines. J Clin Psychiatry 1990;51(12, suppl A):31–37.

76. Pollack MH. Long-term management of panic disorder. J Clin Psychiatry 1990;51(5, suppl):11–13.

77. Lydiard RB, Ballenger JC. Antidepressants in panic disorder and agoraphobia. J Affective Dis 1987;13:153–168.

78. Liebowitz MR. Antidepressants in panic disorders. Br J Psychiatry 1989;155(suppl 6):46–52.

79. Lydiard RB. Desipramine in agoraphobia with panic attacks: An open, fixed-dose study. J Clin Psychopharmacol 1987;7:258–260.

80. Noyes R, Garvey MJ, Cook BL, Samuelson L. Problems with tricyclic antidepressant use in patients with panic disorder or agoraphobia: results of a naturalistic follow-up study. J Clin Psychiatry 1989;50:163–169.

81. Sheehan DV, Paj BA. Panic disorder. In: Dunner DL, ed. Current psychiatric therapy. Philadelphia: Saunders, 1992:275–282.

82. Zitrin CM, Klein DF, Woerner MG, et al. Treatment of phobias: I. Comparison of imipramine hydrochloride and placebo. Arch Gen Psychiatry 1983;40:125–138.

83. Fyer AJ, Liebowitz MR, Gorman JM, et al. Comparative discontinuation of alprazolam and imipramine in panic patients. Presented at the Annual Meeting of the ACNP, Puerto Rico, December 1988.

84. Mavissakalian M, Michelson L. Two-year follow-up of exposure and imipramine treatment of agoraphobia. Am J Psychiatry 1986;143:1106–1112.

85. Zitrin CM, Juliano M, Kahan M. Five-year relapse rate after phobia treatment. Presented at the Annual Meeting of the American Psychiatric Association, Chicago, Illinois, May 1987.

86. Cohen SD, Monteiro W, Marks IM. Two-year follow-up of agoraphobics after exposure and imipramine. Br J Psychiatry 1984;144:276–281.

86a. Mavissakalian M, Perel JM. Protective effects of imipramine maintenance treatment in panic disorder with agoraphobia. Am J Psychiatry 1992;149:1053–1057.

87. Gittleman-Klein R, Klein DF. Controlled imipramine treatment of school phobia. Arch Gen Psychiatry 1971;25:204–207.

88. Gorman JM Liebowitz MR, Fyer AJ, et al. An open trial of fluoxetine in the treatment of panic attacks. J Clin Psychopharmacol 1987;7:329–332.

89. Schneier FR, Liebowitz MR, Davies SO, Fairbanks J, Hollander E, Campeas R, Klein DF. Fluoxetine in panic disorder. J Clin Psychopharmacol 1990;10(2):119–121.

90. Den Boer JA, Westenberg HGM, Kamerbeek WDJ, et al. Effect of serotonin uptake inhibitors in anxiety disorders: a double-blind comparison of clomipramine and fluvoxamine. Int Clin Psychopharmacol 1987;2:21–32.

91. Mavissakalian M, Perel J, Bowler K, et al. Trazodone in the treatment of panic disorder and agoraphobia with panic attacks. Am J Psychiatry 1987;144:785–787.

91a. Black DW, Wesner R, Bowers W, Gabel J. A comparison of fluvoxamine, cognitive therapy, and placebo in the treatment of panic disorder. Arch Gen Psychiatry 1993;50:44–50.

92. Lydiard RB, Ballenger JC. Panic-related disorders: evidence for the efficacy of the antidepressants. J Anx Disord 1988;2:77–94.

93. Buigues J, Vallejo J. Therapeutic response to phenelzine in patients with panic disorder and agoraphobia with panic attacks. J Clin Psychiatry 1987;48:55–59.

94. Kelly D, Guirguis W, Frommer E, Mitchell-Heggs N, Sargant W. Treatment of phobic states with antidepressants. A retrospective study of 246 patients. Br J Psychiatry 1970;116:387–398.

95. Lum M, Fontaine R, Elie R, Ontiveros A. Probable interaction of sodium divalproex with benzodiazepines. Progress in Neuro-Psychopharmacology & Biological Psychiatry 1991;15(2):269–273.

96. Primeau F, Fontaine R, Beauclair L. Valproic acid and panic disorder. Can J Psychiatry 1990;35(3):248–250.

97. Roy-Byrne PP, Ward NG, Donnelly PJ. Valproate in anxiety and withdrawal syndromes. J Clin Psychiatry 1989;50(3, suppl): 44–48.

98. Ontiveros A, Fontaine R. Sodium valproate and clonazepam for treatment-resistant panic disorder. J Psychiatr Neurosci 1992;17(2):78–80.

99. Marks IM. Fears, phobias and rituals. New York: Oxford University Press, 1987.

100. Barlow DH. Anxiety and its disorders: the nature and treatment of anxiety and panic. New York: The Guilford Press, 1988.

101. Clum GA, Borden JW. Etiology and treatment of panic disorders. Prog Behav Modif 1989;24:192–222.

102. Beck AT, Emery G. Anxiety disorders and phobias: a cognitive perspective. New York: Basic Books, 1985.

103. Ost LG. Applied relaxation: Description for a coping technique and review of controlled studies. Behav Res Ther 1987;25: 397–409.

104. Marks I, O'Sullivan G. Drugs and psychological treatments for agoraphobia/panic and obsessive-compulsive disorders. Br J Psychiatry 1988;153:650–658.

105. Mavissakalian M, Michelson L, Dealy RS. Pharmacological treatment of agoraphobia: imipramine versus imipramine with programmed practice. Br J Psychiatry 1983;143:348–355.

106. Telch MJ, Agras WS, Taylor CB, et al. Combined pharmacological and behavioral treatment of agoraphobia. Behav Res Ther 1985;23:325–335.

107. Mavissakalian M, Michelson L. Agoraphobia: relative and combined effectiveness of therapist-assisted in vivo exposure and imipramine. J Clin Psychiatry 1986;47:117–122.

108. Klein DF, Ross DC, Cohen P. Panic and avoidance in agoraphobia: application of path analysis to treatment studies. Arch Gen Psychiatry 1987;44:377–385.

109. Wardle J. Behavioral therapy and benzodiazepines: allies or antagonists? Br J Psychiatry 1990;156:163–168.

110. Sargent M. NIMH Report: Panic disorder. Hosp Comm Psychiatry 1990;41: 621–623.

Obsessive-Compulsive Disorder

Obsessions are persistent anxiety provoking ideas, thoughts, impulses, or images that are recognized as originating internally. They are experienced as intrusive and senseless, prompting the patient to ignore, suppress, and/or neutralize them. Typical obsessive themes include:

- Contamination
- Aggression
- Safety or harm
- Sex
- Religious scrupulosity
- Somatic fears
- An excessive need for symmetry or exactness.

If another illness is present, the diagnosis of obsessive-compulsive disorder (OCD) requires that the content of the obsessions be unrelated to the focus of the other disorder.

Compulsions are repetitive, purposeful, intentional behaviors performed in response to an obsession, typically according to certain rules or in a stereotyped fashion.

These behaviors are designed to neutralize obsessions, but again, the individual recognizes them as unreasonable or excessive. Typical compulsive behaviors include:

- Cleaning
- Washing
- Checking
- Excessive ordering and arranging
- Counting
- Repeating
- Collecting.

An additional requirement for the diagnosis of OCD relates to the severity dimension. Thus, symptoms should cause marked distress, be time consuming (taking up to several hours/day), and interfere significantly with normal functioning. Because patients do not necessarily volunteer their symptoms, screening questions such as "Do you wash your hands over and over?" "Do you have to check things repeatedly?" Do you have thoughts that distress you and cannot get rid of?" may be necessary (1).

EPIDEMIOLOGY

OCD, once thought to be very rare, was found to have a lifetime prevalence of 2.5% by an NIMH Epidemiologic Catchment Area study (2). Other epidemiological surveys, such as in Edmonton, Canada, have found a similar prevalence (i.e., 3.0%) (3). A two-stage survey in adolescents first used a preliminary screening of more than 5000 high school students with an OCD inventory, and then a personal semistructured interview by a team of 13 skilled clinicians. Corrected for age of incidence, this study also yielded figures (i.e., 1.9 ± 0.7%), similar to those in adult populations, further validating the earlier studies (4). About half of OCD patients have their onset before age 21 (mean age 19.8 ± 1.9). In general, onset is in childhood, adolescence, or young adulthood, and although the disorder fluctuates somewhat, it usually persists throughout life (5). Less than 10% become progressive, with the adult manifestation essentially identical to that in childhood, with only the content of the symptoms changing (6).

Rasmussen has suggested three underlying psychological dysfunctions:

- An abnormality of risk assessment
- A pathologic doubt
- A need for certainty or perfection (1).

Cross-cultural studies show that OCD occurs in many different groups and is essentially identical, although the content may differ slightly. For example, the Saudis, with their religious association of body washing and prayers, are often obsessed about these issues. By contrast, Hindus are more concerned about dirt, because it plays a prominent role in their religion (7).

COMORBID DISORDERS

A substantial number of OCD patients, as high as 50%, also have associated *major depression.* Similarly, many have some symptoms of depression, whether it be feeling sad, hopeless, inadequate, having sleep disturbances, or other changing vital functions. This disorder, however, starts at a younger age than depression (i.e., about half of OCD patients present before age 21). There is also a somewhat higher incidence of *phobias, panic disorders,* and *alcohol abuse* with OCD than in the general population.

The association with *Gilles de la Tourette's Syndrome* is particularly important. Although only a few OCD patients have tics, the prevalence is much higher than in the general population. Conversely, obsessive-compulsive symptoms are common in Tourette's patients. Thus, there is a clear association between Tourette's disorder and OCD. Tourette's is familial, and most likely genetically transmitted (8). Less is known about the heritability of OCD, but there is some suggestion that it is, at least in part, genetically determined (9).

There have been several large studies of the prevalence of both Tourette's and OCD in index cases having Tourette's disease (10, 10a). In the cases of Tourette's with OCD symptoms, the age-corrected ratio is 18%, with relatives having Tourette's disease, chronic tics, or OCD (10%). In relatives of patients that have Tourette's symptoms only, 17% have either Tourette's disorder or chronic tic disorder and 14% have OCD. Thus, the incidence of OCD in relatives is identical in index cases of those with Tourette's with OCD and index cases of Tourette's only. Finally, follow-up studies find that a significant percentage of children with OCD develop Tourette's syndrome (11).

A great many OCD patients have movement disorders, and conversely, a wide variety of movement disorders also have OCD symptoms, including:

- Sydenham's chorea
- Postencephalitic Parkinson's disease
- Huntington's disease (12).

There is also an occasional association between OCD and *organic brain syndromes, epilepsy,* and other *disorders of the basal ganglia.*

DIFFERENTIAL DIAGNOSIS OF OCD

We do not know the full spectrum of OCD, but having effective drugs means

that atypical presentations can be treated, and if improvement occurs, this supports the proposition that the variant is a manifestation of OCD (13). Several disorders may be variants of OCD, and similarities to this condition include their obsessional quality, familial patterns, and responsiveness to similar drug therapies (14). They may include:

- *Trichotillomania* (or hair pulling)
- *Nail biting*
- *Bowel or bladder obsessions*
- *Pathological jealousy*
- *Dysmorphophobia* (i.e., obsession that a body part is disfigured)
- *Cancer phobias*
- *Self-mutilation* (e.g., picking at one's face) (15–20)

Schizophrenic Disorders

Although many *schizophrenic patients* demonstrate obsessive-compulsive symptoms, it is relevant to note that this problem has received little systematic investigation. There are conflicting case reports of schizophrenic patients with obsessive-compulsive symptoms who failed to benefit when given an anti-OCD drug in addition to an antipsychotic, and other cases where this strategy was beneficial. There are also reports of certain repetitive behaviors that mimic OCD and are benefited by the addition of clomipramine (21).

Personality Disorders

One study of 17 OCD patients treated with medication found that nine of the 10 responders no longer met criteria for the diagnosis of a personality disorder, whereas five of the seven nonresponders, continued to meet criteria. These data imply that some personality disorders may be secondary to a primary diagnosis of OCD (22).

Anxiety Disorders

Some obsessions or compulsions may masquerade as a simple phobia or agoraphobia; or conversely, anxiety about OCD symptoms may mimic a panic attack. Alternatively, it is possible that the comorbidity is real and has some significance other than definitional.

There are clear biological distinctions between OCD and panic disorder. For example, panic attacks are produced by CO_2 inhalation, lactate infusion, yohimbine administration, psychoadrenergic stimulants, isoproterenol, and mCPP. By contrast, none of these agents, except for mCPP, exacerbates obsessions or compulsions. Further, OCD is benefited most by SRIs, whereas panic attacks are helped by a variety of antidepressants, (e.g., TCAs, SRIs, MAOIs).

BIOLOGICAL CORRELATES OF OCD

Genetics

Studies show that OCD tends to run in families. A study of the NIMH cohort of 70 children with OCD found that 25% of fathers and 9% of mothers had the disorder, and in general there was an increased familial occurrence in first-degree relatives of OCD patients (4). In addition, studies of twins find that two out of three monozygotic twins are concordant for OCD (23).

As noted earlier, there is also a genetic association between OCD and Tourette's syndrome, with many Tourette's patients experiencing OCD symptoms (24–26). Tourette's is thought to be an autosomal dominant disease, and although it has not been localized as yet, studies are actively

in process, with at least 50% of the autosomal genome excluded as the locus (27).

Neuropsychiatric Disorders

As noted earlier, several neurological disorders that involve the basal ganglia (e.g., caudate nucleus, globus pallidus, putamen) also manifest OCD symptoms (27a). They include such varied conditions as:

- Huntington's disease
- Choreoacanthocytosis
- Sydenham's chorea
- Postencephalitic Parkinsonism.

Imaging Studies

Although large numbers of OCD patients have not yet been evaluated with functional (e.g., PET and SPECT) or structural imaging (i.e., MRI and CT), there are suggestions that an abnormality might be located near the head of the caudate nucleus, the globus pallidus, and/or the orbital frontal area. This is consistent with a basal ganglia or frontal cortical-subcortical circuit disorder (28, 29).

Neurotransmitters

Two lines of evidence implicate the serotonin system: it has a significant role at several sites in the circuitry connecting the frontal cortical and the basal ganglia locations; and agents that benefit OCD have potent serotonin effects (e.g., clomipramine, SRIs).

Animal Models

There are also some animal models of OCD, including:

- Lick *granuloma*. Several studies show that large dogs who lick their forepaws repetitively, producing a severe lesion, are benefited by clomipramine or fluoxetine, but not desipramine (30).

- *Feather picking* in parrots and a similar disorder in monkeys are also helped by clomipramine (31, 32).

DRUG TREATMENT OF OCD

Most antidepressants block serotonin (5-HT) and/or norepinephrine (NE) reuptake. Only a few, however, are highly potent and/or selective blockers of 5-HT reuptake. Earlier, amitriptyline was considered a potent serotonin reuptake inhibitor; however, it proved to have only a modest effect in comparison to some of the newer agents (e.g., clomipramine, fluoxetine, sertraline, paroxetine, and fluvoxamine). Although clomipramine is the best-studied SRI for OCD, its active metabolite, desmethylclomipramine, also inhibits NE reuptake. Therefore, in vivo, clomipramine affects both amine systems, making it a distinct high-potency SRI, but not serotonin-specific. By contrast, fluoxetine, sertraline, paroxetine, and fluvoxamine have negligible NE blocking properties, making them both highly potent and highly specific for serotonin.

The fact that clomipramine benefits OCD while other standard tricyclics and MAO inhibitors are relatively ineffective, suggests that only SRIs have the necessary properties to be effective. This argument was countered by Marks et al., who suggested that some OCD patients are depressed, and that antidepressants primarily helped the mood disorder, only secondarily improving OCD (33). Given this controversy, it is important to demonstrate that SRIs are specifically effective in OCD, and this is best accomplished by placebo controlled trials. A second question relates to their specificity, which can be demonstrated by comparing these agents to conventional antidepressants. If the SRIs are found more effective, this would have implications for the biological basis of OCD, as well as the mechanism of action of these "antiobsessive" agents.

Meta-Analysis of SRIs for OCD

The primary question for this meta-analysis was whether the high-potency SRIs are differentially effective in OCD. Further, because we cannot argue for greater efficacy of SRIs over placebo if they are only shown to be superior to standard antidepressants (because we do not know if any antidepressant (AD) would be more effective than placebo), we also performed meta-analyses of those studies comparing individual SRIs (i.e., clomipramine, fluvoxamine) as well as all SRIs to placebo. Indeed, there are several published double-blind, random-assignment studies comparing high potency SRIs to placebo and/or standard antidepressants, including the following comparative agents:

- Placebo
- Desipramine
- Imipramine
- Nortryptiline
- Doxepin
- Amitryptiline
- Clorgyline (34–54)

Ideally, the rating assessment used for our analyses should be predetermined so as not to introduce a bias; however, these studies used a variety of instruments to evaluate efficacy. This created an issue concerning which instrument should be chosen for entry into the meta-analysis. A quantitative rating scale designed specifically to assess obsessive-compulsive symptoms would be the instrument of choice, so we rank-ordered those available, starting with the Yale-Brown Obsessive-Compulsive Rating Scale (YBOCS). This hierarchy was then applied in each study, to choose the best scale(s) available. When more than one scale was used, we also performed separate analyses for each to control for the possibility that investigators chose the rating assessment with the biggest drug-drug or drug-placebo difference. We entered the results into a computer program developed for meta-analyses of crossed designs (Gibbons R, Davis JM, manuscript in preparation).

SRIs versus Placebo

The meta-analysis of all studies comparing SRIs to placebo for the treatment of OCD found that the active drug produced a better result in every trial (Table 13.8). Because most studies compared *clomipramine* to placebo, we also calculated the effect size and statistical significance for this agent alone (Table 13.9). There were

also two studies with *fluvoxamine*, and their combined results showed a highly significant effect for this drug as well (Table 13.10). There was also one study with *sertraline*, which found it superior to placebo (55). *Fluoxetine* is curently under investigation, with early limited controlled trials promising (56, 57).

SRIs versus Standard ADs

Also of interest was the comparison of all SRIs to other standard ADs. For those 11 studies, the effect size was 0.79 and 0.71 for the first two measures. The Z statistic was 8.0 and 7.2, for a significance level of 10^{-15} and 10^{-12}, respectively. These results were highly homogeneous, with the effect sizes consistent over all studies (Table 13.11). If clomipramine alone was considered in the meta-analysis, the effect sizes were essentially unchanged (i.e., 0.79 and 0.70; Z scores = 7.6 and 7.2; probabilities of 10^{-14} and 10^{-12}) (Table 13.12).

Table 13.8.
All Serotonin Reuptake Inhibitors versus *Placebo* for OCD

	Number of Studies	Effect Size	Variance	Z	p Value
Measure 1	12	1.11	0.006	15.0	10^{-50}
Measure 2	12	1.16	0.005	14.7	10^{-49}

Table 13.9.
Clomipramine versus *Placebo* for OCD

	Number of Studies	Effect Size	Variance	Z	p Value
Measure 1	9	1.26	0.007	14.8	10^{-49}
Measure 2	9	1.17	0.007	14.3	10^{-46}

Table 13.10.
Fluvoxamine versus *Placebo* for OCD

	Number of Studies	Effect Size	Variance	Z	p Value
Measure 1	2	0.79	0.04	3.77	0.0001
Measure 2	2	0.85	0.05	3.84	0.0001

Table 13.11.
All Serotonin Reuptake Inhibitors versus *Standard ADs* for OCD

	Number of Studies	Effect Size	Variance	Z	*p* Value
Measure 1	11	0.79	0.01	8.0	10^{-15}
Measure 2	11	0.71	0.01	7.2	10^{-12}

Table 13.12.
Clomipramine versus *Standard ADs* for OCD

	Number of Studies	Effect Size	Variance	Z	*p* Value
Measure 1	10	0.79	0.01	7.6	10^{-14}
Measure 2	10	0.70	0.009	7.2	10^{-12}

In conclusion, whether we considered clomipramine alone or the SRIs combined, the evidence clearly found them to be more effective than standard antidepressants.

AUGMENTATION STRATEGIES FOR OCD

Inasmuch as monodrug treatment can reduce the severity of OCD by up to 67%, but typically does not completely eliminate the disorder, it is pertinent to ask whether other adjunctive therapies (e.g., drugs or psychotherapy) could produce a qualitatively better change.

Drug Augmentation

Case reports suggested that adding *lithium* to the SRIs was beneficial, so several controlled studies compared lithium supplementation to clomipramine and one added lithium or placebo to fluvoxamine (58). Unfortunately, neither provided evidence that adjunctive lithium was helpful.

Another study of nine treatment-resistant patients (despite vigorous treatment with clomipramine plus lithium), found that three patients responded to the addition of *trazodone;* relapsed when tra-

zodone was discontinued; and responded again when it was readministered (59). A recent small, double-blind study comparing trazodone to placebo in 21 patients, however, found no difference in therapeutic benefit between this agent and placebo (60).

Fenfluramine augmentation of SRIs in one open study benefited six out of seven patients (61). Many patients have both Tourette's and OCD symptoms, and one case study found that *pimozide* helped Tourette's symptoms while *fluvoxamine* helped the OCD symptoms, suggesting some specificity for each symptom (62). In a naturalistic study of Tourette's with associated OCD, adjunctive *fluoxetine* produced 81% improvement in the complicating OCD symptoms (63).

There is also some evidence that *buspirone* may be helpful in OCD, with one small study finding buspirone alone equieffective to clomipramine (64). Preliminary data also indicate that buspirone may be an effective augmentation of the SRIs.

In one series of nine patients who received open *antipsychotic* augmentation of fluvoxamine (with or without lithium), those who had comorbid tic disorder or schizotypal personality disorder were further benefited (65). In another nine patients who did not have either of these disorders, only two were helped by anti-psychotic augmentation (65).

Non-Drug Augmentation

Concurrent with the introduction of clomipramine in 1966, Meyer first reported on the benefit of behavioral therapy for OCD (66). Thus, while studies were finding the SRIs possessed antiobsessive properties above and beyond their antidepressant effects, a parallel literature also developed demonstrating the efficacy of behavioral techniques for OCD, especially prolonged in vivo exposure and response prevention (67). Further, and in contrast to the high relapse rate with drug discontinuation, a substantial number of patients continue to demonstrate benefit months to years after behavioral interventions (68, 69). Limited therapist contact time allowing patients the independence to develop and implement their own programs also seems to be a more cost-effective approach (70).

Because significant OCD symptoms often remain or recur, even when there is substantial improvement with a specific therapy, a combined complementary approach seems to be the optimal strategy for most patients.

MAINTENANCE DRUG THERAPY FOR OCD

There is clear clinical evidence that most patients relapse if SRIs are discontinued. For example, in a random assignment study where placebo was substituted for clomipramine, 16 out of 18 patients relapsed on placebo by week 7 (71). A second, 2-month study of patients maintained on clomipramine found that only two relapsed and nine remained well, whereas eight relapsed and only one remained well when desipramine was substituted (72).

CONCLUSION

There is little doubt that the SRIs are better than placebo. All studies also found these agents consistently and significantly more effective than standard ADs; but each had a small sample size, and the results were not striking. Because of the consistency across studies, however, the meta-analysis was highly statistically significant.

It is important to note that this observation is a very rare phenomenon in pharmacology. Meta-analyses of studies comparing various standard antidepressants for major depressive disorder reveal that all are equally efficacious (see also Chapter 5) (73). Similarly, meta-analyses of studies comparing antipsychotics find all equally efficacious for psychotic disorders (see also Chapter 7) (74). It is very unusual to find a subclass of drugs more efficacious than others in the same class. Hence, if some antidepressants are clearly more effective than other ADs in OCD, it is truly noteworthy. In addition to finding that the SRIs are more effective than standard antidepressants, the results are also homogeneous, in that the degree to which these drugs outperform their earlier generation counterparts remains consistent across all studies.

The question of an even more selective efficacy for clomipramine over the SRIs, however, remains unanswered due to a paucity of well-designed studies. One comparison of clomipramine to fluoxetine found no significant difference in efficacy (75). Because clomipramine is not a pure serotonergic drug (i.e., it also inhibits norepinephrine uptake by virtue of an active metabolite), its mechanism of antiobsessive action remains uncertain. Studies designed to address these questions may shed light on a specific biochemical dysfunction or possible aberrant interactions among different neurotransmitter systems.

Two other observations help to differentiate serotonin reuptake inhibitors' antiobsessive from their antidepressive effects, as well as address the concerns raised by Dr. Marks. The first is provided by these agents' differential rate of improvement for depression versus OCD. Generally, the rate of improvement in depression is rapid, the largest change occurring in the first few weeks, and dropping dramatically by the fourth to sixth week, because most patients are then recovered. The rate of improvement with these agents for OCD, however, is much slower than this (taking approximately twice as long), suggesting a different mechanism of action.

The second observation concerns mechanism of action and stems from subgroup analyses. In the collaborative studies of Ciba-Geigy, patients were selected for OCD without depression, and the total improvement was compared to those who had OCD with depression. There was no difference in the antiobsessive effects of these agents in either group. This analysis treated associated depression as a discontinuous variable (i.e., present or absent). An alternate method is to correlate the degree of coexisting depression to improvement in OCD. When this was done, no correlation was evident. Returning to Dr. Marks' hypothesis, if serotonin agents improved OCD as a secondary effect to their antidepressive properties, there should be a high correlation between improvement in a coexisting depression and obsessive symptoms.

Based on our results, we would conclude that:

• Serotonin reuptake inhibitors are more effective than placebo or standard ADs in the treatment of OCD, while equieffective to standard ADs for depression

• Our review was able to distinguish these agents' antiobsessive properties from their antidepressant properties.

Appendices K and L summarize the diagnostic criteria and Figure 13.3 summarizes the treatment strategy we would suggest given the evidence thus far. The concurrent use of drug plus behavioral therapy seems to offer the best chance for improvement in the majority of patients. Finally, in those most severely affected (i.e., manifest an unremitting course despite several adequate trials of drug and behavioral therapies), psychosurgical intervention may offer the only viable chance for relief of this disabling disorder (76, 77).

REFERENCES

1. Rasmussen SA, Eisen JL. The epidemiology and differential diagnosis of obsessive compulsive disorder. J Clin Psychiatry 1992;53(4, suppl):4–10.
2. Karno M, Golding, JM, Sorenson SB, Burnam A. The epidemiology of obsessive-compulsive disorder in five US communities. Arch Gen Psychiatry 1988;45:1094–1099.
3. Bland RC, Orn H, Newman SC. Lifetime prevalence of psychiatric disorders in Edmonton. Acta Psychiatr Scand 1988; 77(suppl 338):24–32.
4. Flament MF, Whitaker A, Rapoport JL, Davies M, Zaremba Berg C, Kalikow K, Sceery W, Shaffer D. Obsessive compulsive disorder in adolescence: an epidemiological study. J Am Acad Child Adolesc Psychiatry 1988;27(6):764–771.
5. Rasmussen SA. Obsessive-compulsive disorder in dermatologic practice. J Am Acad Dermatol 1985;13:965–967.
6. Goodwin DW, Guze SB, Robins E. Follow-up studies in obsessional neurosis. Arch Gen Psychiatry 1969;20:182–187.
7. Mahgoub OM, Abdel-Hafeiz HB. Pattern of obsessive-compulsive disorder in eastern Saudi Arabia. Br J Psychiatry 1991;158:840–842.
8. Comings DE, Comings BG. Hereditary

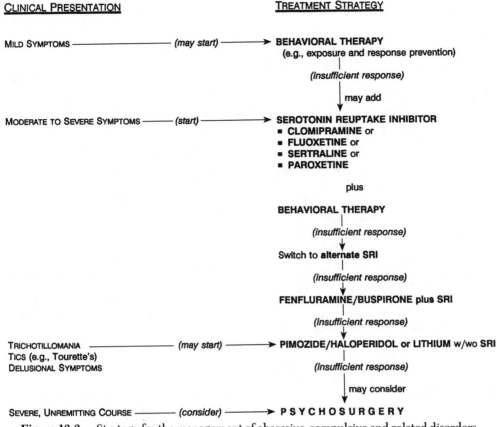

Figure 13.3.   Strategy for the management of obsessive-compulsive and related disorders.

agoraphobia and obsessive-compulsive behavior in relatives of patients with Giles de la Tourette's syndrome. Br J Psychiatry 1987;15:195–199.

9. Pauls DL, Leckman JF. The inheritance of Gilles de la Tourette's syndrome and associated behaviors: evidence for autosomal dominant transmission. N Engl J Med 1986;315:993–997.

10. Pauls DL, Raymond CL, Stevenson JM, Leckman JF. A family study of Gilles de la Tourette Syndrome. Am J Hum Genet 1991;48:154–156.

10a. Shapiro AK, Shapiro E. Evaluation of the reported association of obsessive compulsive symptoms or disorders with Tourette's disorder. Compr Psychiatry 1992;23(3):152–165.

11. Rapoport JL, Swedo SE, Guze BH, et al. Childhood obsessive compulsive disorder.

J Clin Psychiatry 1992;53(4,Suppl.):11–16.

12. Cummings JL, Cunningham K. Obsessive-compulsive disorder in Huntington's disease. Biol Psychiatry 1992;31:263–270.

13. Fallon BA, Liebowitz MR, Hollander E, Schneier FR, Campeas RB, Fairbanks J, Papp LA, Hatterer JA, Sandberg D. The pharmacotherapy of moral or religious scrupulosity. J Clin Psychiatry 1990;51:517–521.

14. Ratnasuriya RH, Marks IM, Forshaw DM, Hymas NFS. Obsessive slowness revisited. Br J Psychiatry 1991;159:273–274.

15. Stein DJ, Hollander E. Dermatology and conditions related to obsessive-compulsive disorder. J Am Acad Dermatol 1992;26:237–242.

16. Fishbain DA, Goldberg M. Fluoxetine for obsessive fear of loss of control of malodor-

ous flatulence. Psychosomatics 1991;32(1): 105–107.

17. Epstein S, Jenike MA. Disabling urinary obsessions: an uncommon variant of obsessive-compulsive disorder. Psychosomatics 1990;31(4):450–452.

18. Jenike MA, Vitagliano HL, Rabinowitz J, Goff DC, Baer L. Bowel obsessions responsive to tricyclic antidepressants in four patients. Am J Psychiatry 1987;144(10): 1347–1348.

19. Lane RD. Successful fluoxetine treatment of pathologic jealousy. J Clin Psychiatry 1990;51(8):345–346.

20. Viswanathan R, Paradis C. Treatment of cancer phobia with fluoxetine [Letter]. Am J Psychiatry 1991;148(8):1090.

21. Pulman J, Yassa R, Ananth J. Clomipramine treatment of repetitive behavior. Can J Psychiatry 1984;29:254–255.

22. Ricciardi JN, Baer L, Jenike MA, Fischer SC, Sholtz D, Buttolph ML. Changes in DSM-III-R Axis II diagnoses following treatment of obsessive-compulsive disorder. Am J Psychiatry 1992;149:829–831.

23. Lenane M, Swedo SE, Rapoport JL. Rates of obsessive compulsive disorder for first-degree relatives of patients with trichotillomania. J Child Psychol Psychiatry 1992;33:925–933.

24. Frankel M, Cummings JL, Robertson MM, Trimble MR, Hill MA, Benson DF. Obsessions and compulsions in Gilles de la Tourette's syndrome. Neurology 1986;36: 378–382.

25. Grad LR, Pelcovitz D, Olson M, Matthews M, Grad GJ. Obsessive-compulsive symptomatology in children with Tourette's Syndrome. J Amer Acad Child Adolesc Psychiatry 1987;26(1):69–73.

26. Robertson MM. The Gilles de la Tourette Syndrome and obsessional disorder. Int Clin Psychopharmacol 1991;6(suppl 3):69–84.

27. Pakstis, AJ, Heutink P, Pauls DL, et al. Progress in the search for genetic linkage with Tourette Syndrome: an exclusion map covering more than 50% of the autosomal genome. Am J Hum Genet 1991;48:281–294.

27a. George MS, Melvin JA, Kellner CH. Obsessive-compulsive symptoms in neurologic disease: a review. Behav Neurology 1992;5:3–10.

28. Baxter Jr LR, Schwartz JM, Guze BH, et al. PET imaging in obsessive-compulsive disorder with and without depression. J Clin Psychiatry 1990;51(4, suppl);61–69.

29. Rapoport JL. Recent advances in obsessive-compulsive disorder. Neuropsychopharmacology 1991;5(1):1–10.

30. Rapoport JL, Ryland DH, Kriete M. Drug treatment of canine acral lick. An animal model of obsessive-compulsive disorder. Arch Gen Psychiatry 1992;49(7):517–521.

31. Roskopf WJ, Woerpel RW, Reed-Blake S, Lane R. Feather picking in psittacine birds. In: Proceedings of the Association of Avian Veterinarians, June 16–22, 1986, Miami, Fla.

32. Levine BS. Psychogenic feather-picking. Avian/Exotic Pract. 1984;1:23–25.

33. Marks IM, Stern RS, Mawson D, Cobb J, McDonald R. Clomipramine and exposure for obsessive-compulsive rituals: I. Br J. Psychiatry 1980;136:1–25.

34. Thoren P, Asberg M, Cronholm B, et al. Clomipramine treatment of obsessive-compulsive disorder 1. A controlled clinical trial. Arch Gen Psychiatry 1980;37:1281–1285.

35. Bick PA, Hackett E, Chouinard G. Multicenter placebo controlled study of sertraline in obsessive-compulsive disorder. Arch Gen Psychiatry 1989;46:23–28.

36. Flament MF, Rapoport JL, Berg CJ, Sceery W. Kitts C, Mellstrom B, Linnoila M. Clomipramine treatment of childhood obsessive compulsive disorder: a double-blind controlled study. Arch Gen Psychiatry 1985;42:977–983.

37. Goodman WK, Price LH, Rasmussen SA, Delgado PL, Heninger GR, Charney DS. Efficacy of fluvoxamine in obsessive-compulsive disorder. Arch Gen Psychiatry 1989;46:36–44.

38. Karabanow O. Double-blind controlled study in phobias and obsessions. J Int Med Res 1977;5(suppl 5):42–48.

39. Marks IM, Stern RS, Mawson D, Cobb J, McDonald R. Clomipramine and exposure for obsessive-compulsive rituals: I. Br J Psychiatry 1980;136:1–25.

40. Marks IM, Lelliott P, Basoglu M, Noshirvani H, Monteiro W, Cohen D, and Kasvikis Y. Clomipramine, self-exposure and therapist-aided exposure for obsessive-compulsive rituals. I. Br J Psychiatry 1988;152:522–534.

41. Montgomery SA. Clomipramine in obsessional neurosis: a placebo controlled trial. Pharm Med 1980;1:189–192.

42. Perse TL, Greist JH, Jefferson JW, Rosenfeld R, Dur R. Fluvoxamine treatment of obsessive-compulsive disorder. Am J Psychiatry 1987;144:1543–1548.

43. Ciba-Geigy Multi-Center Drug Trial Data, Protocol 59.

44. Ciba-Geigy Multi-Center Drug Trial Data, Protocol 61.

45. Goodman WK, Price LH, Delgado PL, et al. Specificity of serotonin reuptake inhibitors in the treatment of obsessive-compulsive disorder. Arch Gen Psychiatry 1990;47:577–585.

46. Leonard HL, Swedo SE, Rapoport JL, Koby EV, Lenane MC, Cheslow DL, Hamburger SD. Treatment of obsessive-compulsive disorder with clomipramine and desipramine in children and adolescents. Arch Gen Psychiatry 1989;46:1088–1092.

47. Swedo SE, Leonard HL, Rapoport JL, Lenane MC, Goldberger EL, Cheslow DL. A double-blind comparison of clomipramine and desipramine in the treatment of trichotillomania (hair pulling). New Engl Med 1989;321(8):497–501.

48. Zohar J, Mueller EA, Insel TR, et al. Serotonergic responsivity in obsessive-compulsive disorder. Comparison of patients and healthy controls. Arch Gen Psychiatry 1987;44:946–951.

49. Lei. Crossover therapy. Chinese J Neurology Psychiatry 1986;19(5): 275–278.

50. Mavissakalian M, Michelson L. Tricyclic antidepressants in obsessive-compulsive disorder. Anti-obsessional or anti-depressant agents. J Nervous and Mental Disease 1983;171(5):301–306.

51. Volavka J. Neziroglu F, Yaryura-Tobias JA. Clomipramine and imipramine in obsessive-compulsive disorder. Psychiatry Res 1985;14:83–91.

52. Cui. Double-blind trial of clomipramine vs doxepine. Chinese J Neurology Psychiatry 1986;19(5):279–281.

53. Ananth J, Pecknold JC, Van Den Steen N, Engelsmann F. Double-blind comparative study of clomipramine and amitriptyline in obsessive neurosis. Prog Neuropsychopharmacol Biol Psychiatry 1981;5:257–262.

54. Insel TR, Murphy DL, Cohen RM, Alterman I, Kitts C, Linnoila M. Obsessive-compulsive disorder: a double-blind trial of clomipramine and clorgyline. Arch Gen Psychiatry 1983;40:605–612.

55. Chouinard G, Goodman W, Greist J, Jenike M, Rasmussen S, White K, Hackett E, Gaffney M, Bick PA. Results of a double-blind placebo controlled trial of a new serotonin uptake inhibitor, sertraline, in the treatment of obsessive-compulsive disorder. Psychopharmacol Bull 1990;26(3):279–284.

56. Pigott TA, Pato MT, Bernstein SE, Grover GN, Hill JL, Tolliver TJ, Murphy DL. Controlled comparisons of clomipramine and fluoxetine in the treatment of obsessive-compulsive disorder. Arch Gen Psychiatry 1990;47:926–32.

57. Turner SM, Jacob RG, Beidel DC, Himmelhoch J. Fluoxetine treatment of obsessive-compulsive disorder. J Clin Psychopharmacol 1985;5(4):207–212.

58. McDougle CJ, Goodman WK, Price LH. Lithium augmentation in fluvoxamine-refractory obsessive compulsive disorder. American College Neuropsychopharmacol Panels and Posters, 28th Annual Meeting, 1989:176.

59. Hermesh H, Aizenberg D, Munitz H. Trazodone treatment in clomipramine-resistant OCD. Clin Neuropharmacol 1990;13:322–328.

60. Pigott TA, L'Heureux F, Rubenstein CS, Bernstein SE, Hill JL, Murphy DL. A double-blind, placebo controlled study of trazodone in patients with OCD. J Clin Psychiatry 1992;12:156–162.

61. Hollander E, DeCaria CM, Schneier FR, Schneier HA, Liebowitz MR, Klein DF. Fenfluramine augmentation of serotonin reuptake blockade antiobsessional treatment. J Clin Psychiatry 1990;51:119–123.

62. Delgado PL, Goodman WK, Price LH, et al. Fluvoxamine/pimozide treatment of concurrent Tourette's and obsessive-compulsive disorder. Br J Psychiatry 1990;157:762–765.

63. Como PG, Kurlan R. An open-label trial of fluoxetine for obsessive-compulsive disorder in Gilles de la Tourette's Syndrome. Neurology 1991;41:872–874.

64. Pato MT, Pigott TA, Hill JL, et al. Controlled comparison of buspirone and clomipramine in obsessive-compulsive disorder. Am J Psychiatry 1991;148:127–129.

65. McDougle CJ, Goodman WK, Price LH, Delgado PL, Krystal JH, Charney DS, Heninger GR. Neuroleptic addition in fluvoxamine-refractory OCD. Am J Psychiatry 1990:147:652–654.

66. Meyer V. Modification of expectations in cases with obsessional rituals. Behav Res Ther 1966;4:273–280.

67. Greist JH. An integrated approach to treatment of obsessive compulsive disorder. J Clin Psychiatry 1992;53(4, suppl):38–41.

68. Pato M, Zohar-Kadouch R, Zohar J, et al. Return of symptoms after discontinuation of clomipramine in patients with obsessive-compulsive disorder. Am J Psychiatry 1988;145:1521–1525.

69. Pato MT, Murphy DL, De Vane CL. Sustained plasma concentrations of fluoxetine and/or norfluoxetine four and eight weeks after fluoxetine discontinuation. J Clin Psychopharmacol 1991;11:224–225.

70. Marks IM, Lelliott P, Basoglu M, et al. Clomipramine, self-exposure and therapist-aided exposure for obsessive-compulsive rituals. Br J Psychiatry 1988;152:522–534.

71. Pato MT, Zohar-Kadouch R, Zohar J, Murphy D. Return of symptoms after discontinuation of clomipramine in patients with OCD. Am J Psychiatry 1988;145:1521–1525.

72. Leonard HL, Swedo SE, Lenane MC, et al. A double-blind desipramine substitution during long-term clomipramine treatment in children and adolescents with ob-

sessive-compulsive disorder. Arch Gen Psychiatry 1991;48:922–927.

73. Davis JM, Barter JT, Kane JM. Antipsychotic drugs. In: Kaplan Hl, Sadock BJ, eds. Comprehensive textbook of psychiatry, vol. 2, Williams & Wilkins, 1989:1591.

74. Glassman AM, Davis JM, Barter JT, Kane JM. Antidepressant drugs. In: Kaplan Hl, Sadock BJ, eds. Comprehensive textbook of psychiatry, vol. 2. Williams & Wilkins, 1989:1627.

75. Piggott TA, Pato MT, Bernstein SE, Grover GN, Hill JL, Toliver TJ, Murphy DL. A controlled comparison of clomipramine and fluoxetine in the treatment of obsessive-compulsive disorder. American College of Neuropsychopharmacology Abstracts of Panels and Posters. 28th Annual Meeting. 1989:173.

76. Birley JLT. Modified frontal leucotomy: a review of 106 cases. Br J Psychiatry 1964;110:211–221.

77. Sykes M, Tredgold R. Restricted orbital undercutting. A study of its effects on 350 patients over the ten years 1951–1960. Br J Psychiatry 1964;110:609–640.

Trichotillomania

This disorder, listed in the DSM-III-R under Impulse Control Disorders Not Elsewhere Classified, is characterized by impulses to pull out one's hair, often involving multiple sites. Some clinicians have proposed that this condition is a variant of OCD, based on similarities in phenomenology, family history, and response to treatment (1). Originally thought to occur more frequently in females, it is now evident that it may affect males just as often. Many victims of this disorder have histories beginning in childhood and refractoriness to all attempted remedies. Comorbidity of trichotillomania with mood, anxiety, substance abuse, and eating disorders is also common (2). Others have noted that trichotillomania may also coexist with mental retardation and psychotic disorders (see also Appendix R).

Clomipramine and *fluoxetine* may reduce the frequency and intensity of this disorder (3–8). *Lithium* may lead to decreased hair pulling, and mild to marked hair regrowth (9). Unfortunately, relapse after initial improvement has also been reported. For children, such treatments should be reserved for only those with the more severe, refractory forms (see also Figure 13.3).

REFERENCES

1. Rapoport JL. The boy who couldn't stop washing. New York: Dutton, 1989.
2. Christenson GA, Mackenzie TB, Mitchell JE. Characteristics of 60 adult chronic hair

pullers. Am J Psychiatry 1991;148:365–370.

3. Swedo SE, Leonard HL, Rapoport JL, et al. A double-blind comparison of clomipramine and desipramine in the treatment of trichotillomania (hair pulling). N Engl J Med 1989;321:497–501.

4. Turner SM, Jacob RG, Bidel DC, Himmelhoch J. Fluoxetine treatment of obsessive compulsive disorder. J Clin Psychopharmacol 1985;5:207–212.

5. Freeman CP, Hampson M. Fluoxetine as a treatment for bulimia nervosa. Int J Obes 1987;II(suppl 3):171–174.

6. Eras GG, Pope GH, Levine LR. Fluoxetine in bulimia nervosa, double-blind study. Presented at the Annual Meeting of the American Psychiatric Association, May 1989.

7. George MS, Brewerton TD, Cochrane C. Trichotillomania (hair pulling) [Letter]. N Engl J Med 1990;322:470–471.

8. Jenike MA. Trichotillomania (hair pulling) [Letter]. N Engl J Med 1990;322:472.

9. Christenson GA, Popkin MK, Mackenzie TB, Realmuto GM. Lithium treatment of chronic hair pulling. J Clin Psychiatry 1991;52:116–120.

Post-Traumatic Stress Disorder

Post-traumatic stress disorder (PTSD) is attributable to an unusual experience that would be very stressful for almost anyone (e.g., serious threat to life or physical integrity, involvement of the person or a loved one in a major catastrophe, such as a serious traffic accident) (1). This largely environmentally-induced disorder has been frequently observed in combat veterans with a history of exposure to overwhelming stress (2). The patient reexperiences the traumatic event by:

- Recollections
- Dreams
- Acting or feeling as if the traumatic event was recurring
- Intense psychological distress on exposure to events that symbolize or resemble the traumatic event.

Other manifestations of the disorder include persistent avoidance of stimuli associated with the trauma and symptoms of increased arousal, neither of which were present before the incident. To qualify for this diagnosis, a symptomatic period of at least one month is required (see Appendices K and L).

Comorbidity is frequent. For example, Shore et al. (1989) found that among his PTSD patients 28% also had GAD; 29% depression; 12% phobias; and 10% alcohol abuse problems (3).

DRUG THERAPY FOR PTSD

Various psychoactive drugs have been prescribed for PTSD patients. Clinical experience has verified the findings of controlled studies, namely that most of the drugs that are effective for PTSD are also useful for both major depression and panic disorder. In particular, symptoms associated with hyperarousal or reexperiencing of the traumatic incident are benefited by drug therapies (4). This is true not only for the tricyclics (i.e., amitriptyline, imipramine, desipramine, and doxepin) and MAOIs (particularly phenelzine); but also perhaps for benzodiazepines (alprazolam), lithium, carbamazepine, valproic acid, buspirone, fluoxetine, propranolol, and clonidine (5).

Some also advocate the use of hypnotic techniques to facilitate a working through of the traumatic event(s) (6). This approach is based on the frequently observed interrelationship of dissociative reactions and physical trauma.

REFERENCES

1. Epstein RS. Posttraumatic stress disorder: a review of diagnostic and treatment issues. Psychiatric Annals 1989;19(10):556–563.
2. Helzer JE, Robins LN, McEvoy L. Posttraumatic stress disorder in the general population. Findings of the epidemiologic Catchment Area Survey. N Engl J Med 1987;317(26):1630–1634.
3. Shore JH, Vollner WM, Tatum EL. Community patterns of post-traumatic stress disorder. J Nerv Ment Dis 1989;177:681–685.
4. Silver JM, Sandberg DP, Hales RE. New approaches in the pharmacotherapy of posttraumatic stress disorder. J Clin Psychiatry 1990;51(10, suppl):33–38.
5. Davidson J. Drug therapy of post traumatic stress disorder. Br J Psychiatry 1992;160:309–314.
6. Spiegel D, Cardena E. New uses of hypnosis in the treatment of posttraumatic stress disorder. J Clin Psychiatry 1990;51(10, suppl):39–43.

Somatoform Disorder

Also called Briquet's syndrome, somatoform disorder (SD) occurs predominantly in women, is often chronic, and tends to run in families (1). It is manifested by:

- Multiple *somatic symptoms* involving several different bodily systems
- *Absence of an organic cause* for these symptoms
- A tendency by the patient to *dramatize complaints,* to *refuse psychological explanations* for them, and to *manipulate* the doctors
- *Menstrual and sexual* complaints
- A history of *repeated hospitalizations* and *multiple operations* starting before age 30
- A tendency to become *dependent on sedatives, anxiolytics and/or analgesics.*

(see also Appendices K and M).

As a rule, SD patients need counseling and support. The objective is to divert patients' focus from their multiple physical complaints toward efforts to cope with their problems in living and the avoidance of unnecessary medical and surgical therapies that may worsen their illness. Some of these patients may also require insight-oriented psychotherapy. Many complain of depressive and anxiety-related symptoms, and these may mask SD or represent comorbid conditions, so the clinician must be alert to these possibilities (2). Misdiagnosis may result in mismanagement, and mutual hostility is common between these patients and their doctors.

Because SD often goes unrecognized, patients are frequently and inappropriately treated with a variety of anxiolytics and antidepressants, which are seldom beneficial and can evoke a host of adverse effects, about which they complain bitterly. Psychotropics and analgesics should not be prescribed for most SD patients, and if they are, their usage should be carefully monitored. As noted above, they often become dependent on sedatives, anxiolytics and/or analgesics. They may also impulsively overdose with these drugs, at times producing a life-threatening crisis or occasionally, a fatal outcome.

REFERENCES

1. Barsky AJ. Somatoform disorders. In: Kaplan HI, Sadock BJ, eds. Comprehensive textbook of psychiatry, 5th ed. Baltimore: Williams & Wilkins, 1989:1009–1027.
2. Barsky AJ, Wyshak G, Klerman GL. Psychiatric comorbidity in DSM-III-R hypochondriasis. Arch Gen Psychiatry 1992;49:101–108.

Dissociative Disorders

Formerly known as hysterical neuroses of the dissociative type, these disorders are now classified into five categories by the DSM-III-R:

- Psychogenic *amnesia*
- Psychogenic *fugue*
- *Multiple personality* (dissociative identity) disorder

- *Depersonalization* disorder
- *Dissociative* disorder not otherwise specified (1) (see also Appendices K and N).

Psychotherapy, with emphasis on the strength of the therapeutic alliance, has been used more often than drugs for such patients, with hypnotherapy specifically employed as an intervention for multiple

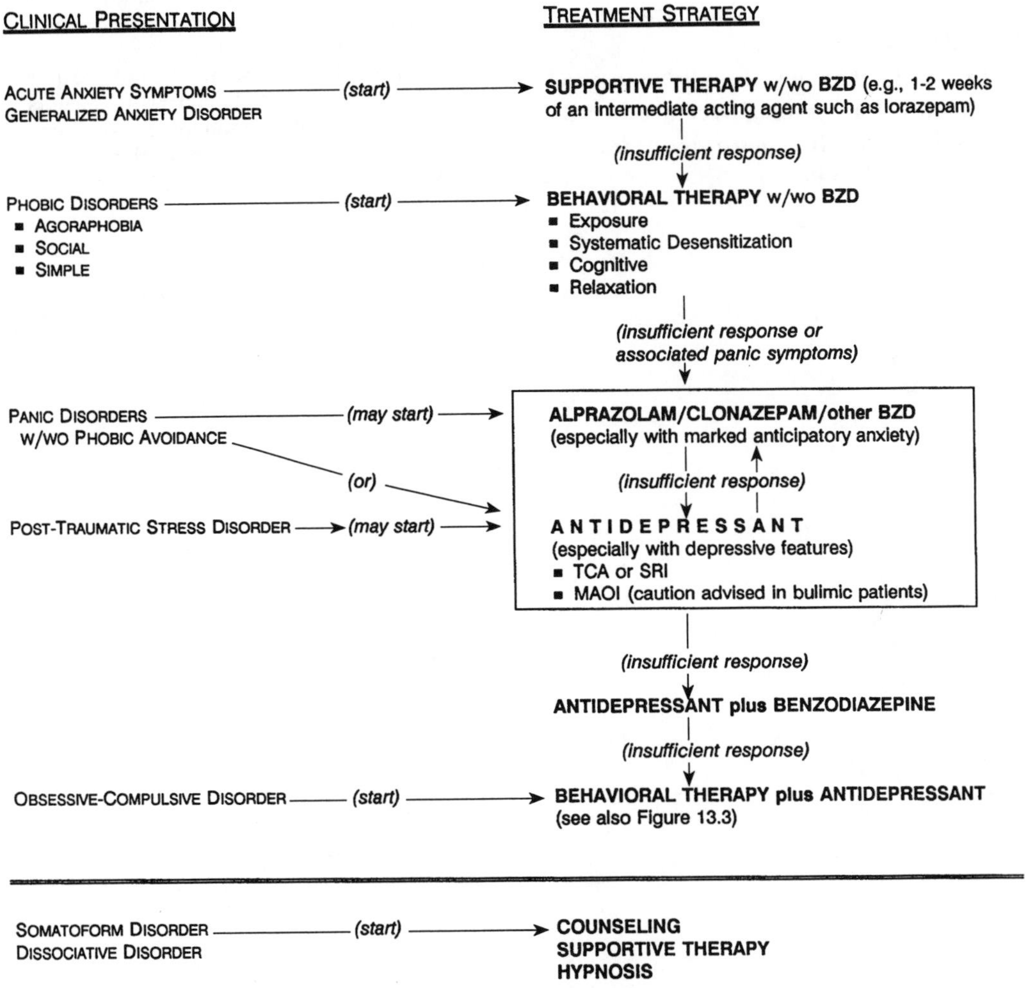

CLINICAL PRESENTATION   TREATMENT STRATEGY

ACUTE ANXIETY SYMPTOMS ——————— (start) ——————→ **SUPPORTIVE THERAPY** w/wo **BZD** (e.g., 1-2 weeks
GENERALIZED ANXIETY DISORDER   of an intermediate acting agent such as lorazepam)

                                                          (insufficient response)

PHOBIC DISORDERS ——————— (start) ——————→ **BEHAVIORAL THERAPY** w/wo **BZD**
  ■ AGORAPHOBIA   ■ Exposure
  ■ SOCIAL   ■ Systematic Desensitization
  ■ SIMPLE   ■ Cognitive
                                                          ■ Relaxation

                                                          *(insufficient response or
                                                          associated panic symptoms)*

PANIC DISORDERS ——————— (may start) ——→   **ALPRAZOLAM/CLONAZEPAM/other BZD**
  w/wo PHOBIC AVOIDANCE   (especially with marked anticipatory anxiety)

                     (or) ——→   *(insufficient response)*

POST-TRAUMATIC STRESS DISORDER ——→ (may start) ——→   **ANTIDEPRESSANT**
                                                          (especially with depressive features)
                                                          ■ TCA or SRI
                                                          ■ MAOI (caution advised in bulimic patients)

                                                          (insufficient response)

                                                          ANTIDEPRESSANT plus BENZODIAZEPINE

                                                          (insufficient response)

OBSESSIVE-COMPULSIVE DISORDER ——————— (start) ——————→ **BEHAVIORAL THERAPY plus ANTIDEPRESSANT**
                                                          (see also Figure 13.3)

SOMATOFORM DISORDER ——————— (start) ——————→ **COUNSELING**
DISSOCIATIVE DISORDER   **SUPPORTIVE THERAPY**
                                                          HYPNOSIS

Figure 13.4.   Overview of treatment strategies for anxiety-related disorders.

personality (dissociative identity) disorder (2, 3).

Despite their common occurrence, there is a paucity of data on the pharmacotherapy of these disorders, with most drug interventions based on symptom manifestation. Thus, anxiolytics are used for associated anxiety, ADs for associated depression, and antipsychotics for any underlying psychosis (e.g., schizophrenia). Generally, pharmacotherapy is low-dose and short-term, prescribed only as long as necessary to alleviate acutely distressing symptoms. Further complicating matters, these patients are often noncompliant and often overreact to the usual pharmacologic effects of these drugs.

In short, they are usually not good candidates for psychopharmacotherapy and seldom derive more than limited symptomatic benefit.

CONCLUSION

Appendices K, L, M, and N summarize the diagnostic criteria and Figure 13.4 overviews our recommended approach to the management of several anxiety-related disorders.

REFERENCES

1. Nemiah JC. Dissociative disorders (hysterical neuroses, dissociative type). In: Kaplan HI, Sadock BJ, eds. Comprehensive textbook of psychiatry, 5th ed. Baltimore: Williams & Wilkins, 1989:1028–1044.
2. Braun BG, ed. Treatment of multiple personality disorder. Washington, D.C.: American Psychiatric Press, 1986.
3. Kluft RP. The treatment of multiple personality disorder (MPD): current concepts. In: Flach FF, ed. Directions in psychiatry. Vol 5. Lesson 24. New York: Hatherleigh, 1985.

CHAPTER 14

Assessment and Treatment of Special Populations

The intent of this chapter is to clarify and to highlight the clinical assessment and drug treatment issues raised by patients whose symptoms occur in the context of specialized circumstances. Thus, this last chapter will cover two major topics:

- Special diagnostic and treatment issues raised during the *life cycle*
- *Medical conditions* complicating psychiatric assessment and drug therapy.

Special life cycle issues concern:

- The pregnant patient
- The child and the adolescent patient
- The geriatric patient
- The personality-disordered patient.

Complicating medical issues can occur in:

- The alcoholic patient
- The seizure-prone patient
- The HIV-infected patient
- The eating-disordered patient.

Since literally volumes have been published for most of these populations, this will not be a comprehensive review of each of these issues. Instead, our purpose is to underscore how complications related to each of these specialized groups may alter the clinician's approach to diagnosis and treatment. Such circumstances will always be considered in the context of alterations in the risk to benefit ratio posed by these patients.

The Pregnant Patient

No other area of psychiatry raises the anxiety of the treating clinician more, than the drug management of the pregnant patient. The risk to benefit ratio must be considered from several important perspectives, including:

- The risk to the *fetus*
- The risk to the *pregnant mother* due to her altered physiology

- The risk of future *behavioral teratogenicity* in the young newborn
- The risk to the mother and the fetus from an *untreated or inadequately managed mental disorder* (1).

These issues are further complicated by an increasing number of pregnancies in women with more severe and chronic mental disorders (2).

We would note that effects on brain morphogenesis may not be apparent for several years. Since psychotropics target the brain, this should be of concern. Further, drugs such as amphetamines and barbiturates have been found to adversely affect the development of laboratory animals. Thus, it is always better to avoid the use of psychotropics during pregnancy, if at all possible.

DRUG THERAPY DURING PREGNANCY

Antipsychotics

The issue of antipsychotics during pregnancy warrants careful scrutiny, given the apparent increasing birth rate in this patient population and the need for chronic drug therapy to maintain optimal functioning (3). Although the literature is unclear regarding the potential for both fetal developmental and later behavioral teratogenicity, it is clear that many patients will require antipsychotic therapy during pregnancy. Miller (1991) has provided specific clinical guidelines, which include:

- *Avoidance of antipsychotics*, if possible, during the period of highest risk for teratogenicity (i.e., 4–10 weeks after conception)
- *Discontinuation of the antipsychotics*, if at all possible, 2 weeks prior to the estimated date of confinement (EDC) to minimize withdrawal effects in the neonate
- The use of *higher potency agents* to minimize sedation, orthostasis, gastrointestinal (GI) slowing, and tachycardia
- If a pregnant patient develops *the neuroleptic malignant syndrome* (NMS), immediate discontinuation of the antipsychotic and the use of bromocriptine to manage symptoms
- Resumption of antipsychotic immediately *postpartum* in chronically psychotic women to minimize development of a postpartum episode
- *Avoidance of routine prophylaxis with antiparkinsonian agents.* If one is necessary, there is no current evidence that any agent is superior to the others (2).

Antidepressants

It is estimated that about 10% of pregnant women will develop a serious depression (4). Most data on teratogenicity involve the tricyclic antidepressants (TCAs), and thus far no major deficits have been identified. Monoamine oxidase inhibitors (MAOIs) are known animal teratogens, but the lack of human data limits any conclusions. Insufficient experience also precludes any firm suggestions about the serotonin reuptake inhibitors (SRIs). Clinical guidelines for the management of depression during pregnancy include the following:

- *Nondrug approaches* (e.g., supportive therapy) are always preferable
- If necessary, *electroconvulsive therapy (ECT) or TCAs* should be given preference
- *Nortriptyline* and *desipramine* may be the TCAs of choice, given their extensive assessment during pregnancy and well-known therapeutic concentrations, which can be checked by therapeutic drug monitoring (TDM)
- If a *TCA* is withdrawn during pregnancy, it should be *gradually tapered* to avoid maternal or fetal withdrawal syndrome
- If possible, *drug tapering* should begin 5–10 days before the EDC (5)
- Those with a prior history may be more susceptible to *postpartum depression*, and maintenance antidepressant (AD) therapy should be carefully considered.

Mood Stabilizers

Bipolar disorder is a recurring illness whose course is even more complicated during pregnancy. Further, most effective drug therapies (e.g., lithium, carbamazepine (CBZ), valproic acid (VPA)) carry significant pharmacokinetic, physiological, and teratogenic risk. The effects of lithium during the first trimester on the developing fetal heart (i.e., Epstein's anomaly) have been well publicized, but are as yet unproven (6). Detailed discussion of these issues can be found in Adverse Effects of Lithium in Chapter 10. Whereas teratogenicity has been well documented for either CBZ or VPA alone, their combined use may be particularly detrimental (7, 8).

Clinical strategies to minimize the risk to mother and fetus, either from drug-induced anomalies or the potential ravages of the disease process include:

* Carefully weighing the *risk to benefit ratio* when contemplating whether to initiate, continue, or withdraw drug therapy
* Considering *alternate therapies* when feasible, such as antipsychotics or ECT
* If lithium is necessary, especially during the first trimester, *sonography* can help evaluate the presence and severity of such anomalies as Epstein's tricuspid valve defect
* If exposed to VPA, the presence of *neural tube* defects should be evaluated
* The increased risk of postpartum psychosis with bipolar disorder warrants the *resumption of medication soon after delivery.* Under these circumstances, the discontinuation of nursing should be considered.

Antianxiety Agents

The experience of pregnancy itself is often anxiety provoking, and symptoms sufficient to warrant drug therapy are common in this group (9). Although this discussion primarily focuses on the benzodiazepines (BZDs), antidepressants and buspirone may also be employed for women of child-bearing age with certain anxiety disorders. Perhaps the best-documented effect of these agents is a neonatal withdrawal syndrome, which has been reported for several of the BZDs (e.g., diazepam, alprazolam, and triazolam).

Clinical issues and approaches should include:

* Alternate, *nondrug management* of anxiety (e.g., behavioral therapies; relaxation techniques; psychotherapy; cessation of stimulants, such as caffeine) whenever possible
* If a BZD is necessary, *lorazepam* may be preferable due to its lower accumulation in fetal tissue; diazepam should be avoided until after the 10th week of gestation to avoid oral defects
* *Gradual tapering of a BZD* before delivery to minimize any neonatal withdrawal phenomena
* *Diphenhydramine* should be avoided due to both fetal teratogenic and withdrawal complications (10).

CONCLUSION

In summary, while it is always preferable to avoid psychotropics during pregnancy, many factors must be weighed before making the best decision for both the mother and the fetus. Because there are very few clear and absolute contraindications to the use of these agents during pregnancy, a carefully informed decision involving the patient, her family, and the physician is the only rational approach.

REFERENCES

1. Coyle I, Wayner MJ, Singer G. Behavioral teratogenesis: a critical evaluation. Pharmacol Biochem Behav 1976;4:191–200.
2. Miller LJ. Clinical strategies for the use of psychotropic drugs during pregnancy. Janicak PG, Davis JM, guest eds. Psychiatr Med 1991;9(2):275–298.
3. Burr WA, Falek A, Strauss LT et al. Fertility in psychiatric outpatients. Hosp Community Psychiatry 1979;30:527–531.
4. Cohen LS, Heller VL, Rosenbaum JF. Treatment guidelines for psychotropic drug use in pregnancy. Psychosomatics 1989;30:25–33.
5. Calabrese JR, Gulledge AD. Psychotropics during pregnancy and lactation: a review. Psychosomatics 1985;26:413–426.
6. Jacobsen SS, Jones K, Johnson K, Ceolin L, Kaur P, Sahn D. Prospective multicentered study of pregnancy outcome after lithium exposure during the first trimester. Lancet 1992;339:530–533.
7. Kaneko S. A rational antiepileptic drug therapy of epileptic women in child bearing age. Jpn J Psychiatry Neurol 1988;42:473–482.
8. Murasaki O, Yoshitake K, Tachiki H et al. Reexamination of the teratological effect of antiepileptic drugs. Jpn J Psychiatry Neurol 1988;42:592–593.
9. Cohen LS. Psychotropic drug use in pregnancy. Hosp Community Psychiatry 1989;40:566–567.
10. Saxen I. Cleft palate and maternal diphenhydramine intake. Lancet 1974;1:407–408.

The Child and the Adolescent Patient

This section will provide an overview of the use of antipsychotics, antidepressants, mood stabilizers, anxiolytics, and psychostimulants in children and adolescents. Because much of the material about the use of these medications in adults is applicable (to the best of our knowledge) to this age range, this section will primarily focus on those areas where there are important differences in terms of efficacy and/or safety.

There is perhaps no area of psychopharmacotherapy where the potential benefits are greater and yet where knowledge and research lag so far behind the rest of the field. Early and effective intervention in a disease process will typically lessen its long-term sequelae. Unrecognized and/or ineffectively treated psychiatric conditions in childhood and adolescence are likely to have profound and lifelong effects on the psychosocial development of the patient, interfering with self-esteem, family and peer relationships, and performance in school. The consequences are likely to persist even after the resolution of an acute episode, profoundly affecting further development and psychosocial adjustment (1). Inadequately treated pediatric psychiatric disorders may lead to:

- Poor self-image
- Poor interpersonal relationships
- Chronic underachievement
- School dropout
- Substance abuse
- Legal problems.

Although the systematic study of the effectiveness of somatic therapies for such conditions should be a national priority, child psychopharmacotherapy is underfunded and thus tragically understudied. Hence, the amount and quality of investigations on children and adolescents are minimal and rather rudimentary by adult standards.

TREATMENT ISSUES

There are many issues that apply to therapies for nonpsychiatric and psychiatric conditions in both children and adults. They bear mentioning, particularly when contemplating the treatment of children, for two reasons. First, the child psychiatric patient often does not present for treatment, but rather is brought to the clinician because someone else (e.g., parent, teacher) is concerned or annoyed by the child's behavior. Thus, the patient may be a passive, if not reluctant, participant in treatment. Second, there is a greater possibility with children than with adults that a beneficial medication may have deleterious effects on growth and development. The clinician therefore needs to consider the following questions carefully prior to initiating treatment:

- Does the child/adolescent have a disorder or syndrome of a type and of *sufficient severity to warrant medication*?
- Do the *needs and the desires of the child and the parent conflict* or are they in synchrony?
- What is the patient's *social and family situation* and how will it influence treatment outcome?
- Will the parent or guardian be able *to assist with the administration and monitoring of the medication*?
- What *other forms of treatment* may be needed (e.g., education about the condition and about better behavioral management techniques, family therapy, and/or individual psychotherapy)?
- *What does the patient think* about his/her condition, the need for treatment, and the treatment that is being recommended?
- How will the treatment affect *the pa-tient's self-concept and relations* with others?
- How is the patient doing *in school* and why? (If there have been any significant changes in level of functioning, then the time course and magnitude of the changes should be carefully assessed.)
- Have *all the options been reasonably discussed* and their relative merits and liabilities weighed?
- What *outcome parameters* will be used to document the potential beneficial and adverse effects of the medication?
- Is the *addition of a second or third medication necessary* (e.g., if the first treatment fails, should it be discontinued rather than resorting to polypharmacy)?

PHARMACOKINETIC ISSUES

Ideally, drug doses in children should be based upon systematic study results, but that is frequently not possible. Dose often has to be empirically determined, after initially extrapolating from adult studies. Unfortunately, there are several pharmacokinetic differences between children and adults that compromise this approach.

Most psychotropic medications are highly lipophilic. The percentage of *total body fat*, which is a reservoir for these lipid-soluble compounds, increases during the first year of life and then decreases until the prepubertal increase (2). Thus, children at different ages have different volumes of deep storage, which can affect the overall residual time a drug remains in the body after its discontinuation.

By 1 year of age, *glomerular filtration rate* and renal tubular mechanisms for secretion have reached adult levels; however, fluid intake may be greater in children. **Thus, lithium has a shorter half-life** and more rapid renal clearance in children as compared with adults (3).

Hepatic enzyme activity by 1 year of age is also fully developed; however, the rate of drug metabolism is also, in part, dependent on liver mass. Relative to body weight, the liver of a toddler is 40–50% greater, and that of a 6-year-old is 30% greater than that of an adult (2). Thus, not surprisingly, children are often much more rapid at clearing drugs than are adults, and frequently they need higher doses on a milligram per kilogram basis to achieve the same plasma levels and clinical effect. Psychostimulants, for example, have been reported to have shorter half-lives in children than in adults. Children also convert tertiary amine TCAs (e.g., clomipramine) to their secondary amine metabolites (e.g., desmethylclomipramine) more extensively than do adults. Nonetheless, children, like adults, have substantial interindividual variability in their rates of biotransformation and elimination; hence, dose must be titrated in reference to the patient's response (4). With some medications, such as TCAs, therapeutic drug monitoring can be used to guide dose adjustment to achieve levels that are more likely to be effective and safe.

TREATMENT OF PSYCHOTIC DISORDERS IN CHILDREN/ADOLESCENTS

Somewhat surprisingly, there have been more systematic data on drug therapies for childhood and adolescent mood disorders, attention deficit disorder, separation anxiety and related conditions than there have been for psychotic disorders. There has been no well-designed study of antipsychotic use in prepubertal children carefully diagnosed with schizophrenia, and only a few in adolescents. In one of the best prospective placebo- and active-drug-controlled studies, haloperidol (2–16 mg/day) and loxapine (10–200 mg/day) were equally effective and superior to placebo (5).

Prevailing clinical opinion is that younger patients with schizophrenia are less responsive to pharmacotherapy than are adult patients (6, 7). Even when the more florid symptoms such as hallucinations and delusions abate with antipsychotics, patients frequently continue to have substantial impairment in social functioning and scholastic performance. Often, thought disorder is the most antipsychotic-refractory of the classic psychotic symptoms.

The recommended dose range for haloperidol in children is 0.5–16.0 mg/day (0.02–0.2 mg/kg/day), but the initial dose should be low, with gradual increments upward as needed and tolerated (6). Advances in the dose should be done no more than twice per week, except in unusual instances. Older adolescents with schizophrenia typically require doses in the adult range, and younger adolescents fall between the recommendations for children and adults. As with adults, the final maintenance dose in children and adolescents must be empirically determined, based upon both benefit and tolerability.

The common adverse effects of low potency antipsychotics (e.g., chlorpromazine, thioridazine) seen in adults also occur in children and adolescents, including: sedation, peripheral anticholinergic effects (e.g., dry mouth, constipation), slowing of intracardiac conduction, and orthostatic blood pressure changes. **Children and adolescents are generally more tolerant of the blood pressure-lowering effects, so that they may develop greater changes before becoming clinically symptomatic. For that reason, it is important to monitor their blood pressure early during the dose titration phase.**

The term "behavioral toxicity" has been used in the child psychiatry literature to describe some of the adverse effects of antipsychotics, specifically:

- Hypoactivity
- Apathy
- Social withdrawal
- Cognitive dulling
- Sedation.

These problems occur most commonly with the low potency antipsychotics (8).

Although similar effects can occur in adults, they are particularly problematic in children and adolescents for three reasons:

- Children and adolescents are more likely to develop *sedation* than adults (7)
- Children and adolescents may *complain less* about these effects, so that the physician must monitor more closely to detect their development
- These effects, if not promptly detected, *may have long-term adverse effects* on the patient's development by interfering at critical psychosocial stages and by compromising the ability to perform in school.

This latter scenario could offset the gains in psychosocial and school performance that should result from effective treatment of the patient's psychotic symptoms.

Acute extrapyramidal side effects (EPSs) (e.g, dystonic reactions, akathisia, and parkinsonism) occur in children and adolescents, just as in adults, especially when treated with high potency antipsychotics (9). The clinical impression is that adolescent boys may be more vulnerable to acute dystonic reactions than are adults. Although these adverse effects can be treated with anticholinergic agents, dose reduction is the preferable first step. For acute dystonic reactions, diphenhydra-mine (25–50 mg) may be given orally or intramuscularly, as can equivalent doses of benztropine. Diphenhydramine has both sedative and anticholinergic properties, with the former helpful in calming the patient while the latter reverses the reaction itself.

One of the principal concerns with neuroleptics for children and adolescents is the development of tardive dyskinesia. While this concern also applies to adult patients, the potential for lifelong exposure to neuroleptics, and the fact that these drugs are being administered during brain maturation, makes this issue even more pertinent in younger patients. Transient withdrawal dyskinesia and tardive dyskinesia have been reported in 8–51% of antipsychotic-treated children and adolescents (6). Unlike adults, there have been reports of dyskinesias occurring within 5 months of initiating treatment in younger patients (10). The problem with such reports is that this population is at increased risk for the spontaneous development of dyskinetic movements because they may also have concomitant autism or a tic disorder. Nonetheless, younger patients may be at increased risk simply because of their age and the fact that their brains are still developing. For this reason, patients should be carefully examined for any baseline movement abnormalities prior to starting a neuroleptic. The use of one of several available scales (e.g., the Abnormal Involuntary Movements Scale (AIMS)) may be helpful in structuring the examination and quantifying the symptoms.

TREATMENT OF MAJOR DEPRESSIVE DISORDERS IN CHILDREN/ADOLESCENTS

Major depressive disorders (MDDs) can occur in children as young as 6 years of age, and diagnosis is based on the same criteria as in adults. In this group, there is a high familial loading for psychiatric disorders, with over 70% of mothers having MDD, either pure or complicated by the presence of another psychiatric syndrome. Fathers, however, are more likely to have alcohol abuse or dependence, as opposed to MDD (11).

Literature Review

Despite considerable efforts, treatment studies in this area have generally been frustrating (11a). Only two studies have demonstrated the superiority of a TCA over placebo for MDD in children, and even these studies have limitations (12, 13). In the Kashani study, there were only nine subjects in the treatment group, the maximum dose of amitriptyline used was low (1.5 mg/kg/day), and the statistical results were modest ($p < 0.05$, based on a one-tail t test, presuming drug would be predicted to be superior to placebo). In the double-blind, placebo-controlled study by Preskorn and colleagues, the group sample sizes were larger (N = 15 per cell) and the imipramine dose was adjusted based on therapeutic drug monitoring to ensure that the patient achieved plasma levels that had previously been found to be safe and effective (14, 15). Nonetheless, imipramine was clearly superior to placebo only through the first 3 weeks of treatment ($p < 0.05$, based on a two-tail t test), but by the end of 6 weeks, the response rates approximated each other.

Similar studies with a variety of other antidepressants, such as SRIs, have also been negative (16, 17). As in adults, SRIs have the advantage of being better tolerated than most tertiary amine TCAs (e.g., amitriptyline) and being safer than all TCAs in terms of overdose. **The latter is particularly important in the adolescent population, where suicide is the second leading cause of death.** Whereas some authorities consider schizophrenia a more frequent antecedent of suicide in adolescents than in adults, MDD remains a critical factor in many cases. Serious and potentially life-threatening suicide attempts in adolescents are often more impulsive than in adults, making the use of medications that are safe from the perspective of overdose especially important.

The principal problem with interpreting AD studies in younger age populations is the high placebo response rate, rather than a failure to respond. Puig-Antich et al. (1979) first reported a substantial placebo response rate (68%) and Hughes et al. (1988, 1990) confirmed this problem, although their placebo response rate was smaller (18–20). Placebo response may be a misnomer in the latter series of studies because all of the patients were hospitalized, and thus treated in a stable and nurturing environment. They also received intensive individual, group, and milieu psychotherapy. Despite the fact that both the imipramine- and the placebo-treated groups received this intensive form of psychotherapy, imipramine had a faster onset of action and produced a higher percentage of full remission, even at the end of 6 weeks of treatment.

In general, drug treatment studies in both children and adolescents with mood disorders have not distinguished drug from placebo, due to the high placebo response rate. Part of this problem is likely due to the heterogenous nature of the population, inasmuch as many patients meet criteria for more than one psychiatric disorder, particularly conduct and oppositional disorders (11). Moreover, patients with these concomitant disorders have a higher response to placebo than to a TCA, whereas the reverse is true for the patients with either MDD only or MDD plus a concomitant anxiety disorder (19). There is also evidence in adults that the duration of the depressive episodes lengthens with subsequent recurrences. While children and adolescents tend to follow a chronic course without treatment, it is not clear that their episodes are stable in terms of the level of symptomatology. Instead, they may have a waxing and waning course, which could compromise the ability to demonstrate treatment effectiveness.

Thus, a considerable amount of research remains to be done to clarify these issues, especially which characteristics predict a preferential response to medications versus placebo. Such work in adults was an important validator of the criteria that are now used to diagnose MDD, as well as to select adult patients for clinical trials of new ADs.

Adverse Effects

While TCAs do not have proven efficacy for MDD in either children or adolescents, they, as well as other forms of AD pharmacotherapy, are employed because no other definitive therapy is available. From the clinical trials already conducted, TDM is important in children and adolescents to assure that the TCA plasma levels are at least safe (14, 15, 21). As in adults, plasma concentrations above 450 ng/ml are associated with an increased risk of potentially serious toxicity, including:

- Delirium
- Seizures
- Slowing of intracardiac conduction, which can lead to heart blocks, arrhythmias, and sudden death (22).

There have been several cases of sudden death in children and adolescents taking desipramine for a variety of indications (23, 24). These cases have raised substantial fears among child psychiatrists, even though the drug was barely detectable at autopsy, indicating that it was unlikely to have been a contributor to the sudden death. Because of the controversy, these cases have led some clinicians to recommend frequent ECG monitoring (baseline and at every dose increase) but without evidence that this would achieve early detection of a problem and avoid a fatal outcome.

Although it is common practice to obtain a baseline ECG prior to initiating a TCA, this practice is also without substantial supporting data regarding its utility or cost effectiveness. In contrast, many clinicians do not routinely obtain at least one steady-state TCA plasma level during treatment, even though inappropriate levels are correlated with adverse central nervous system (CNS) and cardiac effects. Such monitoring, however, is now becoming more common when using these medications in children and adolescents.

The adverse effects of TCAs in younger patients are the same as in adults, except that these agents are more likely to increase blood pressure in the younger age group (15, 25). Serious hypertension is rare, however, with the most common cardiovascular effect being a mild tachycardia. The adverse effects of SRIs and MAOIs in younger patients are also similar to those in adults (26–28).

TREATMENT OF ANXIETY DISORDERS IN CHILDREN/ADOLESCENTS

There is considerable uncertainty in this area, even regarding diagnosis. Such disorders in children often present with features of separation anxiety, phobia, and generalized anxiety. The fact that both adults with panic disorder/agoraphobia and children with separation anxiety can be effectively treated with imipramine suggests some relationship between these two conditions. Furthermore, children with separation anxiety will more often have adult family members with panic disorder, rather than generalized anxiety disorder (Weissman et al., in talk presented on anxiety disorders, Key Biscayne, 1982). On the other hand, separation anxiety (either current or historical) does not predict response to imipramine (29).

This diagnostic uncertainty may help explain why this area has received surprisingly little attention since the study by Gittleman and Klein (1973) that demonstrated a significant benefit over placebo from 6 weeks of treatment with imipramine (mean dose = 159 mg/day) in 45 children with school phobia (30). A subsequent study using lower amounts of clomipramine (40–75 mg/day), was negative but the doses employed make interpretation difficult. Furthermore, because of its relatively poor tolerability and safety profile, clomipramine is no longer a viable option as an anxiolytic agent in adults, much less in children or adolescents.

The medical management of childhood anxiety has also included the use of BZDs, antihistamines, β-adrenergic blockers, and clonidine (31, 32). They are used by clinicians to treat a wide range of anxiety-related disorders, including conditions such as separation anxiety, school phobia, and panic disorder. None of these agents, however, has been the subject of systematic, double-blind, placebo-controlled studies in children or adolescents, and opinions about their effectiveness depend primarily upon anecdotal experience and reports.

The initial doses (in terms of milligrams per kilogram per day) of BZDs used in children and adolescents are the same as in adults. The dose is then titrated based upon a clinical assessment of response rather than empirical data dictating the most appropriate doses, or how long the patient should remain on a given dose before adjusting it or switching to another agent. The safety and tolerability of these medications do not appear to differ significantly whether used by children, adolescents, or adults. Other unstudied issues in this population include the abuse and dependency potential of BZDs, as well as long-term effects on school performance and advancement.

Obsessive-Compulsive Disorder

Obsessive-compulsive disorder (OCD) typically begins in adolescence, but may also become apparent in childhood. Features are the same regardless of the age of onset, with the illness tending to run a chronic course. Until the last few years, there was no specific effective drug treatment, with patients tried on a series of medications, as well as psychotherapy, frequently without substantial improvement. Because of the disability and misery caused by severe forms of OCD, adult patients have even been referred for a variety of psychosurgical procedures, which often produce more significant and long-lasting results than either psychotherapy or medications.

Drug Therapies

That situation has changed with the development of the SRIs, which appear to have unique efficacy in treating OCD when compared with other types of psychotropics (see Obsessive-Compulsive Disorder in Chapter 13). In addition, there has been the development of more effective behavioral approaches, which, in combination with medication, can greatly ameliorate this condition.

The first effective agent, clomipramine, is a TCA rather than an SRI. Although virtually all of the work on clomipramine's effectiveness in OCD has been done in adults, clinicians have also used it to treat children and adolescents. There are, however, several limitations to its use, because this tertiary amine TCA has a number of other potent effects, including:

- Blockade of α_1-adrenergic receptors, which can cause *orthostatic hypotension*
- Blockade of histamine receptors, which can produce *sedation* and possibly *weight gain*
- Blockade of cholinergic receptors, which can result in a variety of peripheral *anticholinergic adverse effects* and *memory impairment*
- Inhibition of $Na^+ : K^+$ ATPase, which inhibits electrically excitable membranes and can produce *intracardiac conduction delays* (33).

For these reasons, clomipramine, like other TCAs, can produce serious toxicity (e.g., delirium, seizures, cardiac arrhythmias, and cardiac arrest) at high plasma drug concentrations (34). These effects are problematic with adults and may be of even greater concern with children and adolescents.

There are other concerns of particular relevance to children and adolescents due to pharmacokinetic differences between this group and adults. While clomipramine is the most potent TCA in terms of inhibiting the neuronal serotonin reuptake pump, it also inhibits the neuronal reuptake of norepinephrine (35). Moreover, its primary metabolite, desmethylclomipramine, is a more potent inhibitor of the norepinephrine than the serotonin reuptake pump. Depending on the patient's hepatic metabolism profile, either des-

methylclomipramine or clomipramine may be the predominant form of the circulating drug. Because children tend to be extensive metabolizers of TCAs, 70% of the circulating drug can be desmethylclomipramine, rather than the parent compound. If serotonin reuptake inhibition is critical to its effectiveness in treating OCD, then clomipramine may be less effective in children due to this pharmacokinetic issue, rather than any fundamental difference in the pathophysiology of the illness between these two age groups.

If clomipramine is used, then TDM can serve several roles. First, it can be used to determine whether the patient is primarily being treated with the parent drug or its metabolite. Second, TDM can be used to guide dose adjustment to ensure equivalent plasma concentrations to those seen in adults successfully treated for their OCD. This approach also ensures that the patient is not reaching concentrations (i.e., >450 ng/ml) that are above the toxic threshold for TCAs (34). Like adults, children and adolescents demonstrate a wide variability in their capacity to metabolize TCAs. As mentioned earlier, children are usually faster metabolizers of these drugs than adults, so they typically need doses of approximately 2.5–3.5 mg/kg. **Once puberty has been reached, the required doses can be reduced by as much as 50%.**

For all of these reasons, there has been considerable interest in the efficacy of specific SRIs (e.g., sertraline, paroxetine, fluoxetine) in the treatment of OCD in both the adult and the pediatric populations. Work is presently ongoing to enlarge the existing database on these agents so that formal Food and Drug Administration (FDA) approval for this indication can be obtained. Specifically, double-blind, placebo-controlled studies of sertraline for the treatment of OCD in children and adolescents are under way, but results are not yet available.

As commonly occurs in this situation, clinicians have been using SRIs to treat OCD in children and adolescents based on their experience in adult patients. This practice is hampered by the fact that the metabolisms of sertraline, paroxetine, and fluoxetine have not been extensively studied in this population. The current wisdom is to adjust the dose on a milligram per kilogram basis in a manner analogous to BZDs. Whereas TDM is not needed for SRIs because of their wide therapeutic index, there is information about what plasma concentrations are typically seen in adult MDD patients who respond to and tolerate these drugs. Thus, another approach would be to titrate the dose of the SRI in children and adolescents to achieve a plasma concentration similar to that seen in depressed adults who respond to these medications. The problem with this recommendation is that it is extrapolating from one condition to another, and while toxic thresholds are probably independent of the disorder being treated, this may not hold for the lower end of the efficacy thresholds. This consideration may, however, be less relevant to the SRIs (in contrast to the TCAs) because they have only one known primary mechanism of action.

TREATMENT OF ATTENTION DEFICIT DISORDER IN CHILDREN/ADOLESCENTS

Unlike the other disorders discussed in this section, Attention deficit disorder (ADD) is a condition that has been better studied in children and adolescents than in adults. In fact, only recently have there been reports on the treatment of adult residual, attention deficit disorder (36). In these cases, treatment has been based on experience in child psychiatry with psychostimulants (e.g., methylphenidate, pemoline, and amphetamines) that have proven to be effective.

In children and adolescents, the decision to medicate is based on problems with inattention, impulsivity, and hyperactivity that are persistent and sufficiently severe to cause functional impairment at school, at home, and with peers. Before treatment with psychostimulants is instituted, however, other treatable causes should be ruled out and behavioral interventions considered. To maximize the likelihood of successful treatment with psychostimulants, parents or guardians should be involved in the treatment plan, including monitoring the administration of the medication, learning new disciplinary techniques, and participating in the patient's appointments for follow-up.

Psychostimulants

Psychostimulants have been studied for the treatment of hyperactivity or attention deficit disorder since 1936. As a group, these agents are moderately to markedly effective in 75% of hyperactive children (37). **Claims that the effects of psychostimulants in children are paradoxical and do not apply to adults are spurious. Moderate doses of these agents improve attention, concentration, and overall cognitive functioning in adults just as they do in children.** It is only at higher doses that psychostimulants cause distractibility and increased psychomotor activity in both children and adults, although the dose needed to produce these symptoms in children may be higher. This appears to be a difference in sensitivity, because by age 3 years, children have similar absorption, distribution, metabolism, elimination, and protein binding of these drugs as do adults (38).

Methylphenidate

This agent is the most widely used and best-studied medication for this condition. It is generally given in divided doses (e.g., in the morning before school and again at lunch time), consistent with its half-life (Table 14.1). This short half-life allows plasma levels to drop before bedtime and thus may explain why insomnia is not more problematic.

The short half-life of methylphenidate can also be a disadvantage in specific patients, however, due to an end-of-dose rebound in dysfunctional behavior. There can also be problems with the child taking the medication at school. For these reasons, a *sustained-release version of methylphenidate* has been developed, but unfortunately, there are several limitations with this product, including:

- Its *pharmacokinetics* are less reliable
- *Onset of action* is frequently delayed
- *Overall effectiveness is less* and more variable from day to day
- *Rapid and high plasma drug concentrations* can result if a child chews the sustained-release capsule rather than swallowing it (39).

Pemoline

This agent has a longer half-life, which further increases with chronic administration (41). It may be given once a day to some children and is generally reserved for cases where the effects of methylphenidate do not persist long enough for optimal control of distractibility and hyperactivity. The longer duration of activity is not consistent across all children, however, and must be individually assessed to determine whether this presumed advantage is being realized. Many clinicians also believe that it has less abuse potential than either methylphenidate or dextroamphetamine. Whereas pemoline's efficacy is based on a double-blind study involving both a placebo and an active (methylphenidate) comparison treatment arm, the magnitude of its effect is generally not thought to be as great as that of either methylphenidate nor amphetamines (41). In addition, the time of onset of activity is appreciably delayed when compared to the other agents (Table 14.1).

Amphetamines

These drugs also have a longer half-life than methylphenidate, but not as long as pemoline (Table 14.1). Proponents of this agent cite the longer half-life as one of the reasons that amphetamines are better agents for the treatment of ADD. It is clearly a useful alternative, because up to 20% of children who respond poorly to one psychostimulant will respond well to an-

Table 14.1.
Psychostimulants Used to Treat Attention Deficit Disorder in Children and Adolescents

Feature	Methylphenidate	Pemoline	Dextroamphetamine
Elimination half-life	2–3[a]	2–12	6–7
Time to peak plasma concentration (T_{max})	1–3	1–5	3–4
Onset of behavioral effect	1	3–4 weeks	1
Duration of behavioral effect	3–4	Not available	4
Daily dose range			
mg/kg/day	0.6–1.7	0.5–3.0	0.3–1.25
mg/day	10–60	37.5–112.5	5–40

[a]All time values are given in hours unless otherwise noted.

other. Dextroamphetamine is also less expensive, but frequently not covered by medical assistance programs. There is also concern about its abuse potential and the possibility of the child's medication being diverted to the illicit drug market. Finally, some researchers have suggested that amphetamines are the most likely psychostimulant to affect the patient's growth. For these reasons, they are less commonly utilized, which may at times be detrimental to the patient.

In summary, the effective drug treatment of ADD does more than simply reduce the child's activity level and increase the attention span, although these effects may be central to the overall improvement (42). Research has also documented improvement in off-task behavior, as well as in arithmetic and language tasks (39, 43). Finally, there is usually an increase in positive social behavior in school, improved teacher-child interactions, and a more positive relationship between the mother and the child (44–48).

Long-Term Psychostimulant Therapy

Children with ADD can remain symptomatic through adolescence and possibly into adulthood (36). Nonetheless, little has been done to assess the effectiveness of psychostimulants in adolescence. One study of 13- to 18-year-old patients, found two different doses of methylphenidate (mean = 15 mg/day and 31 mg/day) to be effective when compared with that of placebo (49). The results fit a dose-response curve, with the higher dose being superior to the lower dose, and both doses superior to placebo, based on rating scores by parents and teachers. The design was not ideal, however, given that the majority of patients were on methylphenidate at the time of referral to the study, thus the population may have been biased in terms

of drug responsiveness. On the other hand, the outcome provides support for continuing methylphenidate in adolescents who responded well as children yet remain sufficiently symptomatic to warrant continued treatment.

There is also evidence that effective treatment during childhood leads to better ultimate outcome as adults. A follow-up study compared the status of children who received at least 3 years of continuous methylphenidate treatment to a group who were diagnosed prior to psychostimulant availability (50). The former had less subsequent psychiatric treatment, fewer car accidents, led more independent lives, had achieved a higher educational level, and demonstrated less aggression than the never medicated group. This group also reported a more positive view of their childhood, higher self-esteem, and better social skills. These findings were also supported by Loney et al. (1981), who reported that children with ADD treated with psychostimulants for 6 months or longer did better, in terms of better parent ratings and less problems with alcohol and drug abuse, than those who were not (51). Inasmuch as these studies were retrospective, there is always the possibility that the ability of the child and the family to stay in treatment was a more critical variable than was medication treatment. The available evidence, however, suggests that effective treatment of ADD may have long-lasting effects on the psychosocial adjustment of the patient. In a related follow-up study, conduct disorders in adolescents almost exclusively occurred in those who retained features of ADD (52). Conceivably, effective intervention early in childhood may alter the course, decreasing the likelihood of developing conduct disorder as an adolescent and antisocial personality disorder with its various complications (e.g., alcohol and drug abuse, criminality) as an adult.

These intriguing findings underscore the fact that drug therapy does not occur in a vacuum. **Effective treatment of psychiatric disorders regardless of the patient's age can significantly affect the ability to interact and master one's environment successfully.** It also affects the way others perceive the patient, and thus, their social relationships. Drug therapy can augment and can be augmented by education about the illness and its treatment, as well as by more formal psychotherapy when necessary. The findings with ADD simply underscore this point, as there are similar findings with childhood depressive disorder (1, 19).

Despite these positive findings, concerns have been raised about the possible long-term deleterious effects of psychostimulant treatment.

Adverse Effects

The most common adverse effects of psychostimulants include:

- Anorexia
- Weight loss
- Irritability
- Insomnia
- Abdominal pain.

These effects are usually self-limited, often disappearing after 2–3 weeks. Less common, but more serious, adverse effects include:

- *Increased blood pressure*
- *Tachycardia*
- Precipitation of a *tic-like movement* disorder
- *Nightmares*
- Hypersensitivity *rash*
- *Hepatotoxicity,* as manifested by elevated liver function tests
- *Psychotic* symptoms.

Blood pressure and heart rate should be monitored at each visit during the dose titration phase to permit early detection of adverse effects on these parameters. To minimize the risk of developing movement disorders or psychotic symptoms, psychostimulants should be used cautiously in any patient with a history of tics, psychotic symptoms, or a family history of Tourette's syndrome or schizophrenia. There is no evidence that psychostimulants can lower the seizure threshold or cause seizures.

Safer et al. (1972) reported a significant decrement in growth velocity in children treated for extended intervals with psychostimulants (53), and multiple investigations followed this report, but their results varied widely. **The emerging consensus is that the growth spurt in adolescence after psychostimulant discontinuation compensates for any earlier effect on growth velocity; thus, eventual height is not compromised.** What is less clear is whether this compensatory growth spurt would hold true for those continued on psychostimulants through adolescence. Hence, clinicians have an increased responsibility to determine whether a medication has had a positive effect, and should only continue it when such an effect has been documented to their satisfaction.

Even when a positive effect has been documented, children are typically given a holiday off the psychostimulant during summer months when demands upon their attention, concentration, and activity levels are usually lessened due to vacation. Whereas the goal is to give the patient as long a holiday off the medication as possible, it should be at least 2 weeks in duration, so the clinician can determine whether the child needs to have the medication reinstituted during the next school year. When the continued need for the medication is equivocal, a holiday off the medication during the school year is also warranted.

Generally, these medications are discontinued when the child reaches puberty. One reason for this practice is that adolescents may be more prone to abuse psychostimulants. Thus, clinical data supporting their necessity must be even more substantial. If the patient relapses to a significant extent, then the clinician may consider reinstituting medication based on the evidence of methylphenidate's beneficial effects in adolescents. In such instances, the clinician must be mindful of the possibility of abuse and monitor growth and development even more closely.

Finally, some researchers have presented data indicating that psychostimulants may be helpful for adult patients with residual ADD (36). Obviously, more information is needed to resolve the question about how long to continue treatment in a patient who has clearly responded.

SPECIAL TREATMENT ISSUES IN CHILDREN/ADOLESCENTS

There are a variety of other conditions that will be mentioned only in a general manner, and the interested reader may pursue further discussions of these topics in various textbooks on child psychiatry or by reviewing the primary literature.

Conduct Disorder

As mentioned earlier, many children with unsuccessfully treated ADD go on to develop conduct disorder. For this reason, there has been interest in the usefulness of psychostimulants. This research has lagged behind even other areas in child psychiatry, however, because of this population's high risk for illicit drug abuse, and by extrapolation, their prescription medications as well.

Tourette's Disorder

Tourette's disease consists of tics (often rapid purposeless movements), noises (grunts, squeals, barks, etc.), and sometimes coarse speech, usually with an onset in childhood. It is inherited by an autosomal dominant mechanism. In some cases, drug treatment is not required, and simply explaining to the parent and child that it is a neurologic condition and does not mean that the child has a mental disorder is often quite reassuring. Indeed, in some cases, enduring the tics is less of a burden that suffering from the dysphoric adverse effects of antipsychotics.

Because of its responsiveness, this condition is one of the clearest childhood indications for treatment with *haloperidol*. In theory, any dopamine blocking agent, particularly any high potency antipsychotic could be used. The typical dose for children 3–12 years old is 0.2 mg/kg/day. *Pimozide* is an alternate agent for those refractory or unable to tolerate haloperidol. *Clonidine* has also been reported to be useful in case reports as well as one controlled study; but although it has the advantage of avoiding acute and chronic extrapyramidal side effects of neuroleptics, its effects on blood pressure have appropriately constrained its use in this age population. There is also the concern about rebound hypertension if this agent is abruptly discontinued (e.g., noncompliance).

Autistic Disorder

Haloperidol has documented efficacy in both the short-term and the long-term treatment of such patients. Specifically, haloperidol can reduce:

- Stereotypic behavior
- Hyperactivity

- Aggressive behavior, including self-abusive behavior
- Social withdrawal
- Temper tantrums.

These patients, however, may be at increased risk for the development of tardive dyskinesia. *Naltrexone* has also been used with reported positive effects, but hepatotoxicity in younger individuals is a concern (54). *Propranolol* can reduce rage outbursts, aggression, and severe agitation (31). *Fenfluramine* reduces hyperactivity in some cases, but it can impair learning and cause bowel dysfunction, weight loss, and possible neurotoxicity (55).

Mania

The differentiation between the emotional vicissitudes of adolescence and mild episodes of bipolar disorder can be quite difficult. Nonetheless, a sizable minority (30%) of adult patients with bipolar disorder report having their first episode during adolescence. Further, manic (Type I) episodes have been observed during adolescence, and the earlier the onset, the more likely the patient will have a psychotic form (3).

Despite these facts, there are few systematic data on the treatment of any psychotic disorder in adolescence, including bipolar disorder. Still, lithium has become popular among clinicians to treat a wide variety of adolescent behavior problems, reformulated as a bipolar disorder, to rationalize the use of this drug. Because of rapid renal clearance, lithium doses may need to be higher to achieve and maintain plasma concentrations in the range of 0.8–1.2 mEq/liter. The adverse effects are similar to those seen in adults, and include: weight gain, decreased motor activity, excessive sedation, gastrointestinal complaints, pallor, headache, and polyuria. The most serious concerns in children and adolescents are the long-term consequences of lithium accumulation in bone, as well as its effects on thyroid and renal function.

When a patient responds to lithium, the inevitable question of duration of therapy arises. The period of highest risk for relapse is at least the first 6 months following remission, but this vulnerable interval may extend up to 18 months (56). Therefore, many clinicians recommend leaving the lithium-responsive patient on medication for at least 2 years after remission.

Alternate Treatments

Like adults, some adolescents do not respond to lithium, and many clinicians will next try an anticonvulsant, such as valproic acid or carbamazepine. Their use is based solely on their antimanic activity in adults; there are only a limited number of case reports about the treatment of bipolar adolescents with carbamazepine (57). Because carbamazepine and valproic acid are labelled and used to treat seizure disorders in children and adolescents, there is more systematic knowledge about their pharmacology in this age group than there is about lithium. Patients in these trials were often on other anticonvulsants at the same time, however, complicating attempts to extrapolate from this experience to the use of these agents as the sole therapy for childhood or adolescence bipolar disorder. For example, the risk of serious and potentially fatal hepatotoxicity with valproic acid appears to occur almost exclusively in children under the age of 10 years who are on multiple anticonvulsants for congenital seizure disorders. How or whether this risk translates to children or adolescents who are on monodrug therapy with valproic acid for bipolar disorder is unknown. Nonetheless, the clinician needs to be aware of this possible risk and take steps to increase the likelihood of early detection should this problem arise. Such steps include:

• Appropriately warning the patient and the family of the *early symptoms of hepatotoxicity*
• *Monitoring* the patient appropriately during follow-up visits by inquiring about these early symptoms
• Performing *periodic liver function tests.*

Other than the question of hepatotoxicity with valproic acid in children and adolescents, there are no other unique toxicity considerations when using anticonvulsants in this age range.

Enuresis

Nonpharmacological management is preferable, with the *bell and pad conditioning paradigm* most helpful. Otherwise, the most common form of drug treatment is *imipramine*. Typically, the initial dose is 25 mg/day administered 1 hour before bedtime, and this may be increased to 50 mg/day in children under 12 and to 75 mg/day for those over 12 years. The dose however should not exceed 2.0 mg/kg/day. After a 7-day trial with an adequate dose, 60% of the patients will have experienced relief from bedwetting. The adverse effects are the same as those seen in children and adolescents treated with imipramine for MDD.

CONCLUSION

While various childhood disorders have been reported to benefit from drug therapies, systematic data to support their use are usually minimal or lacking. An additional complication is the clinically significant pharmacokinetic (and perhaps pharmacodynamic) differences between the adult and younger age groups. Thus, the use of drugs in any treatment plan must be carefully considered and cautiously monitored to maintain the risk to benefit ratio in favor of the child or adolescent patient.

Appendix B summarizes the diagnostic criteria and Table 14.2 outlines the various agents and their dosing regimens commonly used for a variety of childhood psychiatric disorders.

REFERENCES

1. Hughes C, Preskorn SH, Tucker S, Hassanein R, Wrona M. Follow-up of adolescents initially treated for prepubertal onset major depressive disorders with imipramine. Psychopharmacol Bull 1990;26(2): 244–248.
2. Briant RH. An introduction to clinical pharmacology. In: Werry JS, ed. Pediatric psychopharmacology: the use of behavior modifying drugs in children. New York: Brunner/Mazel, 1978.
3. Carlson GA. Bipolar disorders in children and adolescents. In: Garfinkel B, Carlson GA, Weller E, eds. Psychiatric disorders in children and adolescents. Philadelphia: WB Saunders Company, 1990:21–36.
4. Preskorn S, Bupp S, Weller E, Weller R. Plasma levels of imipramine and metabolites in 68 hospitalized children. J Am Acad Child Adolesc Psychiatry 1989;28(3):373–375.
5. Pool D, Bloom W, Mielke DH, et al. A controlled evaluation of Loxitane in seventy-five adolescent schizophrenia patients. Curr Ther Res 1976;19:99–104.
6. Campbell M, Green WH, Deutsch SI. Child and adolescent psychopharmacology. Beverly Hills: Sage Publications, 1985.
7. Realmuto GM, Erickson WD, Yellin AM, et al. Clinical comparison of thiothixene and thioridazine in schizophrenic adolescents. Am J Psychiatry 1984;141:440–442.
8. Campbell M, Spencer E. Psychopharmacology in child and adolescent psychiatry: a review of the past five years. J Am Acad Child Adolesc Psychiatry 1988;27:269–279.
9. Teicher MH, Glod CA. Neuroleptic drugs: indications and rational use in children and adolescents. J Child Adolesc Psychopharmacol 1990;1:33–56.

Table 14.2.
Dosing Guidelines for Commonly Used Drugs in Child Psychiatry

ANXIOLYTICS
   Indications: Various anxiety syndromes
      Alprazolam
         Starting dose: 0.25 mg/day; advanced by 0.25 mg every 3–4 days
         Not to exceed 3 mg/day in three divided doses
      Diazepam
         Starting dose: 0.25 mg/day; advanced by 0.5 mg every 3–4 days
         Usual pediatric dose of 1–10 mg/day in two or three divided doses
      Diphenhydramine or Hydroxyzine
         Maximum pediatric dose: 5 mg/kg/day
         Maximum total daily dose: 300 mg/day in 3–4 divided doses
      Propranolol
         Usual pediatric dose: 2–4 mg/kg/day in two divided doses
         Not to exceed 16 mg/kg/day
         Maximum total daily dose: 300 mg
         Note: Should not be stopped abruptly
ANTIDEPRESSANTS
   Indications: Depressive disorders
      Desipramine, Imipramine, Nortriptyline
         Starting dose: 1.5 mg/kg/day in 2 or 3 divided doses
         Advanced by 1.0–1.5 mg/kg/day every 3–5 days
         Usual range: 0.5–2.5 mg/kg/day
         Not to usually exceed 5 mg/kg/day
         Adjust dose to achieve optimal plasma drug levels in terms of both efficacy and safety:
            Imipramine and Desipramine: 125–250 mg/ml
            Nortriptyline: 75–150 mg/ml
         Note: Flu-like syndrome may result due to cholinergic rebound if abruptly discontinued
ANTIPSYCHOTICS
   Indications: Psychoses and autism
         Usual therapeutic range: 0.5–4.0 mg/day (divided dose)
         Starting dose: 0.01–0.05 mg/kg/day in two divided doses
         Advanced by 0.25 to 0.5 mg every 3–4 days
         Four week trial to establish efficacy
         Four- to six-month duration if psychosis remits
PSYCHOSTIMULANTS
   Indications: Attention deficit disorder with hyperactivity
      Methylphenidate
         Starting dose: 5 mg in A.M.; in 3–5 days, add 5 mg at noon, and then advance by 5 mg qod every 3–14 days
         Usual therapeutic dose: 0.3–0.6 mg/kg/dose
         No single dose >20 mg
         Not to exceed 60 mg/day
      Dextroamphetamine
         Starting dose: 2.5 mg in A.M.; in 3–5 days, add 2.5 mg at noon and then advance by 2.5 mg qod every 3–14 days
         Usual therapeutic dose: 0.15–0.3 mg/kg/dose
         No single dose >10 mg
         Not to exceed 40 mg/day
      Pemoline
         Starting dose: 18.75 mg/day in A.M.; with weekly increase of 18.75 mg/day
         Usual therapeutic dose: 0.5–2.0 mg/kg/day
         Not to exceed 112.5 mg/day

10. Herskowitz J. Developmental toxicology. In: Popper C, ed. Psychiatric pharmacosciences of children and adolescents. Washington, D.C.: American Psychiatric Press, 1987.

11. Hughes CW, Preskorn SH, Weller E, Weller R, Hassanein R. A descriptive profile of the depressed child. Psychopharmacol Bull 1989;25:232–237.

11a. Jensen PS, Ryan NO, Prien R. Psychopharmacology of child and adolescent major depression. Present status and future directions. J Child Adol Psychopharmacol 1992;2(1):31–45.

12. Kashani JH, Shekim WO, Reid JC. Amitriptyline in children with major depressive disorder: a double-blind crossover pilot study. J Am Acad Child Psychiatry 1984;23:348–351.

13. Preskorn S, Weller E, Hughes C, Weller R, Bolte K. Depression in prepubertal children: DST nonsuppression predicts differential response to imipramine versus placebo. Psychopharmacol Bull 1987;23:128–133.

14. Preskorn S, Weller E, Weller R. Depression in children: relationship between plasma imipramine levels and response. J Clin Psychiatry 1982;43:450–453.

15. Preskorn S, Weller E, Weller R, Glotzbach E. Plasma levels of imipramine and adverse effects in children. Am J Psychiatry 1983;140:1332–1335.

16. Simeon JG. Pediatric psychopharmacology. Can J Psychiatry 1989;34:115.

17. Lapierre YD, Ravel KJ. Pharmacotherapy of affective disorders in children and adolescents. Psychiatry Clin North Am 1989; 12:951.

18. Puig-Antich J, Perel J, Luptakin W, et al. Plasma levels of imipramine (IMI) and desmethylimipramine (DMI) and clinical response in prepubertal and major depressive disorder: a preliminary report. J Am Acad Child Psychiatry 1979;18(4):616–627.

19. Hughes C, Preskorn SH, Weller E, Weller R, Hassanein R, Tucker S. The effect of concomitant disorders in childhood depression on predicting treatment response. Psychopharmacol Bull 1990;26(2): 235–238.

20. Hughes C, Preskorn S, Weller E, Weller R, Hassanein R. Imipramine vs placebo studies of childhood depression: baseline predictors of response to treatment and factor analysis of presenting symptoms. Psychopharmacol Bull 1988;24:275–279.

21. Preskorn S, Weller E, Jerkovich G, Hughes C, Weller R. Depression in children: concentration dependent CNS toxicity of tricyclic antidepressants. Psychopharmacol Bull 1988;24:140–142.

22. Preskorn SH, Fast GA. Therapeutic drug monitoring for antidepressants: efficacy, safety, and cost effectiveness. J Clin Psychiatry 1991;52(6):23–33.

23. Riddle MA, Nelson JC, Kleinman CS, et al. Sudden death in children receiving Norpramin: a review of three reported cases and commentary. J Am Acad Sci Adolesc Psychiatry 1991;30:104.

24. Biederman J. Sudden death in children treated with a tricyclic antidepressant: a commentary. Biol Ther Psychiatry. 1991; 14:1.

25. Lake CR, Mikkelsen EJ, Rapoport JL, et al. Effect of imipramine on norepinephrine and blood pressure in enuretic boys. Clin Pharmacol Ther 1979;39:647.

26. Ryan ND, Puig-Antich J, Rabinovich H, et al. MAOIs in adolescent major depression unresponsive to tricyclic antidepressants. J Am Acad Child Adolesc Psychiatry 1988; 27:755.

27. Riddle MA, Hardin MT, King R, et al. Fluoxetine treatment of children and adolescents with Tourette's and obsessive compulsive disorders: preliminary clinical experience. J Am Acad Child Adolesc Psychiatry 1990;29:45.

28. Gwirtzman HE, Guze BH, Yager J, et al. Treatment of anorexia nervosa with fluoxetine: an open clinical trial. J Clin Psychiatry 1990;51:378.

29. Gittelman R, Klein DF. Relationship between separation anxiety and panic and agoraphobic disorders. Psychopathology 1984;17(suppl 1):56–65.

30. Gittelman-Klein R, Klein DF. School phobia: diagnostic consideration in the light of imipramine effects. J Nerv Ment Dis 1973;156(3):199–215.

31. Coffey BJ. Anxiolytics for children and adolescents: traditional and new drugs. J Child Adolesc Psychopharmacol 1990;1: 57–83.

32. Bernstein GA, Garfinkel BD, Borchart CM. Comparative studies of pharmacotherapy for school refusal. J Am Acad Child Adolesc Psychiatry 1990;29:773–781.

33. Preskorn S. Tricyclic antidepressants:

whys and hows of therapeutic drug monitoring. J Clin Psychiatry 1989;50(suppl): 34–42.

34. Preskorn SH, Fast GA. Therapeutic drug monitoring for antidepressants: efficacy, safety, and cost effectiveness. J Clin Psychiatry 1991;52(6):23–33.

35. Rudorfer MZ, Potter WZ. Pharmacokinetics of antidepressants. In: Metzler JV, ed. Psychopharmacology: the third generation of progress. New York: Raven, 1987:1353–1363.

36. Wender PH. The hyperactive child, adolescent, and adult: Attention Deficit Disorder through the lifespan. New York: Oxford University Press, 1987.

37. Dulcan MK. Using psychostimulants to treat behavioral disorders of children and adolescents. J Child Adolesc Psychopharmacol 1990;1:7–20.

38. Coffey B, Shader RI, Greenblatt DJ. Pharmacokinetics of benzodiazepines and psychostimulants in children. J Clin Psychopharmacol 1983;3:217–225.

39. Pelham WE, Bender ME, Caddell J, Booth S, Moorer SH. Methylphenidate and children with attention deficit disorder: dose effects on classroom academic and social behavior. Arch Gen Psychiatry 1985;42(10):948–952.

40. Sallee F, Stiller R, Perel J, et al. Targeting imipramine dose in children with depression. Clin Pharmacol Ther 1985;37:606–609.

41. Conners CK, Taylor E. Pemoline, methylphenidate, and placebo in children with minimal brain dysfunction. Arch Gen Psychiatry 1980;37(8):922–930.

42. Jacobvitz D. Treatment of attentional and hyperactivity problems in children with sympathomimetic drugs: a comprehensive review. J Am Acad Child Adolesc Psychiatry 1990;29:677–688.

43. Douglas VI, Barr RG, O'Neill ME, Britton BG. Short term effects of methylphenidate on the cognitive, learning and academic performance of children with attention deficit disorder in the laboratory and classroom. J Child Psychol Psychiatry 1986;27: 191–211.

44. Whalen CK, Henker B, Swanson JM, Granger D, Kliewer W, Spencer J. Natural social behaviors in hyperactive children: dose effects of methylphenidate. J Consult Clin Psychol 1987;55(2):187–193.

45. Whalen CK, Henker B, Dotemoto S. Methylphenidate and hyperactivity: effects on teacher behaviors. Science 1980;208 (4449):1280–1282.

46. Whalen CK, Henker B, Dotemoto S. Teacher response to the methylphenidate (Ritalin) versus placebo status of hyperactive boys in the classroom. Child Dev 1981;52(3):1005–1014.

47. Barkley RA, Karlsson J, Strzelecki E, Murphy JV. Effects of age and Ritalin dosage on the mother-child interactions of hyperactive children. J Consult Clin Psychol 1984;52(5):750–758.

48. Barkley RA, Karlsson J, Pollard S, Murphy JV. Developmental changes in the mother-child interactions of hyperactive boys: effects of two dose levels of Ritalin. J Child Psychol Psychiatry 1985;26(5):705–715.

49. Varley CK. Effects of methylphenidate in adolescents with attention deficit disorder. J Am Acad Child Psychiatry. 1983;4:351–354.

50. Hechtman L, Weiss G, Perlman T: Young adult outcome of hyperactive children who received long-term stimulant treatment. J Am Acad Child Psychiatry 1984;23(2):261–269.

51. Loney J, Kramer J, Milich RS. In: Gadow KD, Loney J, eds. Psychosocial aspects of drug treatment for hyperactivity. Boulder, Colo.: Westview Press, 1981:381–415.

52. Gittelman R, Mannuzza S, Shenker R, Bonagura N. Hyperactive boys almost grown up. I. Psychiatric status. Arch Gen Psychiatry 1985;42(10):937–947.

53. Safer D, Allen R, Barr E. Depression of growth in hyperactive children on stimulant drugs. N Engl J Med 1972;287(5):217–220.

54. Bernstein GA, Hughes JR, Mitchell JE, Thompson T. Effects of narcotic antagonists on self-injurious behavior: a single case study. J Am Acad Child Adolesc Psychiatry 1987;26:886–889.

55. Campbell M, Spencer EK. Psychopharmacology in child and adolescent psychiatry: a review of the past five year. J Am Acad Child Adolesc Psychiatry 1988;27:269.

56. Strober M, Morrell W, Lampert C, Burroughs J. Lithium carbonate in prophylactic treatment of bipolar illness in adolescents: a naturalistic study. Am J Psychiatry 1990;147:457–461.

57. Hsu LKG. Lithium-resistant adolescent mania. J Am Acad Child Adolescent Psychiatry 1986;25:280–283.

The Elderly Patient

It is a truism that the elderly are exquisitely susceptible to the effects of drugs, and there are many reasons for this. Thus, aging affects:

- The *cardiovascular* system, with cardiac output and perfusion of other organs diminished
- *Kidney* function, which is slowed because of diminished renal blood flow and glomerular filtration rate
- *Liver* function, which is often compromised.

Also associated with these bodily changes may be the development of organic brain disease.

For these reasons, before prescribing any psychoactive drug, clinicians should be familiar with the physical status of the elderly patient, and equally important, the clinician should always take a comprehensive personal drug history. This would include all medicines prescribed for the patient in the prior 6 months, as well as all over-the-counter preparations that the elderly often use to self-medicate. A personal drug history may confirm the use of multiple drugs dispensed by several different physicians, most of whom are unaware that other doctors are also prescribing. A good drug history will help identify:

- Noncompliance
- Potential and/or actual adverse drug interactions
- Inappropriate drug prescription or management.

Finally, a good personal drug history often reveals that iatrogenic polyphar- **macy is often the cause of ill health, both physical and psychiatric, in the elderly.**

PHARMACOKINETIC AND PHARMACODYNAMIC ISSUES

Bodily changes that accompany aging often produce alterations in the pharmacologic actions of drugs. Thus, drug absorption and distribution are often modified because of altered blood flow, bodily composition, hepatic metabolism, protein binding, and renal excretion. In addition, there are also age-related effects in receptor sensitivity (i.e., pharmacodynamic changes). Another factor that should not be overlooked in the elderly is alcohol consumption, given its impact on the clearance of many drugs.

Mindful of the age-related pharmacokinetic changes for all drugs, prescribers of psychotropics should always:

- Initiate therapy with a *low dose*
- *Gradually increase dose* with low increments, days or weeks apart
- Prescribe as *few drugs* as possible
- *Regularly monitor* the patient for therapeutic and adverse drug effects
- Employ *therapeutic drug monitoring* when warranted
- Enlist the patient's collaboration in *individualizing and simplifying the drug regimen* as much as possible (e.g., discontinuing all drugs not absolutely necessary)
- Work with the patient to *ensure compliance* by limiting the total number of drugs and by simplifying dosing schedules.

COMPLIANCE ISSUES

Compliance with psychopharmacotherapy can be enhanced by fully informing the elderly patient about what he or she can reasonably expect from the prescribed drug and by enlisting relatives as informed, knowledgeable helpers. This can be achieved by explaining drug therapy to both patients and their relatives using the guidelines recommended by Blackwell, which include:

- The key to rational and effective treatment often lies in the *explanation of therapy* made to the patient, thus influencing expectations, response, compliance, and the ability to tolerate adverse effects.
- The *ideal discussion* would cover:
  - The *name* of the drug
  - Its *appearance*
  - *Regimen* and *dose*
  - *Reason for prescribing*
  - Anticipated degree and rate of *response*
  - Common or troublesome *adverse effects*
  - *Likely duration* of therapy.
- *Adverse effects can be explained in a matter-of-fact way without arousing alarm.* The precise nature of the explanation should be tempered to match the patient's clinical state, but it should never be entirely overlooked. An acutely disturbed schizophrenic may comprehend little, but will still cooperate more readily if some rapport is obtained; depressed, anxious, or obsessive patients may require reassurance that they will not become addicted to medication; and it may also be necessary to explain that while therapeutic effect is somewhat delayed, adverse effects can be immediate.

- For some schizophrenic or suicidal patients, *explanations should also be given to relatives who may assume responsibility,* but in other instances it may be important for the *patient to assume complete control.* The latter may be particularly true of patients who tend to place the onus for a 'cure' entirely on the physician.
- Finally, it is obviously important to caution the patient about *possible drug interactions* and about *possible interference with activities* such as driving (1).

PRESCRIBING DRUGS FOR THE ELDERLY

Rational psychopharmacotherapy for the elderly requires acknowledging that most of them need few medicines, as Stubbs has emphasized:

> What the elderly need is to be mentally active, socially active, and physically active—and in that order. Their greatest pleasure is to be independent and to be comfortable. The purpose of treatment is to secure these things for them. Too often, it does the reverse. Medication that is not simple may be taken wrongly or may need to be administered by others. Frequent dosage is time-consuming, disturbs social life, and tends in many cases to noncompliance. . . . Ineffective or unnecessary medicines are, to say the least, wasteful. . . . The moment we begin to think about our health, we endanger it, for hypochondriasis has begun. Overtreatment confirms to many people their fears of ill health. The doctor's greatest gift to his patient is courage. To take that away is a poor service indeed. All too often our patients' disabilities are worsened or even due to the very remedies we prescribe.
>
> It is usually possible to discuss with the patient steps proposed in treatment and the gains hoped for. Some will ask for treatment to be simplified. Many are heartened to find they do as well with less. In the case of those already forgetful or

muddled, the doctor might well consider what real gain treatment might achieve. . . . In the old, sedatives and hypnotics are best avoided. When mental capacity or reserve is already reduced these medicines can only reduce it further. In some people memory is worsened and control of the limbs impaired by as little as half a tablet of nitrazepam at night. Its withdrawal may restore their liberty. Confusion, falls, fractures, fear, urinary incontinence, antisocial behavior, and aggression are all seen at times to be due to sedatives and hypnotics (2).

Although these points may seem obvious, too many elderly patients leave their physicians' offices without having received any information at all about the drug(s) prescribed for them. Whenever possible, oral instructions should be accompanied by the same information in writing because elderly patients may seem to understand in the office but forget once they get home or when confronted with a particular situation such as a missed dose or a possible adverse effect. Providing the same information to relatives is also beneficial.

In summary, the presence of medical disease, other, nonpsychotropic agents, expectable changes with aging, and a decreased functional reserve in certain organ systems (e.g., the brain or the kidney) make the elderly a more difficult population for drug treatment.

Antipsychotics

As a general principle, psychotic disorders in the geriatric age group are the same as those experienced earlier in life. Indeed, manic or schizophrenic patients who first present with symptoms in their late teens often have the same disorder in their 70s and 80s. Although the overall treatment strategy is the same, there may be tactical differences. For example, as noted earlier, the elderly often suffer from medical problems, and consequently are

receiving a variety of medications. Thus, drug-drug interactions between psychotropics and other general medical agents are a frequent complicating issue. The medical disease itself may also interfere with the use of a psychotropic. For example, patients with preexisting heart block may be particularly vulnerable to the conduction disturbances induced by certain tricyclics.

Some of the expected changes with age, such as the reduction in cholinergic neurons or the presence of Alzheimer's dementia may accentuate the anticholinergic effects of many antipsychotics and antidepressants. **Thus, the elderly have increased sensitivity to the anticholinergic properties of any drug, often resulting in a central anticholinergic syndrome** (3). This condition is characterized by the loss of immediate memory, confusion, disorientation, and florid visual hallucinations, at times superimposed on other psychoses, such as schizophrenia or psychotic depression.

Elderly patients who suffer from schizophrenia, as well as those who suffer from psychotic depression and mania usually require antipsychotics. In general, however, the dosage requirements are substantially lower than for younger age groups for most of them, but not necessarily all. Thus, many patients may respond to a very small dose and experience excessive adverse effects to doses even lower than that needed when they were younger. Therefore, the clinician should start with a lower dose (often the lowest dose possible) and titrate up at a much more gradual rate. Some elderly patients, however, may require moderate, or even rarely, high doses.

Management of Agitation

Agitation in both the demented and the nondemented elderly represents an important clinical problem that can occur in nursing homes, state hospitals, the patient's own home, or when they are living with their adult children or grandchildren. This phenomenon should not be confused with schizophrenia, mania, psychotic depression, or simple generalized anxiety. Strange as it seems, despite the large number of elderly and the importance of managing this common condition, it has received little scrutiny in either open or controlled clinical investigations.

Experienced geriatric psychiatrists generally recommend low doses of antipsychotics for the agitated elderly (4–6). Because these agents are often effective, some have hypothesized a common physiologic basis between agitation in the elderly and other psychotic processes. While we know that, empirically, antipsychotics are effective, and anxiolytics are usually ineffective, we do not know whether these agents are uniquely indicated for agitation in those elderly individuals who have never previously experienced a psychotic episode. In part, this is because most studies have intermixed schizophrenia, psychotic depression, as well as other major disorders with agitation, with agitated patients who have no previous history of psychosis. Thus, generalizations about appropriate indications are not possible. A properly designed study should only include those who have a psychosis secondary to either aging or a known brain disorder. To our knowledge, there have been only two double-blind, controlled studies, one of which is unpublished (7; Barnes, Finkle, Davis, and co-workers, 1992, unpublished). Both found antipsychotics superior to placebo in treating agitation in the elderly. There have also been five double-blind studies of organic psychosis in state hospital geriatric units (8–12) (see Table 14.3). There have also been a limited number of studies that focused on psychosis secondary to a wide variety of organic brain disorders (13). This population undoubtedly includes some of the agitated, demented elderly, but differs from the nursing home population, at least in part, because psychosis predominates in these patients, while in the nursing home setting, senility is the predominant problem.

These limited data show that antipsychotics are clearly superior to placebo, when either considering the studies individually or pooling them by a meta-analysis.

Therapeutic Calvinism in the Treatment of Nursing Home Agitation. It is certainly true that elderly patients who receive a variety of medications have a greater propensity for drug-drug, drug-disease, and drug-aging interactions. In a

Table 14.3.
Drug Treatment of Organic Psychosis

| Study | Number of Subjects | Responders (%) | | Difference (%) |
		AP (%)	Placebo (%)	
Hamilton L, Bennett J (1962)	27	22	0	22
Sugerman A et al. (1964)	18	56	0	56
Rada R, Kellner R (1976)	42	45	20	25
Petrie W et al. (1982)	59	35	9	26
Stotsky B (1984)	363	79	43	36
	509	66%	35%	31%

Chi square = 64; df = 1; $p = 1 \times 10^{-15}$.

patient with an impaired brain, sedatives may disrupt what little cognitive reserve is left, resulting in a worsening of behavior. Similarly, because anticholinergics may differentially impair memory in a patient with preexisting memory loss, clinicians should avoid using drugs with these properties. For example, because diphenhydramine has substantial anticholinergic properties, it is not the antihistamine or sedative of choice in the elderly. Unfortunately, a therapeutic Calvinism is developing, which suggests that many of these medications are unnecessary, and indeed harmful. Thus, some report that with little expense and effort one can reduce the number of medications prescribed in nursing homes with only a risk of minimal deterioration is some patients (14).

This position has resulted in federal agencies mandating the curtailment of psychopharmacologic agents, especially antipsychotics, based on documentation of their inappropriate use. As a result, an empirical investigation found a 37% reduction in antipsychotic use 1 year after these regulations were implemented, as well as a 20% reduction in dose; however, there was also an increased mortality rate. This last issue was also noted in our empirical study, where four deaths occurred in the placebo group (Barnes et al., unpublished data). Thus, it is possible that untreated agitation may push some elderly patients into a decompensation, ultimately leading to serious morbidity and even death. We would support the intelligent choice of medications based on rational reasons, but avoid the position that all medication is bad, serving only as a substitute for adequate staffing. In this context, there is a great deal of trial and error in dosage adjustment, and there is no substitute for close monitoring in conjunction with frequent feedback from nursing staff.

Antidepressants

Depressive symptoms occur in about 15% of community residents over the age of 65 (14a). The prevalence of major depression in the elderly is estimated to be about 3%. Notably, 13% of patients admitted to a nursing home will develop a depressive episode within 1 year. The elderly are even more predisposed to depression than younger age groups because of:

- Concurrent medical disorders
- Chronic pain
- Increased use of drugs, both prescribed and over-the-counter
- Sadness and bereavement secondary to life cycle issues
- Social isolation.

While depression may be the most common psychological symptom in old age, the appropriate diagnosis is often missed or mistaken for another condition (e.g., dementia). For example, many older patients present with complaints of cognitive impairment or vague somatic symptoms that are compatible with other common suspected or concurrent medical problems, but for which no firm physical basis can be established.

Depression in the elderly can be divided into early-onset and late-onset types (i.e., first episode occurs at age 60 or before versus after 60 years of age, respectively). The distinction has clinical utility, especially for the late-onset type, in that:

- It is usually triggered by medical disorders
- There is a higher frequency of cognitive impairment, cerebral atrophy, white matter changes
- Genetic and developmental factors may play a greater role

- Family history of depression is less frequent
- Early insomnia, agitation, hypochondriasis, delusions, and atypical presentation are also more frequent with this type
- There is a higher mortality rate.

For example, completed suicide rates in 80- to 84-year-olds are more than twice the ratio in the general population (i.e., 26.5 versus 12.4/100,00).

Several factors must be considered if AD therapy is to be optimized in this age group. In addition to a thorough medical evaluation, as outlined earlier in this chapter as well as in Chapter 1, other potential contributing issues must be considered and dealt with if a satisfactory outcome is to be achieved. These may include:

- Social situation and support system
- Level of independence
- Financial status.

For these, as well as other reasons (e.g., altered life roles, chronic medical disorders), psychosocial therapies must always be included as part of a comprehensive treatment stategy for depression in the elderly.

Another major problem is that these patients are often either overtreated or undertreated. The former usually occurs when various age-related pharmacokinetic and pharmacodynamic factors are ignored. The latter is most often due to an overly conservative approach because of the patient's advanced age and/or concurrent medical problems. Finally, an important issue is the frequency of noncompliance (intentional or otherwise) in this group.

Choice of Antidepressant

In contrast to the controlled data available for younger adults, randomized clinical drug trials are quite limited in the depressed elderly. In general, the most important issues in choosing a drug for the elderly are similar to those outlined in Chapter 7. Additionally, increased emphasis should be given to a drug's side-effect profile and the value of TDM to assure adequate versus toxic or subtherapeutic dosing. For example, in a patient with cardiac conduction delay, the TCAs would not be the ideal first choice. In a physically healthy elderly patient, however, *the cautious use of secondary amine TCAs*, such as nortriptyline or desipramine, may be appropriate because of their clearly defined therapeutic plasma levels, proven efficacy, and known side-effect profile. The SRIs may avoid some of the more serious adverse effects seen with the TCAs. Thus, if expense is not a major concern, the *SRIs* are also an appropriate first choice. *Trazodone* and *bupropion* are also appealing because of their milder anticholinergic and cardiovascular effects. With milder mood disturbances, a brief trial with *psychostimulants*, such as methylphenidate, can be attempted.

MAOIs are usually not recommended because of uncertainty about adherence to dietary restrictions and the very real problem of hypotension. When used in selected patients, however, phenelzine has been found to be safe and effective. As noted in Chapter 7, however, the introduction of selective, reversible MAOIs, such as moclobemide, may lead to a greater use of this class of ADs in all age groups.

For more severe forms of depression, characterized by a rapidly deteriorating course or nonresponsiveness to drug intervention, or in patients with serious concurrent medical disorders, *ECT* may be the most appropriate alternative (see also Chapter 8) (15).

Dose. Whatever agent is chosen, a general rule is to start at half the usual adult dose (and even lower if organicity is involved) and to increase the drug at a slower rate. Thus, for a drug like desipramine or nortriptyline, 10–25 mg/day may be the best initial strategy. Fluoxetine can be initially given in doses of 10 mg/day or 20 mg every second or third day. Sertraline (initiated at 25 mg/day) is also an appropriate alternate strategy. If sedation is required, an agent such as trazodone (e.g., starting dose 25 mg at bedtime) may be used as the sole AD or cautiously in combination with one of the other compounds discussed.

Adequate length of treatment may be longer (e.g., 6–12 weeks) in this population due to age-related pharmacokinetic and pharmacodynamic changes. TDM may be helpful to assure levels that are therapeutic and nontoxic. Maintenance doses comparable to acute levels for 6 to 12 months after remission are usually appropriate.

Antimanics

As with depression in late life, mania can be divided into early-onset and late-onset types. It is estimated that 5–10% of elderly affectively disordered patients present with manic symptoms. Presentation tends to be more atypical, with secondary mania caused by an organic factor a much more common phenomenon in the elderly versus younger patient population. As with the younger cohort, mania may be recurrent and disabling in some older patients.

Whereas lithium remains the standard approach, increased complications in the elderly, especially when there is compromise of the CNS, endocrine, or renal systems, makes this agent a less attractive choice. Lower doses (e.g., 150–300 mg)

should be initiated, with many elderly patients achieving adequate response on total daily doses of lithium in the 450–600 mg range. If a more rapid response is necessary, low-dose high-potency antipsychotics can also be used in the early phases. Alternatively, a BZD, such as clonazepam or lorazepam, may be indicated (15a).

An alternate strategy to lithium may be an anticonvulsant, such as CBZ or divalproex sodium. For example, a recent open trial in seven elderly patients found that VPA produced marked-to-moderate improvement in five previously refractory patients. Further, the drug appeared safe in this group of patients who also suffered from several medical disorders as well (16). Clearly, controlled trials in this age group are necessary to clarify the relative risk to benefit ratio of the available mood stabilizers.

Benzodiazepines

As a symptom, *anxiety* appears to be common among elderly patients, and Table 14.4 lists common factors that underlie this symptom (17). Nevertheless, only sparse data are available on the incidence and prevalence of anxiety disorders in this population (18). Simple phobia may be the only anxiety disorder with an onset after age 60 years (19). According to an Epidemiologic Catchment Area Survey, phobic disorders may be the most common anxiety-related condition among those over age 65 years, followed by generalized anxiety disorder. By contrast, panic disorder may be relatively rare (20, 21). As in younger adults, anxiety in the elderly may be due to a variety of causes; however, recent onset of nonphobic anxiety suggests an organic or iatrogenic basis that merits thorough investigation before treatment is initiated (18).

Sleep disturbances are quite common among the elderly. According to a recent National Institutes of Health Consensus Development Conference, disrupted sleep afflicts over half of Americans age 65 years or older who live at home and about two-thirds of those who live in long-term care facilities (22). Although changes in sleep/wake patterns appear to accompany advancing age, disrupted sleep may also be secondary to a wide variety of factors (20). As with anxiety, careful diagnosis is important before any treatment is initiated. Factors that commonly contribute to disturbed sleep are listed in Table 14.5.

Choice of Benzodiazepine

If BZDs are used in the elderly, they should be prescribed at the lowest possi-

**Table 14.4.
Factors That May Cause Anxiety in the Elderly**

Physical illness
  Respiratory disease
  Cardiac disease
  Gastrointestinal syndromes
  Anemia
  Metabolic disorders
  Endocrine disorders
Psychiatric/neurologic illness
  Major depressive disorder
  Alzheimer's disease
  Delirium
  Seizure disorders
  Encephalopathies
  Postconcussion syndrome
Other
  Withdrawal syndromes (alcohol, nicotine,
    caffeine, sedatives, hypnotics)
  Grief and mourning
  Hospitalization
  Institutionalization
  Insomnia
Drugs
  Caffeine
  Alcohol
  Bronchodilators
  Salicylates
  Sympathomimetics
  Antiparkinsonian agents
  Neuroleptics (akathisia)
  Hypotensive agents
  Steroids
  Anorectics
  Diuretics
  Hallucinogens
  Digitalis toxicity
  Anticholinergic toxicity

**Table 14.5.
Factors That May Disturb Sleep in the Elderly**

Physical illness
  Respiratory disease
  Cardiac disease
  Arthritis, pain syndromes
  Prostate disease
  Endocrine disease
  Sleep apnea syndrome
  Restless legs syndrome
Psychiatric/neurologic illness
  Major depressive disorder
  Anxiety disorders
  Alzheimer's disease
  Delirium
Environment
  Situational anxiety
  Hospitalization
  Poor sleep hygiene
  Extensive bed rest
  Lack of appropriate exercise
  Confinement to a nursing home
  Circadian rhythm disturbances
  Noise
  Nondiuretic nocturia
  Light
  Grief and mourning
Drugs
  Alcohol
  Nicotine
  Caffeine
  Long-term use of hypnotics (prescription and
    over-the-counter)
  Diuretics
  Bronchodilators
  Steroids
  Respiratory stimulants
  β-Blockers
  Corticosteroids
  Alerting antidepressants
  Monoamine oxidase inhibitors
  Immunosuppressants
  Methyldopa
  Phenytoin

ble dose for the shortest possible time, and on an intermittent rather than a regular basis. The decision to use these agents should be made with considerable caution, and only after possible underlying causes of the patient's symptoms have been explored and treated appropriately. Although surveys indicate the elderly are frequently prescribed BZDs, the NIH Consensus Development Conference stated that the efficacy and safety of sedatives and hypnotics has not been established for older people, nor has the extent to which they contribute to or alleviate sleep problems (20, 23, 24). Salzman has pointed out that relatively few research studies, most of which are seriously flawed, have examined the therapeutic effect of these agents in the elderly (25). Thus, recommendations for the use of BZDs in the elderly are derived almost exclusively from studies of young adult patients, studies of pharmacokinetics and toxicity in the elderly, and clinical and anecdotal experience.

Age can significantly alter the pharmacokinetics of BZDs metabolized by oxidation, tending to reduce their clearance (see also Chapters 3 and 12). This may lead to drug accumulation and possible toxicity during chronic administration, particularly in elderly men (26). BZDs transformed by conjugation have relatively short half-lives and accumulate less during multiple dosing; in part because the conjugation (as opposed to the oxidation) process appears to be less influenced by age. Age also appears to enhance pharmacodynamic sensitivity to BZDs, so that at any given plasma or brain concentration, the elderly experience an increased intensity of drug effect compared to younger patients (26). In addition, physical or emotional illness (e.g., stroke, Parkinson's disease, dementia, and disorders that impair protein binding, hepatic metabolism, or

renal clearance) may increase sensitivity (25). Finally, concomitant use of other drugs with CNS effects (e.g., ADs, stimulants, steroids, alcohol) may exacerbate BZD toxicity (25).

Adverse Effects

Use of both long and short half-life BZDs in the elderly has been associated with a number of potentially serious unwanted effects, of which the most common are excessive sedation and cerebellar, psychomotor, and cognitive impairment (25) (see Table 14.6).

Although short half-life BZDs are usually recommended for the elderly because they are less likely to accumulate and are rapidly eliminated, there have been few comparisons of their effects on performance in the elderly. In one study of nonanxious elderly volunteers, both diazepam (long half-life, oxidation) and oxazepam (short half-life, conjugation) produced comparable self-rated sedation and fatigue during chronic administration (21). These effects persisted in diazepam subjects during a 2-week washout period, but rapidly returned to baseline in the oxazepam subjects.

Long half-life BZDs may increase the risk of daytime sedation, lethargy, cognitive impairment, delirium, as well as falls and hip fractures (27–29). Long-term use of flurazepam (30 mg/day) has been associated with an increased incidence of ataxia and hallucinations (30). However, short half-life BZDs also may cause serious adverse effects. Ataxia, depression, confusion, amnestic syndromes, and oversedation have been reported in elderly lorazepam users, and there is some evidence that short-acting BZDs may also increase the risk of falls (31–35).

Triazolam. In 1983, the United States Food and Drug Administration

Table 14.6.
Adverse Effects of BZDs in the Elderly

CNS depression
  Excessive sedation
  Drowsiness
  Fatigue
Cerebellar
  Ataxia
  Dysarthria
  Incoordination
  Unsteadiness
  Falls, hip fractures
Psychomotor
  Slowed reaction time
  Diminished motor accuracy
  Impaired eye-hand coordination
CNS stimulation
  Paradoxical excitement
  Nightmares
  Insomnia
  Agitation
  Hallucinations
  Belligerence
Cognitive
  Confusion
  Anterograde amnesia
  Impaired short-term recall
  Increased forgetfulness
  Decreased attention
  Delirium

(FDA) approved triazolam, 0.5 mg (for healthy adults), 0.25 mg (for the elderly and debilitated), and 0.125 mg based on data suggesting these doses would be safe and effective. Five years later, the FDA withdrew the 0.5-mg dose from the United States market, but continued approval of the 0.125-mg dose and the 0.25-mg dose (now the recommended starting dose for nonelderly insomniacs) without new studies to demonstrate its efficacy in such patients. These actions were in response to scientific data indicating the risk of adverse reactions to triazolam is dose dependent, a fact not emphasized by either the manufacturer nor by the FDA.

In late 1991 and early 1992, the Committee on Safety of Medicines of the United Kingdom concluded that the risks of treatment with triazolam at the li-censed doses (0.25 mg and 0.125 mg) outweighed the benefits. The United Kingdom and a few other countries banned triazolam primarily because of persistent reports of adverse reactions. As of the end of February 1992, France, Spain, and New Zealand suspended the 0.25-mg dose of triazolam but allowed continued marketing of the 0.125-mg dose; while Canada and Japan lowered the recommended starting dose for nonelderly insomniacs to 0.125 mg.

In February 1992, the FDA approved new labelling on triazolam. Whereas the prior labelling recommended that triazolam not be prescribed in quantities exceeding a 1-month supply, the label now recommends that prescriptions be written only for short term (7–10 days) treatment of insomnia. It also states that use for more than 2–3 weeks requires a complete reevaluation of the patient. The new labelling also sets definite dose limits, stating that for geriatric or debilitated patients, a dose of 0.25 mg should not be exceeded, being reserved only for exceptional cases.

Between 1980 and 1991, only a few published studies examined the safety and the hypnotic efficacy of the 0.125-mg dose of triazolam in the elderly (36–42). These studies and case reports indicate that with continued use, the initial efficacy of the 0.125-mg dose of triazolam in the elderly begins to wane after 1 week and progressively diminishes to ineffectiveness, usually by the sixth week of continuous administration. During the same period the risk of potentially serious adverse reactions increases.

One study evaluated only the cognitive effects of single doses of 0.125-mg triazolam (42). Although the others assessed hypnotic efficacy, in all but one of these, study duration was 2–14 nights. In the remaining study, with a duration of 3–9 weeks, 5 of 22 elderly subjects (23%) were taken off triazolam between the third and fifth weeks because of serious adverse effects (41). The researchers reported:

> At week 3 significantly more triazolam patients were rated as more restless during the day ($p < 0.05$) and they also appeared more hostile, less relaxed, more irritable, and more anxious. After withdrawal of triazolam, these adverse reports were reduced. . . . Our study suggests that the use of triazolam in older patients, given in conservative doses, may have significant disadvantages.

The investigators who studied only the cognitive effects of triazolam (0.125 mg) stated,

> Elderly persons may remain unaware of or fail to express on standard rating instruments, the sedative effects of triazolam seen by an observer and evident in the results of tests of psychomotor function and memory (42).

Triazolam may cause sedation, learning and memory impairment, confusion, irritability, paranoid delusions, aggression and irrational behavior, reversible delirium, anterograde amnesia, and automatic movements (32, 43–47). In a placebo-controlled study of the pharmacokinetic and pharmacodynamic effects of single doses (0.125 mg and 0.25 mg) of triazolam (short half-life, oxidation) in healthy young and elderly subjects, triazolam caused a greater degree of sedation and greater impairment of psychomotor performance in the elderly than in the young (42). Triazolam also has a narrow therapeutic range in the elderly, and overdosage may occur with as little as 2 mg, an amount only four to eight times the recommended dose (48). Three cases of fatal triazolam overdose have been reported in elderly patients who were debilitated or had taken other psychotropic drugs and alcohol (49).

BZD-induced amnesia, confusion, depression, and oversedation in the elderly may be misdiagnosed as dementia (50).

Sedatives/hypnotics as a group, and BZDs in particular, are frequently implicated in drug-related hospital admissions in the elderly (51, 52). This group are at particular risk for abrupt drug discontinuation when hospitalized, with resulting withdrawal symptoms that may be unrecognized as such and attributed to other health problems (31, 53–55). BZD hypnotics should not be routinely prescribed in the hospital unless the patient has a demonstrated sleep disorder (56). Even then, reassurance that restless sleep is normal in such a situation may obviate the need for a hypnotic (48).

Patients with Breathing Disorders. Some evidence indicates that BZDs may exacerbate breathing difficulties in patients with chronic lung disorders (57, 58). Because flurazepam has been reported to exacerbate sleep apneas in middle-aged and elderly normal volunteers, the possibility of undiagnosed sleep apnea should always be considered before a BZD is prescribed (59).

Demented Patients. As mentioned earlier, in the discussion on APs, although BZDs are commonly used to treat the severe agitation, anxiety, and restlessness that may accompany dementia, response is unpredictable (60). These drugs may exacerbate confusion and agitation, producing mild to severe amnestic syndromes resembling dementia of the Alzheimer's type (61–65). Demented elderly patients may also be at risk for BZD-caused oversedation (64–66). If long half-life BZDs are used, oversedation and aggravation of dementia may become chronic (66). Buspirone, or low doses of a sedative antipsychotic such as thioridazine, are often useful alternatives (12, 67–69).

Although severe disruption in the

sleep-wake cycle is a common feature of dementia, the use of BZDs in such cases may also produce significant behavioral toxicity. Alternative drug approaches include bedtime use of thioridazine in nondepressed patients or nortriptyline in depressed patients (70). Nonpharmacologic techniques involving good sleep hygiene, as well as exercise, restriction of daytime naps, and regulation of morning awakening, may also be helpful (20).

Benzodiazepine Discontinuation in the Elderly

In the elderly, there is evidence that abrupt discontinuation of long-term BZD use may be associated with severe withdrawal symptoms, including confusion, disorientation, and hallucinations (50, 54, 55). Gradual discontinuation, however, appears to be tolerated as well by the elderly as by younger patients (71). The cognitive impairment associated with BZD administration is reversible with drug discontinuation, often improving memory and concentration (24, 25).

Alternate Therapies

Drug Therapy

Despite the serious drawbacks to the use of BZDs in the elderly, there are few pharmacologic alternatives. *Barbiturates* and *meprobamate* have a high incidence of adverse effects and toxicity and should not be used. Small doses of *sedating antidepressants*, though generally well tolerated as hypnotics in younger patients, may produce a higher incidence of anticholinergic effects in the elderly. *Antihistamines*, a common ingredient in over-the-counter sleeping aids, are less effective than BZDs and may cause delirium if dosage is not carefully titrated. Although *chloral hydrate* is contraindicated in patients taking

drugs that may interact adversely with it (e.g., warfarin, phenytoin), it is unlikely to cause habituation or delirium (48). Confusion and hallucinations, however, have been reported (72).

Buspirone may be an effective anxiolytic in the elderly and less likely than BZDs to produce excessive sedation (73–76). Dizziness, however, may be a problem. Whereas *ADs and β-blockers* may be useful alternatives in younger patients, there are no data documenting their effectiveness for anxiety in the elderly (25). Although *antipsychotics* may be helpful in reducing severe agitation, their side-effect profile makes them unsuitable for use in subjective anxiety states (18, 25).

Nondrug Approaches

These include patient education about:

- Good *sleep hygiene* and what constitutes "normal" sleep
- *Avoidance of stimulating substances* (alcohol, caffeine)
- *Reduction of environmental stimuli* that may disturb sleep (noise, light)
- *Reducing worry* at bedtime
- Regular *exercise* (20) (see also Treatment of Sleep Disorders in Chapter 12).

Efforts directed toward helping patients understand and cope with specific problems (bereavement, finances, illness, reduced social interactions, etc.) should be considered whenever possible. Various psychotherapies may also be useful (18).

CONCLUSION

The aging body and mind are in many respects unchartered territory when considering psychopharmacotherapeutic interventions. What we do know is that management with these drugs is often unnecessary, may do more harm than good, and when employed may adversely interact with a host of other medications the elderly require. While the judicious use of psychotropics may be warranted in certain situations, the clinician must remain especially vigilant when choosing this course of action.

REFERENCES

1. Blackwell B. Explaining psychoactive drug therapy to the patient. Int Drug Therapy Newsletter 1986;21:32.
2. Stubbs CM. Medication in the elderly. Therapeutic Notes 186, April 14, 1982, Department of Health, Wellington, Australia.
3. Sunderland T, Tariot, PN, Cohen RM, Weingartner H, Mueller EA, Murphy DL. Anticholinergic sensitivity in patients with dementia of the Alzheimer type and age-matched controls. A dose-response study. Arch Gen Psychiatry 1987;44:418–426.
4. Salzman C. Treatment of the agitated demented elderly patient. Hosp Commun Psychiatry 1988;39(11):1143–1144.
5. Risse SC, Barnes R. Pharmacologic treatment of agitation associated with dementia. J Am Geriatr Soc 1986;34:368–376.
6. Sunderland T, Silver MA. Neuroleptics in the treatment of dementia. Internat J Geriatr Psychiatry 1988;3:79–88.
7. Barnes R, Veith R, Okimoto J, Raskind M, Gumbrecht G. Efficacy of antipsychotic medications in behaviorally disturbed dementia patients. Am J Psychiatry 1982;139(9):1170–1174.
8. Sugerman AA, Williams BH, Adlerstein AM. Haloperidol in the psychiatric disorders of old age. Am J Psychiatry 1964; 120(2):1190–1192.
9. Hamilton LD, Bennett JL. The use of trifluoperazine in geriatric patients with chronic brain syndrome. J Am Geriatrics Soc 1962;10:140–147.
10. Petrie WM, Ban TA, Berney S, Fujimori M, Guy W, Ragheb M, Wilson WH, Schaffer JD. Loxapine in psychogeriatrics: a placebo- and standard-controlled clinical investigation. J Clin Psychopharmacol 1982; 2(2):122–126.
11. Rada RT, Kellner R. Thiothixene in the treatment of geriatric patients with chronic organic brain syndrome. J Am Geriatr Soc 1976;24(3):105–107.
12. Stotsky B. Multicenter study comparing thioridazine with diazepam and placebo in elderly, nonpsychotic patients with emotional and behavioral disorders. Clin Ther 1984;6:564–559.
13. Devanand DP, Sackeim HA, Brown RP, Mayeux R. A pilot study of haloperidol treatment of psychosis and behavioral disturbance in Alzheimer's disease. Arch Neurol 1989;46:854–857.
14. Avorn J, Soumerai SB, Everitt DE, Ross-Degnan D, Beers MH, Sherman D, et al. A randomized trial of a program to reduce the use of psychoactive drugs in nursing homes. N Engl J Med 1992;327:168–173.
14a. NIH Consensus Development Panel on Depression in Late Life. Diagnosis and treatment of depression in late life. JAMA 1992;268:1018–1023.
15. Alexopoulos GS, Young RC, Abrams RC. ECT in the high-risk geriatric patient. Convulsive Ther 1989;5:75–87.
15a. Coppen A. Everyday management of affective disorders. Lancet 1987;i:886.
16. McFarland BH, Miller MR, Straumfjord AA. Valproate use in the older manic patients. J Clin Psychiatry 1990;51:479–481.
17. Gurian BS, Miner JH. Clinical presentation of anxiety in the elderly. In: Salzman C, Lebowitz BD, eds. Anxiety in the elderly. Treatment and research. New York: Springer, 1991.
18. Barbee JG, McLaulin B. Anxiety disorders: diagnosis and pharmacotherapy in the elderly. Psychiatr Ann 1990;20:439–445.
19. Thyer B, Parrish RJ, Curtis GC, et al. Ages of onset of DSM-III anxiety disorders. Compr Psychiatry 1985;23:113–122.
20. Prinz PN, Vitiello MV, Raskind MA, Thorpy MJ. Geriatrics: sleep disorders and aging. N Engl J Med 1990;323:520–526.
21. Salzman C, Shader RI, Greenblatt DJ, Harmatz JS. Long vs short half-life benzodiazepines in the elderly. Arch Gen Psychiatry 1983;40:293–297.
22. Monjan AA. Sleep disorders of older people: report of a consensus conference. Hosp Commun Psychiatry 1990;41:743–744.
23. National Disease and Therapeutic Index (NPDI). Ambler, PA, IMS, 1986.
24. Mellinger GD, Balter MB, Uhlenhuth EH. Prevalence and correlates of the long-term regular use of anxiolytics. JAMA 1984;251:375–379.
25. Salzman C. Pharmacologic treatment of

the anxious elderly patient. In: Salzman C, Lebowitz BD, eds. Anxiety in the elderly. Treatment and research. New York: Springer, 1991.

26. Greenblatt DJ, Shader RI. Benzodiazepines in the elderly: pharmacokinetics and drug sensitivity. In: Salzman C, Lebowitz BD, eds. Anxiety in the elderly. Treatment and research. New York: Springer, 1991.

27. Ray WA, Griffin MR, Schaffner W, Baugh DK, Melton LJ III. Psychotropic drug use and the risk of hip fracture. N Engl J Med 1987;316:363–369.

28. Ray WA, Griffin MR, Downey M. Benzodiazepines of long and short elimination half-life and the risk of hip fracture. JAMA 1989;262:3303–3307.

29. Sorock GS, Shimkin EE. Benzodiazepine sedatives and the risk of falling in a community-dwelling elderly cohort. Arch Intern Med 1988;148:2441–2444.

30. Marttila JK, Hammel RJ, Alexander B, Zustiak R. Potential untoward effects of long-term use of flurazepam in geriatric patients. J Am Pharmacol Assoc 1977;17:692–695.

31. Ancill RJJ, Embury GD, MacEwan GW, Kennedy JS. Lorazepam in the elderly—a retrospective study of the side-effects in 20 patients. J Pharmacol 1987;2:126–127.

32. Robin DW, Hasan SS, Lichtenstein MJ, et al. Dose-related effects of triazolam on postural sway. Clin Pharmacol Ther 1991;49:581–588.

33. Campbell AJ, Somerton DT. Benzodiazepine drug effect on body sway in elderly subjects. J Clin Exp Gerontol 1982;4:341–347.

34. Swift CG, Haythorne JM, Clarke P, Stevenson IH. The effect of ageing on measured responses to single doses of oral temazepam. Br J Clin Pharmacol 1981;11:423P–414P.

35. Doyle CJ. Halcion and bed-related falls. Loss Control Bulletin, 1987;5(7). Insurance Department, Humana Inc, Louisville, KY.

36. Lipani JA. Preference study of the hypnotic efficacy of triazolam 0.125 mg compared to placebo in geriatric patients with insomnia. Curr Ther Res 1978;24:397–402.

37. Day BH, Davis H, Parsons DW. An assessment of two hypnotics in the elderly. Clin Trials J 1981;273–286.

38. Roehrs T, Zorick F, Wittig R, Roth T. Efficacy of a reduced triazolam dose in elderly insomniacs. Neurobiol Aging 1985;6:292–296.

39. Bonnet MH, Dexter JR, Arand DL. The effect of triazolam on arousal and respiration in central sleep apnea patients. Sleep 1990;13:31–41.

40. Woo E, Proulx SM, Greenblatt DJ. Differential side effects profile of triazolam versus flurazepam in elderly patients undergoing rehabilitation therapy. J Clin Pharmacol 1991;31:168–173.

41. Bayer AJ, Bayer EM, Pathy MSJ, Stokes MJ. A double-blind controlled study of chlormethiazole and triazolam as hypnotics in the elderly. Acta Psychiatr Scand 1986;73(suppl 329):104–111.

42. Greenblatt DJ, Harmatz JS, Shapiro L, et al. Sensitivity to triazolam in the elderly. N Engl J Med 1991;324:1691–1698.

43. Patterson F. Triazolam syndrome in the elderly. South Med J 1987;80:1425–1426.

44. Shader RI, Greenblatt DJ. Triazolam and anterograde amnesia: all is not well in the z-zone. J Clin Psychopharmacol 1983;3:273.

45. Schogt B, Conn D. Paranoid symptoms associated with triazolam. Can J Psychiatry 1985;30;462–463.

46. DeTullio PL, Kirking DM, Zacardelli DK, Kwee P. Evaluation of long-term triazolam use in an ambulatory veterans administration medical center population. DICP, the Annals of Pharmacotherapy 1989;23:290–293.

47. Thompson JF, Robinson CA. Triazolam in the elderly. N Engl J Med 1991;325:1743–1744.

48. Moran MG, Thompson TL, Nies AS. Sleep disorders in the elderly. Am J Psychiatry 1988;145:1369–1378.

49. Sunter JP, Bal TS, Cowan WK: Three cases of fatal triazolam poisoning. Br Med J 1988;297:719.

50. Miller F, Whitcup S. Benzodiazepine use in psychiatrically hospitalized elderly patients. J Clin Psychopharmacol 1986;6:384–385.

51. Williamson J, Chopin JM. Adverse reactions to prescribed drugs in the elderly: A multicentre investigation. Age Ageing 1980;9:73–80.

52. Grymonpre RE, Mitenko PA, Sitar DS, Aoki Fy, Montgomery PR. Drug-associated hospital admissions in older medical patients. J Am Geriatr Soc 1988;36:1092–1098.

53. Moss JH. Sedative and hypnotic withdrawal states in hospitalised patients [Letter]. Lancet 1991;338(8766):575.

54. Foy A, Drinkwater V, March S, Mearrick P. Confusion after admission to hospital in elderly patients using benzodiazepines [Letter]. Br Med J (Clin Res) 1986;293 (6554):1072.

55. Speirs CJ, Navey FL, Brooks DJ, Impallomessi MG. Opisthotonos and benzodiazepine withdrawal in the elderly. Lancet 1986;2:1101.

56. Berlin RM. Management of insomnia in hospitalized patients. Ann Intern Med 1984;100:398–404.

57. Model DG, Berry DJ. Effect of chlordiazepoxide in respiratory failure due to chronic bronchitis. Lancet 1974;2:869–870.

58. Rudolf M, Geddes DM, Turner JA, et al. Depression of central respiratory drive by nitrazepam. Thorax 1978;33:97–100.

59. Guilleminault C, Silvestri R, Mondini S, et al. Aging and sleep apnea: Action of benzodiazepines, acetosolamide, alcohol and sleep deprivation in a healthy elderly group. J Gerontol 1984;39:655–661.

60. Salzman C. Treatment of agitation, anxiety, and depression in dementia. Psychopharmacol Bull 1988;24:39–42.

61. Hale WE, Stewart RB, Marks RG. Antianxiety drugs and central nervous system symptoms in an ambulatory elderly population. Drug Intell Clin Pharm 1985;19:37–40.

62. Larson EB, Kukull WA, Buchner D, Reifler BV. Adverse drug reactions associated with global cognitive impairment in elderly persons. Ann Intern Med 1987; 107:169–173.

63. Thompson TL, Moran MG, Nies AS. Psychotropic drug use in the elderly. New Engl J Med 1983;308:134–138.

64. Bartus RT, Dean RL, Beer B, Lippa AS. The cholinergic hypothesis of geriatric memory dysfunction. Science 1982;217: 408–417.

65. Block RI, De Voe M, Stanley M, Pomara N. Memory performance in individuals with primary degenerative dementia: its

66. Salzman C. Treatment of the agitated demented elderly patient. Hosp Commun Psychiatry 1988;39:1143–1144.

67. Colenda CC III. Buspirone in treatment of agitated demented patient [Letter]. Lancet 1988;1:1169.

68. Kirven LE, Montero EF. Comparison of thioridazine and diazepam in the control of nonpsychotic symptoms associated with senility: Double-blind study. J Am Geriatr Soc 1973;21:546–551.

69. Covington JS. Alleviating agitation, apprehension, and related symptoms in geriatric patients: A double-blind comparison of phenothiazine and a benzodiazepine. South Med J 1975;68:719–724.

70. Reynolds CF III, Hock CC, Stack J, Campbell D. The nature and management of sleep/wake disturbance in Alzheimer's dementia. Psychopharmacol Bull 1988;24: 43–48.

71. Schweizer E, Case GW, Rickels K. Benzodiazepine dependence and withdrawal in elderly patients. Am J Psychiatry 1989;146: 529–521.

72. Kramer C. Methaqualone and chloral hydrate: Preliminary comparison in geriatric patients. J Am Geriatr Soc 1967;15:455–461.

73. Napoliello MJ. An interim multicentre report on 677 anxious geriatric outpatients treated with buspirone. Br J Clin Pract 1986;40:71–73.

74. Robinson D, Napoliello MJ. The safety and usefulness of buspirone as an anxiolytic in elderly versus young patients. Clin Ther 1988;10:740–746.

75. Singh AN, Beer M. A dose range finding study of buspirone in geriatric patients with symptoms of anxiety. J Clin Psychopharmacol 1988;8:67–68.

76. Levine S, Napoliello MJ, Domantay AG. Open study of buspirone in octogenarians with anxiety. Human Psychopharmacol 1989;4:51–53.

similarity to diazepam-induced impairments. Exp Aging Res 1985;11:151–155.

The Personality-Disordered Patient

The DSM-III-R currently groups personality disorders into three clusters:

• Cluster A: the odd/eccentric
• Cluster B: the dramatic/erratic

* Cluster C: the anxious (see also Appendices T and U)

Several recent studies have noted that some personality disorders may partially benefit from trials with psychotropic agents. While the majority of trials have involved borderline personality (a Cluster B disorder), no clear specific drug therapy has emerged for this or for that matter any other personality disorder. Instead, most authors suggest that drug therapy should be symptom oriented. Thus, these agents can be targeted to specific symptoms, regardless of the type of personality disorder.

With this approach, a variety of symptom presentations might benefit from the same agents indicated for the full diagnostic syndrome, including:

* *Antipsychotics* (usually in low doses for brief periods of time) for transient psychosis, paranoia, impulsivity, and cognitive disorders, particularly in Cluster A patients
* *Antidepressants* (TCAs, SRIs, MAOIs) for panic attacks, phobias, attention deficit hyperactivity, compulsive symptoms, and of course, depressive syndromes
* *Mood stabilizers* for dyscontrol, rage, violence, affective lability, and impulsivity
* *Anxiolytics* for panic symptoms, social phobia or agoraphobia, and acute conversion symptoms.

Ayd has summarized the critical issues to consider, whenever considering drug therapy in these patients:

* Emphasize that drugs are *not a panacea*
* Address *unrealistic expectations* for therapy
* Always employ *concurrent nonpharmacological therapies* in addition to medication

* Serial drug substitutions are preferable to concurrent multiple drug use (i.e., *avoid polypharmacy*)
* If possible, *avoid drugs that may cause tardive dyskinesia (TD), paradoxical disinhibition,* or *lower the seizure threshold*
* Continually review for *informed consent* (1).

BORDERLINE PERSONALITY DISORDER

Borderline personality disorder (BPD) is characterized by a pervasive pattern of unstable affect, stormy interpersonal relationships, and behavioral dyscontrol. It is estimated that 1–2% of the general population manifest this syndrome. It is also a comorbid condition with major mood disorders (i.e., different studies estimate from 25–75% of these patients have a major depression and 5–20% a bipolar disorder). Furthermore, as many as 25% of bulimics may also suffer from BPD; and about 70% of BPD patients abuse alcohol or drugs. Self-mutilation, suicide attempts, and completed suicides are all too frequent. **Indeed, it is estimated that 3–10% of these patients will kill themselves.**

There is a modest link to mood disorders, but it is weak in magnitude and somewhat inconsistent. For example, some studies suggest that BPD often exists in families with other members who have bipolar disorder (2).

Drug Therapy

There are a limited number of studies investigating drug treatment. Goldberg, in a double-blind study of BPD or schizotypal personality disorder, found drugs superior to placebo. This was particularly true for the schizotypal personality disorder, and to a more modest degree for the BPD patients as well (3). Soloff et al. compared haloperidol, amitriptyline, and placebo, finding the antipsychotic clearly superior to amitriptyline or placebo (4). Cowdry and Gardner, in a multiple crossover design, compared trifluoperazine, tranylcypromine, carbamazepine, alprazolam, and placebo in 16 BPD patients (5). Many in the antipsychotic group either did not tolerate the drug or clinically deteriorated, but the five patients on trifluoperazine who completed the trial experienced modest benefit. The MAOI tranylcypromine seemed to produce the greatest improvement; and 10 of the 11 subjects on carbamazepine also had a modest improvement in mood. Alprazolam was ineffective and, indeed, 7 of 12 patients either attempted suicide or were assaultive.

It is important to note that there is some overlap between BPD and atypical depression as defined by Liebowitz and Klein, who also use the term hysteroid dysphoria to characterize this condition (6). Many of their patients also met the criteria for BPD, and data from several studies by this group have demonstrated that phenelzine produces greater improvement than either imipramine or placebo (7).

ANTISOCIAL PERSONALITY DISORDER

As noted in Chapter 6, there is some evidence that impulsive violence may be related to low brain serotonin, as manifested by low CSF 5-HIAA. This leads to the hope that elucidating the biology of impulsivity may lead to an effective drug treatment. Unfortunately, we know of no clinical trials presently addressing this question.

HISTRIONIC PERSONALITY DISORDER

This personality disorder is also similar to the syndrome that Liebowitz and Klein have termed hysteroid dysphoria or atypi-

cal depression (6). MAOIs have proven to be very helpful in this condition, and these data are reviewed in Chapter 7. Rifkin et al. also investigated the effects of ADs in patients with emotionally unstable personalities, a syndrome characterized by excitability and ineffectiveness when confronted with minor stress (8). This syndrome is primarily found in female adolescents whose moods consist of:

- Short periods of *intense unhappiness*
- *Social withdrawal*
- *Depression* and *irritability*
- Episodes of *impulsivity*
- *Rejection of religious rules*
- *Pleasure* seeking.

They found that imipramine produced improvement in 67%, and chlorpromazine helped in 81% of these cases, with both agents demonstrating a statistically significant greater improvement over placebo.

PARANOID PERSONALITY DISORDER

There have been a few controlled studies and some anecdotal information that low-dose antipsychotics may benefit some of these patients when used in conjunction with psychotherapy (9).

SCHIZOTYPAL AND RELATED PERSONALITY DISORDERS

One single-blind study treated 17 schizotypal patients with a modest dose of haloperidol (i.e., 2–12 mg/day), and produced some benefit, although many were quite sensitive to the adverse effects of this drug (10). Goldberg's study also found that thiothixene benefited both schizotypal disorder as well as BPD (2). Similarly, low dose antipsychotics had a modest effect in patients with both schizotypal and obsessive-compulsive personality disorders (11).

Although the term pseudoneurotic schizophrenia has been dropped from our nomenclature, Klein made an interesting observation regarding the drug treatment of this condition. Specifically, in an investigation comparing the effects of chlorpromazine and imipramine in a wide variety of patients, they observed that imipramine was beneficial (12). Thus, in this controlled study, imipramine produced a positive outcome in 60%, in contrast to placebo, which produced only a 25% positive outcome.

OBSESSIVE-COMPULSIVE PERSONALITY DISORDER

Obsessive-compulsive *disorder* is rare in obsessive-compulsive *personalities*. One study found that only 6% of these personality disorders have OCD, thus it is quite likely that the two conditions are distinct (13). The implication for treatment is that agents helpful for OCD (e.g., clomipramine) may not benefit obsessive-compulsive personality disorder. Definitive studies to address this issue have not been conducted, however.

AVOIDANT PERSONALITY DISORDER

β-Blockers inhibit peripheral autonomic movements in anxiety, and MAOIs benefit social phobias (see Phobic Disorders in Chapter 11). Because such features may also be present in avoidant personality disorder, a trial with these medications may be warranted. Like other personality disorders, however, there have been few controlled clinical trials to test this question.

PASSIVE AGGRESSIVE AND NARCISSISTIC PERSONALITY DISORDERS

We are not aware of any drug treatment studies of these disorders.

CONCLUSION

The drug therapy of personality disorders sorely lacks supportive data from controlled trials. Most positive results occur when medications are targeted for specific symptoms, rather than specific diagnostic conditions. Further, MAOIs may be particularly beneficial for a constellation of symptoms associated with such various conditions as atypical depression, hysteroid dysphoria, as well as histrionic and borderline personality disorders. The propensity for self-destructive impulses in the last group, however, dictates the closest monitoring of these agents and the availability of only limited medication supplies with any given prescription.

REFERENCES

1. Ayd F. Psychopharmacologic treatment of personality disorders. Int Drug Therapy Newsletter 1990;25(4):1–2.
2. Widiger TA, Frances AJ. Epidemiology. diagnosis, and comorbidity of borderline personality disorder. In: Tasman A, Hales RE, Frances AJ, eds. Review of psychiatry. Vol 8. Washington, D.C.: American Psychiatric Press, 1989:8.
3. Goldberg SC, Schulz SC, Schulz PM, et al. Borderline and schizotypal personality disorders treated with low-dose thiothixene vs placebo. Arch Gen Psychiatry 1986;43: 680–686.
4. Soloff PH, George A, Nathan S, Schulz PM, Ulrich RF, Perel JM. Progress in pharmacotherapy of borderline disorders. Arch Gen Psychiatry 1986;43:691–697.
5. Cowdry RW, Gardner DL. Pharmacotherapy of borderline personality disorder. Arch Gen Psychiatry 1988;45:111.
6. Liebowitz MR, Klein DF. Interrelationship of hysteroid dysphoria and borderline personality disorder. Psychiatr Clin North Am 1981;4(1):67–87.
7. Liebowitz MR, Quitkin FM, Stewart JW, McGrath PJ, Harrison WM, Markowitz JS, et al. Antidepressant specificity in atypical depression. Arch Gen Psychiatry 1988;45: 129–137.
8. Rifkin A, Quitkin F, Carrillo C, Blumberg

AG, Klein DF. Lithium carbonate in emotionally unstable character disorder. Arch Gen Psychiatry 1972;27:519–523.

9. Munro A. Monosymptomatic hypochondriacal psychosis. Br J Hosp Med 1980;24:34–38.

10. Hymowitz P, Frances A, Jacobsberg L, et al. Neuroleptic treatment of schizotypal personality disorder. Compr Psychiatry 1986;27:267–271.

11. Schulz SC. The use of low dose neuroleptics in the treatment of "schizo-obsessive"

patients. Am J Psychiatry 1986;143:1318–1319.

12. Klein DF. Importance of psychiatric diagnosis in the prediction of clinical drug effects. Arch Gen Psychiatry 1967;16:118–126.

13. Baer L, Jenike MA, Ricciardi JN, Holland AD, Seymour RJ, Minichiello WE, Buttolph ML. Standardized assessment of personality disorders in obsessive-compulsive disorder. Arch Gen Psychiatry 1990;47:826–830.

The Alcoholic Patient

The World Health Organization defined alcoholism as a chronic behavior disorder manifested by repeated drinking of alcoholic beverages in excess of community norms for dietary and social purposes and to an extent that it interferes with one's health or social and economic functioning (1).

More recently, a committee comprised of representatives from the National Council on Alcoholism and Drug Dependence and the American Society of Addiction Medicine have developed a definition that includes typical behavioral changes as well as the concept of denial (2). Thus, they characterized alcoholism as:

- A *primary chronic disease* with genetic, psychosocial, and environmental factors influencing its development and manifestations
- An often *progressive and fatal* condition
- *Impaired control* over drinking
- *Preoccupation* with this drug
- *Use despite adverse consequence*
- Distortions in thinking, especially *denial*
- *Continuous* or *periodic.*

After heart disease and cancer, alcohol-related disorders are considered the third most important health problem in the United States, estimated to account for at least one-fourth of all hospitalizations in this country. Almost 50% of those who suffer from alcohol dependence also abuse other legal and illicit drugs (see also Appendix D). Alcohol is involved in 25–35% of all suicides and 50–70% of all homicides; it also figures prominently in accidental deaths and domestic violence (3, 4).

Of the approximately 100 million Americans who imbibe, about 10% suffer from alcoholism, while consuming about 50% of all alcoholic beverages in this country. There are also an estimated 10–12 million problem drinkers, with men's risk for developing severe problems three to four times higher than women's. Although the heaviest drinking occurs at an earlier age for men than for women, the abstinence rate for both sexes begins to increase after age 50 years (5). The "end stage" drinker constitutes less than 3% of the alcoholic population and describes an individual who is generally:

- Unemployed
- Transient
- A daily drinker
- Without social and economic support

- In a deteriorated psychological and physical state.

Adolescents abuse alcohol more frequently than any other drug, with an incidence ranging from 15 to 25%. Traffic accidents involving teenagers often involve alcohol, and the number of traffic-related deaths increases or decreases concomitantly with the lowering or raising of the legal drinking age in various states.

The precise incidence of alcoholism in the *elderly* remains unknown, but retired and recently widowed men seem to be at higher risk (6). Physicians and family members often overlook the effects of alcohol on an elderly person's physical and psychological health and may mistake this problem for an organic mental disorder. In the elderly, preexisting organic mental disorders, a decreased volume of distribution, and the concurrent use of other medication may potentiate the effects of alcohol on cognition, affect, and behavior (see The Elderly Patient in this chapter).

There is strong evidence for at least a familial pattern and perhaps a hereditary basis for some types of alcoholism (7).

ALCOHOL-RELATED PSYCHIATRIC COMPLICATIONS

Alcohol abuse is associated with many psychiatric complications, starting with those involving acute consumption or withdrawal. These include:

- *Intoxication* and its complications (e.g., disinhibition, aggressiveness, depression, and suicide)
- *Idiosyncratic* (or pathological) *intoxication*
- *Withdrawal syndrome,* which may include:
  - Tremors
  - Hallucinosis

- Seizures
- Delirium (e.g., delirium tremens).

A patient who is intoxicated or undergoing alcohol withdrawal should be hospitalized for management if any of the following are present:

- History of *severe withdrawal symptoms*
- Recent *seizure* or history of withdrawal seizures
- Recent *head trauma*
- Serious *medical complications* (e.g. pancreatitis, gastrointestinal bleeding, hepatitis, cirrhosis, or pneumonia)
- *Delirium* or hallucinosis
- *Fever* greater than 101° Fahrenheit
- Significant *malnutrition or dehydration*
- The *Wernicke-Korsakoff* syndrome
- Severe *depression or suicide risk* (8).

In regard to this last issue, the question of comorbid depression associated with alcohol dependence can represent a difficult clinical picture. Whereas ADs may be quite appropriate and useful, premature intervention may be unnecessary. For example, Dackis and colleagues (1986) found that 80% of 49 severely depressed alcoholics remitted after 2 weeks of unmedicated sobriety (9). They concluded that many severe depressions are alcohol-induced organic mood syndromes and improve spontaneously with abstinence.

Most intoxicated individuals do not need hospitalization, display none of the above medical problems, and experience minimal withdrawal symptoms. Thus, observing and treating them in the emergency room or a nonmedical detoxification center for 6–12 hours may be all that is required.

Acute Alcohol Intoxication

Alcohol is similar to other general anesthetics in that it depresses the CNS. Clinically, it may appear to be a stimulant because it first suppresses inhibitory control mechanisms, resulting in early disinhibition. In general, the effect of alcohol on the CNS is proportionate to its blood concentration, but the effects are more marked when the concentration is rising.

In the alert intoxicated patient, general management is primarily supportive and protective. Thiamine 100 mg intramuscularly is given initially, and repeated three times a day orally for the next several weeks. A multivitamin preparation should also be given orally each day. If the patient is restless, a short-acting BZD, such as lorazepam (1–2 mg i.m. or orally) may be repeated every 4–6 hours as needed. If the patient is violent or severely agitated, an AP may be necessary with low-dose, high-potency agents, such as haloperidol (5–10 mg i.m. every hour as needed), preferable. If larger doses are necessary, one should reconsider the diagnosis.

Alcohol Idiosyncratic Intoxication

This syndrome has similarities to the paradoxical reaction seen with barbiturates or BZDs, as well as epileptoid syndromes, including temporal lobe seizures and intermittent explosive disorder. Brain injury from trauma or encephalitis may also predispose some to an abnormally excessive response to even small amounts of alcohol.

Clinical signs and symptoms include sudden onset of irrational, combative, or destructive behavior after ingesting relatively small amounts of alcohol. The behavior is atypical of the individual when not drinking, and usually begins within minutes to hours. After the acute outburst, the patient usually lapses into deep sleep and upon awakening will have only fragmentary memory or total amnesia for the episode. Treatment should attempt to diminish stimulation as much as possible, and antipsychotics, such as haloperidol, 2–10 mg orally or intramuscularly, may reduce combative or destructive behavior.

Alcohol Withdrawal or Abstinence Syndrome

This condition may emerge after a period of relative or absolute abstinence, with the cause(s) unknown. The duration of drinking and quantity of alcohol required to produce noticeable symptoms vary widely. Abstinence may also result from intercurrent illness, hospitalization for an unrelated illness, or lack of money to buy alcohol. The full spectrum of this syndrome, which ranges from an early, mild withdrawal picture to delirium is frequently seen in large hospital emergency room settings.

Early withdrawal peaks at about 24 hours and rarely will the syndrome emerge several days after cessation. Symptoms may clear in a few hours or last up to 2 weeks, and may include:

- *Tremulousness,* which is the earliest and most common sign. Associated symptoms may last for 10–14 days, and include nausea, vomiting, tension, and insomnia.
- *Alcoholic hallucinosis,* which usually consists of auditory hallucinations (but may also be visual) in a clear sensorium. They usually emerge within the first few days, and may persist after all other withdrawal symptoms have resolved.
- *Seizures* ("rum fits") are generalized motor events that usually peak 12–48 hours after cessation of alcohol consumption. Partial seizures suggest a focal lesion and require careful neurological evaluation.
- *Withdrawal delirium* (delirium tremens) usually appears 1–4 days after

abstinence and peaks at about 72–96 hours. The mortality rate may be as high as 15% with serious complicating medical problems. Clinical signs and symptoms include profound confusion, illusions, delusions, vivid hallucinations, agitation, insomnia, and autonomic hyperactivity. Death results from infection, cardiac arrhythmias, fluid and electrolyte abnormalities, or suicide (in response to hallucinations, illusions, or delusions).

Treatment

The treatment of alcohol withdrawal incorporates *general supportive measures* as well as management of specific symptoms. Supportive measures include abstinence from alcohol, ample rest, adequate general nutrition, and reality orientation. It is important to treat the syndrome vigorously, and when appropriate, to prevent it by using sufficient doses of medication.

Typically, the *BZDs* are used on an as-needed basis to treat objective signs of withdrawal, such as tremor, tachycardia, or hypertension. The longer-acting BZDs, such as chlordiazepoxide and diazepam, have the advantage of less frequent dosing but the risk of drug accumulation. The intermediate-acting agents, such as lorazepam, are less likely to accumulate but need to be administered more frequently to prevent reemergence of signs and symptoms. One approach might be lorazepam, 2 mg orally every 2 hours as needed, for as long as needed. The acute dose is then tapered over a 1- to 2-week period using a twice-daily or three-times-daily regimen. Total daily doses of more than 10–12 mg are rarely required. A fixed-dose regimen may not work because of the variability in duration and severity of symptoms. In the severely agitated pa-

tient, lorazepam (2 mg intramuscularly every hour) or diazepam intravenously (5–10 mg slowly) may be necessary. *β-Adrenergic blockers*, such as atenolol, have been tried as adjuncts to BZDs to treat autonomic hyperactivity. For example, atenolol (100 mg orally daily) has been given for moderate to severe tachycardia. Occasionally, *APs*, such as haloperidol (2–10 mg i.m. or orally), may be needed.

Treatment of withdrawal seizures depends on whether there is a prior history. If there is no history, prophylactic anticonvulsants will probably not help. Further, BZDs used for sedation also have anticonvulsant properties, so adequate doses should minimize the risk of seizures. One should avoid APs that can lower the seizure threshold and cause extrapyramidal symptoms and hypotension. Patients with a history of withdrawal or other seizure disorders are at greater risk and should be treated with an anticonvulsant, such as *phenytoin*. If the patient is currently receiving a maintenance dose, continue phenytoin, 300–400 mg/day orally. If the patient is not receiving medication or if it was discontinued 5 or more days previously, give a loading dose of phenytoin, 15 mg/kg intravenously in saline, at a rate not to exceed 50 mg/min, and then start maintenance doses 24 hours later. Some withdrawal seizures can be prevented by restoring serum magnesium levels with *magnesium sulfate* (2 ml of a 50% solution, up to three doses), given with intravenous fluids over 8 hours.

Treatment of delirium includes:

- *Reduce environmental stimulation*
- Monitor *vital signs* frequently
- *Restrain* combative or agitated patients
- Monitor *fluid and electrolyte* balance, correcting any imbalance
- Maintain *blood pressure* with intravenous saline and glucose

- Give *thiamine*, 100 mg intramuscularly initially, then 100 mg orally tid
- Replenish other *vitamin stores* with folate, B complex, and multivitamin supplements
- Give a *BZD*, such as diazepam, 5–10 mg orally every 1–2 hours, as needed for sedation, with a maximum of 80–100 mg daily. If the patient is severely agitated, give 5–10 mg diazepam intravenously slowly every 20 minutes, until the patient is sedated
- A low-dose high-potency *AP*, such as haloperidol (2–5 mg intramuscularly every 2–4 hours), may also be necessary to control acute symptoms on an as-needed basis
- *Search for and treat complicating illnesses* such as pneumonia, gastrointestinal bleeding, hepatic decompensation, pancreatitis, subdural hematoma, and fractures.

Alternate strategies with some evidence for efficacy include:

- Clonidine
- β-Blockers
- Anticonvulsants
- Calcium antagonists

COMPLICATING MEDICAL CONDITIONS IN THE ALCOHOLIC PATIENT

Because several major diseases are commonly associated with alcoholism, treatment of alcohol-related psychiatric disorders may have to be modified if one of these conditions is present.

Cirrhosis

Ninety-five percent of all alcohol is metabolized in the liver; the remaining 5% is excreted via the kidneys and the lungs (see Chapter 3). The rate of metabolism increases with fasting and after protracted periods of drinking. Alcohol has a direct toxic effect on the liver, and whereas only 10–20% of long-term heavy drinkers develop significant hepatic damage, BZDs must be used cautiously because they are primarily metabolized by this organ. If there is evidence of disease, oxazepam and lorazepam are the BZDs of choice because they are not metabolized by the liver. When oral drugs cannot be used, lorazepam (2–8 mg intramuscularly daily) is preferred.

As discussed in Chapter 3, the phases of alcohol consumption can have varying effects on the metabolism of concomitantly administered psychotropics. Thus, *acute alcohol ingestion* generally interferes with the metabolism of drugs, increasing plasma concentration. *Ingestion over several weeks* stimulates hepatic enzymes, accelerating the metabolism of many other drugs. Finally, cirrhosis induced by *chronic alcohol* insult will diminish enzyme concentration and liver mass, again increasing plasma levels of various concurrently administered drugs metabolized by this system. Fluid and electrolyte therapy must take into account the development of ascites and the possibility of right-sided heart failure. Salt restriction to 500 mg/day and bed rest are the initial conservative treatments, with medical consultation usually required.

Because heavy cigarette smoking is typically associated with alcohol dependence and may lead to impaired *pulmonary function*, BZDs should be used more cautiously to reduce the risk of oversedation and respiratory depression. Hypoxia can cause agitation and is exacerbated by treatment with sedative drugs. Again, shorter half-life agents and those with fewer active metabolites should by employed (e.g., oxazepam or lorazepam). Alcoholics also have an increased risk of aspiration of gastric contents or infected oropharyngeal material, with resulting aspiration pneumonia.

Erosive *gastritis* caused by recent excessive ingestion of alcohol is the most common cause of gastrointestinal bleeding in alcoholics. Bleeding usually subsides with cessation of drinking and administration of antacids. If the patient has cirrhosis, bleeding from esophageal varices must be suspected.

ALCOHOL-RELATED NEUROLOGICAL DISORDERS

Chronic neuropsychiatric disorders may arise from nutritional deficiencies, gastric malabsorption, and hepatic dysfunction, including (10):

- The *Wernicke-Korsakoff* syndrome
- Cerebral *cortical atrophy* (alcohol-associated dementia)
- *Cerebellar degeneration*
- *Polyneuropathy*
- Alcohol *myopathy*
- *Pellagra syndrome* (e.g., dementia, dermatitis, diarrhea, and death).

Deficiencies of thiamine and B vitamins arising from poor nutrition and malabsorption are usually the basis for these neurological sequelae.

The *Wernicke-Korsakoff* syndrome consists of both an acute (i.e., Wernicke's encephalopathy) and a chronic phase (i.e., Korsakoff's psychosis). The acute encephalopathy may be precipitated or worsened by carbohydrates (including intravenous glucose) unless thiamine is also replenished before or during administration. Wernicke's encephalopathy may first be manifested by:

- *Mental status abnormalities*, especially global confusion, inattentiveness, and a hypokinetic delirium

- *Ataxia*
- *Ocular findings*, including nystagmus (horizontal or vertical), weakness or paralysis of the lateral recti muscles, and weakness or paralysis of conjugate gaze.

Korsakoff's psychosis is most characterized by:

- Anterograde and retrograde *amnesia*
- *Decreased insight*
- *Apathy*
- *Inability to learn.*

Although *confabulation* (unconscious fabrication of facts because of memory impairment) is often considered a key symptom, it is not always present. Thiamine, initially given i.m. and then orally (100–300 mg/day), can reverse many of these symptoms, assuming irreversible changes have not occurred.

Pellagra is often characterized by mental abnormalities such as anxiety, irritability, and depression. The classic symptoms of pellagra are known as the "4 Ds": dementia, diarrhea, dermatitis, and death. Inflammation of mucosal surfaces, weakness, anorexia, and other gastrointestinal disturbances are also seen. Niacin (300–500 mg/day) is the definitive therapy.

Other neurological syndromes (e.g., cerebral cortical atrophy, myopathy, cerebellar degeneration) are also associated with alcoholism, but their pathogenesis is less certain than that of nutritional deficiency disorders. Abstinence from alcohol plus vitamin replacement and physical therapy comprise the standard treatment approach for these conditions.

DRUG THERAPY DURING REHABILITATION

Treatment is best approached by using a disease model in which alcoholism is considered a chronic medical disorder, and not simply a psychological or social problem. As with any other chronic illness, relapse is a normal part of the recovery process. Because the etiology of alcoholism is unknown and it afflicts a heterogeneous population, therapeutic strategies must keep in mind that some will not respond to more accepted forms of management. In this context, agents that reduce one's desire to drink may be important adjuncts (11).

Disulfiram (Antabuse) is an aversive drug that can be prescribed in conjunction with other forms of therapy such as Alcoholics Anonymous and individual counseling. It is recommended only for patients with good compliance and no serious physical condition (e.g., cardiovascular disease). After 6–12 months, disulfiram may be stopped if a patient has been able to remain sober; however, some may require the drug indefinitely to ensure sobriety. The usual loading dose is 250–500 mg/day for 3–5 days, although adverse effects may require a lower dose. Most patients are adequately maintained on 125–200 mg/day. A patient who drinks while taking the agent may experience facial flushing, sweating, headaches, nausea, vomiting, chest pain, dyspnea, weakness, dizziness, blurred vision, and confusion within minutes. Respiratory depression, shock, arrhythmias, seizures, and death are rare. Before disulfiram is prescribed, patients must be informed about these adverse effects, including the possibility of a serious disulfiram-ethanol reaction, and written informed consent should be obtained. Disulfiram may interfere with the action of other commonly prescribed drugs such as anticoagulants, phenytoin, and isoniazid.

Lithium has been reported to be an effective adjunct for maintaining abstinence in the detoxified alcoholic, especially if there is a personal or family history of a mood disorder or a cyclical pattern of impulsive drinking (12). A recent double-blind, placebo-controlled trial, however, found no difference between lithium and placebo (13). If utilized, the same principles of lithium administration for the treatment and prevention of bipolar disorder can be followed (i.e., an average total dose is 900–1200 mg/day, and a blood level of 0.5–1.5 mEq/liter). The patient should be maintained on lithium for at least 1 year before it is discontinued, with treatment reinstituted if affective symptoms or a pattern of impulsive drinking reemerge.

SRIs, such as fluoxetine, and serotonin specific agents, such as buspirone, may be effective in decreasing alcohol craving and consumption. At present, a number of studies have shown some benefit with these agents (14–17).

Naloxone and naltrexone have been shown to reduce alcohol consumption in alcohol-craving animals (18, 19). In addition, several studies have indicated that the opioid system may be involved in the regulation of alcohol intake in various animals. Recently, two well-controlled studies using naltrexone in humans have produced dramatically effective results (20, 21). While these data are not sufficient to make definitive recommendations, ongoing studies should clarify the potential benefit of this agent shortly.

CONCLUSION

To paraphrase William Osler: "If you know alcoholism, you know all of medicine." This observation may be particularly pertinent given alcohol's myriad neuropsychiatric manifestations, comorbid mental disturbances, and complicating medical conditions. The interaction between alcohol and its related physical disturbances requires the careful use of various psychotropics to safely detoxify patients and to help prevent more serious medical or emotional complications. The use of BZDs should only be short-term, given the propensity of many patients to transfer their dependence from alcohol to these agents. Various agents have the ability to decrease alcohol craving by different mechanisms and may benefit selected patients.

REFERENCES

1. DeLuca JR, ed. Fourth special report to the US Congress on alcohol. U.S. Government Printing Office, 1981.
2. Morse RM, Flavin BK. The definition of alcoholism. JAMA 1992;268(8)1012–1014.
3. Goodwin WD. Alcoholism. In: Kaplan HI, Sadock BJ, eds. Comprehensive textbook of psychiatry. 2 vols. 5th ed. Baltimore: Williams & Wilkins, 1989.
4. Black DW, Yates W, Petty F, Noyes Jr R, Brown K. Suicidal behavior in alcoholic males. Compr Psychiatry 1986;27(3):227–233.
5. Vaillant GE. The natural history of alcoholism. Cambridge, MA: Harvard University Press, 1983.
6. Atkinson RM. Alcohol and drug abuse in old age. Washington D.C.: American Psychiatric Press, 1984.
7. Schuckit MA. Biology of risk for alcoholism. In: Meltzter HY, ed. Psychopharmacology: the third generation of progress. New York: Raven Press, 1987.
8. Bean-Bayog M. Inpatient treatment of the psychiatric patient with alcoholism. Gen Hosp Psychiatry 1987;9(3):203–209.
9. Dackis CA, Gold MS, Pottash ALC, Sweeney DR. Evaluating depression in alcoholics. Psychiatry Res 1986;17:105–109.
10. Parsons AO, Butters N, Nathan PE, eds. Neuropsychology of alcoholism: implications for diagnosis and treatment. New York: Guilford Press, 1987.
11. Sellers EM, Naranjo CA, Peachey JE. Drug therapy: drugs to decrease alcohol consumption. N Engl J Med 1981;305:1255.
12. Fawcett J, Clark DC, Gibbons RD, Aagesen CA, Pisani VD, Tilkin JM, et al. Evaluation of lithium therapy for alcoholism. J Clin Psychiatry 1984;45:494–499.
13. Dorus W, Ostrow DG, Anton R, Cushman P, Collins JF, Schaefer N, et al. Lithium treatment of depressed and nondepressed alcoholics. JAMA 1989;262:1646–1652.
14. Naranjo CA, Sellers EM, Sullivan JI, Woodley DV, Kadlec K, Sykora K. The serotonin uptake inhibitor citalopram attenuates ethanol intake. Clin Pharmacol Ther 1987;41:266–274.
15. Gorelick DA. Serotonin uptake blockers in the treatment of alcoholism. Recent developments in alcoholism 1989;7:267–281.
16. Naranjo C, Kadlic K, Sanhueza P, Woodley-Rimus D, Kennedy R, Sellers E. Fluoxetine differentially alters alcohol intake and other consummatory behaviors in problem drinkers. Clin Pharmacol Ther 1990;47:490–498.
17. Gorelick DA, Parendes A. Effect of Fluoxetine or alcohol consumption in male alcoholics. Alcoholism. Clin and Exper Res 1992;16(3):261–265.
18. Myers RD, Borg S, Mossberg R. Antagonism by naltrexone of voluntary alcohol selection in the chronically drinking macaque monkey. Alcohol 1986;3:383–388.
19. Volpicelli JR, Davis MA, Olgin JE. Naltrexone blocks the post-shock increase of ethanol consumption. Life Sci 1986;38:841–847.
20. O'Malley SS, Jaffe A, Chang G, Schottenfeld RS, Meyer RE, Rounsaville B. Naltrexone and coping skills therapy for alcohol dependence: a controlled study. Arch Gen Psychiatry 1992;49:881–887.
21. Volpicelli JR, Alterman AI, Hayashida M, O'Brien CP. Naltrexone in the treatment of alcohol dependence. Arch Gen Psychiatry 1992;49:876–880.

The Seizure-Prone Patient

These individuals have conditions that predispose them to seizures, including:

- Epilepsy
- Alcoholism

- Electroencephalographic abnormalities
- Cerebral arteriosclerosis
- Other CNS degenerative states.

Unfortunately, these patients also often have a comorbid condition warranting psychopharmacotherapy with antipsychotics, anxiolytics, ADs, or other drugs. Selecting the appropriate psychoactive drug for the seizure-prone patient is often problematic because therapeutic doses of some agents may alter thresholds and spark various types of seizures in normal patients, epileptic individuals, and those with predisposing factors (1).

In addition, some psychotropics may adversely interact with concomitantly prescribed anticonvulsants. Thus, certain agents may raise an anticonvulsant's serum level, producing toxicity. For example, imipramine interacts with phenytoin, resulting in a serum elevation of the latter drug, increasing the risk of intoxication (2, 3).

Conversely, other psychoactive drugs may lower the serum level of an anticonvulsant, resulting in a loss of seizure control.

There is also evidence that the metabolism of psychotropics may be altered by anticonvulsants, interfering with therapeutic efficacy. For example, mean steady state plasma nortriptyline concentrations in epileptics on anticonvulsants were found to be 50% less than those of patients not on anticonvulsant therapy (2). If the dose of the AD is then adjusted to achieve higher blood levels, it is possible that this may increase the risk of seizures due to the effect of higher AD doses on the convulsive threshold (1).

TREATMENT WITH VARIOUS PSYCHOTROPICS

ADs and APs can lower the seizure threshold. Studies of the EEG effects and relative epileptogenic potency of tricyclics, as well as other cyclic ADs, however, have found some differences in their seizure-inducing properties. After reviewing the experimental and clinical literature, including his own animal studies, on the convulsive effects of non-MAOI ADs, Trimble concluded: "Of those available, both clinical and experimental data would suggest that the conventional tricyclic drugs, and in particular, clomipramine, imipramine, and amitriptyline, are most likely to exacerbate epilepsy" (1). Other agents likely to provoke seizures are mianserin, maprotiline, and bupropion. At the other end of the spectrum, SRIs and MAOIs have a low propensity to induce seizures. Nomifensine is the only AD to date shown to actually possess anticonvulsant properties in animal models (unfortunately it has been withdrawn from the market due to other adverse reactions).

Although some psychotropics, including certain ADs, may be less likely to provoke seizures than others, it must be stressed that therapeutic doses of even those with a lesser epileptogenic potential may still provoke convulsions in patients with or without predisposing factors. It is important to point out that part of the danger is dose related. For example, epileptic seizures in maprotiline-treated patients have been exceedingly rare when the dosage is 150 mg/day or less. Similarly, doses of bupropion less then 450 mg/day or clozapine less than 600 mg/day reduce the incidence of seizures (4).

At present, knowledge of the effects of most psychoactive drugs, including their epileptogenic potential is somewhat limited. Hence, prudence dictates the reassessment of anticonvulsant blood levels shortly after the initiation of, as well as during drug therapy in the seizure-prone. If there is a significant change in seizure frequency, even in the absence of anticonvulsant plasma level changes, another AD should be considered (5).

CONCLUSION

Psychotropics may affect seizure threshold; therefore they should be prescribed cautiously for the seizure-prone. Treatment should be initiated with lower doses, and dose increments should be gradual. High-dose therapy should be avoided if at all possible, and abrupt discontinuation of long-term high doses (especially of the BZDs) should be avoided, since this is more likely to provoke a seizure (see Chapter 12 also). Anticonvulsants such as CBZ and VPA may serve a dual purpose in certain patients with major psychiatric disorders and a susceptibility to seizure activity.

REFERENCES

1. Trimble M. Non-monoamine oxidase inhibitor antidepressants and epilepsy: a review. Epilepsia 1978;19:241–250.
2. Richens A. Clinical pharmacology and medical treatment. In: Laidlaw J, Richens A, eds. A textbook of epilepsy. London: Churchill Livingstone, 1976.
3. Perucca E, Richens A. Interaction between phenytoin and imipramine. Br J Clin Pharmacol 1977;4:485–486.
4. Davidson J. Seizures and bupropion: a review. J Clin Psychiatry 1989;50:256–261.
5. Schaul N. Psychotropic drugs and seizures. In: Kane JM, Liberman JA, eds. Adverse effects of psychotropic drugs. New York: Guilford Press 1992.

The HIV-Infected Patient

HIV-related psychological complications present a unique challenge to the practicing clinician. Not only do these patients have severe associated psychosocial stressors but also varied neuropsychiatric manifestations that complicate any potential intervention (see Table 14.7).

Acquired immunodeficiency syndrome (AIDS) and AIDS-related complex (ARC) are distinguished by weight loss, chronic fatigue, fevers, night sweats, oral leukoplakia, oral candidiasis, and generalized lymphadenopathy. They also show evidence of neurotropic as well as their better-known lymphotropic features. **Thus, up to 70% of these patients will have clinically apparent mental changes during the course of their disease. Neuropsychological impairment may, in fact, be the first symptom of HIV-related disorders (1).**

Early studies have found that among HIV outpatients 67% manifest adjustment disorder with mixed emotional features, and 80% of inpatients manifest an organic mental disorder. Further, postmortem studies on patients who suffered from AIDS have found that neuropathological abnormalities occur in about 90%. These abnormalities have included:

- *Toxoplasmosis*
- *Fungal* infections
- *Viral* infections
- *Vascular* lesions
- *Neoplasms*.

In the CNS, tumors include primary and secondary lymphomas and rarely, Kaposi's sarcoma. It is also thought that the retrovirus, HIV itself, may be encephalopathic.

Table 14.7.
Etiology of Neuropsychological Disorders in Patients with HIV-1 Infection[a]

Direct CNS infection with HIV virus
Secondary malignancies of the CNS from immunocompromise
   Primary CNS lymphoma
   Burkitt's lymphoma
   Disseminated Kaposi's sarcoma
   Other sarcomas
   Candidiasis
Secondary CNS infections from immunocompromise
   Cerebral toxoplasmosis
   Herpes simplex encephalitis
   Cryptococcosis
   Mycobacterium tuberculosis (rare)
   Atypical mucobacterial infection (rare)
   Progressive multifocal leukoencephalopathy (Papillomavirus)
Systemic complications of HIV infection or side effects of its treatment
   Nutritional deficiencies, especially vitamin B_{12} deficiency
   Drug-related neurotoxicities
   Metabolic encephalopathies
Psychological reactions of the patients to having disease

[a]From Jobe TH. Neuropsychiatry of HIV disease. In: Flaherty J, Davis JM, Janicak PG, eds. Psychiatry: diagnosis and therapy. New York: Appleton and Lange, 1993.

DIAGNOSIS

Because an increasing number of patients with a concurrent psychiatric disorder and HIV infection are requiring intervention, this poses an important challenge to the mental health field. The most common diagnosis given to these patients is an adjustment disorder with mixed emotional features; however, one must always be cognizant of the potential for an underlying, but as yet unrecognized, organic process. The typical neuropsychiatric complications can be divided into four major categories:

- AIDS-related *dementia complex and delirium*
- Organic *psychosis*
- *Mood* disorders
- *Anxiety* states.

Oftentimes, these conditions may coexist, making diagnosis and treatment planning exceedingly complicated.

GENERAL MANAGEMENT OF THE HIV-INFECTED PATIENT

General nonpharmacological therapeutic approaches consist of:

- *Supportive psychotherapy*
- *Psychoeducation*
- *Family therapy*
- *Mobilization of social support systems*
- *Follow-up neuropsychological testing.*

A related issue is the growing number of AIDS-phobic individuals, who often benefit from empathic, informed reassurance, thus avoiding HIV antibody testing or the need for more intensive treatment.

DRUG THERAPY

Because these patients may be exquisitely sensitive to the effects of medication, the general principle is always to start with the lowest dose and increase the medication very slowly. The route of administration may also be problematic, as some patients have very poor absorption, and thus medications may not be adequately assimilated. Parenteral administration is also often complicated by decreased muscle mass, thrombocytopenia, and difficulty in finding veins.

AIDS-Related Dementia and Delirium

Zidovudine (AZT) is the first agent approved for the treatment of HIV infection, and there is also some evidence that it may partially reverse the cognitive disruption associated with AIDS dementia complex (2). This agent, however, may also cause CNS complications, such as headache, insomnia, and restlessness. Some authors have also reported dramatic responses with *methylphenidate*, whether depression was present or not (3).

Psychosis

In cases of organic psychosis or delirium, pharmacotherapy with a moderately potent AP agent such as molindone, which also has limited anticholinergic adverse effects, is indicated. High-potency APs should be avoided because of their tendency to produce unusually severe extrapyramidal side effects or neuroleptic malignant syndrome (4, 5). This may be due to underlying damage in the basal ganglia, secondary to HIV-induced changes. Alternatively, i.m. or i.v. *microdoses* of haloperidol (e.g., 0.5 mg bid) may be helpful, while minimizing the chances for an extrapyramidal side effect reaction.

There are also some commonly used drugs that may induce organic mental syndromes in these patients. For example, medications with anticholinergic properties (e.g., antiparkinsonian agents, tricyclics, low-potency APs, certain antiemetics, such as prochlorperazine, and antihistamines) may all induce a delirium

characterized by visual and/or tactile hallucinations, confusion, and agitation. Treatment is primarily discontinuation of the offending agent and waiting for the symptoms to subside.

If an antiparkinsonian agent is needed to counteract neuroleptic-induced adverse effects, some have recommended amantadine, rather than benztropine. The dose is usually 50 mg, twice a day, with a gradual increase to 100 mg twice daily, if necessary.

In situations characterized by agitation, Gilmer and Busch have recommended lorazepam in small doses (0.5 mg) given intravenously by slow push or intramuscularly (6). In those manifesting psychotic symptoms, who also have difficulty with the extrapyramidal side effects associated with the higher potency agents, loxapine or molindone may be the better choice. These drugs may also be preferable in the seizure-prone patient.

Mood Disorders

Depression

Mood disturbance, primarily depression, can range from mild adjustment phenomena to a major depressive episode with psychotic features. Depression in this group can be categorized as:

- *Reactive* depressive syndromes, including adjustment disorders
- *Concomitant major depressive disorders*, which were either preexisting or recently identified
- *Organic* depressive syndromes.

One problem in making the diagnosis of depression in HIV- or AIDS-related disorders is the lack of specificity of the typical neurovegetative signs and symptoms, since fatigue, insomnia, anorexia, and weight loss are very common in both conditions. Again, if AD therapy is contemplated, one should start with lower doses, increase more gradually, and preferably avoid agents with greater anticholinergic properties. There is virtually no information on the use of SRIs, MAOIs, or bupropion in these patients.

Reactive depression secondary to knowledge of seropositivity or the onset of serious physical symptoms is best managed by supportive therapy and, if necessary, by ADs. The drug of choice is an AD with low anticholinergic potency (e.g., sertraline, trazodone), started more slowly and maintained at a lower level than in non-AIDS patients. Given AIDS-induced altered metabolism, TDM may be helpful in establishing an effective, non-toxic dose. **There has been a growing recognition that psychostimulants may be helpful in HIV- or AIDS-related affective syndromes.** Thus, pharmacotherapy, such as methylphenidate, 10–20 mg/day (up to 40 mg/day), or dextroamphetamine, 5–15 mg/day (up to 60 mg/day), has been helpful in patients with mild depression who also show symptoms of social withdrawal, fatigue, and apathy; as well as mild cognitive impairment. At times, the combination of low-dose AD and psychostimulant may be more effective and less likely to induce adverse CNS effects.

Gilmer and Busch reported on one patient who developed *manic symptoms* associated with AZT therapy, whose affective symptoms remitted when the drug was discontinued, only to return when it was reintroduced (6). In two other patients, Gilmer and Busch were able to continue AZT when lithium was added to control manic symptoms.

Suicide is almost always an issue when a patient is severely depressed, and many with HIV disease will consider this option at one time or another during the course of their illness. The potential for suicide may increase rapidly as the physical symptoms accelerate, because of the patient's fear that they will not be able to act on these thoughts when their debilitation becomes severe. Developing a good rapport is very important if the suicidal desire is to be diminished through counseling or psychotherapy. ECT may be the treatment of choice in more emergent situations.

Mania

While mania in AIDS patients appears to be uncommon, such episodes can pose a serious hazard and require rapid control. Haloperidol (0.5 to 5 mg i.v.) may be an effective strategy, in part because this route of administration may be less likely than oral doses to induce acute EPS (7).

Anxiety

During the initial, asymptomatic period of HIV disease, nearly all patients experience varying degrees of anxiety and bouts of dysphoria. Stress-reducing techniques and supportive psychotherapy may be effective in dealing with such symptoms. BZDs are indicated for those with severe episodic anxiety, often bordering on panic, that is not sufficiently responsive to these nondrug interventions. Patients should be counseled about and discouraged from using over-the-counter hypnotics that contain anticholinergic agents.

In the management of anxiety, the cumulative effects of longer half-life *BZDs* often result in excessive sleepiness, apathetic states, and confusion (with or without paradoxical agitation). Thus, short- and intermediate-acting agents such as oxazepam, lorazepam, and alprazolam are preferable. Lower doses (e.g., 0.5 to 1.0 mg of lorazepam; 0.25 to 0.5 mg of alprazolam) are preferable. Agents with very short half-lives, such as midazolam and triazolam, are not well tolerated, especially in those with more severe neurocognitive disruption.

Small doses of *trazodone* (25–50 mg) at bedtime may be useful as a sedative-hypnotic. More data are required on pain control and analgesia using *low dose opioids* on a short-term basis, which may also benefit anxiety. For example, the use of morphine in patients with advanced disease has been found to be particularly helpful in decreasing their associated anxiety.

CONCLUSION

The utmost sensitivity and constant support are often all we can offer in the face of this devastating illness. Intelligent application of both nondrug and drug therapies must always be complemented by hope and comfort. The aim should not be to simply prolong life, but whenever possible, to improve its quality. When psychotropics are employed, drug-induced delirium is a real and ever-present complication. This is due to CNS sensitivity as well as AIDS-induced gastrointestinal and hepatic compromise, which can alter a drug's metabolism and disposition. Thus, low drug doses, increased very gradually, should be the guiding principle.

REFERENCES

1. Jobe TH. Neuropsychiatry of HIV disease. In: Flaherty J, Davis JM, Janicak PG, eds. Psychiatry: diagnosis and therapy. New York: Appleton and Lange, 1993.
2. Yarchoan R, Brouwers P, Spitzer AR, Grafman J, Safai B, Perno CF, et al. Response of human-immunodeficiency associated neurological disease to 3'-azido-3'-deoxythymidine. Lancet 1987;1:132–135.
3. Fernandez F, Adams F, Levy JK, et al. Cognitive impairment due to AIDS-related complex and its response to psychostimulants. Psychosomatics 1988;29:38–46.
4. Burch EA, Montoya J. NMS in an AIDS patient. J Clin Psychiatry 1989;9:228–229.
5. Ostrow D, Grant I, Atkinson H. Assessment and management of AIDS patients with neuropsychiatric disturbances. J Clin Psychiatry 1988;49(suppl):14–22.
6. Gilmer W, Busch K. Neuropsychiatric aspects of AIDS and psychopharmacologic management. Janicak PG, Davis JM, guest eds. Psychiatr Med 1991:313–329.
7. Menza MA, Murray GB, Holmes, VF, et al. Decreased extrapyramidal symptoms with intravenous haloperidol. J Clin Psychiatry 1987;48:278–280.

The Eating-Disordered Patient

The role of pharmacotherapy in eating-disordered patients has yet to be clearly defined. In those with concurrent disorders, such as dysthymia or psychosis, appropriate psychotropic agents may be beneficial. Further, there is some early promising, albeit preliminary, data that SRIs, such as fluoxetine, may have at least short-term "antibulimic" properties. **In all situations, the clinician must keep in mind the potential for greater adverse effects, due to the malnourished status and/or binging- and purging-related complications.** Furthermore, the propensity toward substance abuse and self-destruction may find a fatal outlet when these patients are prescribed drugs such as the TCAs.

Eating disorders can be divided into:

- Anorexia nervosa
- Bulimia nervosa
- Bulimia nervosa multisymptomatic.

(see also Appendix B)

ANOREXIA NERVOSA

Anorexia nervosa is a heterogeneous and multifactorial eating disorder that

occurs most commonly in prepubertal, adolescent, and young females. It is a relentless pursuit of thinness and a morbid fear of fat. The distortion of body image is considered central to the diagnosis by most experts. It is also characterized by refusal to maintain a normal body weight and obsession with dieting to the point of inducing profound weight loss, with body weights at least 15% below that expected. Most of the weight loss is accomplished in secret.

Anorectic patients often suffer from hypotension, hypothermia, and abnormal ECGs, all of which are consistent with starvation. Like patients with depression, they have high cerebrospinal fluid concentrations of corticotropin-releasing hormone. Amenorrhea is common in menstruating females with this syndrome.

Drug Therapy of Anorexia Nervosa

A plethora of psychotropics has been tried in the treatment of this disorder, including:

- Typical and atypical *antipsychotics* (e.g., chlorpromazine, pimozide, sulpiride)
- Appetite *stimulants* (e.g., cyproheptadine)
- *Antidepressants* such as the tricyclics (e.g., amitriptyline, clomipramine); SRIs (e.g., fluoxetine); and MAOIs
- *Lithium.*

To date, no antipsychotic has been found to be more than minimally or partially beneficial, and most have caused adverse effects that outweigh any therapeutic advantages. The only appetite stimulant shown in controlled double-blind trials to be of some benefit is cyproheptadine, but only in nonbulimic anorexics. Neither TCAs, MAOIs, lithium, nor

fluoxetine have been found to be an effective treatment for anorexia nervosa.

BULIMIA NERVOSA

This eating disorder has an unknown etiology; is common in women; and is characterized by binging and purging, disturbances of mood, and neuroendocrine abnormalities. Bulimics report binge eating ranging from 2 to 20 times per week, with 50% binging daily and one-third binging several times a day. Three-fourths purge daily, and 50% of those purge multiple times a day. Up to one-third of bulimics have a history of anorexia nervosa. Approximately one-third also use laxatives. Each binge may be followed by a depressed mood, self-criticism, and self-induced vomiting. There is also a subpopulation of patients with bulimia nervosa who engage in regular binge eating without purging.

A minority have coexistent anorexia nervosa (anorexia nervosa-bulimia variant), with a worse prognosis than those with bulimia nervosa alone. They present with a low body weight and other typical features such as fear of fatness, vigorous exercising, and amenorrhea. Typically, all types of bulimic patients have a history of numerous strict or fad diets, punctuated by recurrent episodes of binge eating and persistent overconcern with body shape and weight. Major Depressive Disorder, as well as alcohol and drug abuse, often coexist in a large number of these patients.

Drug Therapy of Bulimia Nervosa

Attempts to treat bulimia nervosa with pharmacotherapy have almost been as frustrating as for anorexia nervosa. Most investigations have centered on assessing the possible efficacy of:

- Anticonvulsants (e.g., phenytoin, carbamazepine)
- TCAs (e.g., imipramine, desipramine, amitriptyline)
- Newer HCAs (e.g., bupropion, mianserin, trazodone)
- MAOIs (e.g., isocarboxazid, phenelzine)
- SRIs (e.g., fluoxetine)
- Lithium.

Most studies have been open designs, and neither these, nor controlled double-blind studies, have provided evidence of more than minimal improvement in some patients. A few controlled trials, however, have shown that HCAs are more effective than placebo in reducing the frequency of overeating and the intensity of some of the symptoms of bulimia nervosa (1, 2). There also is some evidence that this may be true for fluoxetine as well. One controlled study suggested that fluoxetine up to 60 mg/day had a significant effect compared to placebo (3). A long-term (more than 3 months) open study also produced data indicating that fluoxetine may significantly reduce the frequency of binges and purges (4). It should be noted that when useful, ADs have been equally effective whether or not the patient is depressed (5, 6). This suggests that the decrease in bulimic symptoms may not be due to the drugs' antidepressant action, but rather an expression of a direct effect on brain mechanisms that control eating. There is no evidence that these drugs have an impact on disturbed attitudes about body shape and weight or extreme attempts to diet (7, 8).

There have been no studies of the extent of lasting improvement following AD therapy for bulimia nervosa and one report is far from encouraging (9). Thus, any benefits may be short lived. **Until it has been shown that ADs have more than a** **selective and transitory effect, their place in the treatment of bulimia nervosa must be questioned** (10).

BULIMIA NERVOSA MULTISYMPTOMATIC

Patients with this disorder not only have a disturbed eating pattern but also problems with impulse control, often resulting in drug and/or alcohol abuse, self-mutilation, kleptomania, and sexual disinhibition. They also may have symptoms of OCD or obsessive-compulsive personality disorder. In these individuals, manipulation of food is associated in varying degrees with alcohol and drug abuse. They are typically poor candidates for pharmacotherapy, and not surprisingly, have been as unresponsive to a variety of psychotropics as their anorexic and bulimic counterparts.

CONCLUSION

Advances in psychopharmacotherapy are occurring at an ever-accelerating pace. These events demand an increasing sophistication on the part of all clinicians working in the mental health field. Whether they prescribe medications or not, knowledge about the role as well as potential benefits and risks of drug therapy is a prerequisite providing the best care possible for our patients. These issues are most evident when caring for the specialized needs of the patients considered in this final chapter. The aim of these discussions is to provide signposts and reasonable courses of action based on the present state of knowledge. The clinician must remain alert to such issues as well as to the inevitable advances that will occur in the assessment and therapeutic management of these special populations.

REFERENCES

1. Freeman CPL, Munro JKM. Drug and group treatments for bulimia/bulimia nervosa. J Psychosom Res 1988;32:647–660.
2. Agras WS, McCann U. The efficacy and role of antidepressants in the treatment of bulimia nervosa. Ann Behav Med 1987;9: 18–22.
3. Foss I, Trygstad O, Jettestad S. Double-blind study of fluoxetine and placebo in the treatment of bulimia nervosa [Abstract]. Presented at the Fourth International Conference on Eating Disorders, New York, April 28, 1990.
4. Fava M, Herzog DB, Hamburg P, Riess H, Anfang S, Rosenbaum JF. A retrospective study of long-term use of fluoxetine in bulimia nervosa [Abstract]. Presented at the Fourth International Conference on Eating Disorders, New York, April 28, 1990.
5. Hughes PL, Wells LA, Cunningham CJ, Ilstrup DM. Treating bulimia with desipramine: A double-blind, placebo-controlled study. Arch Gen Psychiatry 1986; 43:182–186.
6. Walsh BT, Gladis M, Roose SP, et al. Phenelzine vs placebo in 50 patients with bulimia. Arch Gen Psychiatry 1988;45: 471–475.
7. Rossiter EM, Agras WS, Losch M. Changes in self-reported food intake in bulimics as a consequence of anti-depressant treatment. Int J Eating Disorders 1988;7:779–783.
8. Mitchell JE, Fletcher L, Pyle RL, et al. The impact of treatment on meal patterns in patients with bulimia nervosa. Int J Eating Disorders 1989;8:167–172.
9. Pope HG, Hudson JI, Jones JM, Yurgelun-Todd D. Antidepressant treatment of bulimia: a two-year follow-up study. J Clin Psychopharmacol 1985;5:320–327.
10. Fairburn CG. Bulimia nervosa: antidepressant or cognitive therapy is effective. Br Med J 1990;300:485–486.

APPENDIX

INTRODUCTION

Appendices of Axes I and II Diagnostic Criteria

The third edition of the American Psychiatric Association's Diagnostic and Statistical Manual of Mental Disorders marked the beginning of a new era in the classification of mental disorders in the United States (1). The emphasis on phenomenology in DSM-III and its revision, the DSM-III-R, was a significant departure from the impressionistic, theoretically based schema of its predecessors, the DSM-I (1952) and the DSM-II (1968) (2–4). Currently, the DSM-IV is nearing completion and will further emphasize the role of empirical findings as the basis for diagnosing psychiatric disorders (5). The DSM-IV criteria will continue to incorporate the most recent, relevant literature and data from clinical field trials, as well as strive for compatibility to the tenth revision of the International Classification of Diseases (ICD-10), whenever feasible. In addition, a DSM Sourcebook will document the literature reviews that support the changes made for this edition.

To effectively utilize this system, the clinician must carefully consider an extensive array of information before arriving at a diagnostic label. The myriad of possible diagnoses, as well as the exactness of the criteria within each category, can be a challenge to the most experienced clinician and overwhelming to the novice. Thus, an overview highlighting the organization and critical criteria can facilitate assimilation of this information.

Since the general approach to diagnosis in the DSM-III-R is multiaxial:

- *Axes I and II*, for mental disorders
- *Axis III*, to reflect any physical disorders substantively related to Axes I or II
- *Axis IV*, to provide data on any significant psychosocial stressors

- *Axis V*, to reflect the highest level of adaptational functioning in the previous year.

Information should be provided, when possible, in all relevant areas.

In an effort to enhance the discussion in this text on diagnostic indications for pharmacotherapy, we have adapted our original outline of the DSM-III to provide an overview of the critical criteria pertinent to each diagnostic category on Axes I and II (6). Through the use of a series of diagrams, we have designed a quick reference for the practitioner to more readily identify the salient criteria. All diagrams except Appendices E, I, K, and U are adapted from Janicak PG, Andriukaitis SN. DSM-III: seeing the forest through the trees. Psychiatric Annals 1980;10(8):6–30.

Since the DSM-IV will soon replace the current manual, we have also included brief commentary on changes that are presently under advisement and most likely to be included into the new edition. The specific changes and additions proposed for the DSM-IV are primarily demarcated by italics in parentheses and, when appropriate, dashed boxes as well. This will give the reader an opportunity to easily compare and contrast the most likely differences between these two editions. Some of the significant changes likely to be included are:

- The moving of *Eating and Gender Identity Disorders* from Disorders of Infancy, Childhood, or Adolescence into separate categories, expanding the age groups that can be included.
- The replacement of the term *Organic Mental Disorder* with the term Cognitive Impairment Disorder.
- The dispersion of various *organic syndromes* into their respective categories (e.g., Organic Mood Syndrome, now

under Mood Disorders, as a category termed Secondary Mood Disorder Due to a Nonpsychiatric Medical Condition; or Substance-Induced Mood Disorder).

- The addition of *course modifiers for Substance-Related Disorders* (e.g., on agonist therapy; controlled remission; early, sustained, or full remission)
- The possible addition of *Mixed Anxiety-Depression Disorder*, probably in an appendix.

REFERENCES

1. American Psychiatric Association. Diagnostic and statistical manual of mental disorders. 3rd ed. Washington D.C.: American Psychiatric Association, 1980.
2. American Psychiatric Association. Diagnostic and statistical manual, mental disorders. 1st ed. Washington D.C.: American Psychiatric Association, 1952.
3. American Psychiatric Association. Diagnostic and statistical manual of mental disorders. 2nd ed. Washington, D.C.: 1968.
4. American Psychiatric Association. Diagnostic and statistical manual of mental disorders. 3rd ed, revised. Washington, D.C.: American Psychiatric Association, 1987.
5. Task Force on DSM-IV. DSM-IV options book: work in progress. Washington D.C.: American Psychiatric Association, 1991.
6. Janicak PG, Andriukaitis SN. DSM-III: Seeing the forest through the trees. Psychiatric Annals 1980;10(8):6–30.

Appendix A.   An Overview of DSM-III-R, Axes I and II.

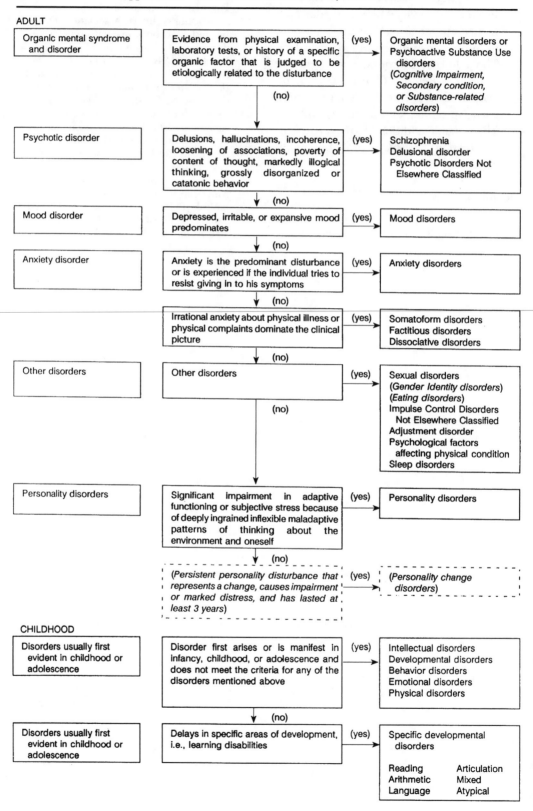

Appendix B.   Disorders Usually First Evident in Infancy, Childhood, or Adolescence.

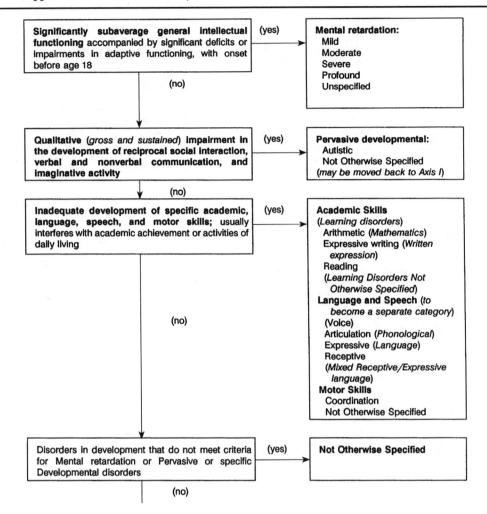

(continued)

Appendix B.—*continued*

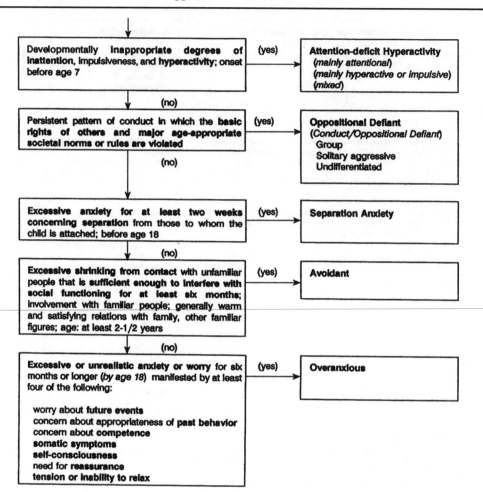

(continued)

Appendix B.—*continued*

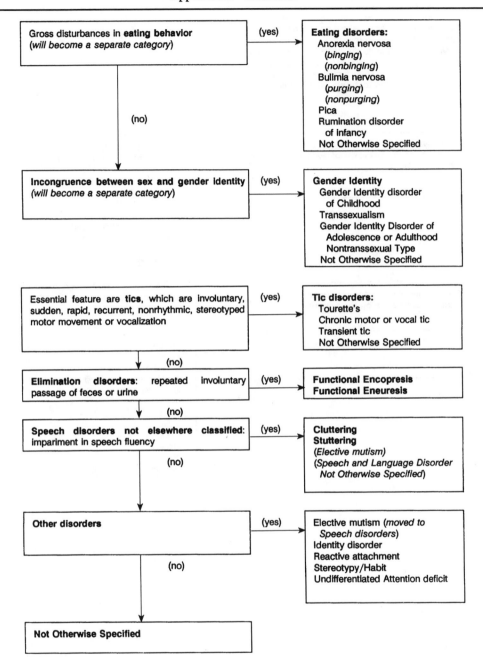

Gross disturbances in **eating behavior**
(*will become a separate category*)

(yes) → **Eating disorders:**
Anorexia nervosa
(*binging*)
(*nonbinging*)
Bulimia nervosa
(*purging*)
(*nonpurging*)
Pica
Rumination disorder
of infancy
Not Otherwise Specified

(no) ↓

Incongruence between sex and gender identity
(*will become a separate category*)

(yes) → **Gender Identity**
Gender Identity disorder
of Childhood
Transsexualism
Gender Identity Disorder of
Adolescence or Adulthood
Nontranssexual Type
Not Otherwise Specified

Essential feature are **tics**, which are involuntary,
sudden, rapid, recurrent, nonrhythmic, stereotyped
motor movement or vocalization

(yes) → **Tic disorders:**
Tourette's
Chronic motor or vocal tic
Transient tic
Not Otherwise Specified

(no) ↓

Elimination disorders: repeated involuntary
passage of feces or urine

(yes) → **Functional Encopresis**
Functional Eneuresis

(no) ↓

Speech disorders not elsewhere classified:
impariment in speech fluency

(yes) → **Cluttering**
Stuttering
(*Elective mutism*)
(*Speech and Language Disorder
Not Otherwise Specified*)

(no) ↓

Other disorders

(yes) → Elective mutism (*moved to
Speech disorders*)
Identity disorder
Reactive attachment
Stereotypy/Habit
Undifferentiated Attention deficit

(no) ↓

Not Otherwise Specified

Appendix C.   Organic Mental Syndromes and Disorders (Cognitive Impairment Disorders).

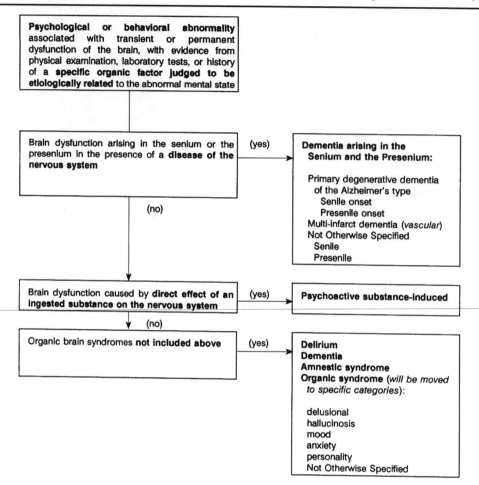

Psychological or behavioral abnormality associated with transient or permanent dysfunction of the brain, with evidence from physical examination, laboratory tests, or history of a **specific organic factor judged to be etiologically related** to the abnormal mental state

Brain dysfunction arising in the senium or the presenium in the presence of a **disease of the nervous system**

(yes) → **Dementia arising in the Senium and the Presenium:**

Primary degenerative dementia of the Alzheimer's type
Senile onset
Presenile onset
Multi-infarct dementia (*vascular*)
Not Otherwise Specified
Senile
Presenile

(no)

Brain dysfunction caused by **direct effect of an ingested substance on the nervous system**

(yes) → **Psychoactive substance-induced**

(no)

Organic brain syndromes **not included above**

(yes) → **Delirium**
Dementia
Amnestic syndrome
Organic syndrome (*will be moved to specific categories*):

delusional
hallucinosis
mood
anxiety
personality
Not Otherwise Specified

Appendix D.   Psychoactive Substance-Use Disorders (Substance-Related Disorders).

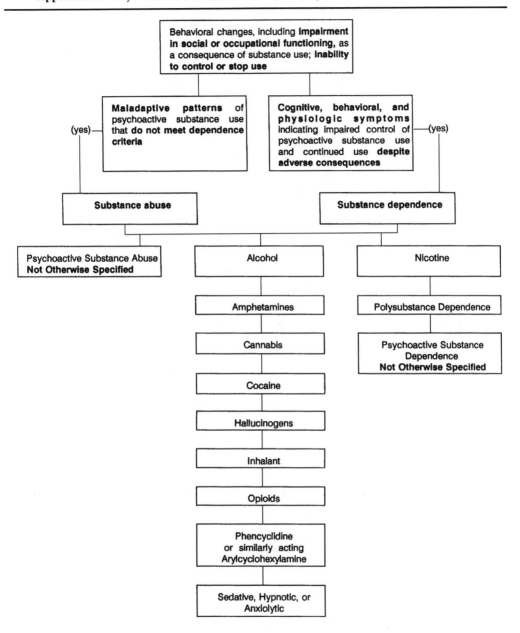

Appendix E. An Overview of Schizophrenic and Other Psychotic Disorders.

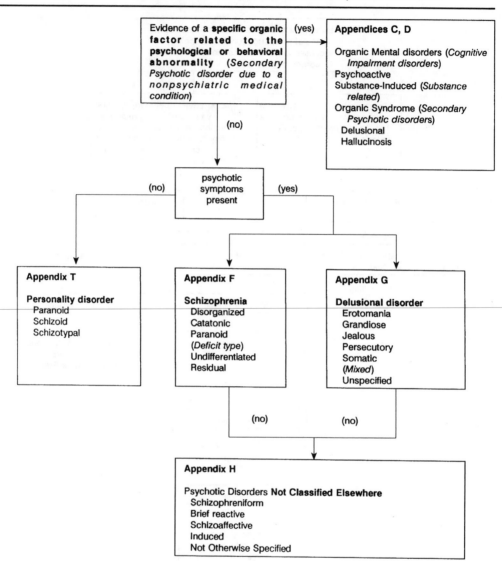

Appendix F.   Schizophrenia.

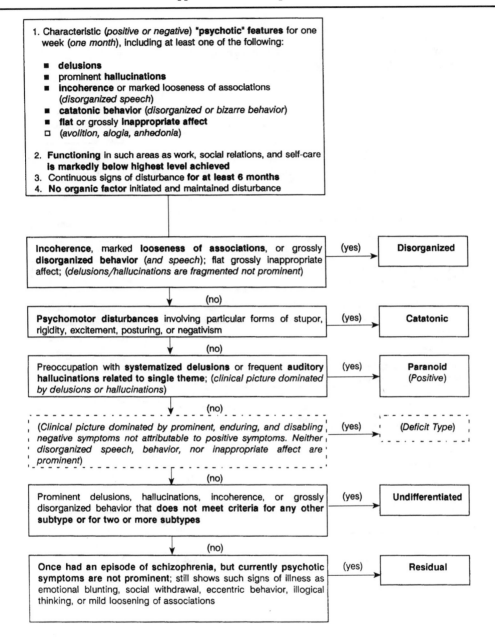

1. Characteristic (*positive or negative*) "**psychotic**" **features** for one week (*one month*), including at least one of the following:

   - **delusions**
   - prominent **hallucinations**
   - **incoherence** or marked looseness of associations (*disorganized speech*)
   - **catatonic behavior** (*disorganized or bizarre behavior*)
   - **flat** or grossly **inappropriate affect**
   - □ (*avolition, alogia, anhedonia*)

2. **Functioning** in such areas as work, social relations, and self-care **is markedly below highest level achieved**
3. Continuous signs of disturbance **for at least 6 months**
4. **No organic factor** initiated and maintained disturbance

---

Incoherence, marked **looseness of associations**, or grossly **disorganized behavior** (*and speech*); flat grossly inappropriate affect; (*delusions/hallucinations are fragmented not prominent*) → (yes) → **Disorganized**

(no)

Psychomotor disturbances involving particular forms of stupor, rigidity, excitement, posturing, or negativism → (yes) → **Catatonic**

(no)

Preoccupation with **systematized delusions** or frequent **auditory hallucinations related to single theme**; (*clinical picture dominated by delusions or hallucinations*) → (yes) → **Paranoid** (*Positive*)

(no)

(*Clinical picture dominated by prominent, enduring, and disabling negative symptoms not attributable to positive symptoms. Neither disorganized speech, behavior, nor inappropriate affect are prominent*) → (yes) → (*Deficit Type*)

(no)

Prominent delusions, hallucinations, incoherence, or grossly disorganized behavior that **does not meet criteria for any other subtype or for two or more subtypes** → (yes) → **Undifferentiated**

(no)

Once had an episode of schizophrenia, but currently psychotic symptoms are not prominent; still shows such signs of illness as emotional blunting, social withdrawal, eccentric behavior, illogical thinking, or mild loosening of associations → (yes) → **Residual**

Appendix G.   Delusional Disorder.

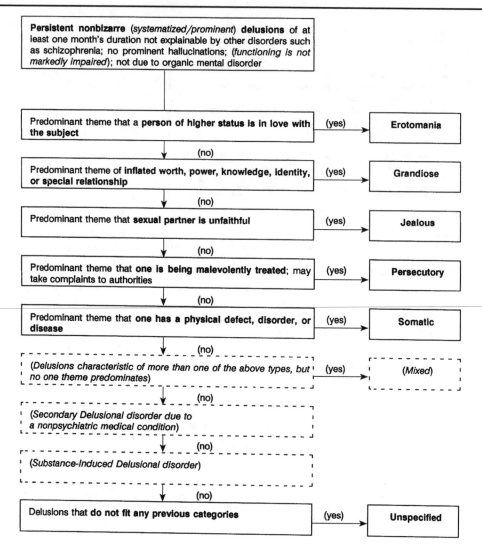

(Adapted from Janicak, Andriukaitis, Psychiatric Annals, 1980)

Appendix H. Psychotic Disorders Not Classified Elsewhere.

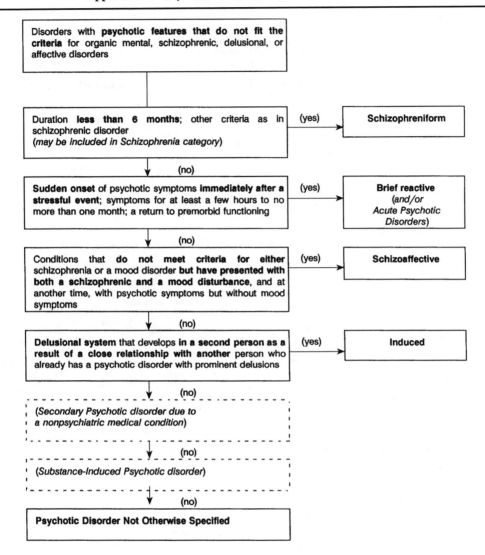

Disorders with **psychotic features that do not fit the criteria** for organic mental, schizophrenic, delusional, or affective disorders

Duration **less than 6 months**; other criteria as in schizophrenic disorder
(*may be included in Schizophrenia category*) → (yes) → **Schizophreniform**

(no)

Sudden onset of psychotic symptoms **immediately after a stressful event**; symptoms for at least a few hours to no more than one month; a return to premorbid functioning → (yes) → **Brief reactive**
(*and/or Acute Psychotic Disorders*)

(no)

Conditions that **do not meet criteria for either** schizophrenia or a mood disorder **but have presented with both a schizophrenic and a mood disturbance**, and at another time, with psychotic symptoms but without mood symptoms → (yes) → **Schizoaffective**

(no)

Delusional system that develops **in a second person as a result of a close relationship with another** person who already has a psychotic disorder with prominent delusions → (yes) → **Induced**

(no)

(*Secondary Psychotic disorder due to a nonpsychiatric medical condition*)

(no)

(*Substance-Induced Psychotic disorder*)

(no)

Psychotic Disorder Not Otherwise Specified

Appendix I.   An Overview of Mood-Related Disorders.

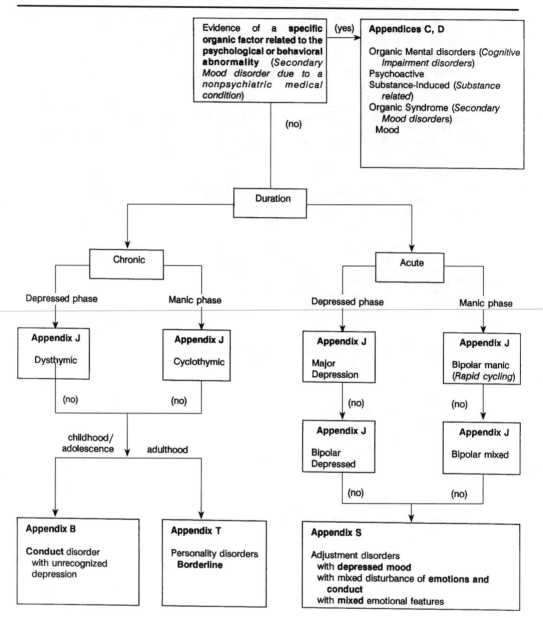

Appendix J.   Mood Disorders.

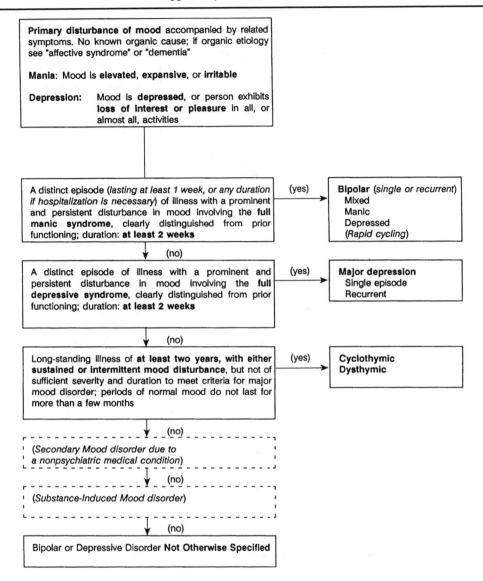

Primary disturbance of mood accompanied by related symptoms. No known organic cause; if organic etiology see "affective syndrome" or "dementia"

Mania: Mood is **elevated, expansive,** or **irritable**

Depression: Mood is **depressed,** or person exhibits **loss of interest or pleasure** in all, or almost all, activities

A distinct episode (*lasting at least 1 week, or any duration if hospitalization is necessary*) of illness with a prominent and persistent disturbance in mood involving the **full manic syndrome,** clearly distinguished from prior functioning; duration: **at least 2 weeks**   (yes) →   **Bipolar** (*single or recurrent*)
Mixed
Manic
Depressed
(*Rapid cycling*)

(no)

A distinct episode of illness with a prominent and persistent disturbance in mood involving the **full depressive syndrome,** clearly distinguished from prior functioning; duration: **at least 2 weeks**   (yes) →   **Major depression**
Single episode
Recurrent

(no)

Long-standing illness of **at least two years, with either sustained or intermittent mood disturbance,** but not of sufficient severity and duration to meet criteria for major mood disorder; periods of normal mood do not last for more than a few months   (yes) →   **Cyclothymic**
Dysthymic

(no)

(*Secondary Mood disorder due to a nonpsychiatric medical condition*)

(no)

(*Substance-Induced Mood disorder*)

(no)

Bipolar or Depressive Disorder **Not Otherwise Specified**

(Adapted from Janicak, Andriukaitis, Psychiatric Annals, 1980)

Appendix K.   An Overview of Anxiety-Related Disorders.

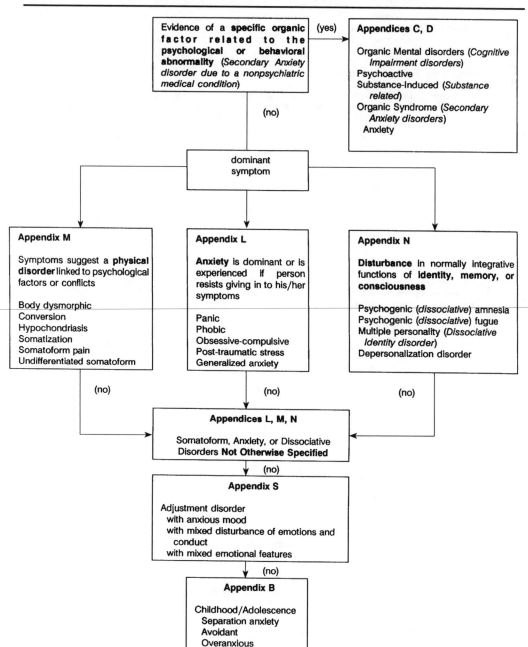

Appendix L.   Anxiety Disorders.

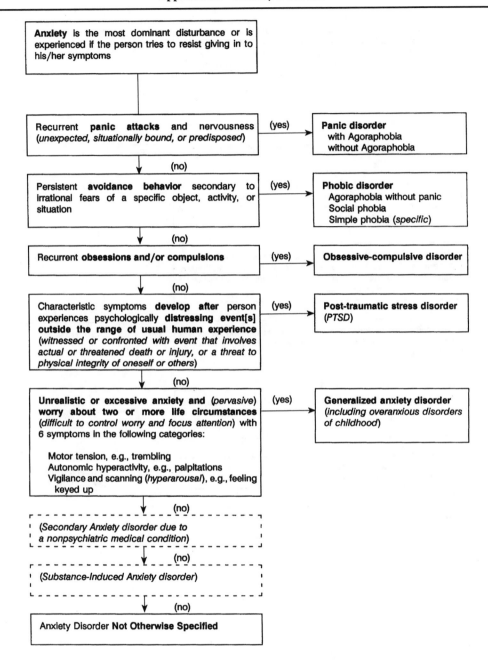

Appendix M.   Somatoform Disorders.

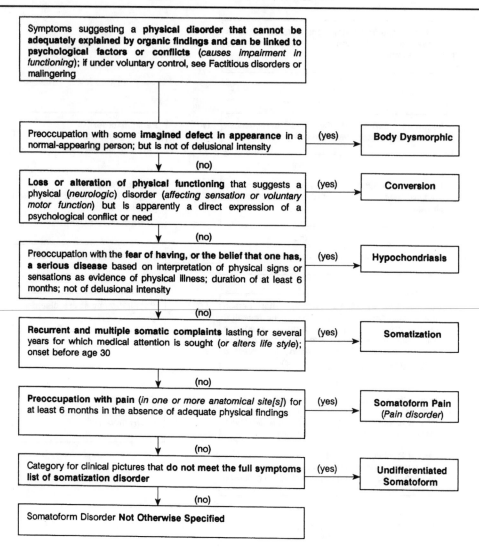

Symptoms suggesting a **physical disorder that cannot be adequately explained by organic findings and can be linked to psychological factors or conflicts** (*causes impairment in functioning*); if under voluntary control, see Factitious disorders or malingering

Preoccupation with some **imagined defect in appearance** in a normal-appearing person; but is not of delusional intensity →(yes)→ **Body Dysmorphic**

(no)

Loss or alteration of physical functioning that suggests a physical (*neurologic*) disorder (*affecting sensation or voluntary motor function*) but is apparently a direct expression of a psychological conflict or need →(yes)→ **Conversion**

(no)

Preoccupation with the **fear of having, or the belief that one has, a serious disease** based on interpretation of physical signs or sensations as evidence of physical illness; duration of at least 6 months; not of delusional intensity →(yes)→ **Hypochondriasis**

(no)

Recurrent and multiple somatic complaints lasting for several years for which medical attention is sought (*or alters life style*); onset before age 30 →(yes)→ **Somatization**

(no)

Preoccupation with pain (*in one or more anatomical site[s]*) for at least 6 months in the absence of adequate physical findings →(yes)→ **Somatoform Pain** (*Pain disorder*)

(no)

Category for clinical pictures that **do not meet the full symptoms list of somatization disorder** →(yes)→ **Undifferentiated Somatoform**

(no)

Somatoform Disorder **Not Otherwise Specified**

Appendix N.   Dissociative Disorders.

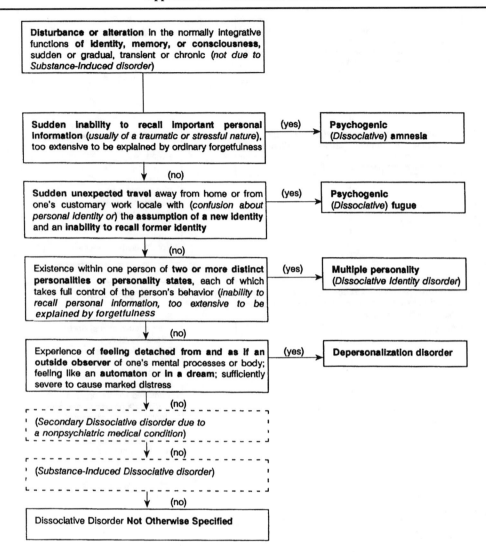

Disturbance or alteration in the normally integrative functions **of identity, memory, or consciousness,** sudden or gradual, transient or chronic (*not due to Substance-Induced disorder*)

Sudden inability to recall important personal information (*usually of a traumatic or stressful nature*), too extensive to be explained by ordinary forgetfulness — (yes) → **Psychogenic** (*Dissociative*) **amnesia**

(no)

Sudden unexpected travel away from home or from one's customary work locale with (*confusion about personal identity or*) the **assumption of a new identity** and an **inability to recall former identity** — (yes) → **Psychogenic** (*Dissociative*) **fugue**

(no)

Existence within one person of **two or more distinct personalities or personality states,** each of which takes full control of the person's behavior (*inability to recall personal information, too extensive to be explained by forgetfulness* — (yes) → **Multiple personality** (*Dissociative Identity disorder*)

(no)

Experience of **feeling detached from and as if an outside observer** of one's mental processes or body; feeling like an **automaton or in a dream**; sufficiently severe to cause marked distress — (yes) → **Depersonalization disorder**

(no)

(*Secondary Dissociative disorder due to a nonpsychiatric medical condition*)

(no)

(*Substance-Induced Dissociative disorder*)

(no)

Dissociative Disorder **Not Otherwise Specified**

Appendix O.   Sexual Disorders.

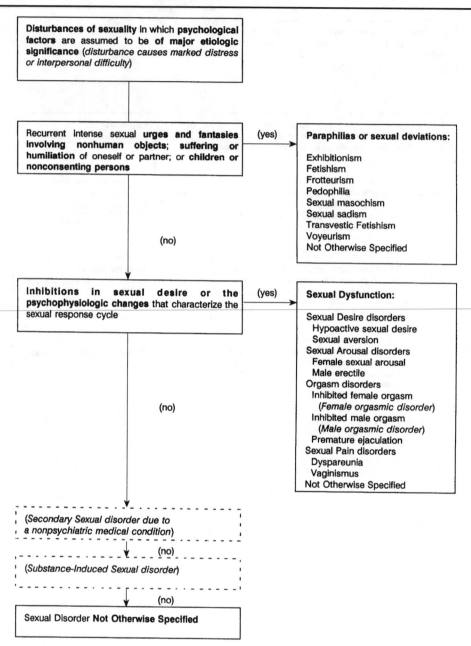

Appendix P.   Sleep Disorders.

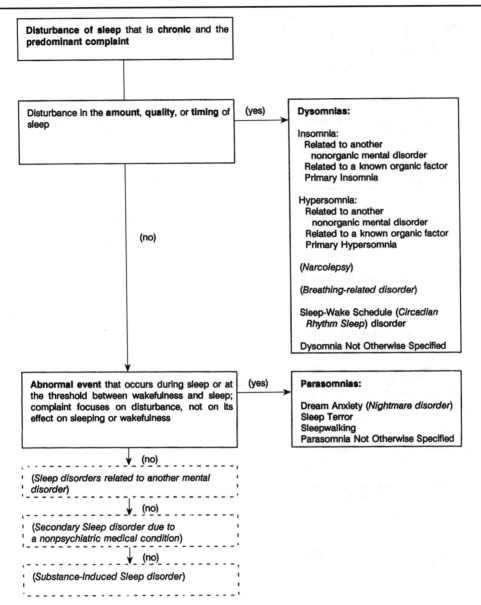

Disturbance of sleep that is chronic and the predominant complaint

Disturbance in the amount, quality, or timing of sleep → (yes)

Dysomnias:

Insomnia:
  Related to another
    nonorganic mental disorder
  Related to a known organic factor
  Primary Insomnia

Hypersomnia:
  Related to another
    nonorganic mental disorder
  Related to a known organic factor
  Primary Hypersomnia

(*Narcolepsy*)

(*Breathing-related disorder*)

Sleep-Wake Schedule (*Circadian Rhythm Sleep*) disorder

Dysomnia Not Otherwise Specified

(no)

Abnormal event that occurs during sleep or at the threshold between wakefulness and sleep; complaint focuses on disturbance, not on its effect on sleeping or wakefulness → (yes)

Parasomnias:

Dream Anxiety (*Nightmare disorder*)
Sleep Terror
Sleepwalking
Parasomnia Not Otherwise Specified

(no)

(*Sleep disorders related to another mental disorder*)

(no)

(*Secondary Sleep disorder due to a nonpsychiatric medical condition*)

(no)

(*Substance-Induced Sleep disorder*)

Appendix Q. Factitious Disorders.

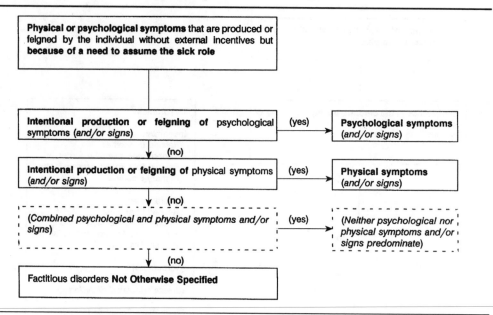

Appendix R. Impulse Control Disorders Not Elsewhere Classified.

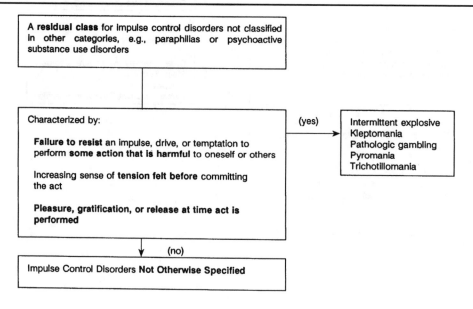

(Adapted from Janicak, Andriukaitis, Psychiatric Annals, 1980)

Appendix S. Adjustment Disorders.

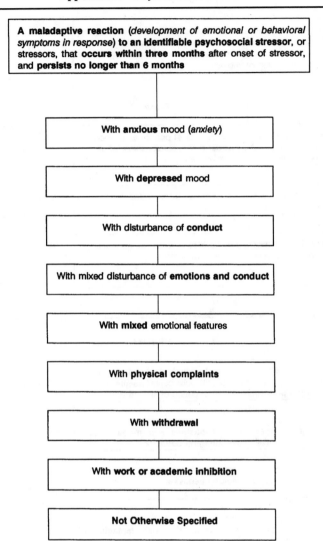

A maladaptive reaction (*development of emotional or behavioral symptoms in response*) to an **identifiable psychosocial stressor**, or stressors, that **occurs within three months** after onset of stressor, and **persists no longer than 6 months**

With **anxious** mood (*anxiety*)

With **depressed** mood

With disturbance of **conduct**

With mixed disturbance of **emotions and conduct**

With **mixed** emotional features

With **physical complaints**

With **withdrawal**

With **work or academic inhibition**

Not Otherwise Specified

Appendix T.   Personality Disorders (Listed on Axis II).

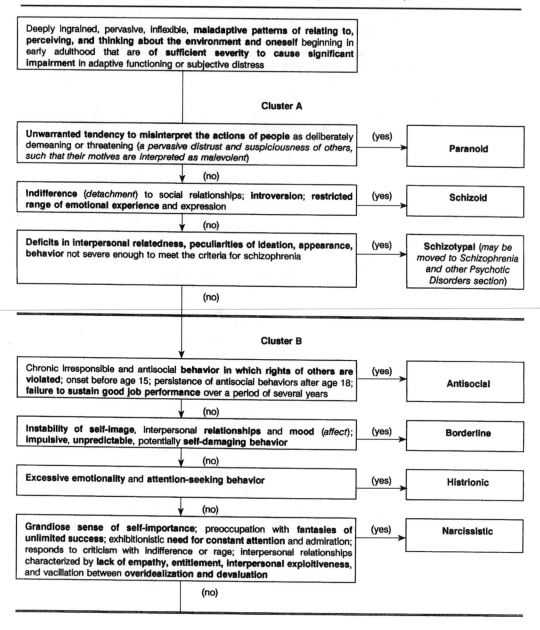

Deeply ingrained, pervasive, inflexible, **maladaptive patterns of relating to, perceiving, and thinking about the environment and oneself** beginning in early adulthood that are **of sufficient severity to cause significant impairment** in adaptive functioning or subjective distress

Cluster A

Unwarranted tendency to misinterpret the actions of people as deliberately demeaning or threatening (a *pervasive distrust and suspiciousness of others, such that their motives are interpreted as malevolent*) — (yes) → **Paranoid**

(no)

Indifference (*detachment*) to social relationships; introversion; restricted range of emotional experience and expression — (yes) → **Schizoid**

(no)

Deficits in interpersonal relatedness, peculiarities of ideation, appearance, behavior not severe enough to meet the criteria for schizophrenia — (yes) → **Schizotypal** (*may be moved to Schizophrenia and other Psychotic Disorders section*)

(no)

Cluster B

Chronic irresponsible and antisocial **behavior in which rights of others are violated**; onset before age 15; persistence of antisocial behaviors after age 18; **failure to sustain good job performance** over a period of several years — (yes) → **Antisocial**

(no)

Instability of **self-image**, interpersonal **relationships** and mood (*affect*); impulsive, unpredictable, potentially **self-damaging behavior** — (yes) → **Borderline**

(no)

Excessive emotionality and attention-seeking behavior — (yes) → **Histrionic**

(no)

Grandiose sense of self-importance; preoccupation with fantasies of unlimited success; exhibitionistic need for constant attention and admiration; responds to criticism with indifference or rage; interpersonal relationships characterized by lack of empathy, entitlement, interpersonal exploitiveness, and vacillation between overidealization and devaluation — (yes) → **Narcissistic**

(no)

(*continued*)

Appendix T.—*continued*

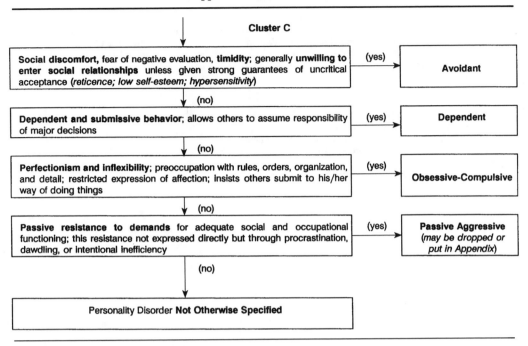

Cluster C

Social discomfort, fear of negative evaluation, **timidity**; generally **unwilling to enter social relationships** unless given strong guarantees of uncritical acceptance (*reticence; low self-esteem; hypersensitivity*)	(yes) →	**Avoidant**

↓ (no)

Dependent and submissive behavior; allows others to assume responsibility of major decisions	(yes) →	**Dependent**

↓ (no)

Perfectionism and inflexibility; preoccupation with rules, orders, organization, and detail; restricted expression of affection; insists others submit to his/her way of doing things	(yes) →	**Obsessive-Compulsive**

↓ (no)

Passive resistance to demands for adequate social and occupational functioning; this resistance not expressed directly but through procrastination, dawdling, or intentional inefficiency	(yes) →	**Passive Aggressive** (*may be dropped or put in Appendix*)

↓ (no)

Personality Disorder **Not Otherwise Specified**

Appendix U.   Personality Change Disorders (DSM-IV).

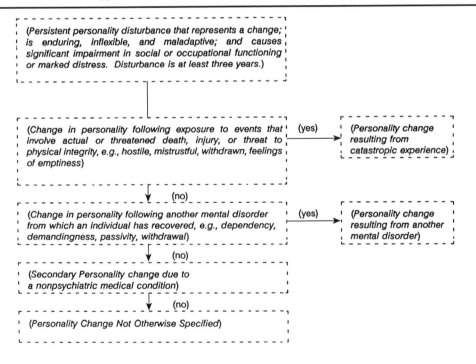

(*Persistent personality disturbance that represents a change; is enduring, inflexible, and maladaptive; and causes significant impairment in social or occupational functioning or marked distress. Disturbance is at least three years.*)

(*Change in personality following exposure to events that involve actual or threatened death, injury, or threat to physical integrity, e.g., hostile, mistrustful, withdrawn, feelings of emptiness*) — (yes) → (*Personality change resulting from catastropic experience*)

↓ (no)

(*Change in personality following another mental disorder from which an individual has recovered, e.g., dependency, demandingness, passivity, withdrawal*) — (yes) → (*Personality change resulting from another mental disorder*)

↓ (no)

(*Secondary Personality change due to a nonpsychiatric medical condition*)

↓ (no)

(*Personality Change Not Otherwise Specified*)

Appendix V.   Other Conditions.

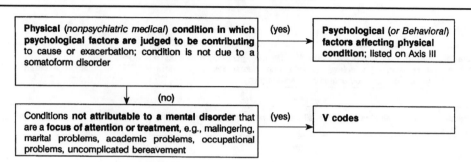

Page numbers followed by *t* or *f* denote tables or figures, respectively.